CARDIOPULMONARY PHYSICAL THERAPY

VOLUME ONE

Cardiopulmonary Physical Therapy

Edited by

Scot Irwin, M.S., P.T.

Assistant Professor, Physical Therapy,
Georgia State University,
Atlanta, Georgia

Jan Stephen Tecklin, M.S., L.P.T.

Assistant Professor of Physical Therapy,
Physical Therapy Department,
Beaver College,
Glenside, Pennsylvania

*with **358** illustrations*

LINE DRAWINGS BY LEINICKE DESIGN
COVER ILLUSTRATION BY JACK TANDY

The C. V. Mosby Company

ST. LOUIS • TORONTO • PRINCETON   1985

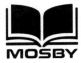

MOSBY

A TRADITION OF PUBLISHING EXCELLENCE

Editor: Rosa L. Kasper
Assistant editor: Connie Leinicke
Manuscript editor: Carl Masthay
Book design: Jeanne Genz
Cover design: Kathy Johnson
Production: Barbara Merritt, Jeanne A. Gulledge

THREE VOLUMES

Printed in the United States of America

The C.V. Mosby Company
11830 Westline Industrial Drive, St. Louis, Missouri 63146

Library of Congress Cataloging in Publication Data
Main entry under title:

Cardiopulmonary physical therapy.

   (Physical therapy; v. 1)
   Includes index.
   1. Exercise therapy.   2. Cardiacs—Rehabilitation.
3. Lungs—Diseases—Patients—Rehabilitation.   4. Physical
therapy.   I. Irwin, Scot.   II. Tecklin, Jan Stephen.
III. Series: Physical therapy (Saint Louis, Mo.); v. 1.
[DNLM: 1. Cardiovascular Diseases—rehabilitation.
2. Physical Therapy—methods.   3. Respiration Disorders—
rehabilitation.   WG 166 C265]
RC684.E9C38   1984   616.2′00462   84-8269
ISBN 0-8016-2512-2

C/VH/VH 9 8 7 6 5 4 3 2 1   01/A/029

CONTRIBUTORS

Susan Enriquez Alvarez, B.S.

Staff Physical Therapist,
St. John's Hospital,
Oxnard, California

Vinod K. Bhutani, M.D.

Research Assistant Professor of Physiology, Department of Physiology, Temple University School of Medicine, Philadelphia; Assistant Professor of Pediatrics, Department of Newborn Pediatrics, Pennsylvania Hospital, Philadelphia, Pennsylvania

Raymond L. Blessey, M.A., P.T.

Assistant Clinical Professor, Department of Physical Therapy, University of Southern California, Los Angeles; Director of Cardiac Rehabilitation, Department of Cardiology, CIGNA Medical Center, Los Angeles, California

Patrice A. Castle, B.S., P.T.

Adjunct Faculty, Department of Physical Therapy, Temple University, Philadelphia; Assistant Director, Department of Physical Therapy, Albert Einstein Medical Center–Northern Division, Philadelphia, Pennsylvania

Linda D. Crane, B.S., M.M.Sc.

Assistant Professor, Department of Pediatrics, School of Medicine, Division of Physical Therapy, School of Community and Allied Health, University of Alabama in Birmingham, Birmingham, Alabama

Jeanne A. DeCesare, M.S., P.T.

Research Physical Therapist, Department of Physical Therapy, The Children's Hospital, Boston, Massachusetts

Joan H. Gault, M.D.

Associate Professor of Physiology, Department of Physiology, Temple University School of Medicine, Philadelphia, Pennsylvania

Kenneth S. Gimbel, M.D., F.A.C.C.

Formerly Director of Coronary Care Unit, The University of Maryland Hospital, Baltimore, Maryland; Clayton General Hospital, Riverdale, Georgia

Willy E. Hammon, B.S., R.P.T.

Director, Rehabilitative Services, Oklahoma Memorial Hospital, Oklahoma City, Oklahoma

David James Henson, M.D.

Fellow, Division of Pulmonary and Critical Care Medicine, Medical College of Pennsylvania, Philadelphia, Pennsylvania

Thomas R. Holtackers, R.P.T.

Supervisor, Chest Physical Therapy, Department of Intensive Care/Respiratory Therapy, Mayo Clinic, Rochester, Minnesota

Nancy H. Humberstone, B.S., M.M.Sc., R.P.T.

Supervisor, Physical Therapy, Department of Physical Therapy, Emory University Hospital, Atlanta, Georgia

Randolph H. Ice, B.S., R.P.T.

President, SCOR Physical Therapy, Inc., Clinical Faculty Member, Department of Physical Therapy, University of Southern California, Los Angeles; Program Director, Department of Cardiac Rehabilitation, Presbyterian Intercommunity Hospital, Whittier, California; Program Director, Cardiac Rehabilitation Program, Sports Conditioning and Rehabilitation Clinic, Orange, California

Scot Irwin, M.A., P.T.

Assistant Professor, Department of Physical Therapy, Georgia State University, Atlanta, Georgia; Director of Physical Therapy and Rehabilitation, Department of Physical Therapy, Clayton General Hospital, Riverdale, Georgia

v

Margaret E. Kleinfeld, B.S., L.P.T.

Adjunct Faculty, Department of Physical Therapy, Temple University, Philadelphia; Director, Department of Physical Therapy, Albert Einstein Medical Center–Northern Division, Philadelphia, Pennsylvania

Brenda Rae Lunsford, M.S.

Supervisor II, Spinal Injury Service, Physical Therapy Department, Rancho Los Amigos Hospital, Downey, California

William L. Morrissey, M.D.

Professor of Medicine, Department of Medicine, Medical College of Pennsylvania, Philadelphia; Medical Director, Respiratory Care Services, Medical College of Pennsylvania, Philadelphia, Pennsylvania

Margery J. Peterson, M.S.

Instructor, Spinal Injury Service, Physical Therapy Department, Rancho Los Amigos Hospital, Downey, California

Thomas H. Shaffer, Ph.D.

Director, Respiratory Physiology Section, Associate Professor of Physiology, Department of Physiology, Temple University School of Medicine, Philadelphia, Pennsylvania

Z. David Skloven, M.D.

Director, Cardiopulmonary Department, Clayton General Hospital, Clayton County, Georgia

Jane Wetzel, B.A.

Supervisor I, Cardiopulmonary Physical Therapy, Physical Therapy Department, Rancho Los Amigos Hospital, Downey, California

Marla R. Wolfson, M.S., L.P.T.

Research Associate in Physiology, Department of Physiology, Temple University School of Medicine, Philadelphia, Pennsylvania

Cynthia Coffin Zadai, M.S., R.P.T.

Director, Chest Physical Therapy, Beth Israel Hospital, Boston, Massachusetts

In memory of

Eli Raymond, Jim Thomas, Robert Gauthier, and Bill Kennedy

from whom we learned so much about life and living

Scot Irwin

To

Randee Lynn, Colby David, Ashley Joy

and in memory of

Coleman

Jan Stephen Tecklin

PREFACE

Cardiopulmonary Physical Therapy is, first and foremost, a text intended for the entry-level physical therapy student and the practicing therapist inexperienced in either cardiac rehabilitation or respiratory care. We, the editors, believe that since such close interaction exists between the cardiovascular and respiratory systems a book about one without the other would have been an incomplete effort. Therefore, the first nine chapters of the book describe the essentials of cardiac rehabilitation—structure, assessment, and program planning—and the following 12 chapters discuss assessment and treatment of patients with a wide variety of acute and chronic pulmonary disorders.

Chapter 1 presents the philosophical approach to and the organizational structure of a rehabilitation program for a patient with coronary artery disease. Chapter 2 examines the pathogenesis of atherosclerosis, which accounts for the majority of cases of heart disease among adults in our society. Hemodynamic considerations of the cardiac patient and pharmacological intervention for this patient group are detailed in Chapters 3 and 4, respectively. Although these two topics are not commonly presented in detail in other physical therapy literature, we strongly believe that an understanding of these topics is critical to developing a scientifically sound rationale for the approach to physical rehabilitation of a person with atherosclerotic coronary artery disease. Aberrant physiological responses to exercise that commonly occur in patients who suffer from impaired myocardial circulation and function are delineated in Chapter 5. A comprehensive and systematic evaluation of patients is described in the following chapter. Using information obtained from the evaluation, a treatment approach is offered in Chapter 7 by which a therapist can plan and implement a comprehensive rehabilitation program that is individualized for each patient. Chapter 8 describes the beneficial effects of aerobic exercise for heart patients. This notion is supported by an extensive review of scientific evidence. The final chapter of this portion of the book is a description of the administrative and management strategies necessary for the effective daily operation of a cardiac rehabilitation program.

The second portion of *Cardiopulmonary Physical Therapy* presents basic science and clinical information regarding the pulmonary system. Chapters 10 through 21 are organized differently from the first nine chapters, in that the bulk of the material in the latter chapters is based on specific groups of patients with pulmonary disease or respiratory dysfunction. Chapter 10 describes the normal structure and function of the lungs and chest wall. Chapter 11 discusses the major patterns of acute respiratory failure and the medical management of patients with each type of failure. Chapters 12 and 13 describe the basic knowledge and skills that the physical therapist needs to both assess and treat patients with varying disorders or diseases of the chest.

Each of the remaining eight chapters discusses in depth a major patient group whose members benefit from physical rehabilitation. Chapter 14 reviews the many common types of thoracic and abdominal operative procedures in which physical therapy plays a major role in both preventing and treating pulmonary complications. Chapter 15 examines the acutely ill patient with medical chest disease who is being treated in the intensive care unit. With the enormous increase in the use of mechanical ventilation during the last two decades, a new patient group with a common problem—ventilator dependency—has arisen. Suggestions for physical rehabilitation of patients with ventilator dependency are presented in Chapter 16. Virtually nowhere in patient care has there been a more rapid advance in technology and care than in neonatology. This topic is succinctly described in Chapter 17. Acute and chronic respiratory problems in toddlers and children is the content in Chapter 18. An approach to rehabilitation of patients with chronic obstructive pulmonary disease is suggested in Chapter 19. Respiratory muscle strengthening is a subject that has been discussed at length in the pulmonology literature in recent years. A concise review of the muscular activities that result in improved pulmonary ventilation is found in Chapter 20. The final chapter of the book examines the management of respiratory complications of acute spinal cord injuries.

Since clients with cardiopulmonary disorders frequently require orthopaedic and neurological intervention, we have provided a detailed index to Volume Two, *Orthopaedic and Sports Physical Therapy,* and Volume Three, *Neurological Rehabilitation.*

Each of the patient-problem chapters presents a review of the basic problems associated with the patient group, suggests an approach to patient assessment, describes treatment procedures, and supports the major assertions with a review of the scientific literature on the subject. This last aspect of these chapters—scientific support—is one of the most important aspects of the pulmonary portion of the text. Most other books and monographs about physical therapy for the patient with respiratory problems provide, as this work does, methods of treatment for various problems. Many other textbooks, especially those from Great Britain, provide little if any scientific support for their recommended treatment approaches. One of the major strengths of *Cardiopulmonary Physical Therapy* is the review of published research that supports the assertions of the contributors regarding approaches to treatment; that is, the contributors not only report what to do but also provide, where such information exists, a reasonable scientific rationale for their suggestions.

Although this book is one of a three-volume series, it is particularly important in concept at this time. Cardiac rehabilitation is a relatively new arena in which physical therapists have been working. There is a constant overlapping of perceived responsibility among the several health professions and technical groups that engage in rehabilitation of the patient with coronary artery disease. It is not our intent or that of the contributors to suggest who does what in cardiac care. Rather, the attempt here is to delineate clearly the knowledge and skill necessary for the physical therapist or other professional to provide exemplary care for the patient with heart disease. As physical therapists become more knowledgeable and skillful in providing an optimal level of care, our importance as members of the cardiac rehabilitation effort will become both obvious and unchallengeable.

There exists a similar scenario within respiratory care.

Physical therapists in the United States have been involved in acute and chronic respiratory care for more than 50 years. In the last two decades, physical therapists, for many reasons, have often voluntarily disassociated themselves from the patient who had respiratory difficulty. During this period, the development of oxygen technicians to inhalation therapists to respiratory therapists has been remarkable. Is it naïve to believe that there is a cause-and-effect relationship. Regardless, there is a clear need and a clear responsibility for each group. In addition, there is some area of overlap that is dealt with differently from hospital to hospital.

Why discuss this issue here? One of the major purposes of the pulmonary section of *Cardiopulmonary Physical Therapy* is to defuse, at least within physical therapy, the notion that "chest PT" is equivalent to bronchial drainage with manual percussion and vibration. Our skills in assessment and treatment of musculoskeletal disorders, our knowledge of exercise, and our ability to remedy movement dysfunction provide physical therapists a large responsibility for the rehabilitation of the varied groups of patients with pulmonary and respiratory disorders. When these skills are combined with the skills needed for provision of bronchial hygiene and prevention of postoperative pulmonary complications, the physical therapist's major contribution to chest patients should be obvious. To deny this contribution and to ignore our role is, in our opinion, a frivolous abdication of our responsibility to these patients. None of us wants to clap chests for 8 hours each day. Rather, we choose to provide judicious and skillful physical assessment and rehabilitation, combined with appropriate use of bronchial hygiene techniques, to offer wide-ranging therapeutic expertise. This expertise can be appropriately employed in settings that range from the intensive care unit to the home and can include every setting along that recovery route.

This book provides the necessary information for the inexperienced therapist to assume the responsibility to the millions of patients in the United States who suffer from some cardiopulmonary disorder that can be treated with physical rehabilitation methods.

Jan Stephen Tecklin
Scot Irwin

ACKNOWLEDGMENTS

I would like to thank the following persons for their support, guidance, editorial assistance, and contributions. The order of names in no way connotes the significance of their contributions. Mr. Don Lassen, Dr. J. Perry, Ms. Brenda Lunsford, R.P.T., Mr. Dennis Scheidt, Mr. Randy Ice, R.P.T., Dr. Z.D. Skloven, Dr. K. Gimbel, Dr. Ron Freireich, Ms. Ellen Hillegess, R.P.T., Ms. Susan Butler, R.P.T., Ms. Sue Ellen Story, R.P.T., Ms. Anne McCullars, Mr. Robert Donatelli, R.P.T., Ms. Colleen Kigin, R.P.T., Mr. and Mrs. V. Irwin, and Stacey, Joshua, and Jacob Irwin.

A very special thank you goes to my colleagues Mr. Ray Blessey, R.P.T., and Ms. Cynthia Zadai, R.P.T., without whom this text would have never been completed.

Scot Irwin

There are a number of persons without whom the pulmonary portion of *Cardiopulmonary Physical Therapy* would have never come to pass. I would like first to thank each of my contributors. Each has major patient care, administrative, or research responsibilities; added to those responsibilities were the additional tasks of reviewing the literature, developing outlines, writing several drafts, searching for figures, developing tables and charts, and compiling reference lists. As editor, I felt at times like a task master, but each contributor complied with my requests cheerfully and no friendships were severed—no mean feat. The staff at The C.V. Mosby Company was most helpful and cheerful and endured my missed deadlines with professional aplomb and only the occasional disgruntled comment.

There are a few other personal thanks that I feel compelled to offer to those who have endured with me during my efforts on behalf of *Cardiopulmonary Physical Therapy:*

To my chairman, George Logue, for his calm unwavering support and understanding of the time, effort, phone calls, mail, and so on, that I invested in this book and that probably detracted from my efforts at Beaver College.

To my dear friend the late G.E. Bud DeHaven, who fostered in me the responsibility of sharing information with my colleagues through publication.

To my mentor, Douglas S. Holsclaw, M.D., who shared with me his vast knowledge of pulmonary medicine and guided my early efforts at writing for publication.

To Randee, my wife, Colby, my son, and Ashley, my daughter, for enduring the long hours of my pouring over manuscripts and revisions when they would much rather have had my interest and time. Although my interest and time might have been periodically in short supply, my love never was.

To all of you "thanks!"

Jan Stephen Tecklin

CONTENTS

PART ONE

CARDIAC PHYSICAL THERAPY AND REHABILITATION

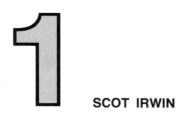

SCOT IRWIN

Philosophy and structure of a cardiac rehabilitation program

The first part of *Cardiopulmonary Physical Therapy* is devoted to the development, implementation, and potential impact of a program of rehabilitation of patients with coronary artery disease. The approach to cardiac rehabilitation that is presented in the forthcoming pages is derived from a philosophy of patient care that incorporates available scientific knowledge of coronary artery disease, specific team and patient goals, and specialized clinical skills into a logically structured program. This philosophy and its programming have been applied successfully in a variety of hospital settings, from large university-based rehabilitation centers to rural community hospitals.

PHILOSOPHICAL FOUNDATION

One key to effective cardiac rehabilitation is thorough understanding of the philosophical principles upon which it is based. The basis of our philosophy rests upon three equally essential principles.

The first principle is that coronary artery disease is a progressive, chronic disease process that is closely aligned with certain epidemiologically documented risk factors. The second is that an exercise program for patients after a heart attack or bypass surgery is beneficial if it is individually designed for each patient and objectively evaluated on an ongoing basis. The final principle is that the process of cardiac rehabilitation requires a team approach. Cardiac rehabilitation requires an enormous amount of patient education, and this education covers a multitude of medical specialty areas. No *one* health care professional can adequately provide all the services needed to conduct an effective program of rehabilitation.

RISK-FACTOR MODIFICATION

Patients with coronary artery disease are suffering from a chronic, generally progressive disease process. The dis-

ease is atherosclerosis. The exact cause of this disease is not well understood, but it is associated with certain well-documented risk factors. These risk factors have been studied extensively and are generally prominent in modern societies where an abundance of high-fat foods and leisure time are available (see Chapter 2).

The program described in this text is continuously directed toward the reduction of those risk factors associated with the atherosclerotic disease process. The goal is to educate all the patients about the various risk factors and to give each patient and his or her families a specific list of those risk factors that apply directly to their case. It is important to convey to patients that a modification of their risk factors does not guarantee that no further disease progression will occur. Risk factor reduction should not be considered a cure. It is simply a logical approach to a poorly understood disease process. The scientific data to support risk factor modification as a means of reducing coronary mortality and morbidity are equivocal at best. However, risk factors increase the chance of developing atherosclerosis, and thus it follows that reduction of these risk factors may decrease the risk of further disease progression.

Risk factor modification often requires major life-style changes for the patient with coronary artery disease. Thus one of the principles of our program is to convey to patients that their program of cardiac rehabilitation requires lifelong application. Our educational programs are directed toward having patients follow through with their program at home.

OBJECTIVE CONTINUOUS EVALUATION OF EXERCISE RESPONSES

An effective, safe exercise program for patients with coronary artery disease must be founded on objective, continuous evaluation of patient responses. Their exercise responses must be assessed by measurement and interpretation of the five available clinical monitoring tools: heart rate, blood pressure, electrocardiogram, heart sounds, and symptoms. Additional elements that must be considered when one is developing an exercise program for cardiac patients include medical history, medications, hemodynamic function, coronary anatomy, extent and time of infarction, and patient goals and psychological condition. Each change in a patient's exercise program should be based on a thorough objective evaluation. Thus progression of a patient's activity level throughout the rehabilitation process can be made objectively. If this principle is followed by a therapist with good clinical skills, there is no need for patients to follow arbitrary step-by-step programs to progress their activity levels. Continuous evaluation of patient exercise responses creates an individualized, safe and effective progression of activity.

TEAM APPROACH

To achieve a unified team approach, the team should be led by a patient care coordinator. It is the role of the coordinator to work with each member of the team to implement team goals and to assure that all team members advocate the same principles of patient care. The coordinator should have a sound background in electrophysiology, pathophysiology, exercise physiology, and patient care concepts. The coordinator should be responsible for educating the various team members in the principles and philosophy of cardiac rehabilitation. An effective team should include a physician, a nurse, a dietician, a physical therapist, a psychologist, and a medical social worker. Variables such as space, equipment, and patient population will govern the composition of teams at different institutions.

Team goals

General team goals should not be equated with the patient treatment goals (discussed later). Team goals should include but are not limited to the following:

1. Creation of an educational environment in which patients are given clear, consistent guidance
2. Agreement that patients should be taught to accept the program goals as part of a lifelong endeavor
3. Delegation of patient problems and questions to the appropriate team member for resolution

Patient goals

A constant assessment of the patient's own goals must be made throughout the rehabilitation program. The physical therapist should always keep the patient's goals in mind. These goals may often change dramatically as the patients begin to understand and accept the seriousness of their disease and the life-style changes that must be made to improve their chances of survival.

Commonly, the patient's initial goals are to get home and back to work. They often feel fine and overtly or covertly deny that they have anything wrong with them at all. They often believe that their physician has made a mistake. As they begin to understand their disease process and accept their condition, their goals begin to change. As the weeks go by, therapists must continually help patients reassess their goals and guide them toward realistic goals.

The patient's own goals supersede any other goals that the team members may have determined. Little patient compliance will be achieved unless the patient's goals are incorporated into the program.

CLINICAL KNOWLEDGE AND SKILLS

To participate effectively in a cardiac rehabilitation program, a physical therapist must possess theoretical knowledge in cardiopulmonary anatomy and physiology, pathophysiology of arteriosclerosis and coronary artery disease, normal and abnormal cardiac hemodynamics, normal and abnormal exercise physiology, pharmacological effects of cardiac medications, and electrophysiology. It is strongly suggested that you explore these areas in depth by reviewing and studying the selected references listed at the end of each chapter in this book.

CLINICAL SKILLS DEVELOPMENT

Effective implementation of a program of cardiac rehabilitation requires the attainment and use of specialized clinical skills. Therapists with an exceptional level of theoretical knowledge may have little impact on their patient's care unless their clinical skills are reliable. The clinical data base that is obtained on every patient must be reproducible and accurate. Without accuracy, physicians will not accept or utilize the information obtained to modify the patient's medical regimen. Physicians will not trust the physical therapist's information, and thus they will be hesitant to refer their patients.

Physical therapists should have the clinical skill and knowledge to rapidly obtain and accurately interpret (1) electrocardiographic changes (ST segments and arrhythmias), (2) blood pressure responses during exercise, (3) breath sounds and heart sounds, (4) heart rate, and (5) symptoms (especially angina).

Incorporation of the philosophical foundation with the theoretical knowledge and clinical skills listed will assist in the creation of a safe, effective, and rewarding program of cardiac rehabilitation.

BASIC PROGRAM STRUCTURE

The structure of a cardiac rehabilitation program should be directed toward those goals that are common to all patients. The initial goals (phase I) include (1) screening patients for the appearance of complications, (2) initiation of low levels of activity, (3) education of the patients and their families, and (4) measurement of the effectiveness of the patient medications in controlling their cardiovascular status during activity. The emphasis during phase I is upon stabilization of the patient's condition and assurance that general daily activity does not produce undesirable effects. Goals one and four are not often recognized or listed as goals for an inpatient cardiac rehabilitation program, but, in fact, they are more important to most referring physicians than any other goal.

In general, physicians have a great deal of information available to them about their patients' cardiovascular status in a resting state, but they have very little data about their patients' cardiovascular responses to activity. A physical therapist with the proper knowledge and clinical skills can provide this information. Phase I of a cardiac rehabilitation program should provide information to the physician about patient responses to progressive increases in activity. This information will frequently cause the physician to make adjustments in their patients' medications.

The long-term goals associated with phases II and III of the cardiac rehabilitation program structure echo the philosophy previously discussed. They include (1) reduction of risk factors, (2) improvement in physical work capacity, (3) return to *safe* vocational and recreational activity levels, (4) decrease in angina, (5) decrease in fear of the disease, and (6) frequent, objective communication to the physician about patient responses to exercise and medications. The most pronounced impact of phases II and III is achieved when goals 1, 3, 5, and 6 have been attained.

Post–myocardial infarction phase I

Phase I, the acute phase, begins with referral to the cardiac rehabilitation program and ends at discharge from the hospital about 10 to 14 days later. Patients should be referred for cardiac rehabilitation when they are medically stable. This is generally from 3 to 6 days after infarction and depends on whether the patient's condition is complicated or uncomplicated.

Patients with complications, as defined by McNeer and others, require more time to recover from their acute infarction. Uncomplicated patients are usually referred to the cardiac rehabilitation program and discharged earlier. Patient rehabilitation programs consist at this stage of a self-care evaluation (see discussions of patient evaluation in Chapter 6 and phase I programming in Chapter 7, patient and family education, Holter monitoring, graduated ambulation, and a predischarge submaximal or low-level treadmill test).

Phase I for patients after bypass surgery is also an inpatient phase, but this usually is only 5 to 9 days in duration. The rehabilitation program is often more directed toward preventing the pulmonary complications of the surgery (see Part Two of this text for the pulmonary aspect).

Phases II and III are the same for patients after bypass surgery and after acute myocardial infarction.

Phase II: after the acute stage

Phase II, the subacute phase, begins with completion of the low-level treadmill test and ends when the maximal treadmill test and cardiac catheterization have been completed. This phase may vary from 5 to 12 weeks after infarction. Six weeks appears to be most common. One may note with some surprise that a cardiac catheterization is included as part of phase II. It has been my experience that proceeding to phase III, high-level exercise training, without catheterization data may be misleading and sometimes unsafe for the patient. The cardiac catheterization gives invaluable and otherwise unobtainable data about patient heart function and disease severity (see Chapters 2 and 3).

Phase III: long-term follow-up

Phase III is the lifetime phase. During this phase, the patient continues on an individually designed exercise program based on periodic, formal reevaluations. These reevaluations are in the form of maximal symptom-limited exercise tests conducted at six months after infarction and annually thereafter. Phase III is the high-level exercise conditioning phase where patients who have appropriate ventricular function and are well controlled medically are encouraged to high levels of aerobic exercise, at 75% to 90% of their maximum heart rate obtained from their treadmill test.

Physical therapy for cardiac patients can be an exciting, rewarding, beneficial experience. Within this text, some key components to developing and conducting a cardiac rehabilitation program are reviewed. Therapists are encouraged to apply the theoretical information and clinical skill descriptions to their individual patient care programs. In this way, the therapist can apply the philosophy, goals, and structure of the cardiac rehabilitation program described within this text.

2

RAYMOND L. BLESSEY

Atherosclerosis: an overview of the basic mechanism of atherogenesis, pathophysiology, and natural history

This chapter is designed to provide essential background information for the chapters that follow. It begins with a review of the coronary anatomy and includes discussion of (1) theoretical mechanisms involved with coronary artery and vein graft atherosclerosis, (2) the pathophysiology of the disease process, and (3) the natural history of the disease within the various subsets of patients with coronary artery lesions.

CORONARY ARTERY ANATOMY

The clinician involved with the coronary artery disease patient must have a thorough understanding of coronary anatomy to evaluate and treat patients appropriately. The information that follows is meant to be a review, and one should refer to other texts for a more complete discussion of coronary artery anatomy.[15,20,23,29,67]

There are two major epicardial or surface coronary arteries, the right coronary artery and the left main coronary artery. They both originate from the root of the aorta and give off several major epicardial branches and multiple endocardial branches, which penetrate the left or right ventricular muscle mass perpendicular to the parent epicardial vessel (Fig. 2-1). The endocardial branches extend to the myocardial wall referred to as the "subendocardial zone." It should be emphasized that the exact course of each major epicardial vessel and its branches and therefore the area of the myocardium it supplies is variable. The most common patterns of coronary artery distribution are discussed below.

Left coronary artery system

The left main coronary artery is usually 2 to 4 cm in length and bifurcates into two major epicardial branches,

the left anterior descending artery and the circumflex artery (Fig. 2-2). In some cases, there are one or two additional intermediate epicardial branches that arise at the bifurcation of the left main artery referred to as a "ramus intermedius."

The left anterior descending artery (LAD) runs along the interventricular groove either up to or around the apex of the heart. In fact, in the majority of cases, the LAD extends beyond the apex and runs up along the posterior interventricular sulcus. The LAD gives off several diagonal branches (epicardial arteries) of varying size. These diagonal branches, along with the parent artery, supply the entire anterior portion of the left ventricle and most of the superior or lateral wall of the left ventricle. In addition, the LAD gives off a series of septal perforators (endocardial vessels) that begin at the proximal segment of the parent vessel and run in an anteroposterior plane. These endocardial vessels off the LAD supply two thirds of the upper or superior portion of the interventricular septum and all of the inferior aspect of the septum. It is not uncommon for the LAD to supply smaller branches (endocardial vessels) to portions of the right ventricle as well. These branches often anastomose with branches from the right coronary artery (RCA).

The left circumflex artery (LCA) usually arises at a perpendicular angle to the left main artery and runs beneath the left atrial appendage and along the atrioventricular groove (Fig. 2-2). In approximately 12% of the cases, the LCA continues along the atrioventricular groove to the crux (junction between the atrioventricular, interatrial, and interventricular sulci) and gives off a posterior descending artery. In the majority of the cases, the LCA terminates at the obtuse margin (edge between apex of the heart and

6

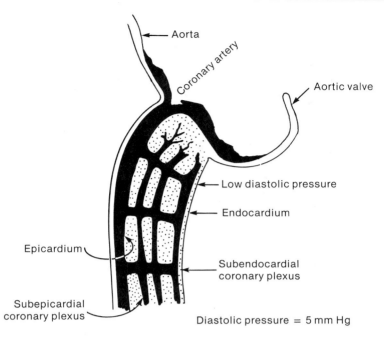

Fig. 2-1. Scheme of epicardial, subepicardial, and subendocardial branches. (From Ellestad, M.: Stress testing, Philadelphia, 1976, F.A. Davis Co.)

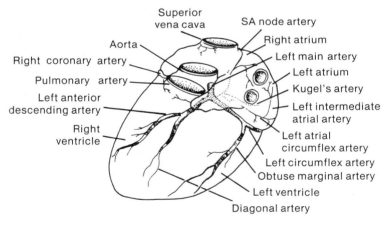

Fig. 2-2. Left anterior oblique view of the heart showing the distribution of both the left anterior descending and circumflex arteries and their major epicardial branches. (From Hamby, R.I., ed.: Clinical-anatomical correlates in coronary artery disease, Mt. Kisco, N.Y., 1979, Futura Publishing Co., Inc.)

pulmonary artery root) and gives off a varying number of arteries referred to as obtuse marginal branches. The number of branches that the circumflex artery gives off to the posterior wall of the left ventricle is indirectly (and reciprocally) related to the distribution of the RCA and its branches.

In summary, the left coronary artery system supplies up to 70% of the left ventricular muscle mass and at least 54% of the right and left ventricular muscle mass. The LAD and its branches supply the entire anterior wall of the left ventricle, most of the superior wall, the majority of the interventricular septum, the anterior wall of the right ventricle, the anterior papillary muscle, the proximal portion of the right bundle branch, the anterior division of the left bundle branch, and the AV node via an anterior septal perforator. The circumflex artery distribution is variable, but it usually supplies portions of the superior and marginal left ventricular wall, portions of the posterior left ventricular wall, the left atrial muscle mass, and the lateral papillary muscle. Forty percent of the time, the circumflex gives off a sinus node artery, and in approximately 10% of the cases, the posterior descending artery off the circumflex (via a posterior septal branch) supplies the AV node.

Right coronary artery system

The right coronary artery (RCA) originates from the right or anterior sinus of Valsalva and runs directly inferior in the atrioventricular groove beneath the right atrial appendage (Fig. 2-3). The length and number of branches of the RCA, and therefore the amount of myocardial and nerve tissue it supplies, is inversely proportional to the distribution of the circumflex and to a certain degree the LAD. In 86% of the cases, the RCA extends around to the crux of the heart. The RCA and its branches supply most of the right ventricle muscle mass and inferior surface of the left ventricle, portions of the posterior wall, the posteroinferior aspects of the interventricular septum, and the right atrial muscle mass. In 60% of the cases the RCA supplies the sinus node artery, and in 90% of the cases, the posterior descending artery off the RCA supplies the AV node. In addition, the RCA supplies the distal portion of the right bundle branch and the posterior division of the left bundle branch.

As discussed earlier, there is a reciprocal distribution pattern between the RCA and circumflex artery. Autopsy studies have demonstrated that there are three basic patterns of coronary circulation in terms of which artery is primarily responsible for the blood supply of the posterior

wall of the left ventricle. In approximately 86% of the cases, the RCA reaches the crux of the heart and gives off the posterior descending area, supplying the majority of the left ventricular posterior wall area (Fig. 2-4). In 12% of the cases, the circumflex artery reaches the crux and

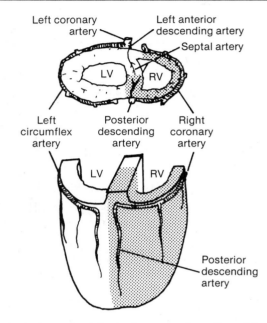

Fig 2-4. Scheme of a right dominant vascular pattern of the posterior aspect of the heart. In the upper portion of the diagram the heart is viewed from above with the atria removed. *Stippled area*, Portion of the heart supplied by the right coronary (RCA). Notice the posterior septal perforator off the RCA supplying the septum and AV node. The clear area of the diagram is supplied by the left coronary artery (left anterior descending and circumflex arteries). (From Hamby, R.I., ed.: Clinical-anatomical correlates in coronary artery disease, Mt. Kisco, N.Y., 1979, Futura Publishing Co., Inc.)

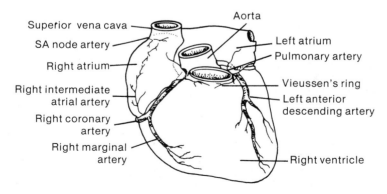

Fig. 2-3. Anterior or front view of the heart showing the distribution of the right coronary artery and the left anterior descending artery. (From Hamby, R.I., ed.: Clinical-anatomical correlates in coronary artery disease, Mt. Kisco, N.Y., 1979, Futura Publishing Co., Inc.)

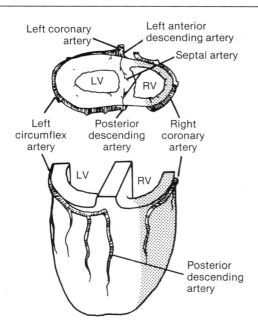

Fig. 2-5. Scheme of a left dominant vascular pattern of the posterior myocardium. Clear area represents portion of the heart supplied by the left coronary artery. See legend in Fig. 2-4 for further explanation. (From Hamby, R.I., ed.: Clinical-anatomical correlates in coronary artery disease, Mt. Kisco, N.Y., 1979, Futura Publishing Co., Inc.)

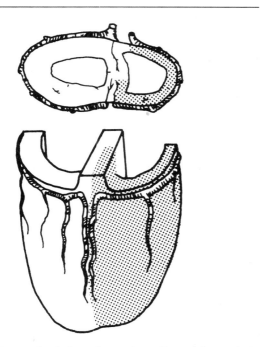

Fig. 2-6. Scheme of a balanced vascular pattern of the posterior myocardium. Note that both the circumflex and the right coronary artery supply equal portions of the posterior myocardium and the posterior aspect of the septum. See legend in Fig. 2-4 for further explanation. (From Hamby, R.I., ed.: Clinical-anatomical correlates in coronary artery disease, Mt. Kisco, N.Y., 1979, Futura Publishing Co., Inc.)

gives off the posterior descending artery (Fig. 2-5), and in 2% of the cases, both the RCA and circumflex arteries reach the crux (Fig. 2-6) and supply an equal portion of the posterior wall (balanced system). The term "dominant" coronary system has been used to designate the coronary artery responsible for the majority of the posterior wall circulation. Based on the above information, 86% of the cases are right dominant, 12% of the cases are left dominant, and 2% of the cases have a balanced coronary system. The term "dominance," however, does not relate to the artery system responsible for the majority of the blood supply, since, as stated previously, the left coronary system always supplies at least 60% to 70% of the left ventricle muscle.

An awareness of the distribution patterns of the coronary arteries as described above and, more thoroughly, in the recommended references is essential to the clinician whose aim is to evaluate and treat each patient as an individual. The significance of this base-line knowledge will be appreciated further after completion of the remaining sections of this chapter.

RISK FACTORS AND THE DEVELOPMENT OF CORONARY ARTERY DISEASE
Framingham study

In 1949, a prospective epidemiological study of 5209 men and women 30 to 62 years of age was initiated in Framingham, Massachusetts, in order to determine the relationship between life-style and antecedent personal attributes to the development of cardiovascular diseases (atherosclerosis).[10] After the initial evaluation, these men and women were followed with biennial examinations including (1) questionnaires dealing with activity level and smoking history, (2) blood chemistry studies, (3) blood pressure evaluation, and (4) resting 12-lead electrocardiogram. The specific design and methods of the study were published in detail in 1963.[10] The study population has been very cooperative, with only 2% of the total population being lost to follow-up and 80% of the subjects having missed none of the biennial examinations. Because Framingham is a relatively small city with only one general hospital, the investigators have been able to monitor accurately cardiac events in their subjects. Gordon[17] and Kannel[31] have recently published papers that update the findings of the Framingham Study and more precisely identify the risk factors for the development of atherosclerosis. Hypertension, smoking, elevated serum cholesterol or triglycerides, abnormal glucose tolerance (diabetes), sedentary life-style, family history of coronary disease, age, and male sex are all factors that individually or in combination with each other, increase the likelihood or risk of developing coronary artery disease and hence are referred to as risk factors. The studies of Rosenman and Jenkins indicate that personality type (type A versus type B) may be associated with risk of coronary disease.[30,54]

Table 2-1. Probability (per 1000) of having cardiovascular disease within 8 years according to specified characteristics in a 45-year-old man. Framingham Study: 18-year follow-up*

Glucose intolerance	Choles-terol	Does not smoke cigarettes							Smokes cigarettes						
		Systolic blood pressure (mm Hg)							Systolic blood pressure (mm Hg)						
		105	120	135	150	165	180	195	105	120	135	150	165	180	195
A. No left ventricular hypertrophy by electrocardiogram															
Absent	185	22	27	35	43	54	68	84	38	47	59	73	91	112	138
	210	28	35	43	54	68	84	104	47	59	73	91	113	138	169
	235	35	44	54	68	84	104	129	59	74	91	113	139	169	205
	260	44	55	68	85	105	129	158	74	92	113	139	170	206	247
	285	55	68	85	105	129	158	192	92	113	139	170	206	247	293
	310	68	85	105	130	158	192	232	114	140	170	206	248	294	345
	335	85	105	130	159	193	232	277	140	171	207	248	295	346	401
Present	185	39	49	61	76	95	117	143	67	83	102	126	154	188	226
	210	49	61	76	95	117	144	175	83	103	126	155	188	227	271
	235	62	77	95	117	144	176	212	103	127	155	189	227	271	320
	260	77	95	118	144	176	213	255	127	156	189	228	272	321	374
	285	96	118	145	176	213	255	303	156	189	228	272	321	375	431
	310	118	145	177	214	256	303	355	190	229	273	322	375	432	490
	335	145	177	214	256	304	356	411	229	273	323	376	433	491	550
B. Left ventricular hypertrophy by electrocardiogram															
Absent	185	60	75	93	115	141	172	208	101	124	152	185	223	266	315
	210	75	93	115	141	172	209	250	124	152	185	223	267	315	363
	235	93	115	142	173	209	251	297	153	186	224	267	316	369	425
	260	116	142	173	209	251	298	349	186	224	268	316	369	426	484
	285	142	173	210	252	298	350	405	225	268	317	370	426	485	543
	310	174	210	252	299	351	406	464	269	318	371	427	485	544	602
	335	211	253	300	351	406	464	523	318	371	428	486	545	602	657
Present	185	105	129	158	191	231	275	324	170	205	246	293	344	399	456
	210	129	158	192	231	275	325	378	206	247	293	344	399	457	516
	235	158	192	232	276	325	379	436	247	294	345	400	457	516	574
	260	193	232	277	326	380	436	495	294	346	400	458	517	575	631
	285	232	277	327	380	437	496	554	346	401	459	518	576	632	635
	310	278	327	381	438	496	555	612	402	459	518	576	633	685	734
	335	328	382	438	497	556	613	667	460	519	577	633	686	734	773

From Kannel, W.B.: Am. J. Cardiol. **37**:269, 1976.

Statistically, the strongest or most predictive risk factors are smoking, elevated cholesterol, and hypertension. The role of genetics and its influence on the individual's resistance to the atherogenic precursors of smoking, hypertension, and so on are not clearly understood. Many experts in the field, most notably Kannel, believe that an adverse family history increases the risk for coronary disease primarily because families share risk factors such as smoking habit, poor diet, sedentary life-style, and tendency to develop hypertension.

Some common misconceptions about the risk factors exist because of the confusion between the so-called normal values, which merely represent the average value for a given population, or because of belief in outdated information. The Framingham statistics indicate that elevation of the systolic blood pressure is as strong a predictor for future coronary disease as elevated diastolic blood pressure for both men and women. Furthermore, the presumably innocuous rise in systolic blood pressure with age is associated with increased risk of future coronary events. The typical "normal" laboratory values for serum cholesterol of 150 to 300 mg/dl are also misleading. The Framingham studies indicate that the risk of developing coronary disease varies with the degree of elevation in the serum cholesterol, with a significant increase in risk when the value exceeds 220 mg/dl. Men who smoke as little as 1 to 9 cigarettes per day have 1.6 times the risk of developing atherosclerosis compared to that of the nonsmoker. The statistics for female light smokers are not much different. On the brighter side, quitting smoking can decrease the future risk of a coronary event as much as 50%.

The presence of other coexisting risk factors alters the

likelihood of developing coronary artery disease dramatically. For example, a 35-year-old man with elevated systolic blood pressure and serum cholesterol who smokes can have up to 38 times the risk of a coronary event within 6 years when compared to an age-matched male without risk factors. Table 2-1 illustrates more completely the probability relationship between multiple risk factors at varying levels of severity.[31]

Cholesterol

Although, as mentioned previously, total serum cholesterol is a predictor of future coronary events, the studies of Gordon[18] and others[1,6,32] indicate that it is important to know more about the various components of the serum cholesterol. Cholesterol does not circulate freely in the plasma because it is insoluble in an aqueous solution. Various plasma proteins bind with cholesterol and therefore facilitate transport from the liver to the target organs. The combination of these protein and cholesterol (or triglycerides) are referred to as ''lipoproteins.'' Refer to the review article by Grundy for more detailed discussion of cholesterol metabolism and transport.[22] There are two major classes of lipoproteins that are responsible for the transport of endogenous cholesterol, low-density lipoprotein (LDL), and high-density lipoprotein (HDL). Approximately 70% to 80% of the total serum cholesterol is bound to LDL, the chief transporter of cholesterol to the body cells. HDL functions to transport cholesterol from the body's cholesterol pools (red blood cells, spleen, muscle, adipose tissue) to the liver for excretion. The work of Gordon[11] and Miller[46] indicate the elevated serum levels of LDL or low serum levels of HDL or both increase the risk for the development of coronary artery disease. Gordon also reported that the ratio of total cholesterol to the HDL (cholesterol value divided by HDL value) is related to the probability of developing coronary atherosclerosis. A high total cholesterol-to-HDL ratio, such as 10, indicates that only a small portion of the total cholesterol is HDL and places the person at approximately two times the normal risk of experiencing a future coronary event.

Risk factor interrelationships

Finally, in consideration of the risk factors, it is important to keep in mind that there is a considerable amount of association or interrelationship between the risk factors. For example, low HDL values are associated with cigarette smoking,[52] sedentary life-style,[39,76] and with diabetes.[19] Diabetes is also associated with abnormally elevated serum triglycerides.[35] Thus the risk of developing coronary artery disease is related to multiple factors that are often associated with one another, and the greater the number of risk factors that exist, the greater the likelihood of developing angina, having a myocardial infarction, or dying suddenly from coronary artery disease.

Venous atherosclerosis

Atherosclerotic changes can and do occur in saphenous vein grafts, and the likelihood of this occurrence relates to the presence or absence of some of the major risk factors. Lie and others reported that 79% of the vein grafts in nine patients with hyperlipidemia who survived for 13 to 75 months after surgery had arteriosclerotic changes.[36] On the other hand, atherosclerosis was found in only 12% of the vein grafts in the patients with normal lipids. Barboriak[4] and Meadows[45] also reported evidence of atherosclerosis in vein grafts of hyperlipidemic patients. The effect of continued smoking, hypertension, and diabetes on vein graft atherosclerosis will require further study.

Mechanisms of atherogenesis: the relationship to risk factors

It is clear from the previous discussion that there are certain factors that increase the likelihood of developing coronary artery disease or vein-graft atherosclerosis. However, a cause-and-effect relationship between the risk factors and atherosclerosis cannot be assumed on the basis of the epidemiological studies alone. Salel and others investigated the relationship between a risk-factor index (score derived from total number of risk factors) to the presence or absence of coronary disease found at the time of angiography.[59] In this study, a significant relationship was found between the risk-factor index and coronary disease. In addition, the study results indicated that patients with multivessel disease had significantly higher risk-factor indexes compared to patients with single vessel disease. The specific relationship between the risk factors and atherogenesis is still undetermined.

A brief review of arterial and venous structure and function is warranted before discussion of the theoretical mechanisms involved with the genesis of the atherosclerotic process (atherogenesis). Arteries consist of three distinct layers (tunicae): intima, media, and adventitia (Fig. 2-7). The intima (inner layer) is lined with endothelial cells and supported by connective tissue. The middle layer, or media, consists mainly of smooth muscle cells, and the outer layer, or adventitia, consists of collagenous elastic fibers and small blood vessels (vasa vasorum). Veins, like arteries, have three layers, but the amount of smooth muscle tissue and elastic tissue is considerably less, most likely because veins function in a low-pressure system.

In addition to their function as conduits or tubes through which blood is transported from point to point, studies have shown that there is selective active transport of plasma proteins through the inner layer, or intima, to the adventitia and eventually to the lymphatic vessels.[41,61] The disturbance of this selective transport is postulated to be one of the key mechanisms involved with the process of atherogenesis.[2] Further discussion of this point follows.

Although all the mechanisms and processes involved with the formation of atherosclerotic lesions are not totally

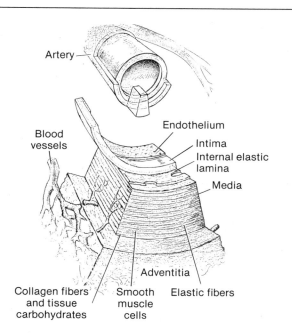

Fig. 2-7. Enlargement of a section of a coronary artery and its structural components, namely, the endothelium, the media consisting primarily of smooth muscle cells, and the adventitia. (From Benditt, E.P.: Sci. Am. **263**(2):74, 1977.)

understood, there is enough evidence from animal and human studies to construct a reasonable theoretical model of the process of atherogenesis.[71] This model relates most of the major risk factors to the basic mechanisms involved with the formation of atherosclerotic lesions. Refer to Braunwald's text for a more detailed discussion of the pathogenesis of atherosclerosis.[25]

There is evidence that the major component of the atherosclerotic plaque is LDL cholesterol and that when LDL cholesterol is allowed to seep into (insudate) the intima, it results in smooth muscle cell proliferation, increased collagen formation, and other reactions that are involved with the pathogenesis of atherosclerosis.[25,33,70,72,73,75] Furthermore, there are several identified factors that are responsible for alteration of the permeability of the arterial endothelial layer. This injury or damage to the arterial endothelial layer allows insudation of several macromolecules, such as LDL and fibrinogen, both of which are believed to be key factors in the atherogenic process. Huper[26,27,28] and others[3,34,50,74] have shown that hypoxia and elevated levels of serum carbon monoxide alters arterial permeability. These data suggest one way in which the risk factor of cigarette smoking plays a direct role in atherogenesis. Hypertension (probably as a result of direct trauma) and angiotensin II also have been shown to damage the endothelial cells and therefore alter permeability of the endothelial layer.[8,60] Catecholamines (epinephrine,

norepinephrine, serotonin, bradykinin), which can be elevated by stress or cigarette smoking, also cause endothelial damage.[63,64]

There is also evidence that certain blood components such as platelets and monocytes play a role in the pathogenesis of atherosclerosis. Mustard's studies demonstrated that platelets tended to adhere to the damaged or injured arterial intimal surfaces, and he and his co-workers speculated that this platelet aggregation contributed to the progression of the atherosclerotic process.[48,49] The more recent work of Ross has confirmed that platelet aggregation and eventually degeneration does occur at the site of intimal injury and that a platelet-derived growth factor (PDGF) is released at these sites.[55-58] Furthermore, this PDGF has been shown to stimulate increased cholesterol synthesis in the smooth muscle cells, increase the tendency for LDL cholesterol to bind to the smooth muscle cells, and stimulate proliferation of smooth muscle cells. All the above processes, including the smooth muscle cell proliferation, stimulated by the PDGF are believed to be important to the overall pathogenesis of atherosclerosis (Fig. 2-8).[56] The process of platelet aggregation is not totally unrelated to the known risk factors for coronary artery disease. In fact, hyperlipidemia, cigarette smoking, and glucose intolerance have been shown to increase the tendency for platelet aggregation.[9,13,48,69]

The role of high-density lipoproteins should be considered when one is examining the role of risk factors in the pathogenesis of atherosclerosis. There is evidence that HDL cholesterol protects against the formation of atherosclerotic plaques by (1) removing cholesterol and cholesterol esters from smooth muscle cells in the arterial wall[7,47,68] and (2) blocking the atherogenic action of LDL on the smooth muscle cells of the intima.[78] Further study is currently underway to investigate the protective mechanisms of HDL cholesterol. Based on what is currently known we can begin to understand why the epidemiological studies referred to earlier have consistently shown low levels of serum HDL to be a strong risk factor for coronary artery disease.

In summary, there is growing scientific evidence relating the major risk factors directly to the pathogenesis of atherosclerosis. These data underscore the importance of therapeutic modalities aimed at risk-factor reduction that are utilized in both primary and secondary prevention programs.

HEMODYNAMICS OF CORONARY ARTERY FLOW IN NORMAL AND DISEASED STATES

It is important to understand the normal determinants of myocardial oxygen supply and demand before attempting to appreciate the consequences of hemodynamically significant atherosclerotic occlusions in the coronary arteries.

The average resting coronary blood flow in man is 75 ml of blood per minute per 100 grams of myocardium and

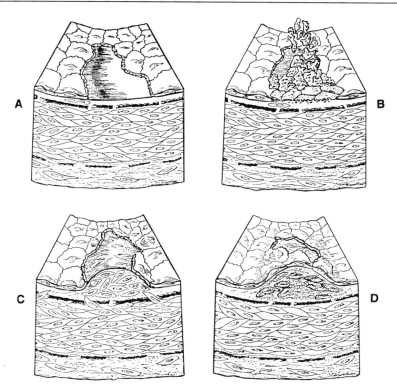

Fig. 2-8. A, Diagram of area of endothelial damage or injury, the major initial phase of atherogenesis. **B,** Secondary phase of atherogenesis involving platelet aggregation, a phase that probably precedes smooth muscle cell proliferation. **C,** Diagram of smooth muscle cell proliferation and migration from the media to the intima. **D,** Insudation of low-density-lipoprotein cholesterol within the inner layers of the arterial wall. (From Ross, R.: N. Engl. J. Med. **295:**420, 1976.)

can increase to as high as 350 ml of blood per minute per 100 grams at maximal exercise. Coronary blood flow or supply is dependent on (1) the driving pressure and (2) the resistance to flow along the coronary vascular bed. Because of the relatively high left ventricular subendocardial pressures (in relation to the distending pressures of the coronary arteries) and of intramyocardial pressure in general during systole, there is virtually no coronary flow to the subendocardial zones and minimal flow to the subepicardial regions.[37] Therefore the driving pressure is essentially the systemic diastolic blood pressure, since effective coronary filling takes place only during diastole. In the normal person the left ventricular end diastolic pressure is low (5 to 10 mm Hg) and therefore has little or no adverse effect on the net driving pressure (systemic diastolic blood pressure minus LV end-diastolic pressure). The vascular resistance to flow is dependent on the tone of the smooth muscle of the arteries and the length of the arteries. A third factor in determining coronary flow is length of filling time. Since the coronary arteries fill during diastole and since diastole comprises two thirds of the entire cardiac cycle at rest, filling time is not a limiting factor. During

exercise, as the heart rate increases, the time of systole remains fairly constant and the diastolic filling time can decrease as much as 35% to 40%. Once again, in the normal person, filling time, even during maximal exercise, is not a limiting factor. The determinants of myocardial oxygen demand are (1) heart rate, (2) systemic systolic blood pressure, (3) myocardial wall tension, and (4) rate of pressure generation in the left ventricle. At rest the average myocardial oxygen demand (MVo_2) is 10 ml of O_2/min/ 100 gm of myocardium, and with exercise the MVo_2 can exceed 50 ml of O_2/min/100 gm. In the normal, since the myocardium extracts 75% of the oxygen (a-$\bar{v}o_2$, or arterial and central venous oxygen difference) from the coronary blood supply both at rest and with exercise, any increase in myocardial oxygen demand is matched by an increase in coronary blood supply. The coronary blood flow is autoregulated as a result of both neural and metabolic influences. The most potent metabolic coronary vasodilator is hypoxia. In fact, it is assumed that the vasodilatory influence of hypoxia overrides the vasoconstricting influence of the alpha-adrenergic fibers that innervate the coronary vessels during exercise. The coronaries are also innervated by beta$_1$ and beta$_2$-adrenergic fibers, which act to vasodilate the vessels but play a relatively minor role in the regulation of coronary blood flow. In summary, the coronary blood flow is determined by (1) mechanical factors such as the driving pressure, extravascular pressure, and diastolic filling time, (2) metabolic factors such as hypoxia and to a lesser degree (3) neural influences resulting from innervation of both alpha- and beta-adrenergic fibers.

The obvious problem that fixed coronary atherosclerotic lesions present is the flow-demand relationship in a reduced coronary flow capacity, since the driving pressure decreases beyond the site of the lesion. What degree of stenosis is sufficient to reduce the capacity for blood or is hemodynamically significant? Logan demonstrated that at low flow rates (10 to 30 ml/min) resistance to flow was minimal; however, at flow rates of 30 to 100 ml/min, resistance increased two- to threefold.[38] More importantly, he demonstrated that lesions involving less than 70% to 80% stenosis had fairly constant curves of flow versus percent stenosis, but that with lesions greater than a range of 70% to 80% stenosis, minimal increases in luminal narrowing resulted in pronounced increases in resistance to flow and decrease in flow beyond the stenosis. The length of a lesion also is a factor in determining the hemodynamic consequence of a lesion.[21] A diffuse 50% lesion could impair coronary flow as much as or more than a discrete 70% lesion, for example. Sequential lesions also can have more of a bearing on flow capacity than a single discrete lesion depending on the percent stenosis.

The concept that all atherosclerotic lesions are fixed and rigid is somewhat misleading, and, in fact, there is evidence that coronary lesions are dynamic and variable, depending on the degree of vasomotor tone at the lesion site. Sharp increases in vasomotor tone leading to a localized or diffuse spasm of a coronary artery (with or without a fixed lesion) have been shown to reduce coronary flow significantly resulting in one of several clinical manifestations including resting angina, myocardial infarction or sudden death.[77] Recent evidence suggests that coronary spasm often occurs in patients with atherosclerotic lesions, and the degree of spasm is more severe at the site of the atherosclerotic lesion compared to adjacent uninvolved areas of the same artery in the same patient.[14] Maseri's work points out that there is a definite interrelationship between the vasomotor tone of an artery and the integrity of the endothelium, the presence of vasoactive substances, and certain components in the blood.[42] Specifically, the vasoactive substances that potentially can lead to coronary spasm include catecholamines, thromboxane A$_2$ (a substance derived from phospholipids of agglutinated platelets), serotonin, and histamine. Insufficient secretion of the prostaglandin prostacyclin (PGI$_2$), a vasodilator, can also allow for either localized or diffuse vasospasm, especially with higher than normal concentrations of the various vasoactive substances. Patients with periodic coronary spasm

that results in myocardial ischemia often exhibit certain characteristic signs or symptoms that include but are not limited to (1) a variant angina pattern often involving discomfort at rest and a variable threshold for exertional discomfort, (2) cyclic symptom patterns such as recurrent nocturnal or early morning discomfort, and (3) ST-segment elevation with or without symptoms. The definitive diagnostic procedure for coronary spasm is coronary angiography in conjunction with ergonovine (potent vasoconstrictor) administration. Medical therapy for patients with coronary spasm is discussed in Chapter 4.

In summary, the hemodynamic consequences of a coronary lesion depend on the degree of luminal narrowing, the length of the stenosis, the coronary blood flow rate and the degree of vasomotor tone of the affected artery. Significant perfusion or driving pressure losses beyond the site of the lesion because the above-mentioned factors leads to inadequate perfusion to the subendocardium, an area that is most sensitive to decreased driving pressures because of its direct contact with the left ventricular cavity. In the resting state the perfusion pressure beyond the stenosis must exceed a certain threshold (50 to 60 mm Hg). In the patient with a hemodynamically significant lesion, exercise with the associated increases in the heart rate and systolic blood pressure results in (1) increased extravascular pressure, (2) insufficient coronary flow, and (3) increased left ventricular filling pressures all of which result in decreased coronary perfusion pressures and eventually myocardial ischemia. In addition, as the myocardium becomes ischemic, there is a series of events that are believed to occur that reduce further the capacity for coronary flow.[11] Specifically, the ischemic myocardium does not relax completely, a condition that leads to (1) prolonged period of systole and thus shorter diastolic filling time, (2) decreased compliance of the left ventricle, and (3) increased left ventricular end diastolic pressure and consequently further decreases in the driving pressure, all of which lead to more severe ischemia.

Aortocoronary venous bypass grafts placed in the patient with advanced coronary lesions are subject to perfusion or driving pressures similar to those in the native coronary arteries, since the proximal origin of the grafts is located just distal to the ostium of the native coronary artery. There is recent evidence that blood flow through the grafts in the postoperative state is not determined by the luminal diameter of the graft provided that it is greater than 3 mm.[65] There is still considerable controversy over the influence of graft-to-host vessel-diameter ratio on graft flow. A more important consideration, however, is the influence of the bypass graft on blood flow beyond the lesion site in the coronary vessel.

The hemodynamic effects of coronary artery bypass grafts were studied in 24 patients with 29 grafts by Smith and others.[66] In general, the bypass grafts improved coronary blood flow by a mean of 268%. The authors also noted that in native coronary arteries with less than 80% obstruction there were minimal pressure gradients (difference in pressure before and beyond obstruction) and high postobstruction flow (mean of 75 ml/min/100 gm). When these lesions were bypassed, there was no significant increase in flow rates. In coronary lesions of 80% or greater, postobstruction flow was greatly reduced, and after bypass surgery, flow rates improved significantly. Although this study demonstrates that there appears to be a percent stenosis "threshold" above which bypass grafts increase flow, the results (in terms of absolute values) should be interpreted cautiously since the flow studies were done at rest and therefore at low demands for coronary perfusion. It is likely that the degree of improvement in coronary blood flow during exercise after aortocoronary bypass graft surgery is dependent on the severity of the bypassed lesion.

The effects of medications on both myocardial oxygen demand and coronary flow is discussed in Chapter 4.

ACUTE MYOCARDIAL INFARCTION

Prolonged ischemia as a result of complete occlusion of a coronary artery or a severe occlusion coupled with increased vasomotor tone will result in myocardial cell death or infarction. The exact pathophysiology of the coronary arteries that leads to infarction is not really known, and, in fact, there are at least four likely mechanisms: (1) progression of the atherosclerotic lesion to complete occlusion, (2) near total obstruction coupled with a thrombosis resulting in total obstruction of the vessel, (3) near total obstruction coupled with coronary spasm, or (4) near total obstruction coupled with prolonged relatively high myocardial oxygen demands. The actual process of infarction appears to involve either a single biological event or in some cases a wave of biological functions through which the infarction gradually progresses. Changes in the myocardial tissue (mitochondria, sarcomeres, and so on) begin to occur within 15 minutes after the tissue becomes hypoxic. The necrotic changes are followed by cell absorption and eventually scar formation.

The exact site and extent of necrosis depends on the anatomic distribution of the artery, the adequacy of collateral circulation, presence and extent of previous infarction, and various factors that could influence the myocardial oxygen demand such as catecholamine-release rates, activity of the autonomic nervous system, the systolic blood pressure, and the left ventricular end-diastolic volume and pressure. There are generally two types of myocardial infarctions: (1) transmural infarction, which extends through the subendocardial tissue to the epicardial layer of the myocardium, and (2) subendocardial infarction, which involves only the innermost layer of the myocardium and perhaps, in some cases, portions of the middle layer of tissue but does not extend to include the epicardial region of the myocardium.

The diagnosis of acute myocardial infarction is made from the combination of several findings including clinical history of symptoms, elevation of specific enzyme levels in the blood, presence of acute injury patterns on the 12-lead electrocardiogram, and, most recently, positive findings of special radioisotope studies. It is important to recognize that all the above-mentioned findings are not necessarily evident in every acute myocardial infarction and that in most cases the changes in enzyme levels and the 12-lead electrocardiogram are relied on most heavily.

The classic symptoms of an acute myocardial infarction involve central chest or retrosternal discomfort, which is severe in intensity. The nature of the discomfort varies among patients but most commonly is described as either pain or a pressure or heaviness that the patient states is "like a heavy weight on my chest." The discomfort often will radiate to several areas including the neck or jaw, one or both upper extremities, and the midscapular region. Infarction symptoms usually persist for prolonged periods of time but may wax and wane and are not relieved by nitroglycerin. Associated signs and symptoms commonly include dyspnea, diaphoresis, light-headedness, nausea, apprehension, weakness, vomiting, and hypotension. The clinician must be aware, however, that the so-called classic symptoms described above do not always accompany the infarction and the nature, location, and intensity of discomfort, along with the associated signs and symptoms, can be quite varied. Finally, myocardial infarctions can occur without symptoms; in fact, based on postmortem and epidemiological studies, 20% to 25% of all infarctions are "silent" or asymptomatic.

The use of serum enzymes levels to diagnose an acute myocardial infarction is based on several assumptions that are still somewhat controversial. First, it is assumed that elevation of the enzyme occurs only with cell death and not in instances of prolonged ischemia. Second, the enzyme rise is not attributable to damage in other major organs. Finally, there is a direct relationship between the amount of rise in the enzyme levels and the size of the infarction.

The three enzymes that are characteristically utilized in the diagnosis of acute myocardial infarction include creatine phosphokinase (CPK), aspartate aminotransferase (AST, formerly called "serum glutamic-oxaloacetic transaminase," SGOT), and lactate dehydrogenase (LDH). The serum levels of all three enzymes will generally increase within the first 36 hours of an infarction. The CPK levels usually elevate within 6 hours of myocardial cell death, followed by rises in the SGOT and LDH levels 6 to 12 hours later. The CPK values gradually return to normal over a period of 3 or 4 days, whereas the SGOT and LDH levels resolve by 7 to 9 days after the event. Although all three enzymes are relatively sensitive indicators of myocardial damage, the specificity of serum changes is poor because there are similar enzyme pools in other major or-

Table 2-2. Twelve-lead ECG changes and areas of infarction

Area of infarction	ECG changes
Anteroseptal	Q or QS in V_1-V_3
Anterior (localized)	Q or QS in V_2-V_4; V_1-V_6
Anterior lateral	Q or QS in I, aV_L; V_4-V_6
Lateral	Q or QS in I, aV_L
Inferior	Q or QS in II, III aV_F
Posterior	Increased R waves V_1-V_3

V_1 to V_6 are chest leads; I to III and aV_R, aV_L, and aV_F are extremity leads.

gans such as the brain, liver, and skeletal muscle. Recently, isoenzymes (different molecular forms of the same enzyme) of LDH and CPK have been found to be more specific to myocardial cell death.[70] The most specific isoenzyme is the CPK-II or what is also referred to as the MB-CPK fraction. It usually becomes elevated in the blood serum within 4 hours after infarction and peaks by 36 hours. False-positive rises in the CPK-II can occur in patients with myositis, muscular dystrophies, and pericarditis.

The acute changes in the 12-lead ECG that occur as a result of a myocardial infarction depend on (1) the type of infarction, that is, transmural versus subendocardial, and (2) the area of infarction. By definition, subendocardial infarctions result in new T-wave inversion or ST-segment depression or both that persist for 48 hours and there are no new Q-wave changes or R-wave losses.[40] Transmural infarctions usually result in convex ST-segment elevation associated with T-wave inversion in leads specific to the area of infarction (Table 2-2). In addition, evolutionary changes in the ECG pattern of a patient with a transmural infarction induce a significant Q wave (greater than 0.04 second in duration and greater than 25% of the amplitude of the R wave) and in some cases decreased R-wave voltage. Reciprocal ST-segment depression often occurs in undamaged areas opposite to the area of infarction. Studies indicate that 85% of the time ECG changes establish the correct diagnosis. Postmortem studies indicate that the sensitivity of acute ECG changes in infarction patients is 60% and the false-positive rate is 42%. The most common causes of "false-positive" 12-lead ECG changes include cardiomyopathies, cerebral vascular accidents, pulmonary emboli, hyperkalemia, idiopathic hypertrophic subaortic stenosis, and 12-lead conduction abnormalities such as left bundle branch block and Wolff-Parkinson-White (WPW) syndrome. Note that it is often 24 or more hours before the acute ECG changes described above appear.

NATURAL HISTORY OF CORONARY ARTERY DISEASE

An understanding of the natural history of coronary artery disease is important to the clinician who desires to identify the various subsets of patients that exist and the prognostic significance of each subset. Ideally, the awareness of these subsets, along with the data base accumulated from clinical monitoring, exercise testing, results from special studies, patient history, and physical exam, and so on, provide the basis for an individually designed serial evaluation plan and treatment program (see Chapters 6 and 7).

Atherosclerotic coronary artery disease is generally considered to be a progressive disease that can develop as early as the second decade of life.[12,43] The natural history of the disease is a bit difficult to document because of the variables of medical and surgical therapy, risk-factor reduction, and the presence or absence of other coexisting illnesses. Yet it is important to have some indication whether there appear to be certain factors, relative to the severity of the disease at the time of initial evaluation, that predict the likelihood of future coronary events such as progression of symptoms, recurrent myocardial infarction, or cardiac death. Unfortunately, most of the studies in the literature are limited by relatively short follow-up periods, except for the work of Bruschke[5,6] and Proudfit[53] from the Cleveland Clinic. The results of the Proudfit study will be discussed, since it involved a 10-year follow-up period of 601 nonsurgical patients. All these patients had evidence of at least 50% narrowing of one coronary artery at the time of entry into the study and were less than 65 years of age. This study used the end point of sudden death (terminal illness that began 1 hour before death) and did not attempt to examine carefully the likelihood of progression of symptoms or recurrent infarction. The number of arteries involved was an important prognostic factor with 10-year survival rates for patients with single-vessel, double-vessel, and triple-vessel disease being 63%, 45%, and 23% respectively. The presence of a 50% or greater lesion in the left main coronary artery was also an important prognostic factor with 10-year survival rates of 22%. Survival rates also related to ventricular function. Patients with large myocardial infarctions and therefore poor left ventricular function had lower survival rates than those with small areas of damage and normal ventricular function. Patients with a definite ventricular aneurysm or with ejection fractions less than 40% had 10-year survival rates of 10% to 18%. This finding is supported by the work of Nelson[51] and Hammermeister.[24] Finally, there were other factors that were prognostically influential and were independent of the number of coronary vessels diseased and ventricular function. These factors included the severity of functional impairment imposed by angina pectoris, ECG evidence of left ventricular hypertrophy or conduction defects, and persistence of risk factors such as cigarette

smoking, diabetes, and hypertension. Most recently, functional performance or time on the treadmill test has been shown to be an important predictor of survival as well.[44] Further discussion of this point appears in Chapter 6.

SUMMARY

There are two major epicardial or surface coronary arteries, the right coronary artery and the left main coronary artery. The left coronary system is the major source of blood supply to the left ventricle (LV) in that it perfuses up to 60% to 70% of the LV muscle mass. The precise perfusion distribution patterns of the coronary arteries vary among persons. The exact etiology of atherosclerosis is not fully understood; however, there are certain factors that have been shown to increase the likelihood of the disease process occurring in a given person. The major risk factors include cigarette smoking, increased serum levels of LDL cholesterol and triglycerides, decreased serum levels of HDL cholesterol, hypertension, diabetes, and sedentary life-style. There is evidence that the above factors play a role in the exact mechanisms of atherosclerosis.

The adequacy of coronary blood flow to the myocardium depends on the balance between supply and demand. Atherosclerotic changes in the coronary arteries can significantly decrease coronary supply because of luminal narrowing. Supply can be further compromised by increased vasomotor tone in the coronaries leading to acute spasm of the artery. The possible consequences of an imbalance between supply and demand include myocardial ischemia with or without symptoms, myocardial infarction, or sudden death. The diagnosis of an acute myocardial infarction is based on a combination of findings. Clinical symptoms, serum enzyme levels and changes in the 12-lead ECG are all used to determine the diagnosis of myocardial infarction.

Coronary artery disease is a progressive process. The prognosis of a patient with coronary disease depends primarily on the number of vessels diseased and the degree of left ventricular dysfunction as a result of infarction or ischemia.

REFERENCES

1. Albrink, M.J., and others: Serum lipids, hypertension and coronary artery disease, Am. J. Med. **31**:4, 1961.
2. Aschoff, L.: Lectures in pathology, New York, 1929, Paul B. Hoeber.
3. Astrup, P., and others: Enhancing influence of carbon monoxide on the development of atheromatosis in cholesterol fed rabbits, J. Atheroscler. Res. **7**:343, 1967.
4. Barboriak, J.J., and others: Atherosclerosis in aortocoronary vein grafts. Lancet **2**:621, 1974.
5. Bruschke, A.V.G., and others: Progress study of 590 consecutive non-surgical cases of coronary disease followed 5-9 years. I. Arteriographic correlations, Circulation **47**:1147, 1973.
6. Bruschke, A.V.G., and others: Progress study of 590 consecutive non-surgical cases of coronary disease followed 5-9 years. II. Ventriculographic and other correlations, Circulation **47**:1154, 1973.
7. Carew, T.E., and others: A mechanism by which high density lipoproteins may slow the atherogenic process, Lancet **1**:1315, 1976.
8. Constantinides, P., and Robinson, M.: Ultrastructural injury of arterial endothelium. II. Effects of vasoactive amines, Arch. Pathol. **88**:106, 1969.
9. Carvalho, A.C., and others: Platelet function in hyperlipoproteinemia, N. Engl. J. Med. **290**:434, 1974.
10. Dawber, T.R., and others: An approach to longitudinal studies in a community: the Framingham Study, Ann. N.Y. Acad. Sci. **107**:539, 1963.
11. Ellestad, M.H.: Ischemic ST segment depression: hemodynamic, electrophysiologic and metabolic factors in its genesis. In Stress testing: principles and practice, Philadelphia, 1976, F.A. Davis Co.
12. Enos, W.F., and others: Coronary disease among United States soldiers killed in action in Korea, J.A.M.A. **152**:1090, 1953.
13. Forbiszewski, R., and Worowski, K.: Enhancement of platelet aggregation and adhesiveness by beta lipoproteins, J. Atheroscler. Res. **8**:988, 1968.
14. Friedman, B., and others: Pathophysiology of coronary artery spasm, Circulation **66**:705, 1982.
15. Gensini, G.: Coronary arteriography, New York, 1975, Futura Publishing Co., Inc.
16. Gofman, J.W., and others: Ischemic heart disease, atherosclerosis and longevity, Circulation **34**:679, 1966.
17. Gordon, T., and Kannel, W.B.: Predisposition to atherosclerosis in the head, heart and legs: the Framingham Study, J.A.M.A. **221**:661, 1972.
18. Gordon, T., and others: High density lipoproteins as a protective factor against CHD, Am. J. Med. **62**:707, 1977.
19. Gordon, T., and others: Diabetes, blood lipids, and the role of obesity in coronary heart disease risk for women: the Framingham Study, Ann. Intern. Med. **87**:393, 1977.
20. Gorlin, R.: Coronary anatomy. Chapter 3 in Gorlin, R.: Coronary artery disease, vol. 11, Major problems in internal medicine series, Philadelphia, 1976, W.B. Saunders Co.
21. Gorlin, R.: Physiology of myocardial blood flow and metabolism. Chapter 5 in Gorlin, R.: Coronary artery disease, vol. 11, Major problems in internal medicine, series, Philadelphia, 1976, W.B. Saunders Co.
22. Grundy, S.M.: Cholesterol metabolism in man, West. J. Med. **128**:13, 1978.
23. Hamby, R.I.: Clinical-anatomical correlates in coronary artery disease, New York, 1979, Futura Publishing Co., Inc.
24. Hammermeister, K.E., and others: Variables predictive of survival in patients with coronary disease: selection by univariate and multivariate analyses from the clinical, electrocardiographic, exercise, arteriographic and quantitative angiographic evaluations, Circulation **59**:421, 1979.
25. Hanig, M., and others: Flotational lipoproteins extracted from human atherosclerotic aortas, Science **124**:176, 1956.
26. Huper, W.C.: Arteriosclerosis, Arch. Pathol. **38**:162, 1944.
27. Huper, W.C.: Arteriosclerosis, Arch. Pathol. **39**:57, 1945.
28. Huper, W.C.: Pathogenesis of atherosclerosis, Am. J. Clin. Pathol. **26**:559, 1956.
29. James, T.N.: Anatomy of the coronary arteries, New York, 1961, Harper & Row, Publishers, Inc.
30. Jenkins, C.D., and others: Prediction of clinical coronary heart disease by a test for the coronary-prone behavior pattern, N. Engl. J. Med. **290**:1271, 1974.
31. Kannel, W.B.: Some lessons in cardiovascular epidemiology from Framingham, Am. J. Cardiol. **37**:269, 1976.
32. Kannel, W.B., and others: Serum cholesterol, lipoproteins, and the risk of coronary heart disease: the Framingham Study, Ann. Intern. Med. **24**:1, 1971.
33. Kao, V.C.Y., and Wissler, R.W.: A study of the immunohistochemical localization of serum lipoproteins and other plasma proteins in human atherosclerotic lesions, Exp. Mol. Pathol. **4**:465, 1965.
34. Kjeldsen, K., and others: Ultrastructural intimal changes in the rabbit

aorta after a moderate carbon monoxide exposure, Atherosclerosis **16:**67, 1972.

35. Levy, R.J., and Glueck, C.J.: Hypertriglyceridemia, diabetes mellitus and coronary vessel disease, Arch. Intern. Med. **123:**220, 1969.

36. Lie, J.T., and others: Aortocoronary bypass saphenous vein graft atherosclerosis: anatomic study of 99 vein grafts from normal and hyperlipoproteinemic patients up to 75 months postoperatively, Am. J. Cardiol. **40:**906, 1977.

37. Little, R.C.: Circulation to special areas. In Little, R.C., editor: Physiology of the heart and circulation, Chicago, 1977, Year Book Medical Publishers, Inc.

38. Logan, S.E.: On the fluid mechanics of human coronary artery stenosis, IEEE Trans. Biomed. Eng. **22:**327, 1975.

39. Lopez, A., and others: Effect of exercise and physical fitness on serum lipids and lipoproteins, Atherosclerosis **20:**1, 1974.

40. Madigan, M.P., and others: The clinical course, early prognosis and coronary anatomy of subendocardial infarction, Am. J. Med. **62:**634, 1976.

41. Mancini, R.E., and others: Extravascular distribution of fluorescent albumin, globulin and fibrinogen in connective tissue structures, J. Histochem. Cytochem. **10:**194, 1962.

42. Maseri, A.: Coronary artery spasm and atherosclerosis. In Santamore, W.P., and Boe, A., editors: Coronary artery disease, Baltimore, 1982, Urban & Schwarzenberg, Inc.

43. McNamara, J.J., and others: Coronary artery disease in combat casualties in Vietnam, J.A.M.A. **216:**1185, 1971.

44. McNeer, J.F., and others: The role of the exercise test in the evaluation of patients for ischemic heart disease, Circulation **57:**64, 1978.

45. Meadows, W., and others: Risk factors related to progressive narrowing in aortocoronary vein grafts studied 1 and 5 years, Circulation **64**(Suppl. 4):292, 1981. (Abstract.)

46. Miller, G.J., and others: Plasma high-density lipoprotein concentration and development of ischemic heart disease, Lancet **1:**16, 1975.

47. Miller, N.W., and others: Relationship between plasma lipoprotein cholesterol concentrations and the pool size and metabolism of cholesterol in man, Atherosclerosis **23:**535, 1976.

48. Mustard, J.F., and Murphy, C.A.: Effect of smoking on blood coagulation and platelet survival in man, Br. Med. J. **1:**846, 1963.

49. Mustard, W.P., and others: The role of thrombogenic factors in atherosclerosis, Ann. N.Y. Acad. Sci. **149:**848, 1968.

50. Myaskinov, A.L.: Influence of some factors on the development of experimental cholesterol atherosclerosis, Circulation **17:**99, 1958.

51. Nelson, G.R., and others: Prognosis in medically treated coronary artery disease: influence of ejection fraction compared to other parameters, Circulation **52:**408, 1975.

52. Pozner, H., and Bellimoria, J.D.: Effect of smoking on blood clotting and lipid and lipoprotein levels, Lancet **2:**1319, 1970.

53. Proudfit, W.L.: Natural history of obstructive coronary artery disease: ten year study of 601 non-surgical cases, Prog. Cardiovasc. Dis. **21:**53, 1978.

54. Rosenman, R.H., and others: Coronary heart disease in the Western Collaborative Group Study: final follow-up experience of 8½ years, J.A.M.A. **233(8):**872, 1975.

55. Ross, R.: Atherosclerosis and the arterial smooth muscle cell, Science **180:**1322, 1973.

56. Ross, R: The pathogenesis of atherosclerosis. In Santamore, W.P., and Boe, A., editors: Coronary artery disease, Baltimore, 1982, Urban & Schwarzenberg, Inc.

57. Ross, R., and Glosmet, J.A.: The pathogenesis of atherosclerosis, N. Engl. J. Med. **295:**420, 1976.

58. Ross, R., and others: A platelet dependent serum factor that stimulates the proliferation of arterial smooth muscle cells in vitro, Proc. Natl. Acad. Sci. (USA) **71:**1207, 1964.

59. Salel, A., and others: Risk factor profile and severity of coronary artery disease, N. Engl. J. Med. **296:**1447, 1977.

60. Schwartz, S.M.: Assessment of angiotensin endothelial injury by incident light microscopy, Fed. Proc. **35:**208, 1976.

61. Scott, P.J., and Hurley, P.J.: The distribution of radio-iodinated serum albumin and low-density lipoprotein in tissues and the arterial wall, Atherosclerosis **11:**77, 1970.

62. Shell, W.: Specificity of cardiac enzymes in clinical strategies. In Swan, G., and Corday, E., editors: Ischemic heart disease: new concepts and current controversies, Baltimore, 1979, The Williams & Wilkins Co.

63. Shimamoto, T.: The relationship of edematous reaction in arteries to atherosclerosis and thrombosis, J. Atheroscler. Res. **3:**87, 1963.

64. Shimamoto, T.: Contraction of endothelial cells as a key mechanism in atherogenesis. In Weigel, A., editor: Atherosclerosis III: proceedings of the third international symposium, Berlin, 1974, Springer-Verlag.

65. Simon, R., and others: Blood velocity and dimensions of aortocoronary venous bypass graft in the postoperative state, Circulation **66**(Suppl. I):34, 1982.

66. Smith, S.C., and others: Myocardial blood flow in man: effects of coronary collateral circulation and coronary artery bypass surgery, J. Clin. Invest. **51:**2556, 1972.

67. Sokolow, M., and McIllroy, M.B.: Clinical cardiology, Philadelphia, 1979, Lange Medical Publications.

68. Stein, Y., and others: The removal of cholesterol from aortic smooth muscle cells in culture and Landschutz ascites cells by fractions of human high-density lipoproteins, Biochem. Biophys. Acta **390:**106, 1975.

69. Sullivan, J.M., and others: Studies of platelet adhesiveness, glucose tolerance and serum lipoprotein patterns in patients with coronary artery disease, Am. J. Med. Sci. **264:**475, 1972.

70. Tracy, R.E., and others: On the antigenetic identity of human serum beta and alpha-2 lipoproteins, and their identification in aortic intima, Circ. Res. **9:**472, 1961.

71. Walton, K.W.: Pathogenetic mechanism in atherosclerosis, Am. J. Cardiol. **35:**542, 1975.

72. Walton, K.W., and Burkerley, D.J.: Studies on the pathogenesis of corneal arcus formation. II. Immunofluorescent studies on lipid deposition in the eye of the lipid-fed rabbit, J. Pathol. **111:**97, 1975.

73. Walton, K.W., and others: The pathogenesis of xanthoma, J. Pathol. **109:**271, 1973.

74. Wanstrup, J., and others: Acceleration of spontaneous intimal-subintimal changes in rabbit aorta by prolonged moderate carbon monoxide exposure, Acta Pathol. Microbiol. Scand. **75:**353, 1969.

75. Wissler, R.W.: Principles of the pathogenesis of atherosclerosis. In Braunwald, P., editor: Heart disease: a textbook of cardiovascular medicine, Philadelphia, 1980, W.B. Saunders Co.

76. Wood, P.D., and others: Plasma lipoprotein distributions in male and female runners. Ann. N.Y. Acad. Sci. **301:**748, 1977.

77. Yasue, H.: Pathophysiology and treatment of coronary arterial spasm, Chest **78:**216, 1980.

78. Yoshida, Y., and others: Effects of normolipemic HDL on proliferation of aortic smooth muscle cells induced by hyperlipemic LDL, Circulation **56**(Suppl. 3):100, 1977.

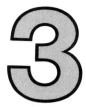

Z. DAVID SKLOVEN

Hemodynamics

This chapter presents a broad description of the cardiovascular system in exercise. Neither the length of the chapter nor its intent permits a highly detailed discussion of central or peripheral vascular physiology and, in particular, of hemodynamics. However, for development of a coherent concept of the exercise cardiovascular response, a reasonable understanding of the fundamental properties of cardiac function and the integration of these properties with the peripheral vascular response are essential. Within this framework, the basic properties governing cardiac function are introduced to provide a basis for discussion of the integrated cardiovascular response to exercise.[7]

CARDIAC MUSCLE MECHANICS

Any discussion of cardiac behavior during exercise requires that one have a clear understanding of the basic principles of cardiac muscle mechanics and pump function. Of fundamental importance are the concepts of (1) preload, (2) afterload, and (3) contractile state—three mechanisms that can be defined first in terms of the structural and chemical properties of the cardiac contractile proteins and then form the cornerstone for further study of the behavior of the heart during exercise.

The sliding-filament model of muscular shortening identifies the fundamental mechanism of muscular contraction as the cross bridging and subsequent force generation that develops between actin and myosin polypeptides in the contractile motor unit (the sarcomere) during the "active state." The magnitude of the force generated is, in large part, a function of the number of actin-myosin cross bridges that can link during a single contraction. This, in turn, is determined by the extent of actin-myosin contraction (Fig. 3-1). Preload, defined within this context, is a stretching force that elongates the resting sarcomere before activation and, as a consequence, governs the extent of cross bridging and ultimately the magnitude of sarcomere force generation during each contraction cycle.

At each instant during contraction, the total force generated by all the left ventricular sarcomeres compresses the blood-filled ventricular cavity, raising intraventricular pressure to aortic pressure level. This, in turn, opens the semilunar valves, and ejection begins. Afterload is conceptualized as the total instantaneous force within the myocardial wall required to elevate intraventricular pressure to aortic pressure level. Afterload, at the sarcomere level, is thus the force required, per sarcomere, to generate this total instantaneous wall force. Afterload is, in effect, a force opposing sarcomere shortening that must be overcome for shortening to occur.

The energy used for force development in the actin-myosin cross bridge is derived from the splitting of ATP by ATPase located on the myosin polypeptide. The rate and intensity of the cross-bridge reaction is largely a function of the specific kinetics of myosin ATPase. The contractile state is a measure of the innate intensity and rate of force development in the contractile unit and is thus a reflection of the reaction kinetics that release energy for force development from ATP.

The three properties of myocardial muscle just described have been studied extensively by use of the papillary muscle strip preparation.[1,2] Brief consideration of this model will enable us to translate fundamentals of muscle mechanics at the sarcomere level to the intact part. In this model (Fig. 3-2), one end of a papillary muscle strip is affixed to a strain gauge so that the force produced can be measured. The opposite end is attached to a movable lever. The lever can be locked so that the muscle strip is permitted to contract, but it prevents any shortening resulting in an isometric contraction. With the lever unlocked and free to pivot about its fulcrum, the muscle strip can both contract and shorten against some load attached to the opposite end of the lever—isotonic contraction. By attachment of different weights (loads) to the lever before stimulation, the muscle can be prestretched to varying initial lengths; that is, pre-

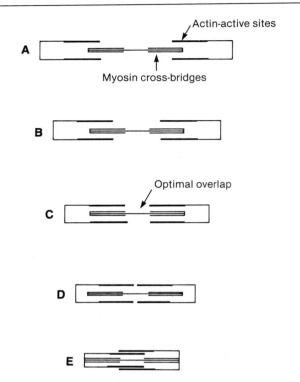

Fig. 3-1. Excessive preload overstresses the sarcomere, **A** and **B**, resulting in suboptimal cross-bridge formation. Inadequate preload, **D** and **E**, results in overlap of actin peptides and suboptimal actin-myosin bridging. Optimal sarcomere length, **C.**

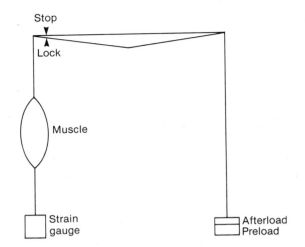

Fig. 3-2. A model of fundamental muscle mechanics. Papillary muscle is affixed to a strain gauge and a movable lever that can be locked. Variations in loading sequence and locking the lever simulates the hemodynamic effects of preload and afterload.

load can be varied. Once the initial resting length has been obtained with the preload, a stop allows additional load to be added to the lever—the afterload. The afterload does not affect the muscle, however, until it attempts to shorten and lift the applied load. For shortening to occur, the muscle strip must generate a force equal to the load it must lift, that is, the afterload.

Stimulation of the muscle strip with the lever fixed produces an isometric contraction in which force is generated but no shortening occurs. A plot of force developed versus initial muscle length (the force-length relation, Fig. 3-3, A reveals that a maximal developed force occurs at a specific initial length (L_0), whereas less force is obtained at lengths less than or greater than L_0. L_0 has been shown to correspond to a sarcomere length of 2 to 2.2 μm, with the length yielding optimal actin-myosin overlap. With the lever free to move, force rises in the stimulated muscle and shortening starts when the force developed equals the afterload. Once shortening starts, the force remains constant (equal to afterload) until relaxation occurs, thus the term "isotonic contraction" (Fig. 3-3, B). The initial velocity of shortening and the total extent of shortening at a given preload can be determined relative to afterload (Fig. 3-3,

B). From these results, it is apparent that both the velocity and the extent of shortening diminish as the afterload rises. At afterload P_0, the maximal force the muscle can generate, shortening ceases and the model behaves as an isometric contraction. In Fig. 3-4, the initial velocity of shortening is plotted versus afterload to give a velocity-force relation. The force intercept at zero velocity defines P_0. Extrapolation to zero afterload yields a theoretical maximal velocity of shortening that has been shown to reasonably reflect the intrinsic rate and intensity of force development, that is "contractile state." This extrapolated peak velocity is termed "V_{max}." Fig. 3-4 illustrates the effect of varying the preload on the velocity-force curve. At higher preloads, greater force is generated at each velocity except at the V_{max}; conversely, except for V_{max}, the velocity of shortening is higher for any given afterload. This behavior is consistent with the concept that preload affects the muscle through a mechanism that does not alter contractile state (i.e., V_{max} is unchanged).

In Fig. 3-4, the result of adding an inotropic agent to the muscle strip bath is seen. Here, in addition to shifting the curve to the right (as with increased preload), the zero load intercept V_{max} is also higher, reflecting a rise in the muscle's contractile state. Thus, at a given preload, raising the contractile state yields greater force-generating capacity or conversely a higher velocity of shortening at a given preload and afterload.

Translation of the concepts of afterload and preload to the intact heart is expedited by use of a thick-walled sphere as a model for the ventricle. During diastole, venous-blood return passively distends the ventricle, and both diastolic

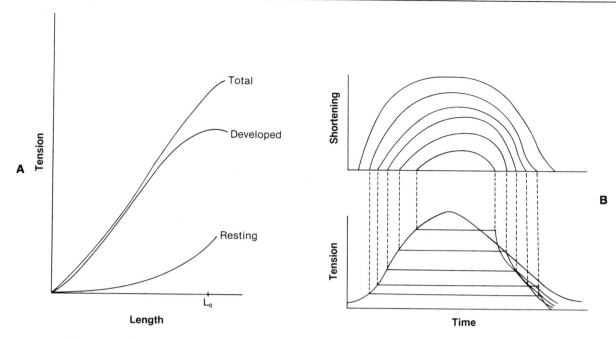

Fig. 3-3. A, Total measured force minus resting from a given initial length. Maximal force develops from length, L_0 (see text). **B,** Shortening is measured at increasing afterloads. The initial slope (shortening per time) defines shortening velocity for each afterloaded contraction. Preload is held constant.

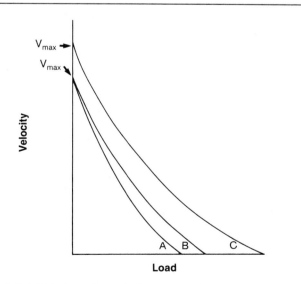

Fig. 3-4. Initial shortening velocity versus afterload, *A.* Increased preload, *B.* Increased contractile state, *C.*

volume and pressure rise. The relation of passive diastolic resting pressure to distending blood volume is determined by the passive elastic properties of the myocardial wall and is depicted in Fig. 3-5 as the diastolic compliance curve for the ventricle. As intraventricular pressure rises, the circumferential force or wall tension (depicted in Fig. 3-6) (as midwall resting tension) increases according to the equation for circumferential tension in a thick-walled sphere:

$$\textbf{(1)} \qquad\qquad T = PR/h$$

where T is mid-wall tension, P is intraventricular pressure, R is radius at the midwall, and h is the wall thickness.

The circumferential tension in the myocardial wall is, strictly speaking, the force that stretches the sarcomeres before contraction. Since T is proportional to intraventricular pressure, P, by equation (1), preload can be more conveniently defined in terms of intraventricular pressure, specifically end-diastolic pressure, in the intact heart. Moreover, through the compliance curve, diastolic pressure and volume are directly related; thus we are able to interchange end-diastolic pressure or end-diastolic volume for preload, whenever either parameter is more applicable to use.

During systole, force or tension developed in the myo-

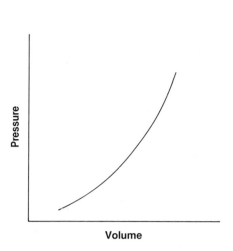

Fig. 3-5. Diastolic pressure versus volume defines the elastic property or "compliance" of the ventricle. The slope of the curve dp/dV represents compliance at a given volume.

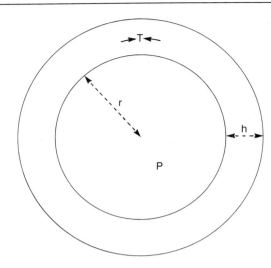

Fig. 3-6. Circumferential wall tension, T, is a function at any instance of ventricular size, R, intraventricular pressure, P, and wall thickness, h.

cardial wall raises intraventricular pressure until central aortic pressure is reached, at which point the aortic valve opens and ejection ensues. The instantaneous systolic wall tension required to elevate intraventricular pressure to aortic levels is given by equation (1) again under the assumption of a thick-walled, spherical model. In this instance, midwall tension is actively developed force resulting from sarcomere force generation, and rigorously defined, this tension represents afterload. From equation (1) afterload, T, is a function of central aortic pressure, P, ventricular size, R, and wall thickness, h. If we assume a constant wall thickness and integrate instantaneous afterload throughout all of systole, the following equation

$$(2) \quad \int_{R_D}^{R_s} P dr = P \times R \qquad (R = \text{average systolic radius})$$

yields a simplified average afterload that is primarily a function of aortic blood pressure and intraventricular radius, R. By adding a further constraint, that R be assumed constant, we obtain afterload proportional to aortic pressure. By equation (3) average aortic blood pressure is a function of flow (cardiac output, CO) and total peripheral resistance (TPR):

$$(3) \quad \overline{P} \propto CO \times TPR = \overline{HR} \times \overline{SV} \times TPR$$

Finally, assuming constant cardiac output, afterload can be shown to be dependent on the level of peripheral vasoconstrictor tone (TPR). Keeping in mind the more rigorous definition of afterload, either mean aortic blood pressure or TPR will be used as a reasonable approximation for this variable in the discussion that follows.

Utilizing the ventricular pressure-volume loop (Fig. 3-7, A), one represents the preload by points along the passive ventricular filling curve (A-C) as end-diastolic volume, whereas afterload in this framework is depicted as intraventricular pressure. The counterpart to the isometric muscle strip contraction in the intact heart is the isovolumic contraction depicted in Fig. 3-7, A. Here, cross-clamping the aorta prevents ejection, and the ventricle can thus develop only force without shortening. From a given end-diastolic volume (A) contraction begins and pressure rises isovolumic to B, peak isovolumic pressure. Repeating the contraction from several end-diastolic volumes (varying preload) defines the isovolumic pressure curve (B-D), which is analogous to the muscle strip force-length relation discussed earlier. The isovolumic pressure line defines the maximum force or pressure that the ventricle can generate from each preload. Line B_1-D_1 illustrates the effect of a positive inotropic intervention where raising contractile state yields greater peak force or pressure development from any given end-diastolic volume. This is analogous to the increase in P_0 resulting from increased inotropy in the papillary muscle model.

A normal contractile cycle is illustrated in Fig. 3-7, B, with the aortic cross-clamp having been removed. At the onset of contraction, intraventricular pressure rises isovolumically from point A until aortic pressure is reached at B, where the aortic valve opens. Ejection then occurs along the line B-C until the isovolumic pressure line is reached. Further ejection is impeded, since any further loss of ventricular volume will occur along the isovolumic pressure line, thus reducing developed intraventricular pressure below aortic blood pressure resulting in closure of

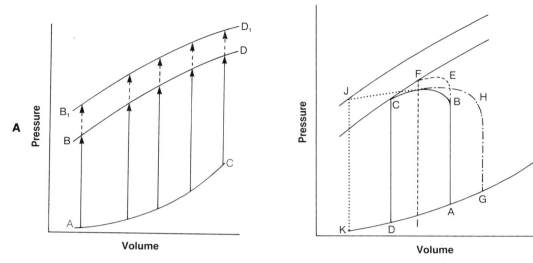

Fig. 3-7. A, Isovolumic contraction from several preloads *(end-diastolic volume, EDV)* yields a peak force curve, the isovolumic pressure curve, *B-D.* Increased contractile state raises the isovolumic pressure curve, B_1-D_1. **B,** Auxotonic contraction (normally ejecting cycle). Control cycle, *A-B-C-D.* Increased preload, *G-H-C-D.* Increased afterload, *A-E-F-I.* Increased contractile state, *A-B-J-K.*

the aortic valve. From C the ventricle relaxes; at first, isovolumically to D and then refills during diastole along its passive compliance curve (D-A).

B-C, the volume change during ejection, is the stroke volume (end-diastolic minus end-systolic volume). The effect on stroke volume (SV) of increasing the preload (greater end-diastolic volume, EDV) is shown by loop (G-H-C-D). Here the ventricle contracting from a higher EDV ejects a larger stroke volume, with the ejection ending at the same point on the isovolumic pressure line as the previous contraction did. That the increment in the stroke volume exactly matches the increment in the end-diastolic volume implies that the heart is capable of increasing its forward output by whatever rise in venous return occurs. Loop A-E-F-I reflects the effect of increasing the afterload (aortic blood pressure) on stroke volume. In order to open the aortic valve, intraventricular pressure must now rise to the higher aortic blood pressure level (E) after which ejection occurs along a new path (E-F) intersecting the isovolumic pressure line at a higher end-systolic volume and pressure. The net result is a reduction in stroke volume concomitant with elevation of aortic blood pressure or afterload. As shown in later sections, the converse is true as well; that is, an increase in stroke volume can be affected by afterload reduction. Fig. 3-7, *B*, illustrates the effect of adding an inotropic agent to the intact heart causing an increase in the contractile state. Since the increased contractile state yields greater force-generating capacity at any ventricular volume, the

entire isovolumic pressure line is shifted leftward and upward, and, assuming constant preload and afterload, stroke volume is enhanced (B-J).

If the data contained in the pressure-volume loops are replotted as stroke volume versus end-diastolic volume (or pressure) a "ventricular-function curve" (Fig. 3-8) is obtained. Here an increase or decrease in preload is depicted by when one moves rightward or leftward along the curve, whereas different levels of contractile state are represented by members of a whole family of ventricular-function curves. Using this convention, one may readily see that the net result of increasing the contractile state compared to reducing the afterload is identical in terms of stroke volume within the context of the ventricular function curve.

Normal cardiac function at rest and during exercise implies that the heart must be capable of maintaining adequate systemic blood flow (cardiac output, CO) to sustain any level of bodily activity throughout this wide range.

The exercise cardiovascular response is complex and not yet fully elucidated, however, all the myriad circulatory changes that occur have, as their final common pathways, modification of preload, afterload, contractile state, and heart rate. A brief consideration of these mechanisms in the context of the ventricular function curve serves as a cornerstone on which to develop a more elaborate cardiovascular response to exercise.

The simplest modality to elevate the cardiac output (CO) is an increase in heart rate (HR), which, up to between

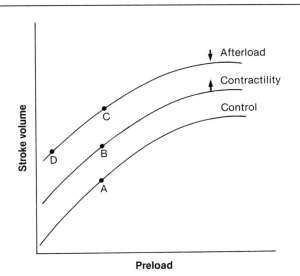

Fig. 3-8. The ventricular function curve. Control SV, *A*, rises to *B* with increased contractile state. Reduction of afterload further augments SV, *C*. Failure of venous return to rise as these events occur would result in a severe limitation in the extent of increase in SV, *D*.

170 to 190, provides a linear rise in the cardiac output according to the equation:

$$CO = HR \times SV$$

At some limiting upper rate, any further increase in heart rate will begin to encroach on diastolic ventricular filling time and the cardiac output will begin to fall. An increase in the heart rate is, in general, accompanied by an increase in the contractile state, and thus the heart shifts to a higher ventricular function curve (Fig. 3-8, point *B*). Concomitant afterload reduction further augments ventricular function (Fig. 3-8, point *C*), the result of both of these mechanisms being higher stroke volume from a given end-diastolic volume. During upright exercise, it is doubtful that an increase in preload occurs; however, the importance of venous return is paramount for were the end-diastolic volume (preload) not maintained at resting levels, the extent of cardiac output augmentation by the preceding mechanisms would be severely compromised (Fig. 3-8, point *D*).

CIRCULATORY RESPONSE TO EXERCISE

"Exercise" without additional qualifications is a nonspecific term encompassing a broad range of types and intensity of muscular activity. This chapter discusses specifically the type of exercise that is categorized as "dynamic" or "aerobic." In particular, dynamic exercise is characterized by the following properties: (1) repetitive, rhythmic muscular movement, generally involving large muscle groups (arms, legs) that can be sustained over a

period of several minutes to hours; (2) the muscles contract in a range far below their maximal capacity for force generation (10% to 30% of maximal strength is utilized); (3) the muscular energy conversion pathways involved are, to all extents, completely aerobic. Common examples of this exercise type include walking, jogging, cycling, swimming, or rowing.

Oxygen consumption

The utilization of entirely aerobic metabolic processes for energy production in this form of exercise provides a convenient and clinically applicable method by which to quantify exercise level or work load. In effect, the intensity of aerobic work is a direct determinant of total body oxygen uptake per unit time, a value that is easily measured in the experimental laboratory and in the clinical setting.

Minute oxygen consumption, or $\dot{V}O_2$, is the product of two complex variables:

(A) $$\dot{V}O_2 = CO \times \text{a-}\bar{v}O_2 \text{ diff}$$

Cardiac output (CO), the volume of O_2-carrying blood pumped per minute, can be thought of as the "delivery" component of the equation; whereas a-$\bar{v}O_2$ diff (arterial and central venous oxygen difference) is the measure of the oxygen "extraction" capacity at the working muscle level. The a-$\bar{v}O_2$ diff is related to the extensiveness of the muscle vascular bed and the level of activity of the cellular oxidative enzyme systems. Since CO = HR × SV, equation (A) can be rewritten as:

(B) $$\dot{V}O_2 = HR \times SV \times \text{a-}\bar{v}O_2 \text{ diff}$$

If testing (in this case, treadmill) is performed with $\dot{V}O_2$ measured at progressively more intense exercise levels, a point is reached where no further increment in HR, SV, or a-$\bar{v}O_2$ diff can occur and exhaustion will ensue within moments. This plateau level of O_2 consumption is a reproducible measure of the subject's total aerobic work capacity and is termed $\dot{V}O_{2\ max}$. Equation (B) then becomes:

(C) $$\dot{V}O_{2\ max} = HR_{max} \times SV_{max} \times \text{a-}\bar{v}O_{2\ max}$$

Aerobic work at the submaximal level can thus be defined in terms of relative work intensity, that is, submaximal $\dot{V}O_2$ as a percent of $\dot{V}O_{2\ max}$:

$$\dot{V}O_{2\ rel} = \frac{\dot{V}O_{2\ actual}}{\dot{V}O_{2\ max}}$$

Cardiovascular response

The immediate adaptive response of the circulatory system to exercise involves virtually every component of the circulation. The essential and unifying features of the circulatory changes accompanying exercise are an augmentation and redistribution of cardiac output, such that the working musculature receives a greatly enhanced blood flow while nonworking areas maintain sufficient flow for normal homeostatic function during even prolonged exercise. The main elements of the circulatory response are (1) generalized vasoconstriction, mediated by the sympathetic nervous system (SNS), (2) greatly increased cardiac pump function attributable to combined (SNS) and peripheral vascular affector mechanisms, and (3) profound locally mediated, reduction in resistance in the working muscle vascular bed.

Vasodilation/vasoconstriction. The systemic vascular system consists of organ-associated arterio-capillary-venous circuits connected in a parallel arrangement (Fig. 3-9). Total resistance to blood flow through this system (total peripheral resistance, or the pressure gradient per unit of blood flow between the aorta and the right atrium) is given by the equation:

(E) $$1/R_t = 1/R_i + \ldots + 1/R_n$$

where R_t is TPR, R_i is resistance in each circuit, and n is total number of circuits.

During exercise, equation (E) can be simplified to $1/\text{TPR} = 1/R_w + R_{nw}$, where R_w represents resistance in the working muscle bed and R_{nw} represents net resistance in all other nonworking organ vascular circuits (Fig. 3-9).

At the onset of exercise (actually beginning even before exercise starts), the resistance (arteriolar) and capacitance (venous) components of the working muscular vascular bed dilate profoundly resulting in a large reduction in resistance to blood flow through the working muscle. At the same time, resistance in nonworking areas increases because of a generalized vasoconstrictive stimulus to be discussed in a later section. The net result of these two opposing vascular phenomena is a characteristic feature of the behavior of total resistance across parallel circuits; that is, despite a widesperad rise in resistance in many beds, a significant drop in resistance in one area can effect a net lowering of resistance across the entire circuit. Table 3-1 illustrates that because of the behavior of resistance across a parallel circuit even a doubling of nonworking resistance during exercise can be offset by a modest (30% to 40%) reduction in resistance in the working muscular bed to yield net reduction in TPR. The situation in the exercising person is, of course, far more complex, but the general principles derived above still hold. If one assumes that $R_w = R_{nw} = 10$ units and TPR = 5 units at rest and a rise in R_{nw} to 20 units with exercise, TPR is calculated as a function of changing R_w (Fig. 3-10).

The vasodilatation response is a profoundly important hemodynamic event that is unique to exercise. Local vasodilatation, by reduction of TPR and thus afterload, can augment the cardiac output independently of any change in heart rate or inotropic state. Thus a portion of the rise in the cardiac output with exercise is directly proportional to the magnitude of the local vasodilatory reaction. Coincident with the reduction in the afterload, the enhanced

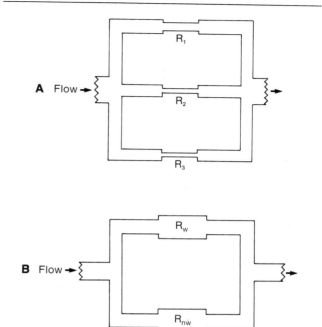

Fig. 3-9. A, *R1, R2, R3:* resistance in specific vascular beds

$$1/R\ total = \sum_{1}^{n} 1/R_i$$

B, During exercise, resistance can be partitioned between working R_w and nonworking R_{nw} vascular compartments.

Table 3-1. Net reduction in total peripheral resistance (TPR)

TPR	Working resistance (R_w)	Nonworking resistance (R_n)
At rest, 5	10	10
6.7	10	20
6.2	9	20
5.7	8	20
5.2	7	20
4.6	6	20
4	5	20
3.3	4	20

flow through the working muscle augments venous return, which serves to maintain preload—a prerequisite for augmented stroke volume. In the absence of this increase in venous return, preload would fall displacing the heart leftward along the ventricular function curve and thus curtailing the rise in stroke volume (Fig. 3-8, point *D*).

The complete mechanism underlying the local vasodilator response has not yet been fully elucidated; however, it is clear that the reaction is entirely locally mediated and

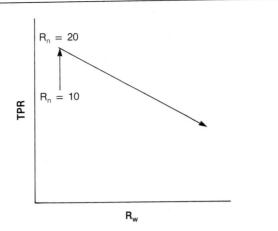

Fig. 3-10. TPR plotted as a function of R_{nw} and falling R_w (see text).

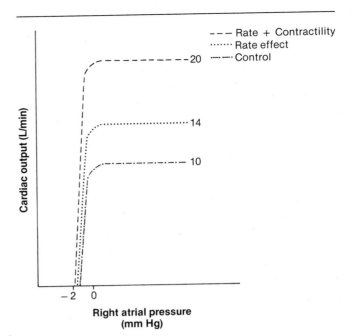

Fig. 3-11. At constant right atrial pressure (RAP), increases in heart rate and contractile state can augment the cardiac output, *CO*, three- to fourfold. Notice the steep drop in the cardiac output with slight reductions in RAP. This is attributable to collapse of the central veins and severely impaired venous return at negative right atrial pressures relative to atmospheric pressure.

independent of the autonomic nervous system. No matter what the specific mediator may be, the local response is directly coupled to the rate and intensity of aerobic work being performed. Thus the extent of local vasodilatation has been repeatedly shown to be linearly proportional to relative work load, that is, $\dot{V}o_2/\dot{V}o_{2\ max}$.

Sympathetic nervous system. A greatly augmented frequency of impulse traffic along sympathetic nervous pathways to the heart and the systemic vascular beds is a characteristic finding in exercise. Concomitantly, there is a general withdrawal of parasympathetic nervous tone. The target organ effects of increased sympathetic nervous system activity can be divided into "central" cardiac and "peripheral" vascular responses.

Cardiac effects. Cardiac autonomic nervous receptors, particularly in the sinus node, the conduction system, and the myocardium, respond in a characteristic fashion to increased sympathetic nervous system stimulation. The frequency of sinoatrial node depolarization increases (cardioaccelerator response) and heart rate rises as exercise begins. The chronotropic (affecting heart rate) response is mediated largely by sympathetic nervous system stimulation; although to some extent the rise in the heart rate is a consequence of diminished parasympathetic (vagal) tone. In addition to the chronotropic response, a strong increase in the rate of force development in the myofibers is seen, a direct result of the inotropic effects of sympathetic nervous system stimulation. Thus the intrinsic pattern of cardiac behavior in exercise is a rise in heart rate and in contractile state. Fig. 3-11 depicts graphically the effects of heart rate and contractile state on cardiac output. It is evident that the combined effects of heart rate and increased contractile function are much more effective in increasing cardiac output than heart rate alone. Note also the critical

importance of maintaining right atrial pressure at or above 0 mm Hg relative to atmospheric pressure (the importance of venous return and maintenance of a preload). The heart rate alone is capable of raising cardiac output about two and a half times basal levels up to a heart rate of about 170 to 190. Beyond this range, inadequate time for ventricular filling will become a limiting factor.

Peripheral effects. Exercise induces a global increase in sympathetic nervous system impulse traffic to all vascular beds, both nonworking and working. Until the higher stages of exercise, when heat loss becomes a major factor, the target organ response in all nonworking vascular beds is vasoconstrictive with increased vascular tone in both resistive and capacitance elements. In the working muscle, however, the local vasodilator mechanisms override the total sympathetic nervous system–mediated vasoconstrictor influence. Thus resistance to blood flow rises in all nonworking beds, whereas vasodilatation and increased flow is seen in the working muscle beds. It is, in fact, this dual pattern of vascular changes that forms the basis for the integrated functional circulatory response to exercise.

Were it not for vasoconstriction in nonworking beds, the otherwise unopposed local vasodilator response would produce, right at the onset of exercise, a sudden and profound fall in blood pressure. In general, the balance between vasoconstriction and vasodilatation results in a graded fall in the total peripheral resistance (TPR) described by

(F) $$1/TPR = 1/R_w + 1/R_{nw}$$

An essential feature of the sympathetic nervous system response to exercise is the linear relationship between sympathetic nervous system outflow and the relative intensity of work load; that is, the sympathetic nervous system activity level is proportional to $\dot{V}_{O_2}/\dot{V}_{O_2\ max}$. Thus, any parameter modulated by sympathetic nervous system tone would be expected to behave similarly and this has been shown to be true for vasoconstriction in nonworking areas; that is, the rise in nonworking resistance is a direct function of relative $\dot{V}_{O_2}$. TPR, which reflects the balance between vasodilatation and vasoconstriction, both of which are directly proportional to relative work load, has also been shown to be a linear function of $\dot{V}_{O_2}$ as a fraction of $\dot{V}_{O_2\ max}$.

The intense constriction of the nonworking capacitance beds (venoconstriction) results in a translocation of up to 40% of the blood contained in them centrally and ultimately to working muscle. Here it is important to emphasize the difference between increased flow rate through a vascular bed and net redistribution of blood volume from one part of the circulatory system to another as a result of relative changes in size or capacity of the various vascular compartments.

Venous return to the heart depends on the pressure gradient from the peripheral veins centrally to the right atrium. Venoconstriction alone by raising peripheral venous pressure can roughly double venous return. In Fig. 3-12, venous return is plotted against right atrial pressure, the graphic representation being such that the intersection of the venous return curve and the abscissa represents peripheral venous pressure. A twofold rise in venous return is seen as the peripheral venous pressure rises from a control of about 8 mm Hg to a maximum of 20 mm Hg. The plateau in each curve occurs because of the tendency for central venous collapse at right atrium pressure (RAP) below atmospheric pressure (less than 0 mm Hg).

Combined cardiac and peripheral responses. The circulatory system is a "closed" circuit; that is, except for minor beat-to-beat imbalances, cardiac input or venous return must be equal to cardiac output. A direct corollary to this is that in order for cardiac output to rise with exercise, venous return must rise to an equal extent. Graphically, the equilibrium point between venous return and cardiac output is represented by the points in Fig. 3-13 where these curves intersect. In the normal resting control, the cardiac output and venous return intersect at a unique point *(A)* where the right atrium pressure (RAP) is near zero and the cardiac output (venous return) is about 5 liters per minute. The effect of maximally raising the contractile state, but with no change in the heart rate or any peripheral vas-

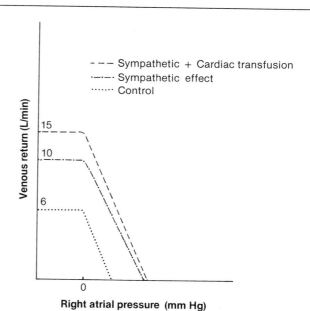

Fig. 3-12. Vasoconstriction (sympathetic effect) increases the peripheral venous to right atrial pressure gradient augmenting venous return. Additional translocation of "cardiac" blood volume to the peripheral vascular system, and ultimately the venous bed, further augments peripheral venous pressure and thus the venous–right atrial gradient. The cardiac transfusion effect results from augmented cardiac emptying (increased stroke volume) because of increased contractile state.

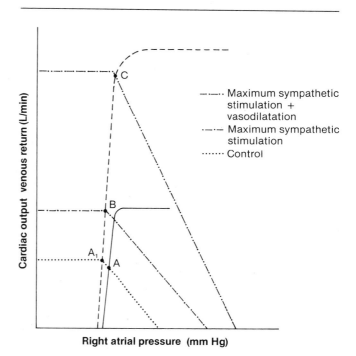

Fig. 3-13. The intersection of the cardiac output and venous return curves (A, A₁, B, C) determines the maximal cardiac output attainable under the conditions defined for each curve.

cular parameter, shifts the intersect to A_1, yielding about a 20% increase in cardiac output.

Further rise in the cardiac output is obviated by the plateau in venous return at A_1 because of the tendency for the central veins to collapse if the right atrium pressure falls below atmospheric pressure. The essential feature is that the required equilibrium between input and output holds the cardiac output to the maximal possible level of venous return, which is only nominally above basal value in the absence of any peripheral adjustments.

Point B (Fig. 3-13) is reached when the maximal peripheral vasoconstriction is achieved, with the elevated venous tone enhancing venous return about twofold. At this point, it is important to recognize that with maximum inotropic cardiac stimulation and peripheral sympathetic nervous system venoconstrictive effects, only a modest rise in the cardiac output is attained because of the limiting level of venous return. In this context then, the profound importance of the local vasodilator response becomes apparent. Point C (Fig. 3-13) represents the intact circulatory response to exercise at a cardiac output of about four times the control value. The difference between the cardiac output at points B and C is entirely attributable to the large drop in resistance to blood flow resulting from vasodilatation in the working muscle bed. Resistance to venous return in Fig. 3-13 is defined as the slope of the venous-return curve, the slope being steeper as resistance falls. The fall in resistance attributable to the local vasodilator response significantly steepens the venous return slope, resulting in a considerably higher return for any given right atrium pressure and enables the input-output equilibrium (point C) to rise to the high level needed to sustain intense exercise.

Blood pressure response to exercise. Ultimately, the peripheral and central circulatory adjustments just described translate into corresponding alterations in preload, afterload, contractile state, and heart rate. Thus, as sympathetic nervous system stimulation of the cardiac inotropic and chronotropic receptors increases, heart rate and contractile state rise and are governed by the relative intensity of the work load. Afterload reduction comes about from the fall in the total peripheral resistance because of local vasodilatation, and the preload is maintained by enhancement of venous return. These functional adaptations thus enable the heart to pump a substantially larger stroke volume at a high minute frequency, resulting in a four- to fivefold increase in cardiac output. Along with the rising cardiac output is a major redistribution of this flow from nonworking beds to the working muscle. Blood pressure (BP) is modulated by the interplay of generalized vasoconstriction and local vasodilatation to avoid a precipitous early drop in pressure and subsequently to yield a progressive net rise in pressure according to the relation $\overline{BP} = CO \times TPR$. Since flow through each parallel circuit is inversely related to that circuit's resistance, the augmented

cardiac output is directed entirely to where it is needed, the working muscles, while the increased perfusion pressure (BP) maintains normal flow rates through the constricted nonworking vascular beds.

Phases of cardiovascular dynamics

The dynamic pattern of circulatory adjustments to exercise can be divided into four fairly distinct phases: (1) the anticipatory phase, in which neurological, humoral, and perhaps mechanical factors prepare the cardiovascular system for exercise; (2) an initial phase encompassing the first few minutes of exercise in which large changes in cardiovascular variables occur as the system rapidly adapts to the requirements of exercise; (3) a period of relative "steady state," during which equilibrium is maintained through minor adjustments in the various cardiovascular parameters; (4) the stage of "cardiovascular drift," characterized by progressively less efficient delivery of oxygen and metabolic needs and increasing demands on the cardiovascular system to dispose of bodily heat.

Anticipatory phase. The earliest changes in response to exercise begin before the onset of actual muscular work. There is frequently a mild increase in the heart rate and in the cardiac output along with a modest elevation in systolic blood pressure in anticipation of exercise. Venous tone throughout the body increases slightly, raising peripheral venous pressure, and thus blood volume is shifted centrally from the periphery. These changes are all consistent with an anticipatory increase in sympathetic nervous system outflow—the intensity and extent of the changes seen being highly variable, suggesting a major element of higher cortical modulation of this early response. Thus the physiological changes preceding a routine jog in the park are, not surprisingly, of much lesser magnitude than those preceding the start of an important race.

Initial phase. The period, usually lasting from 2 to 4 minutes from the onset of exercise until the attainment of a relatively steady state, is termed the "initiation phase." Throughout this stage, the major alterations in circulatory function occur that, in effect, bring about the integrated circulatory response. The principle effector mechanism is the rapid and intense rise in sympathetic nervous system stimulation that modulates the central and peripheral circulatory activity and the locally mediated muscular vasodilator response.

Although by no means completely delineated, a mechanism appears to be operative by which the intensity of the sympathetic nervous system stimulation is a reflection of the level of aerobic exercise defined in terms of percentage of maximum work capacity ($\dot{V}O_{2\ max}$). In turn, all variables that are affected by sympathetic nervous system activity, that is, heart rate, contractile state, and vasoconstriction, have also been shown to be linearly related to the fraction $\dot{V}O_2/\dot{V}O_{2\ max}$. In the working muscle as well, the extent of vasodilatation is directly proportional to local metabolic needs, which in turn correspond in a linear manner to $\dot{V}O_2/\dot{V}O_{2\ max}$. The total peripheral resistance (TPR) is the net result of opposing vasoconstriction and vasodilatation, and since the latter two terms are proportional to relative workload, TPR too varies in an inverse linear relation to $\dot{V}O_2/\dot{V}O_{2\ max}$.

Within seconds of onset of exercise, the heart rate begins to rise and may double within 15 seconds. Because it is easily measured, the heart rate response to exercise has been extensively studied and has been found consistently to bear a linear relation to relative work load. In fact, measurement of heart rate alone provides a reliable, reproduceable measure of exercise intensity in a given subject.

Blood pressure is not a directly controlled parameter, but rather reflects the net interaction of rising cardiac output and falling TPR (BP = CO × TPR).

Typically, systolic blood pressure increases initially rapidly and then more gradually until a plateau level is reached. The final "set" point of blood pressure, not surprisingly, is a direct function of the relative work-load intensity (see Chapter 5).

The rise in cardiac stroke volume results from changes in multiple variables, rather than from any single direct alteration of cardiac function. Thus stroke volume depends on the level of venous return (preload), the blood pressure and TPR (afterload), the contractile state, and the heart rate. In general, in mild to moderate exercise, the stroke volume increases by about 50%, the increase ultimately being proportional to relative work intensity. At more severe levels of exercise, further increases in the stroke volume up to about twofold over resting values may occur.

Although all the parameters that determine the cardiac output are seen to be functions of relative work load, the cardiac output itself is a function not of the relative but of the absolute level of aerobic work. This reflects the requirement that as absolute $\dot{V}O_2$ rises, the O_2 supply or cardiac output must keep pace. In fact, the limiting factor in exercise capacity ($\dot{V}O_{2\ max}$) is, in most cases, specifically the ability to elevate cardiac output. Thus the circulatory pattern that emerges during the initial phase is a rise in the cardiac output directly proportional to $\dot{V}O_2$ and brought about by rapid alterations in multiple hemodynamic parameters that are proportional to the relative level of work, that is, $\dot{V}O_2/\dot{V}O_{2\ max}$.

Steady state. After the initial rapid adjustment phase, if the level of exercise is submaximal, a stage is reached where the major hemodynamic parameters plateau and, except for minor variations, remain relatively constant for up to several hours. The duration of "steady state" depends largely on the intensity of exercise, such that work levels of 50% to 70% of $\dot{V}O_{2\ max}$ can be sustained for hours, whereas near-maximal exertion leads rapidly to exhaustion within minutes. During the steady state, the needs of the exercising muscle are being adequately met be the cardiovascular system, and any major variation in circulatory variables will occur only in response to a change in exercise level itself—homeostasis has been achieved. The unifying factor with which all the cardiovascular variables measured correlate is oxygen uptake as a fraction of $\dot{V}O_{2\ max}$. Adjustments for minor variations in metabolic need are through two mechanisms—one local and one central. Locally, if flow becomes inadequate for metabolic needs, local vasodilatation increases, reducing resistance and directing larger flow to the working muscular bed. Venous return, further enhanced by the additional fall in resistance, augments the cardiac output. Thus a finely tuned system emerges in which minute-to-minute changes in working muscle vascular tone, probably through highly sensitive muscle afferent reflexes modulated by the metabolic milieu, can quickly alter the magnitude and distribution of the cardiac output. At the same time, processing of these signals in sympathetic nervous system centers modulates sympathetic nervous system tone, producing a synergism between the locally mediated effects of vasodilatation and the sympathetic nervous system–related factors of the heart rate, contractile state, and peripheral vasoconstriction.

Cardiovascular drift. As exercise continues, at some variable point in time, a progressive change begins in the cardiovascular functional pattern just described. This final phase is characterized by a gradual increase in heart rate, accompanied by a progressive fall in venous return, stroke volume, and blood pressure. Cardiac output, a function of the absolute exercise level, remains unchanged, however, and a progressive redistribution of flow is seen in the final stage of exercise. A major factor taking precedence as exercise continues is the progressive buildup of body heat produced by working muscles, which must be dissipated largely through the skin. Before this stage, sympathetic nervous system peripheral influence is vasoconstrictive, but now sympathetic nervous system–mediated vasodilatation in the skin begins and becomes a progressively more important factor. As increased blood volume and flow is directed to the skin, splanchnic and nonworking blood flow approaches a minimum. Underlying these changes is a progressive rise in sympathetic nervous system tone, accompanied by a rising heart rate and intense vasoconstriction (except in skin and working muscle) in an effort to meet increasing circulatory demands. At some point, no further effective rise in the heart rate, venous return, or contractile state can occur and now, as further skin vasodilatation occurs, less flow is available to working muscles. Soon, the metabolic and hemodynamic counterparts of exhaustion ensue.

EXERCISE IN THE SUBJECT WITH CORONARY DISEASE: COMPARISON TO THE NORMAL

In the recent past, programs to "rehabilitate" the patient with cardiac disease (usually but not exclusively coronary disease) utilizing as a basic modality some form of aerobic exercise have gained major acceptance and support from the medical profession. This "therapeutic" approach is particularly noteworthy in view of the nearly complete absence of demonstrable effect aerobic training has on the heart in the setting of coronary artery disease. In general, the physiological responses to exercise in the normal subject and the person with coronary disease are qualitatively the same. In contrast, there are however, certain quantitative differences in exercise parameters that are characteristic of the response in coronary disease. In particular, as a group, the coronary subjects have a statistically significant reduction in $\dot{V}O_{2\ max}$ compared to normals. In the coronary subject, as in the normal, the $\dot{V}O_{2\ max}$ depends on two main components, cardiac output (delivery) and a-$\bar{v}O_2$ diff (extraction). Various comparative studies between normals and coronary subjects have shown no difference in a-$\bar{v}O_2$ diff, a not-surprising finding, since a-$\bar{v}O_2$ diff is a function of peripheral vascular and metabolic factors. Thus the basis for the quantitative reduction in $\dot{V}O_{2\ max}$ in coronary disease resides in the impairment of left ventricular function that limits augmentation of stroke volume and cardiac output. Coronary subjects tend to have lower SV_{max}, lower HR_{max}, and lower peak levels of contractility, compared to normals. From equation (C), a reduction in $\dot{V}O_{2\ max}$ is readily understood. Moreover, it has been found that at any given submaximal $\dot{V}O_2$, the contribution to $\dot{V}O_2$ from the cardiac output tends to be less and from a-$\bar{v}O_2$ diff higher in the coronary subject than in the normal. Thus the characteristic finding in the coronary subject during exercise is a greater reliance on peripheral oxygen extractive factors rather than central delivery mechanisms to sustain $\dot{V}O_2$ during exercise.

The major implication of limited $\dot{V}O_{2\ max}$ in coronary disease becomes apparent when a given exercise level and its corresponding $\dot{V}O_{2\ actual}$ are considered as a percent of $\dot{V}O_{2\ max}$; specifically, for any given submaximal work load, the relative work intensity, that is, $\dot{V}O_2/\dot{V}O_{2\ max}$, is greater in the coronary subject, and consequently all the cardiovascular parameters that vary with $\dot{V}O_2/\dot{V}O_{2\ max}$ achieve higher plateau values during steady state. Thus, for the same level of exercise heart rate, the vasoconstriction and blood pressure are more intense in a coronary subject than in the normal.

Exercise capacity in coronary disease

In the absence of angina, the coronary subject's major determinant of exercise capacity, as in the normal, is maximal $\dot{V}O_2$. The subject with angina is unique; his exercise capacity is limited not by $\dot{V}O_2$ augmentation to some maximum, but usually well before this is reached by the development of pain (angina). Thus the distinction is made between limitation of maximal aerobic capacity ($\dot{V}O_{2\ max}$) and limitation attributable to symptoms coming from oxygen lack at the myocardial level.

Myocardial oxygen consumption

Myocardial work, that is, the pumping of blood, is essentially a completely aerobic process, with the myocardial contractile energy requirements being met by oxidative metabolic pathways only. Moreover, at basal conditions, myocardial oxygen extraction is much higher than in resting skeletal muscle and there is no effective myocardial extractive reserve. Increased oxygen supply depends then entirely on increased delivery by greater coronary blood flow. The atherosclerotic process in the coronary subject places an often severe limitation on augmentation of coronary flow; thus with rising myocardial work an imbalance between O_2 delivery and demand occurs. Myocardial oxygen consumption is related linearly to pumping work. Clinically, it has been repeatedly shown that the product of the heart rate and the systolic blood pressure (HR $\times$ BP) closely follows myocardial work load and accurately reflects myocardial O_2 consumption or demand ($M\dot{V}O_2$). Since both HR and BP are functions of relative total body work load, one is not surprised that $M\dot{V}O_2$ has been found to be a linear function of $\dot{V}O_{2\ max}$. In the normal subject, coronary blood flow rises with rising $M\dot{V}O_2$ and $\dot{V}O_2$. In the patient with coronary disease, coronary blood flow is limited and can increase no further at some level of $M\dot{V}O_2$. Beyond this point, a further rise in $M\dot{V}O_2$ requirements is inadequately met and the myocardium becomes ischemic. In practice, the product of HR and BP, when angina begins, has been found to be a sensitive and reproduceable marker of the ischemic limit of exercise capacity.

Training effect

One of the primary aims of the cardiac rehabilitation program is to improve exercise capacity in the patient with heart disease. In the normal subject, endurance training of sufficient intensity and duration leads to an improvement in $\dot{V}O_{2\ max}$ by raising maximal stroke volume and a-$\bar{v}O_2$ diff. The major change in most normal persons appears to involve primarily an enhancement of a-$\bar{v}O_2$; however, improvement in the specific (cardiac) parameters occurs as well, though to a lesser extent. The chronic adjustments to exercise are complex, and thorough discussion of this area is beyond the scope of this chapter (see Chapter 8). In contrast to the normal, in the subject with coronary disease virtually all improvement in $\dot{V}O_{2\ max}$ comes from a rise in a-$\bar{v}O_2$, and no change in cardiac function is seen in response to endurance training. Thus the training effect incurred in the cardiac rehabilitation program is, in effect, a result of enhanced peripheral vascular and working muscle function in exercise and not attributable to any change in cardiac function. The reasons for the lack of cardiac effect are not completely known, but inability to exercise at sufficient intensity (percent of $\dot{V}O_{2\ max}$) and the pathophysiological limitations of coronary disease on ventricular function probably play a major role.

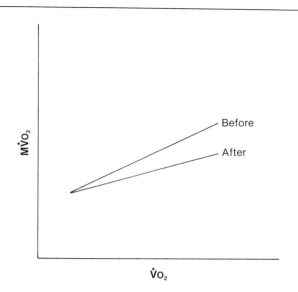

Fig. 3-14. Training effect on myocardial oxygen consumption, or demand ($M\dot{V}O_2$), as a function of the total body oxygen consumption ($\dot{V}O_2$). After training, $M\dot{V}O_2$ rises less for a given absolute level of aerobic exercise ($\dot{V}O_2$).

Table 3-2. Normal values at cardiac catheterization in the resting supine subject

Right atrium (mean)	5 mm Hg
Right ventricle (S/D)	30/5 mm Hg
Pulmonary artery (S/D)	30/20 mm Hg
Pulmonary arterial wedge (mean)	12 mm Hg
Aorta (S/D)	140/90 mm Hg
Left ventricle (S/D)	140/12 mm Hg
Ejection fraction	Greater than 60%
Cardiac index	2.5 L/min/m^2

S/D, Systolic/diastolic.

Nevertheless, symptomatic improvement is seen. This occurs because at any given submaximal $\dot{V}O_2$, the relative exercise intensity after training is lower compared to pretraining performance; that is, $\dot{V}O_2/\dot{V}O_{2\ max}$ is lower because of the training-induced rise in the denominator $\dot{V}O_{2\ max}$. As a consequence, the heart rate and the blood pressure are lower at the given exercise level compared to their pretraining levels, since they are both directly related to $\dot{V}O_2/\dot{V}O_{2\ max}$. Thus the resulting rate-pressure product at a given exercise level is lower after training, reflecting a reduced $M\dot{V}O_2$. In effect, training by increasing $\dot{V}O_{2\ max}$ entirely by peripheral mechanisms yields a reduction in the slope of the line relating $M\dot{V}O_2$ to $\dot{V}O_2$ (Fig. 3-14). As a result, the trained coronary subject can exercise to a higher level before reaching pain threshold, rate pressure product, and symptomatic limitation.

CARDIAC CATHETERIZATION

Table 3-2 lists the normal values obtained at cardiac catheterization in the resting supine subject. Although highly accurate and sophisticated data are obtained at catheterization, translation of these results into exercise capacity and potential for symptomatic improvement through exercise are not at all clear cut. Thus most studies up to now have shown a general lack of correlation between conventional hemodynamic and angiographic data obtained during cardiac catheterization and subsequent performance in a rehabilitation program for a large subset of coronary subjects with mild to moderate disease. This divergence stems in part from errors inherent in extrapolation of resting supine subject data to the upright exercise state. Moreover, exercise performance reflects the interplay of numerous cardiovascular, muscular, and other system variables, as well as compensatory mechanisms that partially mitigate functional impairment in various areas. This complex interaction is by no means interpretable through analysis of catheterization results. Despite its shortcomings, catheterization does provide useful data in formulating reasonable therapeutic goals and demonstrates as well the hemodynamic and anatomic substrate with which the patient must function. In general, it can be shown that a rough concurrence exists between the extent and severity of the coronary atheromatous process and the degree of left ventricular dysfunction and either exercise capacity or potential for improvement. Thus a semiquantitative estimate of coronary stenosis in terms of the number of vessels involved and the severity of individual stenoses has been shown to correlate roughly with exercise capacity and symptom level. Currently, the most widely used measure of total left ventricular pump function is the ejection fraction, and here too a general relation exists between extent of reduction in ejection fraction and exercise performance. Thus the subgroup with normal left ventricular function, in terms of ejection fraction, and single vessel coronary involvement, will, as a whole, have a better chance to exercise to a higher capacity and derive greater benefit from training than the subgroup with advanced three-vessel disease and severely impaired ejection fraction. Unfortunately, the degree of overlap within these subgroups, in terms of symptoms and catheterization findings, significantly reduces the sensitivity and specificity of catheterization data. Moreover, in the largest subset of subjects with "moderate" disease, the lack of statistical validity of most measures derived from catheterization data is most apparent.

Despite their shortcomings, treadmill testing and catheterization data provide the basis for exercise prescription and rehabilitation planning. The therapist should utilize these data as part of a more general evaluation that includes factors such as age, sex, weight, general muscular strength, and previous level of conditioning (exercise habits). Thorough evaluation requires consideration of the significance of concomitant diseases such as chronic obstructive pulmonary disease or peripheral vascular disease, orthopaedic or neurological limitations and a host of other clinical factors too numerous to list here. (see Chapter 6). General physical examination remains the foundation upon which all other modes of physical assessment are built. In particular, the presence of gallop rhythm or cardiac murmurs should be noted and correlated with other known clinical and laboratory data to assess ventricular function or recognize important limitations because of mitral or aortic valvular abnormality. The electrocardiogram may reveal patterns of old infarction, bundle-branch block, ventricular hypertrophy, or rhythm or atrioventricular conduction disturbance, which must be recognized and incorporated into the overall assessment of capacity.

SUMMARY

From this brief overview, it is clear that assessment of physical capacity in its broadest sense is complex and inexact. This is true even in the healthy, highly trained athlete, where it has been shown that the subject with the highest measured $\dot{V}O_{2\ max}$ is by no means the invariable winner of the marathon. Most programs utilize some form of team approach where the final evaluation derives from a variety of medical and paramedical disciplines.

REFERENCES

1. Braunwald, E.: Assessment of cardiac performance in heart disease. In Braunwald, E., editor: A textbook of cardiovascular medicine, Philadelphia, 1980, W.B. Saunders Co.
2. Braunwald, E., and others: Contraction of the normal heart in heart disease. In Braunwald, E., editor: A textbook of cardiovascular medicine, Philadelphia, 1980, W.B. Saunders Co.
3. Clausen, J.P.: Circulatory adjustments to dynamic exercise and effect of physical training in normal subjects and in patients with coronary artery disease, Prog. Cardiovasc. Dis. 18:459, 1976.
4. Neill, W.A.: Regulation of cardiac output in clinical cardiovascular physiology, Prog. Cardiovasc. Dis. 18:121, 1976.
5. Skelton, C.L., and Sonnenblick, E.H.: Physiology of cardiac muscle. In Levine, H.J., editor: Clinical cardiovascular physiology, New York, 1976, Grune & Stratton.
6. Smith, E.E., and others: Integrated mechanisms of cardiovascular response and control during exercise in the normal human, Prog. Cardiovasc. Dis. 18(6):421, 1976.
7. Vatner, S.F., and Pagani, M.: Cardiovascular adjustments to exercise: hemodynamic and mechanisms, Prog. Cardiovasc. Dis. 19:91, 1976.

4

KENNETH S. GIMBEL

Pharmacological considerations

Pharmacological agents provide the foundation for the medical management of cardiovascular disease. This chapter addresses four clinical problems:

1. Angina pectoris
2. Cardiac arrhythmias
3. Congestive heart failure
4. Hypertension

These topics are quite extensive, and by necessity discussion of them will be brief. You are encouraged to supplement this chapter with the references provided.

All the drugs to be discussed may result in adverse or untoward reactions. The risk and the severity of undesirable effects increase when multiple agents are used in combination. The therapist must constantly be alert to the possibility that clinical deterioration is the consequence of too much medication rather than not enough. Changes in clinical status are often accompanied by alterations in drug sensitivity or responsiveness, which may require adjustment of drug dosage.

Note also that the apparent success of a particular therapeutic regimen in a patient at rest or in the "basal state" may not carry over into more active circumstances. Both psychological and physical stresses must be evaluated.

DRUG THERAPY: ANGINA PECTORIS
Causes of angina[6]

Angina pectoris is the subjective expression of myocardial ischemia and signals an imbalance between myocardial oxygen consumption ($M\dot{V}O_2$) and myocardial oxygen delivery. Angina is the cardial symptom of coronary heart disease (CHD) though it may occur in the presence of normal coronary arteries. Other cardiac diseases that may be associated with angina include the following:

1. Aortic valve disease, particularly aortic stenosis
2. Mitral valve prolapse
3. The cardiomyopathies, particularly the hypertrophic varieties
4. Severe systemic hypertension

5. Pulmonary hypertension

In the absence of structural heart disease, angina may be experienced during severe tachycardia or because of severe hypoxemia, or anemia.

$M\dot{V}O_2$ reflects the metabolic work of the myocardium.

Determinants of myocardial oxygen demand[1]

The major determinants of $M\dot{V}O_2$ include the following:

1. Contractile state
2. Heart rate
3. Systolic wall stress

Systolic wall stress varies directly with intracavitary systolic pressure and radius and inversely with wall thickness. Those interventions that increase contractile state, heart rate, and wall stress result in increased $M\dot{V}O_2$. Increasing ventricular volume or systolic pressure result in increasing ventricular wall tension and stress. Additional minor determinants of $M\dot{V}O_2$ include the following:

1. Basal O_2 (energy required to maintain cell membrane integrity, basal metabolic processes, and so on)
2. Activation energy (depolarization-repolarization, electromechanical coupling, relaxation)
3. External work (fiber shortening)

Determinants of myocardial oxygen supply[10,11]

Assuming normal red blood cell mass, normal hemoglobin-oxygen dissociation, and normal arterial blood oxygen content, one can determine the myocardial oxygen supply by the coronary blood flow. The principal determinants of coronary blood flow consist of the following:

1. Aortic diastolic pressure
2. Diastolic period (duration of diastole)
3. Coronary arterial resistance
4. Collateral circulation

Blood flow to the left ventricular myocardium occurs mainly during diastole. During systole, the intramural coronary arteries are compressed by the contracting myocardium. The duration of diastole is inversely related to heart

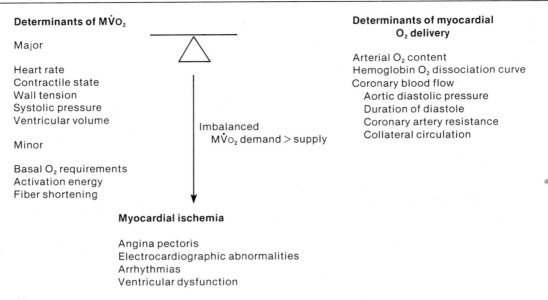

Fig. 4-1. Principal determinants of the myocardial oxygen demand (MVO₂), myocardial oxygen supply, and the consequences of ischemia.

rate; as heart rate is accelerated, less time is available for coronary blood flow. A pressure gradient exists between the aorta and large epicardial coronary arteries and the smaller intramural branches extending from the subepicardial to the subendocardial surfaces of the ventricle. This transmural pressure gradient is the driving force responsible for coronary flow. Flow is opposed by coronary arterial resistance, which is primarily determined by luminal cross-sectional diameter and to a much lesser extent by blood viscosity. During vasodilatation, as cross-sectional area increases, coronary resistance decreases, and blood flow is augmented. In the normal heart, coronary blood flow is responsive to the metabolic needs of the myocardium. The cost of increased myocardial work, expressed as increased MVO_2, is accommodated by an increase in myocardial oxygen delivery mediated through coronary vasodilatation.

Manifestations of ischemia

The presence of obstructive atherosclerotic coronary disease or the appearance of abnormal vascular reactivity in the form of spasm may disrupt this critical autoregulatory mechanism. The resulting imbalance between MVO_2 and myocardial oxygen delivery produces tissue ischemia. Angina pectoris is the subjective expression of this imbalance. Myocardial ischemia may also be manifested as electrocardiographic abnormalities (ST-segment shift, T-wave changes), arrhythmias, and hemodynamic disturbances (see Chapter 3) reflecting left ventricular dysfunction during systole (hypotension, acute left heart failure) and abnormal myocardial relaxation (S₄ gallop, reduced ventricular compliance). Moreover, the electrocardiographic and hemodynamic consequences of ischemia may occur in the absence of angina or its clinical equivalent.

Therapeutic goals

The therapeutic goals in the management of angina pectoris include the following:
1. Termination of the acute attack
2. Reduction in the frequency and severity of subsequent attacks
3. Reduction of the risk of myocardial infarction and sudden death

The first two goals may be achieved with currently available pharmacological agents. Whether contemporary medical therapy favorably influences the incidence of myocardial infarction and sudden death is subject to considerable debate.

Classification of drugs

Three classes of drugs will be considered:
1. Nitrates
2. Beta adrenergic receptor–blocking drugs
3. Calcium antagonists

The efficacy of these agents relates to their ability to restore the balance between myocardial oxygen supply and demand. This is achieved through a reduction in myocardial oxygen demand ($M\dot{V}O_2$), enhancement in myocardial oxygen availability, or a combination of the two. A summary of the principal determinants of $M\dot{V}O_2$ demand, myocardial oxygen supply, and the consequences of ischemia is provided in Fig. 4-1.

Nitrates

Nitroglycerin (NTG, glycerol trinitrate) has been the drug of choice for the treatment of angina pectoris for over a century. Various other organic nitrate esters have been developed and share nitroglycerin's fundamental pharmacological activity, though differing in their route of administration, speed of absorption, and duration of action. The nitrates are potent smooth muscle relaxants though the specific mechanism responsible for this effect is unknown. Their principal cardiovascular activity relates to relaxation of vascular smooth muscle resulting in vasodilatation. This is a nonspecific response demonstrable on both the arterial and venous sides of the systemic and pulmonary circulations. Direct coronary vasodilatation is demonstrable in normal subjects and in patients exhibiting abnormal coronary vascular reactivity (coronary spasm). It is uncertain whether such a direct action contributes to the efficacy of the nitrates in patients with coronary heart disease. In this group, the peripheral vascular effects of the nitrates predominate. Relaxation of smooth muscle within the walls of arteriolar resistance vessels results in a reduction of mean arterial pressure and diminished resistance to left ventricular ejection (that is, afterload reduction). Relaxation of smooth muscle within the large capacitance veins results in venous pooling, diminished venous return to the heart (that is, reduced preload), and reduced ventricular volume. The sum of these alterations is a reduction in left ventricular wall stress and $M\dot{V}O_2$. The changes on the venous side of the circulation dominate, producing a significant fall in cardiac output, which contributes to the hypotension observed during nitrate administration.

Nitrates alter the distribution of coronary blood flow within the walls of the left ventricle, favoring increased flow to the subendocardial region. The subendocardium is in greatest jeopardy during conditions associated with myocardial ischemia, and as such redistribution may be beneficial. There is also some suggestion that nitrates enhance the development of coronary collateral vessels though this is unproved.

In patients with vasospastic (Prinzmetal's or variant) angina, and particularly in the subgroup of patients without demonstrable (atherosclerotic) obstructions, the nitrates act principally by reversing coronary artery spasm and directly dilating the large epicardial coronary vessels. Both coronary blood flow and myocardial oxygen delivery are enhanced, and ischemia is alleviated.

Nitroglycerin is administered sublingually and is rapidly absorbed through the sublingual mucosa and distributed systemically, escaping metabolic degradation by the liver. Its onset of action is approximately 1 minute, with peak activity becoming evident in 3 to 5 minutes, and total duration of action being less than 30 minutes. Nitroglycerin may lose its activity rapidly when exposed to air and must be kept in a tightly closed glass container. The typical burning sensation noted when the tablet is placed beneath the tongue is a useful indication of its continued potency. Nitroglycerin remains the drug of choice for terminating the acute anginal attack. It may also be employed prophylactically before those activities that by experience the patient regularly associates with angina. Isosorbide dinitrate (Isordil, Sorbitrate) is available for sublingual use and in a chewable form. Its onset of action may be slightly delayed and its duration of action is more prolonged than that of nitroglycerin, hence its value when employed for angina prophylaxis. Isosorbide dinitrate is also available in an oral preparation as is erythrityl tetranitrate (Cardilate) and pentaerythritol tetranitrate (Peritrate). Nitrates absorbed from the gastrointestinal tract undergo extensive metabolic degradation in the liver, and therefore large dosages must be given to ensure systemic distribution and the desired effects. When sufficiently large oral dosages are administered, prolonged anginal protection may be realized. These preparations are not designed to abort the acute anginal attack, however. Nitroglycerin ointment (Nitrobid, Nitrol) has regained its popularity, and because of its prolonged duration of action (up to 6 hours), it is particularly useful in the management of nocturnal angina. Two other cutaneous preparations (Transderm-Nitro, Nitrodur) employ a controlled-release system that provide therapeutic levels for up to 24 hours.

The nitrates, as a group, are characterized by a number of side effects related to vasodilatation. These include the following:

1. Vascular headache
2. Cutaneous vasodilatation, flushing, and pallor
3. Hypotension
4. Nausea and vomiting

The incidence and severity of these side effects are determined by the absolute dosage employed and the rapidity with which the drug enters the circulation. The latter is determined primarily by the route of administration. Ranked according to speed of onset of action are amyl nitrate (inhalation), nitroglycerin (sublingual), chewable isosorbide dinitrate, nitrate esters (oral), and nitroglycerine ointment (cutaneous). Hypotension is related to both arteriolar and venous dilatation. The former results in diminished peripheral resistance, whereas the latter reduces ventricular diastolic filling thus limiting forward cardiac output. When the hypotension is mild, these changes may result in dizziness, particularly when the patient is immobile (further aggravating venous pooling) or in association with alcohol consumption. More severe hypotension may elicit symptoms of cerebrovascular ischemia, syncope and complete vascular collapse. Hypotension is usually associated with sympathetically mediated reflex tachycardia, which, if severe, may aggravate myocardial ischemia. Although hypotension diminishes myocardial work, and therefore reduces $M\dot{V}O_2$, severe hypotension impairs coronary flow. In view of their potential for eliciting considerable changes in peripheral vascular tone, nitrates must be employed with great caution within the setting of acute myocardial infarction. On occasion, nitrate-induced hypotension is accompanied by profound bradycardia further compromising cardiac output, sometimes severely.

Beta adrenergic receptor–blocking drugs

The sympathetic and parasympathetic limbs of the autonomic nervous system exert profound effects upon the heart, the peripheral vasculature, and integrated cardiovascular function in the intact organism. The sympathetic neurotransmitter norepinephrine and the adrenal hormone epinephrine released during sympathetic stimulation interact with specific receptor sites distributed within the heart, in vascular and other smooth muscle, and in liver, adipose, and glandular tissues of the body. Two types of receptor sites have been characterized, based upon the activity of a series of adrenergic compounds. In general, alpha-receptor stimulation results in smooth muscle contraction, whereas beta-receptor stimulation results in smooth muscle relaxation. Norepinephrine interacts primarily with alpha receptors, whereas isoproterenol interacts primarily with beta receptors. Epinephrine exhibits both alpha- and beta-adrenergic activity. The beta receptors can further be subdivided into cardiac (beta$_1$) and noncardiac (beta$_2$) categories.

Cardiac beta$_1$ receptors are distributed about the sinoatrial and atrioventricular nodal tissue, along the specialized conduction system, and throughout the atrial and ventricular myocardium. The cardiac consequences of sympathetic stimulation are summarized in Table 4-1. Heightened adrenergic activity results in sinus node acceleration (increased heart rate) and augmented myocardial contractility (positive inotropic effect), two major determinants of $M\dot{V}O_2$. Accordingly, the increased sympathetic activity that regularly accompanies ordinary physical and emotional stress may provoke myocardial ischemia in patients with limited coronary flow. Enhanced adrenergic activity may precipitate ectopic tachyarrhythmias, which may further aggravate ischemia through a combination of increased $M\dot{V}O_2$ and diminished coronary flow, the latter a consequence of an abbreviated diastolic flow period. Arterial hypertension resulting from stimulation of alpha receptors within arteriolar smooth muscle cells or mediated through sympathetic activation of the renin angiotensin system may contribute to increased cardiac work.

Table 4-1. Cardiac response to sympathetic stimulation

Beta$_1$-receptor site	Physiological response	Effect of $M\dot{V}O_2$
Sinoatrial node	Increased automaticity	+ + + +
	Sinus acceleration	
Atrioventricular node	Increased conduction velocity	
	Increased automaticity	
	Acceleration of junctional escape pacemakers	
His-Purkinje system	Increased conduction velocity	
	Increased automaticity	
	Acceleration of ventricular escape pacemakers	
	Enhanced ectopic activity	
Atrial myocardium	Increased contractility	
	Increased conduction velocity	
Ventricular myocardium	Increased contractility	+ + + +
	Increased conduction velocity	

Propranolol (Inderal) was the first beta adrenergic receptor–blocking drug to be marketed in the United States and remains the most widely prescribed at present. It is a noncardioselective competitive antagonist that reversibly combines with beta$_1$- and beta$_2$-receptor sites to inhibit the activity of intrinsic and extrinsic catecholamines. It possesses quinidine-like "membrane-depressant" effects but no intrinsic agonist activity. The cardiac response to beta blockade with propranolol in the intact organism includes the following[13]:

1. Blunted heart rate response to exercise, resting bradycardia at higher dosage levels
2. Reduced myocardial contractility and blunting of sympathetically mediated inotropic support in response to exercise
3. Reduction of normal exercise–induced increase in cardiac output, reduction of resting cardiac output at high dosage levels
4. Blunting of normal hypertensive response to exercise, reduction of resting blood pressure at higher dosages

Although the alterations described impair maximal cardiovascular performance and limit peak external physical work capacity, most patients remain capable of carrying out their ordinary activities without difficulty. The negative chronotropic and inotropic effects of propranolol diminish $M\dot{V}O_2$. This is partially offset by an increase in ventricular volume secondary to bradycardia (increased diastolic filling time) and reduced systolic emptying, which

Table 4-2. Summary of adverse reactions to propranolol

Organ system	Reaction
Cardiovascular	Sinus bradycardia first-, second-, third-degree AV block, systole hypotension, syncope, vascular collapse, shock, worsening congestive heart failure
	(?) "Rebound phenomena" after abrupt withdrawal including increasing angina, myocardial infarction, and sudden death
	Precipitation or aggravation of coronary artery spasm
	Peripheral vascular insufficiency, Raynaud's syndrome
	Impairment of sympathetically mediated reflex activity
Respiratory	Bronchospasm
Central nervous system	Depression, insomnia, vivid nightmares, weakness, fatigue, lassitude, disorientation, hallucination, visual disturbances, short-term memory loss, emotional lability
Gastrointestinal	Nausea, vomiting, abdominal pain, diarrhea, constipation, ischemia, colitis
Miscellaneous	Reversible alopecia, fever, thrombocytopenic purpura, laryngospasm, agranulocytosis

act to increase wall stress. The antihypertensive effects of propranolol further contributes to the favorable reduction in cardiac work. It has also been suggested that beta blockade interferes with catecholamine-mediated platelet aggregation. Platelet aggregates or vasoactive substances or both released during platelet aggregation may play a fundamental role in the pathogenesis of coronary disease.

A number of beta adrenergic blocking drugs are currently available, and several more are under development. Their fundamental pharmacological activity is similar to propranolol. Metoprolol (Lopressor) and atenolol (Tenormin) exhibit relative cardiac selectivity (beta$_1$ blockade) at low dosage levels, but this advantage is lost at higher dosages. Nadolol (Corgard) and atenolol have an extended half-life permitting a regimen of a single dose per day.

The more commonly encountered adverse reactions reflect the physiological changes resulting from beta adrenergic blockade. These are outlined in Table 4-2. The therapeutic range for these agents is quite variable and is influenced by age, general health status, level of background sympathetic tone, and the presence of hepatic and renal disease. Adverse reactions may not be strictly dose related. Particular care must be taken in patients with greatly impaired cardiac function who are dependent on the inotropic support provided by heightened adrenergic tone, in patients with abnormal vascular reactivity (that is, coronary spasm), and in patients with severe bronchospastic pulmonary disease. Following are contraindications to the use of beta blockers:

1. Severe sinus bradycardia, second and third degree AV block unless patient protected by pacemaker
2. Cardiogenic shock
3. Overt congestive heart failure (unless it is secondary to propranolol-responsive arrhythmia)
4. Pulmonary hypertension
5. Bronchial asthma
6. Allergic rhinitis during pollen season

7. Concomitant therapy with adrenergic-augmenting psychotropic drugs

Special precautions include the following:

1. Avoid abrupt withdrawal; may precipitate "rebound" reaction including increasing angina, arrhythmia, infarction, and sudden death
2. May aggravate coronary spasm in patients with vasospastic angina (variant or Prinzmetal's angina)
3. May mask reflex sympathetic response to insulin-induced hypoglycemia and aggravate hypoglycemia
4. May precipitate congestive heart failure in patients with advanced ventricular dysfunction, dependent on inotropic support provided by adrenergic mechanisms
5. May mask symptoms of thyrotoxicosis
6. May aggravate anesthetic-induced myocardial depression

Calcium antagonists[2,3]

The inward flow of extracellular calcium ions across the cell membranes of smooth muscle and myocardial cells is essential to the process of muscular contraction. Electrical depolarization results in conformational changes within the myocardial membrane unblocking specific calcium channels allowing extracellular calcium ions to enter to cardiac cell under the influence of existing concentration gradients. Other stimuli are responsible for similar changes in the permeability of vascular smooth muscle. When intracellular calcium ions achieve a critical concentration, interaction with protein complexes (troponin, tropomyosin) allows the formation of cross bridges between interdigitated actin and myosin filaments resulting in muscular contraction. The calcium-blocking drugs inhibit this inward calcium current, resulting in vascular smooth muscle relaxation, vasodilatation, and diminished myocardial contractility.

The slow inward calcium current contributes to the cardiac monophasic action potential. It is responsible for the initial depolarization phase (phase 0) of cells in the sinoatrial and atrioventricular nodes and contributes to the plateau phase (phase 2) of ordinary myocardium and the specialized cells of the His-Purkinje system. Predictably, the calcium-blocking drugs may have important effects upon cardiac rhythm.

Following are the observed cardiovascular responses to the calcium antagonists:

1. Decreased sinoatrial nodal automaticity, sinus slowing, bradycardia
2. Decreased atrioventricular nodal conduction velocity, P-R interval prolongation, atrioventricular block
3. Decreased myocardial contractility (although demonstrable in isolated muscle preparations, usually not of clinical importance at commonly employed dosage levels)
4. Vascular smooth muscle relaxation, peripheral vasodilatation, hypotension
5. Coronary vascular smooth muscle relaxation, reversal of coronary spasm

Following is a list of potential therapeutic applications:

1. Vasospastic angina (Prinzmetal's variant angina)
2. Angina pectoris
3. Idiopathic hypertrophic subaortic stenosis
4. Hypertension
5. Congestive heart failure (afterload reduction)
6. Arrhythmias
7. Myocardial preservation (cardiac surgery)
8. Other vasospastic syndromes

Currently, two calcium-channel blockers are available for clinical use, and several more are under active development. Verapamil (Isoptin, Calan), in parenteral form is considered by some to be the drug of choice for terminating paroxysmal supraventricular tachycardia. Its usefulness in the management of other arrhythmias is quite limited. Nifedipine (Procardia, Adalat), in contrast, has no important antiarrhythmic activity.

Nifedipine and verapamil are potent vasodilators. Both are extremely effective in reversing and preventing coronary spasm in patients with variant (Prinzmetal's) angina. Similarly, both drugs have proved efficacious in the management of angina complicating coronary heart disease. In this latter group of patients, the calcium antagonists may favorably influence the balance between myocardial oxygen supply and demand through a combination of peripheral arteriolar vasodilatation (diminished afterload) and reduced myocardial contractility. Whether or not a direct coronary artery vasodilating effect is of importance is uncertain. It has been suggested that coronary vasomotion contributes to the functional caliber of vessels in areas of atherosclerotic stenosis. The inhibition of such superimposed dynamic narrowing by the calcium antagonist agents may contribute to their antianginal activity.

The common side effects shared by both verapamil and nifedipine relate to their vasodilatory activity and include hypotension, dizziness, syncope, flushing, and headache. Reflex tachycardia is more common with nifedipine, which lacks significant influence upon the SA and AV nodes. Verapamil, on the other hand, has been associated with bradycardia secondary to sinus node slowing or AV node conduction delay, or both. Because of their negative inotropic activity, both agents may aggravate congestive heart failure in patients with severely compromised ventricular function or in those concomitantly receiving a beta blocker. In practice, however, this has not been a major problem.

DRUG THERAPY: ARRHYTHMIAS
Review of electrophysiology

Cardiac cells are electrically excitable; that is, they are capable of generating an action potential in response to an appropriate stimulus. Once initiated, the excitatory wave propagates along the cell membrane as a regenerative response. The heart is a functional syncytium of cells. The excitatory stimulus generated by the pacemaker cells within the SA node spreads to adjacent atrial myocardium and then, sequentially, to the AV node, His bundle, right and left bundle branches, distal Purkinje system, and ventricular myocardium. The envelopment of the heart by this excitatory process, and the subsequent restoration of the resting equilibrium are responsible for the familiar characteristics of the surface electrocardiogram (ECG).

In the resting state, myocardial cells are polarized; that is, the inner aspect of the cell membrane is negatively charged with respect to the outside. The resting potential is the result of electrochemical gradients established because of the selective permeability of the cardiac cell membrane. Stimulation of the cell provokes specific changes in membrane permeability and ion conductance, alterations in transmembrane voltage, and changes in the internal ionic composition of the cell. These changes in cellular electrical activity are responsible for the monophasic action potential (MAP) registered utilizing microelectrode techniques. The surface ECG represents the summation of the MAP's generated by all the cells of the heart.

Ordinary atrial and ventricular myocardial cells maintain a stable resting potential (phase 4) unless stimulated. Cells within the SA node differ in that resting potential is unstable; that is, these cells spontaneously depolarize. This characteristic of pacemaker cells is termed "automaticity." Automaticity is not unique to SA-node pacemaker cells and may be observed in specialized cells within the atria, around the AV node, and throughout the His-Purkinje system.

Mechanisms of cardiac arrhythmias[8,15-17]

Cardiac arrhythmias reflect disordered electrical activation of the heart. Three phenomena observed during microelectrode studies of myocardial cell preparations may be operative in the genesis of clinical arrhythmias:

1. Abnormal automaticity
2. Reentry
3. Afterpotentials

Ordinarily, the pacemaker cells of the SA node exhibit the fastest intrinsic rate. Pacemaker cells situated elsewhere are suppressed by the depolarization wave originating from the SA node (overdrive suppression). Disease, metabolic derangement, hypoxia, drugs, mechanical stresses, and altered sympathetic nervous activity may permit normally dormant pacemakers to assume dominance. This may become manifest as single or multiple extrasystoles, or as sustained ectopic tachycardia. The specific type of arrhythmia will depend on the location of the ectopic pacemaker and its frequency and regularity.

Two types of reentry phenomena have been described.[15,17] Circus-movement reentry (macroreentry) involves the passage of an electrical wave front around a loop of excitable tissue. Two prerequisites for circus-movement reentry are (1) unidirectional block and (2) slow conduction.

Many "loops" of excitable tissue exist in the normal heart. Slow conduction is characteristic of SA nodal and AV nodal tissue in the normal heart and is regularly observed elsewhere as a result of injury, ischemia, drug effect, or disturbed ionic environment. Unidirectional block is readily induced in both the healthy and diseased heart. Circus-movement reentry may underlie atrial flutter, AV nodal reentrant tachycardia, and some instances of ventricular tachycardia.

Microreentry represents focal reexcitation between myocardial cells in proximity. It is favored by those conditions characterized by asynchronous excitation and repolarization. Ischemia shortens the duration of the monophasic action potentials, and the boundary between healthy and ischemia myocardium may be the site of arrhythmia caused by microreentry. Bradycardia increases the temporal dispersion of refractoriness, increasing the likelihood of focal reexcitation.

Afterpotentials are fluctuations in transmembrane potential observed during the plateau or at the end of the monophasic action potentials. The precise mechanisms responsible for their appearance is unknown. Afterpotentials may be provoked or exaggerated by certain toxins and drugs, including the cardiac glycosides, and may play a causative role in the genesis of the arrhythmias associated with these agents.

Classification of antiarrhythmic drugs

The antiarrhythmic drugs[15,17,22,23] may be categorized according to their dominant electrophysiological effects.

Membrane-depressant agents

1. Quinidine, procaine amide, disopyramide
2. Lidocaine, phenytoin

Quinidine, procaine amide (Pronestyl, Procan SR), and disopyramide (Norpace) exert prominent effects upon phase 0 of the monophasic action potential (MAP). The effectiveness of marginal stimuli (e.g., potential differences attributed to asynchronous repolarization, afterpotentials) may be diminished as a result. These three drugs prolong the duration of the MAP and prolong an effective refractory period. Electrocardiographically, this is manifest as QT_c-interval prolongation and repolarization abnormalities. They also suppress diastolic depolarization in normal and ectopic pacemaker cells. Rhythm disturbances related to abnormal pacemaker activity are often responsive to these agents. In accordance with their extensive electrophysiological effects, these drugs are useful in the management of a variety of arrhythmias. Quinidine, in particular, and, to a lesser degree, procaine amide and disopyramide, may convert atrial fibrillation and flutter to normal sinus rhythm. All three effectively suppress atrial and ventricular premature complexes and may prevent the reoccurrence of atrial and ventricular tachycardias. The direct effects of these drugs is to slow AV nodal conduction. Quinidine and disopyramide, however, may indirectly accelerate AV conduction through vagolytic anticholinergic mechanisms. In the setting of atrial flutter or fibrillation, a dangerous acceleration in ventricular response may be observed, necessitating the simultaneous administration of digitalis or a beta blocker. Combined therapy with quinidine and digoxin has resulted in serum glycoside levels higher than observed when the same dosage of digoxin is given alone. Thus the dosage of digoxin must be diminished when quinidine is added to the therapeutic regimen.

Because of their extensive electrophysiological activity, quinidine, procaine amide, and disopyramide are potentially arrhythmogenic. Suppression of normal automaticity may result in sinus arrest or asystole. Preexisting atrioventricular and intraventricular conduction disturbances may be aggravated when large dosage levels of these drugs are utilized. Particular caution is demanded in patients with evidence of impaired sinus node function, that is, sick sinus syndrome. Quinidine, disopyramide, and, less frequently, procaine amide have been associated with a paradoxical increase in ventricular ectopic complexes, recurrent ventricular tachycardia, and recurrent ventricular fibrillation ("quinidine syncope"). This reaction is usually observed in patients who demonstrate pronounced QT-interval prolongation. A list of other common side effects associated with these agents is provided in the boxed material on the next page.

Beta adrenergic receptor–blocking drugs

The antiarrhythmic potential of the beta blockers may be attributed to one or more of their pharmacological effects:

1. Direct membrane depressant ("quinidine-like") activity

ADVERSE REACTIONS TO COMMON ANTIARRHYTHMIC DRUGS

DISOPYRAMIDE

1. Congestive heart failure may be worsened or be precipitated in patients with greatly impaired cardiac function
2. Severe hypotension, in patients with borderline cardiac function or overt congestive heart failure
3. Severe bradycardia, AV block, asystole; careful monitoring required in patients with sinus node dysfunction and preexisting conduction system disease; increase in ventricular ectopic activity, including ventricular fibrillation, ventricular tachycardia
4. Acceleration of ventricular response in patients with atrial fibrillation and atrial flutter
5. Anticholinergic effects including blurred vision, dry mouth, urinary retention, constipation, impotence
6. Hypoglycemia (rare), rash, pruritus, jaundice, abdominal pain, nausea, vomiting
7. Dizziness, headache, fatigue, depression, malaise, insomnia, paresthesias

PROCAINE AMIDE

1. Hypotension, particularly when administered intravenously
2. Severe bradycardia, AV block, asystole; careful monitoring required in patients with sinus node dysfunction, and preexisting conduction system disease; increase in ventricular ectopic activity, including ventricular fibrillation, and ventricular tachycardia (rare, usually with intravenous therapy)
3. Systemic lupus erythematosus–like syndrome associated with positive ANA (antinuclear antibodies)
4. Contraindicated in patients with myasthenia gravis
5. Anorexia, nausea, vomiting, diarrhea, bitter taste
6. Weakness, mental depression, hallucinations, psychosis
7. Hypersensitivity reactions including rash, angioneurotic edema

QUININE

1. Hypotension, particularly when administered parenterally
2. Severe bradycardia, AV block, asystole; careful monitoring required in patients with sinus node dysfunction, and preexisting conduction system disease; increase in ventricular ectopic activity, including ventricular fibrillation, and ventricular tachycardia
3. Acceleration of ventricular response in patients with atrial fibrillation and atrial flutter
4. Increased serum digoxin concentration, and digitalis intoxication in patients receiving digoxin therapy
5. Cinchonism; tinnitus, headache, nausea, visual disturbances
6. Nausea, vomiting, abdominal pain, diarrhea
7. Hemolytic anemia, hypoprothrombinemia, thrombocytopenia, agranulocytosis
8. Cutaneous flushing, pruritus

LIDOCAINE

1. Apprehension, paresthesias, tinnitus, drowsiness, somnolence, coma, convulsions, respiratory depression, respiratory arrest
2. Nausea, vomiting
3. Hypotension, vascular collapse
4. Severe bradycardia, increasing AV block, asystole; careful monitoring required in patients with sinus node dysfunction and preexisting AV conduction system disease

2. Prevention or reduction of myocardial ischemia
3. Inhibition of arrhythmogenic effects of catecholamines

Commercially available propranolol is a mixture of both D and L isomers. The D isomer lacks beta blocking activity while retaining membrane depressant effects. Propranolol reverses catecholamine-induced acceleration of diastolic depolarization. Sinus node slowing and prolongation of AV nodal conduction are observed at low dosages and are a function of beta blockade. These effects explain the drugs' usefulness in controlling ventricular response during atrial fibrillation and flutter, and in slowing the sinus rate in patients with excessive adrenergic drive (e.g., hyperkinetic heart syndrome). Excessive adrenergic activity or increased sensitivity to circulating catecholamines may also contribute to arrhythmias associated with thyrotoxicosis, general anesthesia, digitalis intoxication, and myocardial infarction.

Higher concentrations of propranolol produce alterations in the monophasic action potential (MAP) of Purkinje cells, suppression of spontaneous diastolic depolarization, and decreased membrane responsiveness. The importance of these direct membrane effects has been questioned, since the plasma concentrations achieved with the customary dosages employed are considerably smaller than the concentrations required to alter MAP properties in microelectrode preparation.

Bretylium tosylate

Bretylium (Bretylol) exhibits distinct electrophysiological effects that set it apart from other antiarrhythmic agents. It is available for parenteral use only.

Bretylium has no effect upon the action potential of atrial muscle. Accordingly, it is ineffective in controlling supraventricular arrhythmias. Bretylium does not suppress and may actually enhance the slope of phase 4 depolarization (pacemaker potential) in Purkinje fibers. Nevertheless, its therapeutic utility is confined to the ventricular arrhythmias. Its predominant effect appears to be on the repolarization phase of the action potential in Purkinje and ventricular myocardial fibers. Bretylium may indirectly hyperpolarize cells by eliciting a transient release of catecholamines, resulting in enhanced membrane responsiveness in abnormally depressed fibers. It also exhibits some adrenergic blocking activity, which may contribute to the hypotension observed during rapid intravenous administration. Bretylium's clinical usefulness is confined to control of recurrent or refractory ventricular tachycardia and fibrillation, particularly in the setting of acute myocardial infarction. It is contraindicated in the presence of digitalis intoxication.

Calcium antagonists

Cardiac fibers may be classified as fast or slow depending on the speed at which they conduct electrical impulses. Fast fibers are characterized by rapid conduction velocity, high resting potential, high threshold potential, rapid rate of depolarization, and large spike amplitude. Fast fiber depolarization (phase 0) is dependent on activation of a "fast" membrane sodium channel. Cell types included in this group include ordinary atrial and ventricular myocardium and Purkinje fibers. Slow cardiac fibers are characterized by their slow conduction velocity, low resting potential, slow rate of depolarization, and small spike amplitude. Depolarization (phase 0) of slow fibers is carried by an inward calcium current. Myocardial cells with these characteristics are located in the sinoatrial and atrioventricular nodes.

The calcium antagonist drugs retard depolarization in slow fibers resulting in sinus bradycardia and AV conduction delays. These drugs also interfere with the calcium current responsible for the plateau phase (phase 2) of the MAP of "fast" fibers as discussed elsewhere.

At present, only two calcium antagonists are available for clinical use—verapamil and nifedipine. Verapamil is considered by some the drug of choice for terminating paroxysmal supraventricular tachycardia. This arrhythmia is often secondary to AV nodal reentry, which is presumably interrupted by blockade of calcium-dependent nodal depolarization. Nifedipine has no important antiarrhythmic activity.

DRUG THERAPY: CONGESTIVE HEART FAILURE
Description of heart failure

The performance of the heart as a pump is primarily dependent on the contractile activity of the myocardium. Myocardial contraction, in turn, is determined by the summated and integrated activity of the individual contractile elements, the sarcomeres. The term "heart failure" indicates that cardiac performance is inadequate for the needs of the body. Congestive heart failure refers to a constellation of signs and symptoms reflecting the heart's inability to meet the metabolic requirements of the peripheral tissues and the various compensatory mechanisms brought into play in an effort to maintain circulatory adequacy.

A variety of structural, metabolic, and toxic conditions may overwhelm the intrinsic reserve capacity of the heart, resulting in congestive heart failure. These may be categorized as follows:

1. Segmental loss of contracting myocardium, e.g., acute myocardial infarction, chronic coronary heart disease
2. Diffuse myocardial dysfunction, e.g., cardiomyopathy, myocarditis
3. Mechanical overload
   a. Systolic overload, e.g., hypertension, aortic stenosis
   b. Diastolic overload, e.g., aortic and mitral regurgitation

Abnormal myocardial contractility (inotropic state) to varying degrees is demonstrable in most failing hearts. This may be expressed as limited cardiac output in response to stress despite high ventricular filling pressure with preservation of basal flow. At the opposite end of the clinical spectrum there is reduced cardiac output at rest and finally cardiogenic shock.

Hemodynamic considerations

Cardiac output represents the quantity of blood expelled from the left ventricle during systole (stroke volume) multiplied by the frequency of cardiac contraction (heart rate). Stroke volume is defined as the difference between left ventricular diastolic and systolic volumes and is determined by the extent of myocardial fiber shortening during systole. In the intact heart, the major determinants of myocardial fiber shortening are the following:

1. Preload: Preload determines diastolic fiber length and at the ultrastructural level the number of active sites available for interaction between actin and myosin filaments. Increased preload results in increased force of contraction.
2. Afterload: Resistance to fiber shortening, determined mainly by resistance to ventricular ejection, which in turn varies directly with peripheral arterial resistance.
3. Inotropic state: Contractile state, measured as the maximal velocity of fiber shortening independent of preload and afterload.

(See Chapter 3 for further explanations.)

Compensatory adjustments

As cardiac pump performance deteriorates, compensatory adjustments are recruited to maintain adequate tissue perfusion. These are as follows:

1. Enhanced adrenergic nervous activity
2. Frank-Starling mechanism
3. Ventricular hypertrophy

Activation of the sympathetic nervous system produces the following changes:

1. Tachycardia (and therefore increased cardiac output)
2. Inotropic support to the failing ventricle
3. Redistribution of peripheral blood flow, including altered patterns of intrarenal blood flow responsible for salt and water retention

The Frank-Starling mechanism is utilized immediately because depressed myocardial contractility results in impaired systolic emptying of the ventricle and increased ventricular end-diastolic volume. On a more chronic basis, salt and water retention expands the intravascular blood volume, maintaining the increase in ventricular dimension. Ventricular dilatation results in greater diastolic fiber stretch (enhanced preload) and force of contraction. These alterations are achieved at the expense of elevated ventricular end-diastolic pressure, which is transmitted backwards to the pulmonary and systemic venous circulations producing symptoms of pulmonary congestion (dyspnea, orthopnea, cough, hemoptysis, etc.) and signs of systemic vascular engorgement (jugular venous distention, hepatomegaly, peripheral edema, etc.).

Over a period of time, mechanical and perhaps ischemic stress stimulates myocardial hypertrophy. The development of additional contractile elements enhances the pumping capabilities of the failing ventricle, reducing the need for other compensatory adjustments. As with other compensatory changes, hypertrophy exacts a price; the increased metabolic requirements of the augmented myocardial cell mass.

Categories of pharmacological agents

The medical management of congestive heart failure includes accurate characterization of underlying pathology, identification of precipitating and aggravating factors, including physical and emotional stresses. It must be emphasized that drug therapy is only one part of this comprehensive approach. Three categories of pharmacological agents currently employed in the management of heart failure are discussed below:

1. Inotropic agents
   a. Cardiac glycosides (digitalis)
   b. Catecholamines
2. Preload-reducing agents
   a. Nitrates
   b. Diuretics
3. Afterload-reducing agents
   a. Sodium nitroprusside
   b. Prazosin
   c. Hydralazine
   d. Phentolamine

Inotropic agents

At the present time, the cardiac glycosides are the only inotropic agents available for chronic oral administration. A number of catecholamines are employed for short-term parenteral inotropic support (e.g., epinephrine, isoproter-enol, dopamine, dobutamine), but up to now no safe and reliable adrenergic compounds given orally are available.

Several digitalis preparations are in clinical use (Table 4-3). They differ with respect to routes of administration, rapidity of action, duration of action, and excretory pathway. Considerable variation in bioavailability has been observed among representative samples of the same drug produced by different manufacturers.

All the cardiac glycosides share the same fundamental pharmacological activity.[5,14,18-21] Three aspects of the pharmacology of digitalis are briefly reviewed:

1. Inotropic activity
2. Electrophysiological effects
3. Autonomic nervous system interactions

The cardiac glycosides bind to specific receptor sites on the myocardial cell membrane and inhibit a membrane Na^+/K^+-ATPase. During myocardial depolarization, extracellular sodium enters, and intracellular potassium is lost from the cardiac cell. Unopposed, repetitive depolarizations would drastically alter the internal ionic environment and disrupt the electrochemical gradients responsible for normal myocardial excitability. Membrane Na^+,K^+-ATPase restores the intracellular ionic balance by actively exchanging intracellular sodium for extracellular potassium against their respective concentration gradients. Digitalis inhibits this Na^+/K^+ "pump." One result is an increase in the concentration of unexchangeable calcium, that is, the fraction available for interaction with the contractile apparatus, within the cell. The calcium-sensitive actinomyosin system consists of at least four proteins: actin, myosin, tropomyosin, and troponin. Troponin inhibits actin/myosin interaction in the absence of calcium. Binding of calcium to troponin releases this inhibitory effect. Digitalis-mediated augmentation of intramyocardial exchangeable calcium results in increased myocardial contractility, expressed as both increased maximal tension development and increased maximal fiber shortening velocity (V_{max}).

Improvement of myocardial contractility at the cellular level is accompanied by improvement of cardiac pump performance as indicated by increased cardiac output despite diminished ventricular diastolic volume (preload). $M\dot{V}O_2$ increases in direct proportion to the magnitude of the inotropic effect, but this may be offset by opposite changes in ventricular wall stress as chamber size diminishes.

The electrophysiological effects of digitalis are principally attributable to inhibition of Na^+/K^+-ATPase and the associated alterations in intracellular ionic composition. More indirectly, the cardiac glycosides influence the electrical properties of the heart through interaction with both the sympathetic and parasympathetic divisions of the autonomic nervous system. Digitalis evokes characteristic changes in the cardiac action potential that are responsible for the familiar repolarization abnormalities noted on the surface electrocardiogram. The direct effects upon myo-

Table 4-3. Digitalis preparations and their actions

Cardiac glycoside	Proprietary name	Route of administration	Gastrointestinal absorption	Average half-life	Total duration of action	Excretory pathway
Digitoxin	Crystodigin Purodigin Digitoxin USP	Oral and par-enteral	90% to 100%	4 to 6 days	2 to 3 weeks	Hepatic-renal
Digoxin	Lanoxin Digoxin USP	Oral and par-enteral	60% to 85%	36 hours	3 to 6 days	Renal
Lanotoside C	Cedilanid	Oral		36 hours	3 to 6 days	Renal
Deslanoside	Cedilanid D	Parenteral	Unreliable	33 hours	3 to 6 days	Renal
Digitalis leaf	Various manu-facturers	Oral	40%	4 to 6 days	2 to 3 weeks	Hepatic-renal
G-strophanthin	Ouabain	Parenteral	Unreliable	21 hours	1 to 3 days	Renal

Table 4-4. Cardiac glycosides: major electrophysiological effects

Electrophysiological property	Effect with low dose	Effect with toxic dose
Automaticity		
SA node	D	I
AV node	–	I
Purkinje	D, then I	I
Excitability		
Atrium	–	D
Ventricle	variable	D
Purkinje	I	D
Effective refractory period		
Atrium	D	
Ventricle	D	
AV node	I	
Purkinje	–, I	
Conduction velocity		
Atrium	I	D
Ventricle	I	D
AV node	D	D
Purkinje	D	D

D, Decreased; *I,* increased; –, no change.

cardiac excitability, membrane responsiveness, automaticity, conduction velocity, and refractoriness are not uniform throughout the heart. Notable variations exist among the specialized cells comprising the pacemaker tissue, AV node, conduction system (His-Purkinje), and ordinary atrial and ventricular myocardium. The principal electrophysiological effects are summarized in Table 4-4.

Digitalis-induced retardation of AV nodal conduction is the most important therapeutic electrophysiological change. This is mediated through a direct prolongation of AV nodal cell refractoriness, in association with increased vagal and diminished adrenergic nervous activity. During atrial fibrillation and atrial flutter, digitalis inhibits the number of atrial impulses traversing the AV node to stimulate the ventricles, slowing ventricular response. Digitalis often causes a termination of paroxysmal supraventricular tachycardia secondary to AV nodal reentry mechanisms.

Inhibition of the Na^+/K^+-ATPase also accounts for the electrophysiological derangements responsible for the most common and serious adverse effects of the cardiac glycosides—the toxic arrhythmias. The list of arrhythmias attributable to digitalis intoxication is quite extensive, and the spectrum varies from asystole to ventricular fibrillation. The more commonly encountered rhythm disturbances include sinus bradycardia, various degrees of AV block, and frequent premature ventricular complexes. The arrhythmogenic potential of the cardiac glycosides attests to their prominent electrophysiological effects. The frequency of toxic arrhythmias encountered in clinical practice underscores the relatively narrow toxic-therapeutic range that exists. Increased parasympathetic (vagal) discharge contributes to digitalis-induced bradyarrhythmias, which may be responsive to vagolytic agents such as atropine. Increased adrenergic activity may contribute to digitalis-induced tachyarrhythmias and may be responsive to beta adrenergic blockade. A summary of commonly encountered side effects is provided in Table 4-5. Special precautions are listed on the next page.

Preload-reducing agents

Ventricular end-diastolic volume is determined by the residual quantity of blood remaining in this chamber at the completion of systole, and the increment added during the subsequent diastolic filling period. A nonlinear, direct relationship exists between ventricular end-diastolic volume and ventricular end-diastolic pressure. As diastolic volume increases, diastolic cavity pressure rises, and this pressure

Table 4-5. Cardiac glycosides: toxic effects

System	Effect
Cardiac	Bradyarrhythmias—sinus bradycardia, sinus arrest, SA exit block; first-, second- (Wenckebach), and third-degree AV block; asystole
	Tachyarrhythmias—premature ventricular complexes, ventricular tachycardia, ventricular fibrillation; atrial tachycardia with AV block; nonparoxysmal junctional tachycardia
Gastrointestinal	Anorexia, nausea, vomiting, abdominal pain, diarrhea, mesenteric insufficiency
Central nervous system	Color vision (purple, yellow), scotoma, headache, malaise, fatigue, confusion, delerium, psychosis, neuralgia
Miscellaneous	Allergic and idiosyncratic reactions, thrombocytopenia, gynecomastia

CARDIAC GLYCOSIDES: SPECIAL PRECAUTIONS

1. Decrease maintenance dosage at the extremes of age, in the presence of advanced myocardial disease, during acute myocarditis, and during the acute phase of myocardial infarction. Reduce dosage in patients with hypothyroidism and myxedema.
2. Decrease maintenance dosage in presence of renal insufficiency (except digitoxin). Reduce digitoxin dosage in presence of hepatic dysfunction.
3. Increased risk of toxic arrhythmia in presence of hypokalemia, hypomagnesemia, hypercalcemia, acidosis, alkalosis, and hypoxia.
4. Arrhythmias may be aggravated by concomitant administration of sympathomimetic agents, or in association with increased adrenergic tone.
5. Bradyarrhythmias may be aggravated by heightened cholinergic tone and by concomitant administration of other cardiodepressant medications.
6. Use with great caution in patients with sick sinus syndrome, or preexisting second- or third-degree AV block. Usually contraindicated in these circumstances unless patient protected by pacemaker.
7. Contraindicated in patients with idiopathic hypertrophic subaortic stenosis; may aggravate left ventricle outflow tract obstruction.
8. In patients with Wolff-Parkinson-White syndrome or with suspected AV nodal bypass tracts, they may accelerate ventricular response during atrial fibrillation or flutter.
9. Reduce maintenance dosage in patients receiving quinidine; combined therapy is associated with increased serum digoxin levels.
10. Increased risk of arrhythmia during electrical manipulation of the heart including pacemaker manipulation, and DC cardioversion.
11. Rarely, rapid intravenous administration may evoke pronounced hypertension.
12. Risk of toxicity greatest during rapid parenteral administration, least during slow oral administration.
13. In patients with severe coronary heart disease, may aggravate angina by increasing MVo_2.

is transmitted backwards into the pulmonary and systemic venous systems. Preload-reducing agents act by limiting venous return to the heart, reducing right and left ventricular end-diastolic volumes and pressures and thus alleviating signs and symptoms of systemic and pulmonary vascular congestion.

Morphine sulfate, a primary drug in the emergency management of pulmonary edema, reduces venous tone, increases venous capacitance, and diminishes venous return to the heart. Similarly, sublingual nitroglycerin, because of its prominent relaxant effects on venous smooth muscle, is often effective in the initial treatment of acute left heart failure. More recently, a number of long-acting nitrate preparations have been successfully used in the long-term management of chronic congestive heart failure. The predominant hemodynamic changes observed include reduction of left ventricular end-diastolic pressure and reduction of pulmonary capillary wedge pressure, with little change in cardiac output or heart rate. Hypotension is the most frequently observed side effect, and it is secondary to a fall in cardiac output caused by ventricular underfilling. Fortunately, patients with congestive heart failure exhibit relatively flat Frank-Starling curves so that modest changes in filling pressure are accompanied by only minor alterations in cardiac output.

The enhanced salt and water losses and increased urine flow induced by diuretic agents results in diminished intravascular volume and reduced ventricular filling pressures. Diuretics therefore may be considered to be chronic preload-reducing agents. Numerous diuretic agents are currently available, differing with respect to their site or sites of action along the nephron, potency, duration of action, and associated metabolic changes. They all may be responsible for signs and symptoms of impaired tissue perfusion consequent to critical reductions in cardiac output. The more frequently observed side effects are summarized in the outline on the next page.

Afterload-reducing agents

Afterload refers to those factors opposing myocardial fiber shortening (contraction). In the intact heart, it de-

---

DIURETICS: SIDE EFFECTS AND PRECAUTIONS

1. May result in metabolic derangement including hypokalemia (except spironolactone and triamterene, which may cause hyperkalemia), hypochloremic alkalosis, dilutional hyponatremia.
2. Increased serum uric acid levels; may provoke acute gouty arthritis.
3. Hyperglycemia; may increase insulin or oral hypoglycemic requirements in previously controlled patients.
4. Azotemia, particularly in patients with preexisting renal disease.
5. Hypercalcemia may be observed particularly with thiazide diuretics; hypocalcemia with furosemide.
6. Use with caution in patients receiving cardiac glycosides; associated electrolyte imbalance increases risk of toxic arrhythmias.
7. ECG abnormalities related to electrolyte imbalance may result in "false-positive" exercise test.
8. May activate or exacerbate systemic lupus erythematosus.

---

scribes the resistance to ventricular ejection. Left ventricular afterload is determined primarily by the integrity of the aortic valve, arterial elasticity, and peripheral arteriolar resistance. Afterload determines the magnitude of left ventricular systolic pressure that must be generated before ejection of blood can proceed. It is therefore an important determinant of ventricular wall stress and of $M\dot{V}O_2$. When preload and contractile state are held constant, reduction in afterload results in increased forward cardiac output and more complete systolic emptying of the ventricle. In the failing heart the improvement in peripheral perfusion and the reduction of central congestion may be achieved with little change or indeed a decrease in MVo_2.

The afterload-reducing agents in current use are vasodilators, and their principal activity is mediated through a relaxation of vascular smooth muscle. They differ from one another with respect to vascular selectivity (i.e., predominant arterial effects, venous effects, or balanced arterial and venous), basic mechanism of action, and incidence of specific adverse effects.

Approximately two thirds of patients with congestive heart failure will respond favorably to vasodilator therapy.[4] Hemodynamic improvement may be noted with one but not another agent in any particular patient. Although careful clinical observation may permit accurate assessment of drug efficacy, invasive hemodynamic monitoring at the onset of treatment is advocated by some clinicians. Although all these drugs have demonstrated short-term effectiveness during acute administration, the maintenance of long-term improvement is still controversial.

Particular benefit has been realized in patients exhibiting pronounced peripheral vasoconstriction, and in the treatment of congestive heart failure complicating specific mechanical problems including mitral regurgitation, aortic regurgitation, and post–myocardial infarction ventricular septal defect.

Hypotension with or without reflex tachycardia is the most common nonspecific side effect and is the usual indication for cessation of therapy. Hypotension may be accompanied by nausea, diaphoresis, dizziness, apprehension, mental confusion, increasing angina, or evidence of deteriorating renal function. Fortunately, these drugs are usually well tolerated, even in patients with normal or low basal blood pressure. This may be attributed to the high resting sympathetic tone that is observed in the presence of heart failure. Nevertheless, particular care must be exercised in patients with evidence of cerebrovascular, coronary artery, and peripheral vascular disease.

Sodium nitroprusside (Nipride) is administered by continuous intravenous infusion. Its onset of action is almost immediate, and its duration of action is quite brief. Nitroprusside is active on both the arterial and venous sides of the circulation, effectively diminishing left ventricular end-diastolic pressure, and pulmonary capillary wedge pressure. Cardiac output and heart rate are either unchanged or increase slightly, whereas mean arterial pressure is either unchanged or diminishes slightly. Nitroprusside reacts with red blood cell sulfhydryl groups and is rapidly converted to cyanide ion and then to thiocyanate. Thiocyanate accumulation may produce hypothyroidism; therefore plasma levels should be monitored in patients receiving high dosages or prolonged infusions.

Prazosin (Minipress) is an orally effective antihypertensive agent that exhibits direct smooth muscle relaxant activity and alpha adrenergic receptor–blocking effects. The hemodynamic response is similar to that of nitroprusside; both left ventricular end diastolic and pulmonary capillary wedge pressures (PCWP) are reduced, with little change in heart rate, cardiac output, and mean arterial pressure. The most common side effect is orthostatic hypotension, sometimes presenting as syncope. This is observed more frequently in hypertensive patients in the absence of congestive failure.

Hydralazine (Apresoline) is an orally effective antihypertensive agent that has been in clinical use for over 30 years. It is a direct smooth muscle relaxant and vasodilator and predominantly affects the arterial side of the circulation. When administered to patients with congestive heart failure, the principal hemodynamic alterations are reduced peripheral arterial resistance with a concomitant increase in cardiac output. Reductions in left ventricular end-diastolic pressure and pulmonary capillary wedge pressure are less impressive than with either nitroprusside or prazosin. Hydralazine is most effective in patients with intense vasoconstriction and reduced cardiac output and less effective in reducing symptoms of pulmonary congestion.

A more balanced effect may be achieved by combined therapy with long-acting nitrates.

When employed as an antihypertensive agent, the most troublesome side effects are tachycardia, flushing and headache from peripheral vasodilatation, and reflex increase in sympathetic activity. A delayed syndrome resembling systemic lupus erythematosus is occasionally observed after prolonged, high-dosage therapy. Hydralazine undergoes hepatic acetylation, and this significantly reduces the concentration of active drug entering the systemic circulation after intestinal absorbtion. Hepatic *N*-acetyltransferase activity is a genetically determined trait. "Slow acetylators" experience a greater incidence of untoward reactions.

Phentolamine (Regitine) is an alpha adrenergic blocking agent. When given to patients with congestive heart failure, it induces a reduction in peripheral arteriolar resistance accompanied by increased cardiac output. Both left ventricle end-diastolic pressure and pulmonary capillary wedge pressure may decrease, but not to the same extent as observed with nitroprusside. This agent is not tolerated as well as the other vasodilator agents described, the most troublesome side effects being hypotension and tachycardia.

DRUG THERAPY: HYPERTENSION
Antihypertensive drugs

Hypertension is the most common chronic cardiovascular disorder recognized in the United States. Despite remarkable advances in our understanding of circulatory physiology, the fundamental mechanism or mechanisms underlying essential or idiopathic hypertension remain enigmatic.[7] Nevertheless, effective antihypertensive agents are available, and successful blood pressure control is achievable in most patients. A detailed discussion of the medical management of hypertension is beyond the scope of this chapter. Several important principles of treatment are mentioned:

1. Before the diagnosis of hypertension is established, repeated, accurate blood pressure determinations should be made.
2. Known secondary causes of hypertension (renal artery stenosis, pheochromocytoma, aldosteronoma, aortic coarctation, oral contraceptive therapy) should be excluded with appropriate diagnostic tests.
3. Once the diagnosis is established, medical therapy should not be delayed or withheld.
4. Patient evaluation should include assessment for evidence of target organ damage (retinal, cardiac, renal, peripheral vascular).
5. Aggravating factors including dietary indiscretion, stress, exercise habits, and medications should be recognized.
6. Effective pharmacological therapy should be instituted with careful medical follow-up to monitor drug efficacy and patient adherence and to minimize adverse reactions.
7. The goal of therapy should be normalization of blood pressure, protection of target organs, and prolongation of life.
8. Patient education is an essential ingredient to successful therapy.

Diuretics

Diuretics exhibit weak antihypertensive activity and are usually prescribed as the initial drug in patients with mild hypertension. The diuretics potentiate the antihypertensive action of more powerful agents and are often used in combination with them in patients with severe hypertension. The numerous thiazide diuretics share approximately equivalent antihypertensive effects when comparable dosages are employed. Furosemide is more effective in patients with impaired renal function and in those with refractory edema. Triamterene exhibits minimal antihypertensive activity and is usually combined with another diuretic to limit potassium loss. Spironolactone is approximately as potent as the thiazides and is often given in combination with them to take advantage of its potassium-sparing activity. It is particularly effective in patients with high plasma renin levels and in patients with aldosteronism.

The mechanisms responsible for the antihypertensive effects of the diuretics are uncertain. Proposed mechanisms include the following:

1. Contraction of plasma volume
2. Direct vasodilator activity
3. Altered vasopressor receptor sensitivity
4. Alterations in vascular wall compliance

Vasodilators

Prazosin (Minipress) exerts direct smooth muscle relaxant and alpha adrenergic receptor–blocking activities. Unlike other vasodilators, it usually does not provoke reflex tachycardia or increase peripheral renin activity. The most frequent and troublesome side effect is postural dizziness and occasionally syncope secondary to orthostatic hypotension. Less commonly observed side effects include nausea, vomiting, diarrhea, constipation, male impotence, blurred vision, dry mouth, and urinary frequency. Prazosin is moderately effective when employed alone and often used in combination with a diuretic and an adrenergic blocking agent.

Hydralazine (Apresoline) is a potent direct smooth muscle relaxant that acts predominantly upon the peripheral arterial resistance vessels. When administered alone, it is usually associated with pronounced reflex tachycardia, which may aggravate myocardial ischemia in patients with coronary heart disease. For this reason, it is contraindicated in the setting of acute myocardial infarction. The hypotensive actions of hydralazine may be counteracted by activation of the renin-angiotensin system with subsequent salt and water retention. These undesirable effects may be minimized by the concomitant administration of a beta adrenergic blocking agent and a potent diuretic.

Minoxidil (Loniten) is the newest and most potent oral vasodilator. It is reserved for patients with severe or malignant hypertension unresponsive to other available drugs. Reflex tachycardia and salt and water retention are prominent side effects, and the concurrent administration of a beta adrenergic blocking agent and diuretic is usually required. Less frequent side effects include excessive body hair growth, pericardial effusion, and electrocardiographic abnormalities.

Adrenergic receptor–blocking drugs

Beta blocking drugs. Five beta adrenergic receptor–blocking drugs are currently available—propranolol (Inderal), metoprolol (Lopressor), nadolol (Corgard), atenolol (Tenormin), and timolol (Blocadren). Their fundamental pharmacological properties are similar. Metoprolol and atenolol exhibit relative beta$_1$ receptor selectivity at low dosages; however, this advantage is lost at the higher dosages commonly employed. Nadolol is four times as potent as propranolol and has a much longer half-life permitting once daily dosage. All these drugs share a spectrum of side effects related to beta blockade, as already described elsewhere.

The beta blockers exhibit moderate antihypertensive activity when employed alone. They are particularly useful in patients with labile hypertension, hyperkinetic heart syndrome, and other conditions associated with heightened adrenergic activity. Beta blockers are often prescribed along with vasodilators to augment the antihypertensive activity of the latter and to prevent the tachycardia that usually accompanies their use.

The antihypertensive action of the beta blockers is attributable to a reduction in cardiac output secondary to their negative chronotropic negative inotropic effects. Reduction of renin secretion and inhibition of the renin-angiotensin axis contributes to their efficacy in hyperreninemic states such as malignant or accelerated hypertension.

Alpha-methyldopa

Alpha methyldopa (Aldomet) is an intermediate-strength antihypertensive available for oral and parenteral use. When administered alone, it effectively controls a majority of patients with mild to moderate hypertension. It is often employed in combination with vasodilator and diuretics in the management of more severe hypertension. In therapeutic doses, methyldopa does not diminish renal blood flow. For this reason, it is of particular value in the treatment of hypertension complicated by renal insufficiency.

Its mechanism of action is not entirely understood. Part of its antihypertensive activity is mediated through central stimulation of alpha adrenergic receptor inhibitors. Reduc-

tion of peripheral plasma renin concentration may contribute. A more peripheral site of action has not been excluded.

Sedation is the most frequently encountered side effect. This may vary from fatigue, to lethargy, to somnolence. These symptoms often abate with continued therapy. Dizziness secondary to orthostatic hypotension is not uncommon. Other nonspecific side effects include headache, dry mouth, sleep disturbances, nasal congestion, depression, and sexual dysfunction.

As many as one third of patients receiving prolonged therapy at high dosage develop a positive direct Coombs' test. Only a small fraction have evidence of hemolysis. Hyperpyrrhexia is seen in 1% to 3% within the first 3 weeks of therapy and may be accompanied by abnormalities of hepatic function. Methyldopa may also be responsible for a viral hepatitis–like syndrome, granulomatous hepatitis, and cholestatic jaundice.

Clonidine

Clonidine (Catapres) is an oral agent effective in the control of mild, moderate, and severe hypertension. It may be employed alone, or in combination with diuretics, vasodilators, or other adrenergic blocking agents. Clonidine is believed to act through stimulation of medullary alpha adrenergic receptors with reduction in sympathetic outflow. Inhibition of the renin-angiotensin system may contribute to its hypotensive effects. Clonidine does not reduce renal blood flow, increasing its usefulness in patients with impaired renal function. Because the drug is excreted by the kidneys, dosage must be adjusted downwards in such patients.

Sedation is the most frequently encountered side effect and may result in fatigue, lethargy, and somnolence. It often diminishes or disappears with continued therapy. By administration of a larger fraction of the total daily dose at night before sleep, the sedative effects can be partially avoided. Orthostatic hypotension is usually less severe than with other antihypertensive drugs. In contrast to the vasodilators, clonidine often induces cardiac slowing rather than tachycardia. An acute withdrawal syndrome consisting of tachycardia, nervousness, sweating, hypertension, and headache has been described. Although abnormal adrenergic activity has been implicated, excessive catecholamine secretion has not been demonstrated. Increased adrenergic receptor sensitivity to normal levels of catecholamines cannot be excluded. Although the withdrawal syndrome is quite uncommon, abrupt discontinuation of the drug should be avoided.

Reserpine

Reserpine is one of a number of rauwolfia alkaloids that exert modest antihypertensive effects. Their widespread pharmacological actions are believed to be secondary to catecholamine and 5-hydroxytryptamine depletion within the central nervous system, peripheral nerves, myocardium, and blood vessels. Reserpine is commonly prescribed as the sole agent in patients with mild hypertension, or in combination with diuretics for moderately hypertensive patients. In large doses, administered parenterally, it is useful in the management of some hypertensive emergencies. The high incidence of toxic side effects associated with high dosages limits its applicability to short-term therapy. Because of its pronounced sedative activity, reserpine is useful in the management of the agitated hypertensive patient. It is contraindicated in patients with a history of mental depression. Other common side effects include nasal stuffiness, lethargy, drowsiness, and appetite stimulation.

Guanethidine

Guanethidine (Ismelin) is a potent antihypertensive usually reserved for patients with moderately severe or severe hypertension and patients who have not responded adequately to other agents. Guanethidine is an adrenergic blocking agent that localizes to postganglionic sympathetic nerve endings depleting the norepinephrine pools and inhibiting the release of neurotransmitter during sympathetic stimulation. The most troublesome side effect is orthostatic hypotension secondary to generalized sympathetic blockade. Guanethidine also depletes myocardial catecholamines and may aggravate preexisting congestive heart failure. Muscular weakness, sexual dysfunction, headache, nasal stuffiness, and bradycardia are other common side effects.

Renin-angiotensin antagonists

Many antihypertensive drugs interact with the renin-angiotensin system. In general, diuretics and vasodilators stimulate renin secretion, and this may blunt the antihypertensive effects of these drugs. The beta blockers, methyldopa and clonidine, inhibit renin secretion, and this may contribute to the antihypertensive effects of these drugs. Captopril (Capoten) is the first of a series of drugs whose antihypertensive activity is specifically related to interference with the renin-angiotensin axis.

Renin, secreted by the kidney, converts circulating angiotensinogen to angiotensin I.[12] Angiotensin I is acted upon by converting enzyme and is transformed into angiotensin II. Angiotensin II is a potent vasoconstrictor and, in addition, stimulates the release of aldosterone from the adrenal cortex. Captopril inhibits angiotensin-converting enzyme, blocking the formation of angiotensin II. Captopril is a potent antihypertensive, reserved for patients with severe or refractory hypertension not responsive to combined therapy with appropriate doses of diuretics, vasodilators, and adrenergic blocking agents. Side effects frequently encountered with other agents including orthostatic hypotension, impotence, tachycardia, and cardiac depression are infrequent with captopril. Serious adverse effects include proteinuria, sometimes associated with the nephrotic syndrome, agranulocytosis, and neutropenia.

SUMMARY

The effects of medications on the cardiovascular system at rest and during exercise cannot be overstated. Physical therapists involved with patients with coronary artery disease should know the types of medications, their effects, and their side effects if their goal is an effective well-monitored cardiac rehabilitation program.

This chapter reviews four classifications of medications commonly used with patients. These medications are used to control (1) angina pectoris, (2) arrhythmias, (3) congestive heart failure, and (4) high blood pressure.

Control of angina is achieved by restoration of the proper balance between $M\dot{V}O_2$ and myocardial oxygen demand. Three categories of drugs have been discussed: nitrates, beta blockers, and calcium channel blockers.

Nitrates reviewed include nitroglycerin, isosorbide dinitrate (Isordil, Sorbitrate), and topical nitroglycerin (Nitrobid, Nitrol, Transderm-Nitro, and Nitrodur).

Beta-adrenergic blockers reviewed included propranolol (Inderal), metoprolol (Lopressor), atenolol (Tenormin), and nadolol (Corgard).

Calcium antagonists reviewed included verapamil (Isoptin, Calan) and nifedipine (Procardia).

The control of arrhythmias primarily involves an effect on the cardiac conduction system and the monophasic action potential (MAP). Mechanisms for cardiac arrhythmias are theorized to result from (1) abnormal automaticity, (2) reentry, and (3) afterpotentials.

Antiarrhythmic drugs classified as membrane-depressant agents include quinidine, procaine amide (Procan SR, Pronestyl), and disopyramide (Norpace). Additional antiarrhythmics include beta adrenergic receptor blockers, calcium antagonists, and bretylium tosylate (Bretylol).

For appreciation of the medications used to control congestive heart failure, a brief review of the causes of heart failure and the hemodynamic considerations involved was given. Drug therapy for congestive heart failure was reviewed in three general categories: (1) inotropic agents, (2) preload-reducing agents, (3) afterload-reducing agents. Inotropic agents include cardiac glycosides, digitoxin, digoxin (Lanoxin), deslanoside, digitalis leaf, lanotoside C (Cedilanid), and G-strophanthin (ouabain). Preload-reducing agents include morphine sulfate, nitrates, and diuretics. Afterload-reducing agents include sodium nitroprusside (Nipride), prazosin (Minipress), hydralazine (Apresoline), and phentolamine (Regitane).

Principles of hypertensive treatment were reviewed, and this included discussion of the causes of hypertension, initiation of drug therapy, evaluation of organ damage, aggravating factors, medical follow-up, goals of therapy, and patient education. A wide range of antihypertensive medications was reviewed. They included diuretics, vasodilators, beta adrenergic blockers, alpha-methyldopa (Aldomet), clonidine (Catapres), reserpine, guanethidine (Ismelin), and renin-angiotensin antagonists.

The pharmacological approach to patients with coronary artery disease is an integral part of their medical management and thus a key component in the construction and implementation of their program of rehabilitation.

REFERENCES

1. Braunwald, E.: Control of myocardial oxygen consumption, Am. J. Cardiol. **27**:416, 1971.
2. Braunwald, E., editor: Introduction: calcium channel blockers, Am. J. Cardiol. **46**(6):1045, 1980; **47**(1):157, 1981.
3. Calcium, calcium antagonists and cardiovascular disease, Chest **78**(suppl.):121, 1980.
4. Chatterjee, K., and Parmley, W.W.: The role of vasodilator therapy in heart failure, Prog. Cardiovasc. Dis. **19**:301, 1977.
5. Doherty, J.E., and others: Clinical pharmacokinetics of digitalis glycosides, Prog. Cardiovasc. Dis. **21**(2):141, 1978.
6. Epstein, S., and others: Angina pectoris: pathophysiology, evaluation and treatment, Ann. Intern. Med. **75**(2):263, 1971.
7. Frolich, E.D.: Newer concepts in antihypertensive drugs, Prog. Cardiovasc. Dis. **21**(3):159, 1978.
8. Gettes, L.S.: The electrophysiologic effects of antiarrhythmic drugs, Am. J. Cardiol. **28**:526, 1971.
9. Goodman, L.S., and Gilman, A., editors: The pharmacological basics of therapeutics, New York, 1975, The Macmillan Co., Inc.
10. Gorlin, R.: Regulation of coronary blood flow, Br. Heart J. **33**(suppl.):9, 1971.
11. James, T.N.: The delivery and distribution of the coronary collateral circulation, Chest **58**(3):183, 1970.
12. Laragh, J.H.: The renin system in high blood pressure, Prog. Cardiovasc. Dis. **21**(3):159, 1978.
13. Lucchesi, B.R., and Leighton, W.S.: The pharmacology of the beta adrenergic blocking agents, Prog. Cardiovasc. Dis. **11**(5):410, 1969.
14. Mason, D.T.: Digitalis pharmacology and therapeutics: recent advances, Ann. Intern. Med. **80**(4):520, 1974.
15. Rosen, M.R., and Gelband, H.: Antiarrhythmic drugs, Am. Heart J. **81**(3):428, 1971.
16. Singer, D.H., and others: Cellular electrophysiology of ventricular and other dysrhythmias, Prog. Cardiovasc. Dis. **24**(2):97, 1981.
17. Singh, B.N., and others: New perspectives in the pharmacologic therapy of cardiac arrhythmias, Prog. Cardiovasc. Dis. **22**(4):243, 1980.
18. Smith, T.W., and Haber, E.: Digitalis, N. Engl. J. Med. **289**(18):945, 1973.
19. Smith, T.W., and Haber, E.: Digitalis, part 2, N. Engl. J. Med. **289**(19):1010, 1973.
20. Smith, T.W., and Haber, E.: Digitalis, part 3, N. Engl. J. Med. **289**(20):1063, 1973.
21. Smith, T.W., and Haber, E.: Digitalis, part 4, N. Engl. J. Med. **289**(21):1125, 1973.
22. Zipes, D.P., and Troup, P.J.: New antiarrhythmic agents: amiodarone, aprindine, disopyramide, ethmozin, mexiletine, tocainide, verapamil, Am. J. Cardiol. **41**(6):1005, 1978.
23. Zipes, D.P.: Introduction: miles to go, Am. J. Cardiol. 41(6):975, 1978.

5

SCOT IRWIN

Abnormal exercise physiology

The information contained in this chapter is another aspect of the knowledge base required by a physical therapist to conduct a cardiac or pulmonary rehabilitation program. To understand the clinical observations discussed, one needs a sound understanding of normal human responses to exercise.[1]

To the purist, the concept of abnormality is truly a misnomer because a clear-cut definition of normality has not been established. Normal values may range from less than average to superaverage. This makes it difficult to determine normal variations from abnormal aberrations. However, to describe some peculiar exertional responses found in patients with cardiac or pulmonary disease, I will use the term ''abnormal.'' These aberrant responses resulting from the pathophysiology of disease highlight the need for individualized programs of patient care.

There are several well-documented and accepted physiological responses to exercise. For example, heart rate and systolic blood pressure rise with increases in work load, and a majority of references on exercise physiology support the argument that cardiac output is the limiting factor for increasing oxygen consumption and determining maximal physical work capacity. Furthermore, numerous articles describe angina threshold (point at which a patient first perceives angina) as a fixed phenomenon based on myocardial oxygen demand, which is strongly correlated to the product of heart rate and systolic blood pressure.[21] Each of these well-established norms has an abnormal counterpart. Varied pathological conditions and treatments (including medications) create demonstrable changes in normal heart rate, blood pressure, and anginal responses during exercise. These abnormal responses and the occurrence of respiratory limitations to maximum oxygen consumption are discussed using a similar format. The format is to define the abnormal response, cite the supporting literature, and then present clinical examples that illustrate the abnormality, followed by a brief theoretical discussion of possible causation and finally summarization of the clinical implications of the abnormal phenomenon.

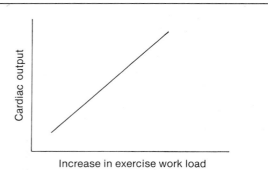

Fig. 5-1. Cardiac output is linearly related to work load. When the work load is progressively increased, cardiac output matches the demand until maximum cardiac output is achieved. (Normal.)

HEART RATE RESPONSE
Normal

Normally, cardiac output and heart rate increase linearly with increases in work load and oxygen consumption demands[34] (Fig. 5-1). At submaximal levels of exercise, the heart rate response is normally linear. At near-maximal and maximal levels of exertion, the heart rate response becomes less linear and increases disproportionately to the work load imposed (Fig. 5-2).

An additional phenomenon that the clinician may observe is that a person's maximum attainable heart rate decreases with age. A useful but limited formula for predicting a maximum heart rate is to subtract 220 from the patient's age (Fig. 5-3). This formula is limited because of the effects of medications (see Chapter 4), abnormal heart rate responses, and the wide range of individual variations in maximum heart rate response ($\pm 10\%$). It is preferable

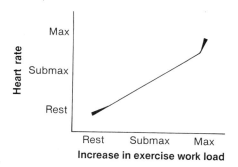

Fig. 5-2. Heart rate response to increases in work load. Submaximal effort is closely related to heart rate response, but at the extremes of exertion the relationship is generally less linear.

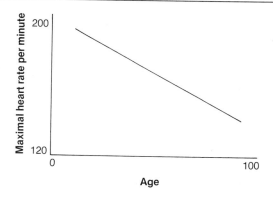

Fig 5-3. Maximal heart rate decreases with an increase in age.

to obtain a patient's true maximum heart rate by performing a maximum symptom-limited exercise test (see Chapter 6).

Abnormal

In the clinical setting a small subset of patients with coronary artery disease demonstrate a clearly abnormal heart rate response to exercise. This phenomenon has been described by Ellestad[13] and by Blessey and others.[3] Although each of them describe slightly different criteria for the response and thus a slightly different population of patients, they do agree that this response represents a sign of an advanced pathological condition. Generally the following criteria are observed:

1. Low resting heart rate (50-70)
2. Poor physical condition (untrained)
3. Advanced coronary artery disease
4. Maximum symptom-limited heart rate achieved during exercise testing is well below the person's predicted maximal heart rate (PMHR) (PMHR is obtained by subtraction of 220 from the individual's age.)
5. Men between the ages of 40 and 60
6. Not on chronotropic inhibiting medications (chronotropic means "influencing the rate of the heart beat")
7. Poor, slow heart rate increase to incremental increases in exercise work load
8. Poor exercise tolerance

A classic example of this phenomenon in the same patient before and after bypass surgery is presented in Figs. 5-4 and 5-5. A summary interpretation of each of these tests follows the graph. Each exercise test was performed in the same manner according to the protocol described in Appendix A.

It is extraordinary that patient A's exercise tolerance was unchanged despite a 42-beat-per-minute increase in his maximum heart rate between the first test before surgery and the second test 8 weeks after surgery. In effect, this patient had a 36% increase in his heart rate reserve but essentially no change in his physical work capacity.

The following findings were recorded on patient A's catheterization: (1) 25% narrowing of the left main coronary artery, (2) less than 50% narrowing at the junction of the proximal and middle thirds of the left anterior descending artery plus a somewhat narrowed appearance throughout its length, (3) about 75% stenosis at the origin of the second posterolateral branch of the circumflex and mildly irregular throughout, (4) right coronary artery 75% stenotic at the ostium and midpoint, (5) hemodynamically the right ventricle and atrium have greatly elevated end diastolic and systolic pressures, (6) left ventricular end-diastolic pressure was greatly elevated, (7) ejection fraction was normal, and (8) the left ventricular contractile pattern was normal. An additional test example is presented to demonstrate this abnormality in somewhat less severe forms. See Fig. 5-6 and the accompanying test description.

Mechanisms

There appears to be a close relationship between patient A's heart rate response and ischemia. (Note that there were no ST-segment changes on either test.) The first test, which vividly demonstrates chronotropic incompetence, also demonstrates the need to watch all the factors involved in exercise testing, not just ST segments.

Neither Ellestad[13] nor Blessey[3] has presented a consistent explanation for this abnormal heart rate response. Hinkle, Carver, and Plakum[17] believe that this response was attributable to ischemia of the sinoatrial node. On the other hand, the work of Jose[19] indicates that as myocardial contractility decreases, as occurs with increasing levels of ischemia, the intrinsic heart rate response decreases; Ellestad has found that this response is an ominous sign of advanced coronary artery disease associated with accelerated rates of mortality and morbidity (Fig. 5-7), especially

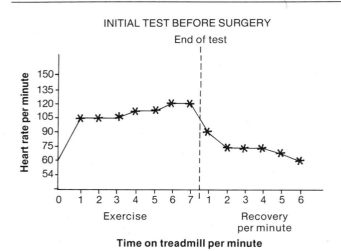

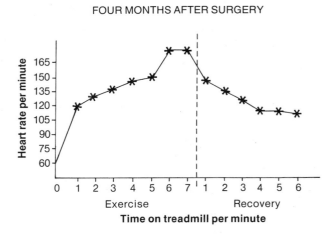

Fig. 5-4. Heart rate response to Bruce Protocol Treadmill Test in patient A, a 45-year-old male patient before surgery. Patient completed 6 minutes and 6 seconds of the Bruce Protocol. He was limited by angina. Resting heart rate was 54, and maximum heart rate was 118. Resting blood pressure was 164/98, and maximum blood pressure was 244/126. He demonstrated moderate systolic and severe progressive diastolic hypertension with exercise. No ST-segment changes were found in any of the six leads: V_1, V_5, V_6, X, CM_4, Y. There were no arrhythmias. His medications were nitroglycerin as needed and Dyazide (triamterene and hydrochlorothiazide). A fourth heart sound was auscultated.

Fig. 5-5. Heart rate response to Bruce Protocol Treadmill Test in patient A (Fig. 5-4) 8 weeks after bypass surgery. Patient completed 6 minutes and 7 seconds of the Bruce Protocol. He was limited by leg pain. Resting heart rate was 62, and maximum heart rate was 160. Resting blood pressure 176/110 and maximum blood pressure was 292/120. He demonstrated severe systolic and diastolic blood pressure response throughout the test. He had no angina or ST-T–segment changes. There was one premature ventricular contraction during exercise. He was not using medications. Fourth heart sound was auscultated.

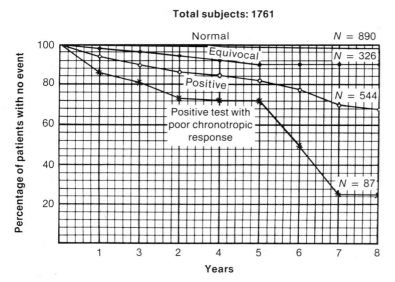

Fig 5-6. Abnormal rate response. Life table display of incidence of myocardial infarctions. Notice the higher incidence of infarction in those with poor chronotropic response to exercise. (Redrawn from Ellestad, M.H.: Stress testing, ed. 2, Philadelphia, 1981, F. A. Davis Co.)

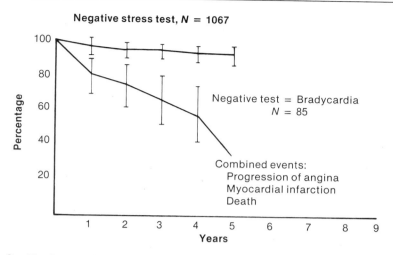

Fig. 5-7. Combined-events bradycardia. Those with bradycardia (pulse fell below 95% confidence limits for age and sex) and normal ST segments have a high incidence of combined events (similar to those with ST-segment depression). (Redrawn from Ellestad, M.H.: Stress testing, ed. 2, Philadelphia, 1981, F. A. Davis Co.)

when compared with patients with normal heart rate responses.[13]

The exact cause of this response is unknown; however, one may speculate that these patients have a neurological, vascular, or humoral reflex that works through the autonomic nervous system to keep their heart rates down. Another possibility is that the ischemia causes a reflex inhibition of the electrical activation in the sinoatrial node, thus decreasing the rate at which the sinoatrial node can fire.

If ischemia is the cause of this decreased heart rate response, the body's defense mechanism is appropriate because a lower heart rate certainly facilitates improved coronary blood flow and decreases myocardial oxygen demand. A lower heart rate lengthens the diastolic period, and thus the coronary artery filling time is lengthened so that an improved perfusion can be achieved. A lower heart rate also decreases myocardial oxygen requirements. Alternatively, an increased diastolic filling time may, especially during exercise, cause large increases in end-diastolic volume. Volume increases are well tolerated by a normal, well-perfused myocardium but in the ischemic myocardium volume changes are associated with increased pressures and thus decreased subendocardial perfusion (see Chapter 2). As you may note from the patient example, his end-diastolic pressure was greatly elevated, 20 mm Hg, at rest. One could speculate that the rising end-diastolic pressures that undoubtedly occur with increased venous return during exercise may somehow be the impetus to a reflex inhibition in heart rate.[19]

Further speculation and research into the probable causes of abnormal heart rate responses to exercise should focus on all the factors that normally control heart rate. This would be an exhaustive review and not within the purview of this text. Perhaps future clinicians and researchers will determine the exact cause of this abnormal response.

The normal heart rate response to increasing levels of exercise in a well-trained athlete is to have a slow resting heart and a gradual but linear rise to a normal maximal rate. The pathological chronotropic incompetence exhibited by the nonathlete is truly an abnormal response that should not be taken lightly by therapists but instead interpreted as a highly abnormal response to exercise.

Summary of clinical significance

1. Less than symptom-limited maximum-exercise tests may mask the patient with abnormal heart rate responses.
2. A slow heart rate at rest and a slow heart rate response to exercise is not always a sign of a good state of fitness.
3. Abnormal heart rate response to exercise may be an ominous sign, predictive of severe coronary artery disease and all its manifestations.
4. Patients who exhibit an abnormal heart rate response to exercise should be monitored carefully and medically supervised closely if they are enrolled in a cardiac rehabilitation program.

BLOOD PRESSURE RESPONSE
Normal

In normal adult males blood pressure response to increasing levels of exertion is not nearly so clearly de-

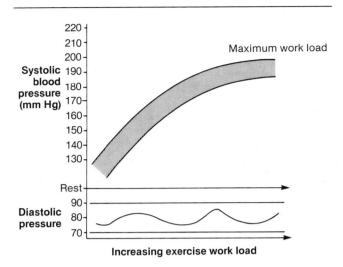

Fig. 5-8. Normal systolic and diastolic blood responses to exertion.

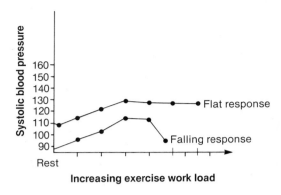

Fig. 5-9. Abnormal systolic blood response to exertion. *Top graph,* Flat response. *Bottom graph,* Poor response with an abnormal fall at peak exercise.

scribed as a heart rate response. All that clinical experience and the scientific literature allow is that systolic pressure rises with increasing levels of work and diastolic pressure rises slightly (less than 10 mm Hg), remains the same, or drops slightly (less than 10 mm Hg) (Fig. 5-8).

Generally, in adult women the systolic blood pressure response to exercise is flatter than that found in men.

The primary reason that blood pressure responses are difficult to categorize is that the auscultatory method of obtaining blood pressure during exercise may be highly inaccurate. An arterial indwelling pressure sensor in the arm would be the most accurate means of obtaining blood pressures but highly impractical. Auscultation of blood pressures during exercise is inaccurate and poorly reproducible. It requires good clinical skill to obtain any blood pressure readings when someone is exercising on a treadmill. It is difficult to obtain reliable blood pressure readings because of the excessive extraneous noise of the treadmill and the arm movement that occurs during an exercise test. At low levels of exercise it is possible to get fairly reliable and reproducible data, but at high levels of exercise it is not at all accurate.[22] This limitation in accuracy of blood pressure recording should be kept in mind as you read this next section because only major changes in blood pressure are considered significant.

Systolic blood pressure rises during exercise because of an increase in cardiac output greater than the decrease in peripheral vascular resistance (see Chapter 3 for specifics). In well-conditioned athletes and younger persons, the diastolic blood pressure may fall precipitously during exercise creating a wide pulse pressure. This phenomenon is rarely seen in patients or older persons (40 or more years of age).

Abnormal

Significant abnormalities in blood pressure responses to increasing levels of exertion occur both in systolic blood pressure and diastolic blood pressure. Both abnormalities often represent the existence of significant pathological conditions and should be recognized, interpreted, and incorporated into each patient's data base.

Systolic abnormality

There are three different abnormal systolic blood pressure responses that occur during increasing levels of exertion. One is a response in which the systolic pressure is low to begin with (less than 110 mm Hg), rises little, and then begins to fall despite increases in work load (Fig. 5-9). The second is the flat response in which the pressure may rise slightly but fails to continue to rise and remains generally below 140 mm Hg (Fig. 5-9). The third and clinically more common response, especially in patients after having an infarction, is a normal submaximal response with a precipitous fall in systolic pressure at higher work loads (Fig. 5-10). This response is often associated with pronounced ST-T depression or elevation changes in the patient's electrocardiogram.

Bruce,[6] Irving,[18] and others have found that this response is highly indicative of a serious pathological condition. They found that patients with poor systolic blood pressure responses and peak pressures less than 140 mm Hg and not on medications had a much higher incidence of sudden death. In addition, they found that this response was most commonly found in three patient groups: patients with severe obstructive coronary artery disease, which caused pronounced ischemia with exertion but with normal ventricular function, patients with cardiomegaly or gross myocardial damage and poor ventricular function, and patients with a combination of those two variables.

Two patients case examples, patients B and C, including

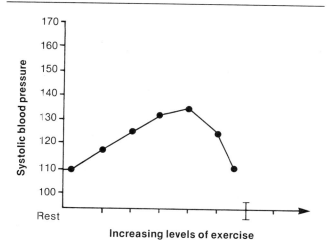

Fig. 5-10. Abnormal systolic blood pressure response to exertion. Striking fall in systolic pressure with exercise despite a normal response at submaximal levels at exertion.

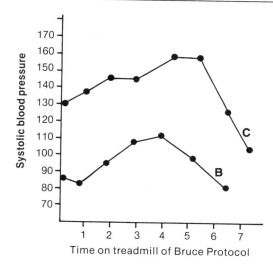

Fig. 5-11. Systolic blood pressure response to a modified low level Bruce Protocol Treadmill Test in patient B, a 67-year-old man, 2 weeks after anteroseptal myocardial infarction. Initial pressure was taken standing. Resting heart rate was 63; maximum heart rate 82. Test stopped because of blood pressure response and shortness of breath. Patient developed a third heart sound. He had frequent ventricular arrhythmias after exercise. His medications were Inderal (propranolol), Procardia (nifedipine), and nitroglycerin, and they may have played a role in his abnormal blood pressure response. ST elevation throughout showed no change. C, Abnormal systolic blood pressure to a Bruce protocol symptom-limited maximal-exercise test. Patient C was a 50-year-old man taking no medications and having no previous history of infarction. Maximum heart rate was 155, no arrhythmias, positive ST-segment depression of 2.0 mm horizontal change during and after exercise, and positive for angina. S₄ after exercise. Resting pressure was 132/84; maximum pressure was 162/90.

the patients' blood pressure response during exercise testing and their catheterization data are presented to provide examples of this abnormal phenomenon (Fig. 5-11).

The abnormal systolic blood pressure response should not remove a patient for consideration in a cardiac rehabilitation program, but the patient's exercise prescription must be adjusted to accommodate this abnormality. Patients with these responses must be monitored closely.

Mechanisms. When we look at the normal systolic blood pressure response, it is common to see a person's blood pressure flatten or fall at peak exercise. Theoretically, as heart rate exceeds 190 beats per minute, the filling time for the ventricle decreases to a point at which stroke volume actually falls. As stroke volume falls, cardiac output levels off but peripheral vascular resistance normally should continue to fall so that a decrease in systolic pressure results. This normal response gives us a clear, logical sequence to explain the mechanism of abnormal responses.

The documentation and descriptions given to us by Bruce,[6] Irving,[18] Benz,[2] and their associates reveals what the cause of this response may be. An ischemic ventricle or a ventricle with a large scar will quickly achieve a maximum stroke volume. Normally, during progressive incremental increases in exercise work loads, venous return rises, causing elevation in the end-diastolic volume. In the normal heart, this elevation in volume is met by increased contractility with a resultant increase in ejection fraction (see Chapter 3). On the other hand, patients with severe pathological conditions (ischemia, large infarcts) are not able to increase contractility. Stroke volume does not increase and in fact may fall. A decreasing stroke volume places severe restrictions on increases in cardiac output.

Since systolic pressure is a result of the relationship between cardiac output and peripheral vascular resistance, an abnormal cardiac output response with a normal fall in peripheral vascular resistance during exercise may be the cause of a falling systolic blood pressure.

As with all of the responses described in this text, a single abnormality such as a fall in systolic blood pressure should not be acted upon unless additional abnormalities are noted. A fall in systolic pressure is often associated with shortness of breath, deep ST-T–segment depression or elevation, angina, and pallor. After exercise, patients frequently will exhibit a third heart sound. The clinician should look for these additional signs and symptoms to confirm the significance of a fall in systolic pressure (Fig. 5-11, B). Be careful not to overinterpret a flat or falling systolic response in middle-aged women or on any patient on antihypertensive or beta blocking medications. These patients may exhibit this response, but unless there are additional signs or symptoms, it may not be significant.

The clinician should be sure that the blood pressure fall

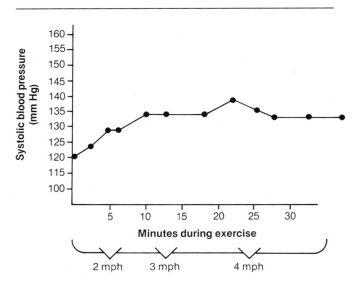

Fig. 5-12. Normal flattening of systolic blood pressure to prolonged exercise at the same work load.

occurs with an increase in work load. In Fig. 5-11 the work loads were increased at minutes 3 and 6. Systolic pressure fell 20 mm Hg or more with an increase in work load. Patient B also became dyspneic, had some angina, and became palloric during the test. Patient C exhibited angina and 2.0 mm of horizontal ST-segment depression.

It is common and normal for systolic pressure to flatten and fall with prolonged (30 to 45 minute) bouts of exercise at the same work load (Fig. 5-12). This should not be considered an abnormal response.

Summary of clinical significance
1. Abnormal systolic blood pressure responses are exhibited by patients with severe ischemia, poor ventricular function, or a combination of these pathological conditions.
2. This abnormality is commonly associated with other significant signs and symptoms.
3. Patients who demonstrate falling systolic blood pressure have higher annual morbidity and mortality.
4. These patients are still candidates for exercise conditioning but must be closely monitored.

Diastolic abnormality

The second less commonly cited, abnormal blood pressure response is a persistent rise in diastolic pressure with increases in exercise work loads. There are numerous articles in the literature that describe normal diastolic blood pressure responses.[22] Many of these contradict one another, but generally the normal diastolic blood pressure response to exercise is to fall slightly (10 to 20 mm Hg) in younger persons and to rise slightly, fall slightly, or remain the same in older persons.

A common sequel to a progressive rise in diastolic pressure with exercise is for the diastolic pressure to remain elevated several minutes after exercise. There is no literature that describes the significance of this finding, but in my clinical experience it is an abnormal finding.

For the purposes of this discussion, an abnormal diastolic blood pressure response occurs when the pressure rises 15 to 20 mm Hg or more. A patient's actual abnormal response and the generally accepted normal response are depicted in Fig. 5-13. Patients who exhibit this response may have coronary artery disease even in the absence of ST-segment changes.[31] Patient D (Fig. 5-13) exhibited the following findings upon cardiac catheterization: All atrial and ventricular pressures were mildly to moderately elevated. The left ventricular end-diastolic pressure was 22 mm Hg at rest. Ejection fraction was normal, and his contractile pattern was normal. His right coronary was irregular throughout its course but without severe stenosis; the left main and circumflex were normal. The left anterior descending artery (LAD) is normal to its midpoint where a 95% to 100% lesion appears to end the LAD, but a large diagonal branch takes off at this same point. This branch and the remnants of the LAD continue to be irregular throughout the rest of their course, but without significant stenosis.

Mechanisms. The cause or causes for progressive diastolic response to exercise are open to speculation. Once again, any of the humeral, neurological, or hemodynamic factors could be the cause of this response. It is of interest, though, to speculate that patients exhibiting the progressive diastolic response to exercise may have a mechanism that senses a need for increased coronary blood flow. This as yet unidentified mechanism may exert an influence on the peripheral vascular tree to increase diastolic pressures and thereby cause an increase in coronary artery driving pressure. The cause or causes may also be simple coincidence. Patients with severe coronary disease generally have some additional peripheral vascular disease, which can dramatically effect systolic and diastolic pressures.

Again, progressive diastolic pressure rise with exercise is a clinical sign that adds to each patient's data base and should be recognized and incorporated into exercise test interpretations and individualized exercise training programs.

Summary of clinical significance
1. Progressive rise in diastolic blood pressure with exercise may indicate severe coronary artery disease.
2. The rise should be at least 20 mm Hg or more and persist after exercise.

ANGINAL RESPONSES

Angina is classically described as a discomfort caused by an impaired blood supply to cardiac muscle. This impairment results in an imbalance between myocardial oxygen supply and demand (see Chapter 2). It is a well-

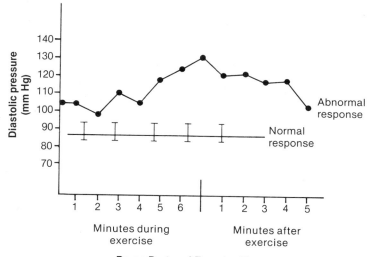

Bruce Protocol Exercise Test

Fig. 5-13. Abnormal diastolic blood pressure response to Bruce protocol symptom-limited exercise test. Patient D was a 47-year-old man who completed 7 minutes and was limited by leg fatigue and shortness of breath. Resting blood pressure (BP) standing was 176/104, and maximum BP was 246/126. He exhibited 2.0 mm of ST-segment depression in four leads and mild angina 4 minutes after exercise. He had frequent multifocal premature ventricular contractions throughout the test and an S_4 after exercise.

documented finding that a patient's threshold for angina is roughly equivalent to a fixed, clinically recordable product of heart rate multiplied by the systolic blood pressure. This multiple is referred to as the "rate pressure product" and is linearly correlated with myocardial oxygen demand.[21] Numerous texts, articles, and scientific papers have been written to describe nicely the reproducibility of a patient's angina at the same rate pressure product.[9,28,33,34] The purpose of this section is to discuss how patients can increase their angina threshold and even eliminate their angina completely.

Angina threshold

Most current practitioners and authors will state that patients with stable angina can improve their exercise tolerance and maximum preangina working capacity, but patients with angina are unable to exceed their anginal rate pressure product.[8,28] An example of this is given below.

Preexercise training (HR, heart rate; SBP, systolic blood pressure)

Work load	2.5 mph	12% grade
Angina threshold	HR 120 angina	SBP 150
Rate pressure product	1.8×10^3	

Postexercise training

Work load	2.5 mph HR 110 no angina	12% grade SBP 150

Rate pressure product	1.65×10^3	
Work load	3.0 mph	12% grade
Angina threshold	HR 120 angina	SBP 150
Rate pressure product	1.8×10^3	

The patient in this example has increased his maximum preangina work load, but his angina threshold and rate pressure product are unchanged since his pretraining status.

One of the most rewarding clinical improvements in a patient is when a patient exceeds his angina threshold by raising the rate pressure product he can attain before experiencing angina. There is even a small percentage of patients who actually eliminate their angina completely. Patients who are capable of increasing or eliminating their angina threshold commonly have the following characteristics:

1. Inoperable coronary artery disease or patients who refuse surgery
2. Highly motivated to exercise
3. Chronic, stable angina
4. Capable of walking through their angina within the first 3 months of their training program

Walk-through angina is angina that occurs during a training session at a specific work load but gradually diminishes and finally goes away despite the fact that the work load is the same or even slightly higher. It is common for patients with angina to get angina when they first

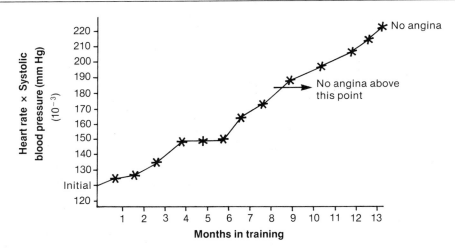

Fig. 5-14. Patient E. Improvement of anginal threshold (by increasing rate pressure product) in a patient over a 13-month period of exercise training.

initiate an exercise session, but with a prolonged warm-up this can be avoided. When they do get angina, walk-through angina occurs when the patient's work load is maintained and the angina abates.

Increasing or eliminating angina thresholds in patients with coronary artery disease is not a quick process. It often takes 12 to 24 months of training (see Chapter 7).

The following actual patient example dramatically demonstrates the phenomenon of increasing a patient's angina threshold and then eliminating the discomfort completely.

Brief medical history (patient E)
　Inferior myocardial infarction, July 1976
　Subsequent stable but frequent exertional angina
　Two-year documented history of hypertension
　Family history of atherosclerosis and diabetes
　Thirty-year 2-pack-a-day smoker who quit July 1976
　Entered outpatient program, 4/17/78
　Age 55, 5'7", 155 lb
　Newspaper publisher
　Medications: propranolol (Inderal) 160 mg/day, furosemide (Lasix), nitroglycerin (see Chapter 4)

Initial exercise test results (R, resting; M, maximum)
　Exercise tolerance 30% below predicted for a sedentary man
　Limited by level 2 angina
　RHR 52, MHR 96, RBP 140/100, MBP 150/100
　Angina began at HR 90, BP 140/100
　No ST-segment depression
　Exercise tolerance 30% below predicted for a sedentary man

Exercise training began at 2.5 mph 0% grade for 30 minutes. He experienced level 1 angina at a heart rate of 90 early in the exercise period, but this gradually abated during the exercise training session without a decrease in work load. Over the next 6 months, the patient progressed to a work load of 4.0 mph with the same angina threshold,

but he experienced frequent walk-through phenomena. At this point, the patient's physician began to reduce his Inderal gradually (see Chapter 4). The patient's maximum heart rate before the onset of angina rises steadily over the next 6 months. He begins a walk-jog program of 3 miles in 45 minutes 5 times a week. His revised exercise training heart rate is 126. A repeat treadmill test is performed 13 months after beginning the program, and the patient is off all medications.

Completed 9 minutes of Bruce Protocol
MHR 145, MBP 158/86
Limited by leg fatigue
No angina
ST-segment depression 2.5 to 3.0 mm
Initial ST shift occurred at HR of 120. Exercise tolerance is 8% below predicted for a sedentary man

Fig. 5-14 graphically depicts the change in this patient's angina threshold.

This patient was well-motivated and compulsive and continued to exercise four or five times a week for 45 to 60 minutes of jogging 4 to 5 miles per session. The reader should realize that this patient is used as an example of an extraordinary phenomenon and is not the common patient, nor would his unusual success easily be reproduced in other patients. This example does, however, demonstrate that angina thresholds are not fixed at immovable rate pressure products.

Mechanisms. As with the other abnormal findings, it is difficult to explain how a person's angina threshold can be increased or eliminated. These patients still exhibit ST-segment depression at the same rate pressure product as they did before their exercise training program and the depth of the depression is unchanged. This indicates that ischemia is still present, but the discomfort that previously accompanied it is gone.

There are numerous possible explanations for the occurrence of this phenomenon, but none of them has been scientifically proved in humans. Following is a list of possible explanations:

1. Increased oxidative enzymes in the heart muscle
2. Improved coronary blood flow through the development of collateral arteries
3. Accomodation of the pain stimulus created by the ischemia via the central nervous system

Any argument that proposes methods to improve coronary blood flow or decrease myocardial oxygen demands should be considered. For the three arguments listed above, neither the first nor second adequately explains why ST changes still occur at the same rate pressure product.[34]

Regardless of the cause for increasing or eliminating angina thresholds, the therapist conducting a cardiac rehabilitation program for patients with reproducible angina thresholds should consider this threshold as a symptom that can be successfully treated and, in some cases, eliminated completely.

Summary of clinical significance

1. Angina may be successfully treated by exercise training.
2. Angina threshold measured by multiplication of the heart rate and systolic blood pressure is not a fixed value.
3. Extensive research into the mechanisms of elimination of angina in humans through exercise training is necessary.

RESPIRATORY LIMITATIONS TO MAXIMUM OXYGEN CONSUMPTION
Normal oxygen consumption limitations

The basis of exercise physiology is derived from the formula for oxygen consumption, $\dot{V}O_2 = CO \times (aO_2 - \bar{v}O_2)$, or the volume of oxygen consumed per minute ($\dot{V}O_2$) is equal to the cardiac output (CO) multiplied by the difference in arterial (a) and central venous $(\bar{v})$ oxygen content. When the components of this formula are analyzed, a wealth of clinically useful information becomes available. Oxygen consumption is one of the foundations of human life. Exertion is dependent on oxygen transport, either during the activity (aerobic or after the activity as a means of repayment of oxygen deficits created during anaerobic activities. Oxygen is essential for normal cell function, and the primary function of our cardiopulmonary system is to maintain a continuous adequate supply.

Cardiac output has been discussed in this chapter and in previous chapters. For our purposes, those discussions will suffice. Instead I will now concentrate the discussion on the second part of the formula, the a-$\bar{v}O_2$ difference.

Arterial oxygen content, a, is normally equal to 20.1 vol%. This number is obtained by multiplication of he-

moglobin concentration in grams per 100 ml of blood by 1.34 ml of O_2 per gram of hemoglobin and then multiplication of that by the percent saturation of the hemoglobin. For example, 15 grams of hemoglobin per 100 ml of blood (a normal value for males) times 1.34 ml of O_2 per gram of hemoglobin equals 20.1 ml of O_2 per 100 ml of blood, or 20.1 vol% (15 gm of Hb $\times$ 1.34 ml of O_2 = 20.1 vol%). This would be true if the hemoglobin was 100% saturated. Normal percent saturation ranges from 95% to 100%.[24]

Changes in arterial oxygen content are dependent on many variables, including but not limited to percent saturation, oxygen content of the atmosphere, ph of the blood, temperature of the blood, minute ventilation, carbon monoxide concentration in the atmosphere, and the pulmonary ventilation/perfusion ratio. To appreciate some abnormal responses found with pulmonary patients, a sound understanding of the effects of these variables is essential. For the purpose of this text, only the variables of ventilation and ventilation perfusion ratio are discussed.[30]

The normal, accepted limitation to maximum oxygen delivery is considered to be attainment of a maximum cardiac output. Patients with chronic obstructive pulmonary disease do not appear to be limited by achieving their maximum cardiac output. They are limited by respiratory mechanics that appear to be intimately associated with ventilation, respiratory muscle oxygen cost, and oxygen saturation.

Ventilation responses
Normal

Ventilation, specifically alveolar ventilation, is one of the keys to the determination of the percent saturation and oxygen content of arterial blood. Alveolar ventilation, V_A, is determined by the total expired volume, V_T, which is equal to the alveolar ventilation plus the dead-space ventilation, V_D: $V_T = V_A + V_D$. Thus alveolar ventilation is $V_A = V_T - V_D$. For the patient with chronic obstructive pulmonary disease, dead-space ventilation inflicts major restrictions on their alveolar ventilation capacity and thus oxygen content of arterial blood. Patients with obstructive pulmonary disease have severely limited tidal volume reserves. In other words, they are unable to increase their tidal volume appreciably. Åstrand states that normal persons can rarely achieve tidal volumes in excess of 50% of their vital capacities during maximal exercise[1] (Fig. 5-15). All patients do not have the same capacity. In fact, many patients have tidal volumes that are relatively fixed. For example, a patient with a fixed or nearly fixed tidal volume is totally dependent upon the frequency of respiration to increase pulmonary ventilation (V_E). In healthy people, it is the tidal volume (V_T) that accounts for a majority of the increase in ventilation at low levels of exertion. It is not until higher levels of exertion that healthy people require increases in the frequency of respiration.

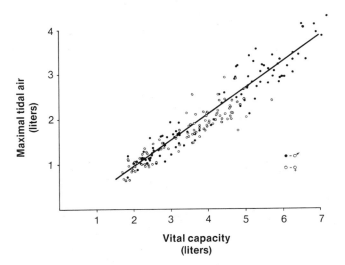

Fig. 5-15. Highest tidal volume measured during running at submaximal and maximal speed (work time about 5 minutes) related to the person's vital capacity measured in the standing position. (From Åstrand, P.-O., and Kaare, R.: Textbook of work physiology, ed. 2, New York, 1977, McGraw-Hill Book Co.)

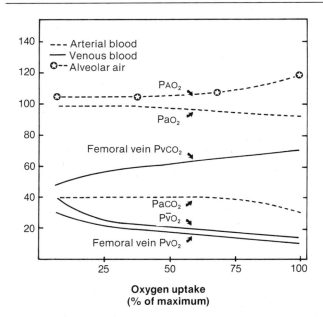

Oxygen uptake
(% of maximum)

Fig. 5-16. Normal oxygen and carbon dioxide tensions in blood and alveolar air at rest and various levels of work up to and exceeding the load necessary to achieve maximum oxygen uptake. (From Åstrand, P.-O., and Kaare, R.: Textbook of work physiology, ed. 2, New York, 1977, McGraw-Hill Book Co.)

Abnormal

Because patients with obstructive pulmonary disease depend on frequency to improve their ventilation, they also ventilate a greater amount of dead space. For example, if we assume that dead space is the same amount and fixed in both cases, it is apparent that the net alveolar ventilation is decreased in obstructive disease. Thus a normal person who has a ventilation of 10 liters per minute and a dead space of 0.20 liter and a respiratory frequency of 10 has an alveolar ventilation that is $10 - (0.20 \times 10) = 8$ liters per minute. The same level of ventilation, 10 liters per minute, achieved by a patient with pulmonary disease through a higher respiratory rate (20) has an alveolar ventilation that is $10 - (0.20 \times 20) = 6$ liters per minute. The alveolar ventilation is the ventilation where gaseous exchange takes place and thus is one of the key components to determine arterial oxygen saturation.

Another key to oxygen saturation is the ventilation/perfusion ratio. This is the ratio that matches the lung ventilation to the perfusion of blood from the right side of the heart. Briefly, when one is at rest sitting, the apex of the lung is well ventilated but poorly perfused, the midportions of the lungs have nearly equal ventilation to perfusion, and the lower lobes have high perfusion and moderate ventilation. The net effect is very close to an equal match between ventilation and perfusion.

The person with obstructive pulmonary disease not only is ventilated poorly, but also often has a very poor ventilation/perfusion ratio. Areas that are poorly ventilated are matched with good perfusion and well-ventilated areas are underperfused. The result of this mismatching is that venous blood may pass through the lungs without coming into contact with fresh air. This blood is then mixed with oxygenated blood in the left atrium and ventricle. As the venous blood and arterial blood gases attain equilibrium, the oxygen concentration decreases.

Normal oxygen consumption response to exercise

During maximal levels of exertion a normal person progressively matches his cardiac output (to the lungs) to the ventilation of his alveoli. This remains true up to near-maximal levels of exertion when alveolar oxygen tension may continue to increase but arterial P_{O_2} may diminish slightly. Arterial CO_2 pressure tends to fall gradually as maximal levels of exertion are achieved (Fig. 5-16). Thus normal arterial oxygen content is essentially unchanged at maximal levels. This argument strongly supports the theory that maximum cardiac output, not respiration, is the limiting factor to maximal oxygen uptake. It is apparent from the work of Åstrand that increases in pulmonary ventilation at maximum oxygen uptake does not increase oxygen uptake in normal persons.[1]

In healthy persons, the respiratory muscles utilize from 0.5 to 1.0 ml of O_2 per liter of ventilation. It is estimated that this unit of oxygen cost per liter of ventilation increases linearly with heavy work loads. The respiratory

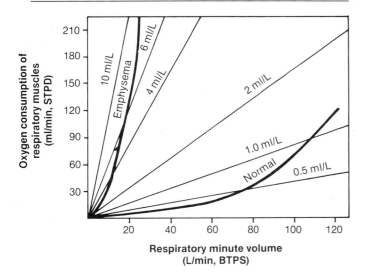

STPD = Standard temperature pressure, dry
BTPS = Barometric temperature pressure, saturated

Fig. 5-17. Oxygen cost of breathing in normal subject and in subject with emphysema, measured as increase in whole-body oxygen consumption during respiratory response to added dead space. Cost of breathing in normal men over usual range of activity is less than 0.5 ml of O_2 per liter of air breathed. (Adapted from Mountcastle, V.B., editor: Medical physiology, ed. 14, St. Louis, 1980, The C.V. Mosby Co.)

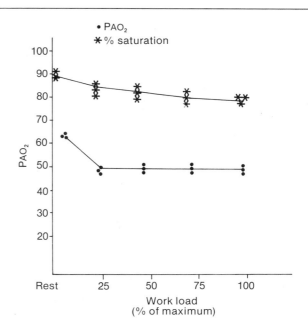

Fig. 5-18. Pao_2 tension and arterial oxygen saturation falling with exercise in three patients with obstructive pulmonary disease. Tests were limited by dyspnea.

muscles may utilize as much as 10% of the total oxygen uptake in normal persons at maximum levels of work.[1]

Abnormal oxygen cost of ventilation

There are only estimates of respiratory muscle costs for the patient with chronic obstructive disease. The mechanical patterns that develop with the various disease processes make any absolute measures limited. Fig. 5-17 does demonstrate the extreme difference in oxygen cost of respiration between a healthy subject and a subject with emphysema. This high cost of breathing is directly related to the patient's (1) high dead-space ventilation, (2) frequency-dependent breathing, and (3) hyperexpanded chest wall, which decreases diaphragmatic function and demands that accessory muscles of respiration be aggressively employed.

Mechanism. When cardiac output rises but ventilation does not improve, the ventilation/perfusion mismatch worsens. The result is a fall in arterial oxygen pressure and saturation. Their arterial oxygen tension drops precipitously (Fig. 5-18) with exertion with the resultant decrease in oxygen saturation and thus oxygen content of their blood. This puts great limitations on their oxygen extraction reserve, (a-$\bar{v}o_2$ differences, which should cause a strong increase in cardiac output as a compensatory mech-

anism for improving oxygen consumption. At rest, many pulmonary patients have greatly elevated resting heart rates. But, it is clear from the exercise arterial graph (Fig. 5-19) that maximum heart rates are not attained before termination of exercise. If we surmise that less than maximum cardiac outputs are achieved and that these patients exercised to their maximum symptom limits (which they all did), then cardiac output was not their limiting factor. In fact, dyspnea appears to be the limiting factor in all these tests. They were all limited by their abnormal ventilation and not by achievement of maximal cardiac output as in the normal state.

Summary of clinical significance

1. Poor respiratory mechanics combined with limited tidal volume reserves may lead to hypoxia and desaturation with exertion.
   a. Pronounced hypoxia as seen in each case is a significant finding. Hypoxia causes the pulmonary vasculature to constrict. The exact neurochemical cause can be examined in Åstrand.[1] The ultimate effect is an increase in pulmonary artery pressure. In turn, constant elevation in pulmonary artery pressures (pulmonary hypertension) leads to right ventricular hypertrophy. Chronic hypertension often leads to right-sided heart failure, a common complication of obstructive pulmonary disease.
   b. The implication to the clinician involved in pul-

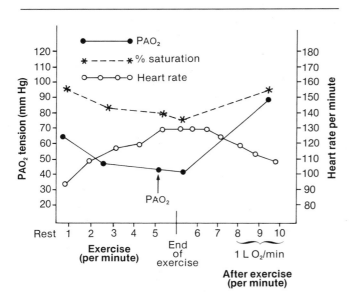

Fig. 5-19. Oxygen tension and saturation compared to heart-rate response to maximal exercise in patient F, a 46-year-old woman. Note heart-rate levels off at 130 at the same time oxygen tension and saturation fall to their lowest levels.

monary rehabilitation is to identify those patients who become hypoxic during even submaximal levels of exertion. A progressive exercise program with a pulmonary patient suffering from exercise-induced hypoxia may quickly be to the patient's detriment.

2. Respiration can be the limiting factor to maximal exertion, specifically in patients with obstructive pulmonary disease.

3. Clinicians should be working to devise treatment techniques that result in improved respiratory mechanics and thus decreased costs of breathing.

4. Controlled research of the exercise responses of pulmonary patients is needed.

SUMMARY

This chapter contains a clinician's view of some abnormal responses to exercise. One should not accept these simple examples as scientific proof of the cause and effect of certain pathological conditions on human exercise response. On the other hand, physical therapists should understand that these phenomena: abnormal heart rate response, bradycardia, abnormal blood pressure responses, hypotension, increased or unlimited angina threshold through exercise training, and oxygen desaturation during exercise all occur. They are indications in some cases of certain severe pathological conditions and often poor prognosis for the patient. It is with this in mind that physical therapists working with cardiac and pulmonary patients

should carefully assess their patients' conditions and interpret their findings against the predicted normal responses that have been scientifically delineated by Åstrand, Mountcastle, and others.[1,5,22,24]

REFERENCES

1. Åstrand, P.-O., and Kaare, R.: Textbook of work physiology, ed. 2, New York, 1977, McGraw-Hill Book Co.
2. Benz, H., and Sambrano, J.: The significance of a hypoadaptive blood pressure response during maximal stress testing in patients with coronary artery disease, master's thesis, Los Angeles, 1977, University of Southern California.
3. Blessey, R., and others: Aerobic capacity and cardiac catheterization results in 13 patients with exercise bradycardia, Med. Sci. Sports Exerc. 8:50, 1976. (Abstract.)
4. Brouha, L., and Harrington, M.E.: Heart rate and blood pressure reactions of men and women during and after muscular exercise, Lancet 77:79, 1957.
5. Bruce, R.A., and others: Maximal oxygen intake and nomographic assessment of functional aerobic impairment in cardiovascular disease, Am. Heart J. 85:546, 1973.
6. Bruce, R.A., and others: Noninvasive predictors of sudden death in men with coronary heart disease, Am. J. Cardiol. 39:833, 1977.
7. Campbell, E.J.M., and others: Simple methods of estimating oxygen and efficiency of muscles of breathing, J. Appl. Physiol. 11:303, 1957.
8. Clausen, J.P., and others: Heart rate and arterial blood pressure during exercise in patients with angina pectoris: effects of training and of nitroglycerin, Circulation 43:436, 1976.
9. Cokkinos, D.V., and Voridis, E.M.: Constancy of pressure-rate product in pacing-induced angina pectoris, Br. Heart J. 38:39, 1976.
10. Conn, E.H., and others: Exercise responses before and after physical conditioning in patients with severely depressed left ventricular function, Am. J. Cardiol. 49:296, 1982.
11. Ehsani, A.A., and others: Effects of 12 months of intense exercise training on ischemic ST-segment depression in patients with coronary artery disease, Circulation 64(6):1116, 1981.
12. Ehsani, A.A., and others: Cardiac effects of prolonged and intense exercise training in patients with coronary artery disease, Am. J. Cardiol. 50:246, 1982.
13. Ellestad, M.H.: Stress testing, ed. 2, Philadelphia, 1981, F.A. Davis Co.
14. Ferguson, R.J., and others: Effect of physical training on treadmill exercise capacity collateral circulation and progression of coronary artery disease, Am. J. Cardiol. 34:764, 1974.
15. Fraser, R.S., and Chapman, C.B.: Studies on the effect of exercise on cardiovascular function: blood pressure and pulse rate, Circulation 9:193, 1954.
16. Henschel, A., and others: Simultaneous direct and indirect blood pressure measurements in man at rest and work, J. Appl. Physiol. 6:506, 1954.
17. Hinkle, L.E., and others: Slow heart rates and increased risk for cardiac death in middle-aged men, Arch. Intern. Med. 129:732, 1972.
18. Irving, J.B., and others: Variations in and significance of systolic pressure during exercise (treadmill) testing, Am. J. Cardiol. 39:841, 1977.
19. Jose, A.D., and Taylor, R.R.: Autonomic blockade by propranolol and atropine to study the intrinsic muscle function in man, J. Clin. Invest. 48:2019, 1969.
20. Kariv, I., and Kellermann, J.J.: Effects of exercise on blood pressure, Malattie Cardiovasc. 10:247, 1969.
21. Kitamura, K., and others: Hemodynamic correlates of myocardial oxygen consumption during upright exercise, J. Appl. Physiol. 32:516, 1972.

22. Loskutoff, D.W.: Study of the relationship of arterial blood pressure response to Bruce Protocol Exercise Tolerance testing, master's thesis, Atlanta, Ga., 1981, Emory University.

23. Metheny, E., and others: Some physiological responses of women and men to moderate and strenous exercise: a comparative study, Am. J. Physiol. **137:**318, 1942.

24. Mountcastle, V.B., editor: Medical physiology, ed. 14, St. Louis, 1980, The C.V. Mosby Co.

25. Nagle, F.J., and others: Comparison of direct and indirect blood pressure with pressure-flow dynamics during exercise, J. Appl. Physiol. **21:**317, 1966.

26. Neill, W.A., and others: Respiratory alkalemia during exercise reduces angina threshold, Chest **80**(2):149, 1981.

27. Ricci, B.: Physiological basis for human performance, Philadelphia, 1967, Lea & Febiger.

28. Robinson, B.F.: Relation of heart rate and systolic blood pressure to the onset of pain in angina pectoris, Circulation **35:**1073, 1967.

29. Schwarz, F., and others: Coronary collateral vessels: their significance for left ventricular histologic structure, Am. J. Cardiol. **49:**291, 1982.

30. Shapiro, B.A., and others: Clinical application of blood gases, ed. 2, Chicago, 1977, Year Book Medical Publishers, Inc.

31. Sheps, D.S., and others: Exercise-induced increase in diastolic pressure: indicator of severe coronary artery disease, Am. J. Cardiol. **43:**708, 1979.

32. Sim, D.N., and others: Investigation of the physiological basis for increased exercise threshold for angina pectoris after physical conditioning, J. Clin. Invest. **54:**763, 1974.

33. Wahren, J., and Bygdeman, S.: Onset of angina pectoris in relation to circulatory adaptation during arm and leg exercise, Circulation **44:**432, 1971.

34. Wilmore, J.H.: Acute and chronic physiological responses to exercise. In Amsterdam, E.A., and others, editors: Exercise in cardiovascular health and disease, New York, 1977, Yorke Medical Books.

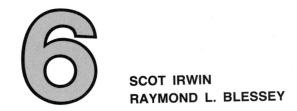

SCOT IRWIN
RAYMOND L. BLESSEY

Patient evaluation

The purpose of this chapter is to describe the evaluation of a patient with coronary artery disease in terms of the significant data available in the medical record; the information that can be obtained from an initial evaluation process; and the methods for obtaining useful clinical data from a patient's response to exercise. An additional objective of this chapter is to communicate that no single piece of patient information has relevance exclusively. Each informational item relates to the others, and the incorporation of all findings completes the patient assessment.

There are two precepts to our evaluation process:

1. The therapist should understand the scientific principles underlying the clinical data observed and recorded.
2. The data obtained are accurate and interpretable.

The basis for this approach is that the selection of appropriate evaluation techniques is attributable to an understanding and application of the sciences, and the validity of the assessment is dependent on the accuracy of the data collection.

Objective patient information is obtained from the medical record including historical data, diagnostic tests performed, laboratory values recorded, and patient interview findings.

The initial evaluation of the coronary patient should begin with a review of the medical record followed by the patient interview and examination. The general purpose of these three preliminary tasks is to allow the therapist to formulate an accurate assessment of the clinical status of the patient, including the severity of the disease, the stability of the symptoms, and the presence of significant medical problems other than the primary diagnosis. Once these tasks have been completed an informed decision can be made to proceed or not proceed with definitive evaluation procedures. These procedures include assessment of the patient's responses to activities of daily living, ambulation, aerobic exercise, and low-level exercise testing. The following is a suggested evaluation and program planning sequence for patients with coronary artery disease beginning with the acute stage of the hospital course:

1. Medical records review and extraction of pertinent data
2. Patient interview and examination
3. Preliminary assessment of clinical status
4. Determination of candidacy for further evaluation
5. Functional activity evaluations (if indicated)
6. Activities-of-daily-living evaluation
7. Monitored ambulation
8. Low-level exercise test
9. Definitive assessment regarding candidacy for exercise therapy
10. Individually monitored aerobic exercise and strengthening program (phase II)
11. Maximal exercise test
12. Additional invasive and noninvasive testing as indicated
13. Group aerobic and strengthening program (phase III)
14. Monitored job simulation evaluation as indicated
15. Serial follow-up testing
16. Additional noninvasive testing as indicated
17. Serum lipid profile
18. Maximal exercise test

Table 6-1. Points of interest and specific evaluation tasks involved with the preliminary and definitive assessment of the patient

Preliminary assessment	Major concerns and points of interest	Evaluation tasks
	Primary diagnosis	Medical record review
	Additional significant medical problems	Physical exam
	Clinical subset	Patient interview
	Complicated versus uncomplicated hospital course	
	Etiology and stability of symptoms	
	Medical therapy	
	Psychosocial status	
	Indications versus contraindications for mobilizing	
	Monitoring needs and protocol	
Definitive assessment	**Major concerns and points of interest**	**Evaluation tasks**
	Signs and symptoms of myocardial ischemia	Functional evaluation of activities of daily living
	Good or poor ventricular function	Monitored ambulation
	Appropriateness of cardiovascular response to activity	Exercise test
	Candidacy for exercise therapy	Individually monitored exercise therapy

MEDICAL RECORD REVIEW

The underlying purpose for extracting clinical information from the medical record is to formulate a basis for the development of both the definitive evaluation sequence and the treatment plan. The therapist should focus his attention on at least the following major areas of interest when reviewing the medical record:

1. Primary diagnosis
2. Additional significant medical problems
3. Medical therapy
4. Clinical subset of the patients based on the number of diseased coronary arteries and left ventricular function
5. Stability of the patient's clinical course and indications versus contraindications for proceeding with the functional evaluation
6. Priorities for cardiovascular monitoring with activity
7. Risk factors for coronary disease
8. Classification of the postevent hospital course into

either complicated or uncomplicated according to the criteria of McNeer and others[25]

The recommended points of interest or concerns in both the preliminary and the definitive aspects of the evaluation, along with the specific evaluation tasks, are listed in Table 6-1. The use of an initial evaluation form that is designed with the above considerations in mind will encourage the therapist to extract the key information from the medical record. Fig. 6-1 is an example of the initial evaluation form currently used at our facilities.

It is not within the scope of this chapter to discuss in detail how the clinician would utilize the medical record review to obtain data and insight related to all the major points of interest listed in Table 6-1. The selected case examples and discussions below are designed to illustrate both the methods of obtaining the pertinent data base and the way in which the information taken from the medical record can be utilized in developing the subsequent evaluation and treatment plan.

INITIAL EVALUATION AND PLAN

Name _____ Hospital No. _____

Age _____ Sex _____ Height _____ Weight _____

Referring physician _____ Date _____

Patient address (home) _____ Phone No. _____

Patient address (work) _____ Phone No. _____

I. MEDICAL HISTORY:

II. RISK FACTORS: Family history _____

Cholesterol _____ Triglycerides _____ HDL ____ LDL _____

Smoking (pk/yr) ____ Hypertension _____ Diabetes _____

Sedentary _____ Obesity _____ Type A _____

Uric acid level _____ PFT's

III. MEDICATIONS (dosage and frequency) _____

_____

_____

IV. CARDIAC CATHETERIZATION: Date ____ LVEDP ____ Ejection fraction _____

Ventricular function _____

Vessels involved—Degree of occlusion _____

_____

_____

V. CORONARY ARTERY BYPASS SURGERY: Date _____ Hospital _____

Grafts _____

Surgeon _____ Complications (if any) _____

VI. MUSCULOSKELETAL EXAM _____

Orthopedic or foot problems _____

Strength and range of motion _____

Chest wall exam _____

VII. EXERCISE TEST RESULTS: Date _____ Duration _____

Limiting factors _____ MHR _____ MBP _____

Blood pressure response _____ Angina _____

ST change _____ Arrhythmia _____

Physical work capacity _____ Heart sounds _____

Fig. 6-1. An example of initial evaluation form designed with major points of interest in mind.

```
┌─────────────────────────────────────────────────────────────────────┐
│              INITIAL EVALUATION AND PLAN—cont'd                       │
│                                                                       │
│  VIII.  PATIENT'S GOALS                                               │
│         _____      │
│         _____      │
│                                                                       │
│    IX.  ECG:  Date _____ Interpretation _____      │
│     X.  INITIAL PHYSICAL FITNESS STAGE _____      │
│    XI.  SOCIAL HISTORY:  Marital status _____      │
│         Occupation _____      │
│         Leisure time activy _____      │
│   XII.  ASSESSMENT:                                                   │
│         _____      │
│         _____      │
│         _____      │
│  XIII.  PLAN:                                                         │
│         _____      │
│         _____      │
│         _____      │
│         _____      │
│                                                                       │
│                              _____ Date _____     │
│                              Registered physical therapist            │
│                                                                       │
│   Copyright Blessey, Huhn, Ice, Irwin, Oschrin, Physical Therapy      │
│   Inc., 1982.                                                         │
└─────────────────────────────────────────────────────────────────────┘
```

Fig. 6-1, cont'd.

Primary diagnosis
CASE EXAMPLE A

Fifty-seven-year-old man with a documented myocardial infarction 10 years ago. A cardiac catheterization at that time revealed multiple vessel disease and that the patient was not a candidate for bypass surgery because of the diffuse nature of his disease. The patient has been asymptomatic up until 2 months ago when he noted onset of retrosternal pain associated with neck and jaw discomfort precipitated by vigorous activity, such as running to catch the bus and climbing numerous flights of stairs rapidly. In the last few weeks the patient noted onset of similar symptoms with mild activity, such as casual walking and carrying packages for short distances. The evening before admission to the hospital, the patient had 3 hours of moderate-to-severe retrosternal discomfort while at rest. These symptoms were not relieved by one nitroglycerin tablet.

Reason for referral to cardiac rehabilitation. To evaluate effectiveness of antianginal medications during functional activities.

Time of entry to program. Four days after hospital admission.

Discussion. The medical history shows that the patient has documented coronary artery disease by angiography and he has had a prior myocardial infarction. The key question after reviewing the medical history of case example A is, Has this patient suffered a second infarction or is the current primary diagnosis unstable angina (also referred to as coronary insufficiency or coronary intermediate syndrome)? To answer this question, the clinician must review the results of at least two other tests contained in the medical record. First, the serum enzyme (CPK, LDH, SGOT) results should be examined to see if there has been a significant rise above the normal level in these values since the patient has been admitted. If, in fact, there has been a rise in the enzymes, review of the more precise isoenzyme results should be obtained. Additionally, a review of the serial ECG interpretations made from studies taken since the patient has been admitted should be completed. Only then will the therapist know whether a myocardial infarction has been ruled out or documented. Presuming that the primary diagnosis in this case is coronary insufficiency, a careful review of the ECG and enzyme values just before mobilization of the patient should be completed to ensure that the clinical status of the patient has not changed since the order for rehabilitation was issued.

In addition to the above, the medical record should be reviewed in an attempt to uncover the presence of other medical problems that may have precipitated the unstable angina. Is there evidence that the patient has recent onset of poorly controlled hypertension based on the admitting note and the nurses' notes? Does the patient have significant anemia based on the complete blood count results? Is there evidence of a valve lesion that may contribute to the unstable pattern of symptoms based on review of the echocardiogram? Has the patient recently demonstrated findings consistent with congestive heart failure based on chest radiograph findings and results of the physician's physical exam and interview?

Having a clear understanding of the patient's primary diagnosis is essential in formulating both the evaluation and treatment plan. In this case the primary diagnosis of coronary insufficiency should encourage the clinician to build into his evaluation protocol careful questioning regarding the stability of the patient's symptoms and regular review of pertinent lab and ECG results when available. In terms of program planning the diagnosis in this case should influence the therapist to schedule the patient for relatively frequent visits as an outpatient, such as three times per week, and to educate the patient regarding a method for quantifying the intensity of his angina, documenting his anginal symptoms, and what action to take in event his symptoms become unstable again.

CASE EXAMPLE B

Forty-two-year-old woman with several hospital admissions secondary to chest pain and frequent premature ventricular contractions. Approximately 1 week ago, patient was readmitted to hospital because of crushing chest pain, which had started while she was doing housework. ECG studies and enzyme levels were negative, and therefore a myocardial infarction was ruled out. An echocardiogram done at the time of this most recent admission suggested mitral valve prolapse. The patient continued to have chest discomfort, and so she was sent for a cardiac catheterization, which revealed normal coronary arteries and moderate mitral regurgitation.

Reason for referral to cardiac rehabilitation
1. To improve exercise tolerance
2. To evaluate rhythm response to exercise
Time of entry to program. Two weeks after hospital admission.
Discussion. Based on the medical history, this is a patient with organic heart disease and chest discomfort; however, the chest discomfort is not related to myocardial ischemia, but, instead, it is attributable to a valvular lesion.

Awareness of the primary diagnosis of mitral valve prolapse (with significant mitral regurgitation) should encourage the clinician to examine the echocardiogram and catheterization results to determine whether there is evidence of the following:
1. Additional valve dysfunction
2. Ventricular or atrial enlargement
3. Compromised resting left ventricular function.

In addition, one should review the rhythm strips and results of the 24-hour Holter monitor to become aware of the frequency and complexity of dysrhymias and the association of the rhythm disturbance to activities. Finally, the clinician should be aware of the medical therapy for rhythm control so that responses to exercise can be interpreted appropriately, an adequate data base can be accumulated documenting the degree of effectiveness of the medication, and potential side effects of the medications can be recognized and reported to the patient's physician.

The primary diagnosis in this case should influence the therapist's approach toward the patient education aspect of the treatment plan. In this case, it would be important to point out the cause of the chest discomfort and its benign nature to the patient. In addition, in terms of further evaluation procedures for this patient, it would be important not to "overmonitor" and thereby encourage this patient to exercise only in a supervised environment.

In summary, the primary diagnosis of the patient obtained from the medical chart should alert the therapist to the additional priority areas of the medical record review that must be completed and should help the therapist begin to formulate the subsequent evaluation plan and treatment plan.

Additional medical problems
CASE EXAMPLE C

Sixty-eight-year-old man with documented myocardial infarction 2 years ago. Patient had onset of exertional chest pressure and shortness of breath in the last 3 months and reports that his exercise tolerance has diminished. A recent treadmill test was done with the major findings: very poor exercise capacity (with functional aerobic impairment, FAI, at 45%) with 2.0 mm ST depression at the maximum heart rate. The major limiting factor on the test was dyspnea. The patient has a 120-pack-per-year smoking history and has been diagnosed as having bronchitis. Other medical problems include adult-onset diabetes mellitus and peptic ulcer disease. The patient has had two previous admissions because of bleeding ulcers.

Reason for referral to cardiac rehabilitation. Patient was referred to the cardiac rehabilitation program as an outpatient for the purpose of improving his exercise tolerance and reducing his risk factors.

Discussion. From the medical history, it is clear that the patient has coronary artery disease and appears to be experiencing exertional symptoms consistent with angina. The key points, though, are to begin considering:
1. What other medical problems are identified in the history that may have an impact on the patient's acute and chronic response to exercise.
2. Which other portions of the medical record may contain additional information documenting the severity of these problems.

Chronic obstructive pulmonary disease (chronic bronchitis) may be at least partly responsible for the patient's poor exercise capacity. Review of the results from the chest radiograph, pulmonary function test, arterial blood gas analysis at rest and with exercise (if available), and 12-lead ECG should give the clinician a better idea of this patient's pulmonary dysfunction.

The history of peptic ulcer disease with recurrent bleeding ulcers should encourage the therapist to review the results of the complete blood count (hemoglobin and hematocrit levels) to rule out anemia, which if severe enough could have a profound effect on this patient's exercise tolerance.

Finally, the history of adult-onset diabetes mellitus should lead to review of serum glucose levels and the urinalysis to determine how well-controlled the patient's glucose levels are. In addition, there should be periodic repeat values to be sure the patient's glucose levels remain normal.

Medical therapy
CASE EXAMPLE D

Forty-eight-year-old man had "flu-like" symptoms for approximately 2 weeks. Primary complaint was weakness and shortness of breath. The patient reported that it was not uncommon to wake up feeling short of breath. Patient finally sought medical attention and was found to have evidence of a anterior myocardial infarction on the 12-lead ECG.

Physical findings
Lungs: rales at both bases
Heart: S_3, S_4, no murmur
Extremities: $1+/4+$ pretibial edema
Medications
Digoxin, 0.25 mg/a day
Furosemide (Lasix), 40 mg/day
Quinadine gluconate (Quinaglute), 200 mg 4 times a day

Discussion. The combination of digoxin and furosemide should be a "red flag" to the clinician that the patient has probably had evidence of congestive heart failure at one time. The clinician needs to review the medical chart to see if there is or has been evidence of congestive failure. The physical findings in case example D of S_3 and pedal and pulmonary edema, along with the medical history, are compatible with heart failure. In addition, the clinician should be alerted to the fact that the patient has had significant arrhythmias (even though there is no mention of it in the history) since the medical therapy includes Quinaglute. Further review of the medical record and discussion with the physician is indicated in order to identify the exact nature of the rhythm disturbance.

CASE EXAMPLE E

Fifty-seven-year-old male with a long history of hypertension and premature ventricular contractions. Patient had onset of exertional chest discomfort and was referred for exercise testing. The exercise test was positive for ischemia and angina, and the patient was referred for coronary angiography. Just before the cardiac catheterization the patient suffered a myocardial infarction. The patient became stabilized and eventually had coronary angiography and subsequent bypass surgery. After surgery, the patient had recurrent pericarditis and frequent premature ventricular contractions that did not respond to class I antiarrhythmics (quinidine, procaineamide, disopyramidephosphate [Norpace]; refer to Chapter 4). During a maximal exercise test done postoperatively, the patient had a sustained run of ventricular tachycardia. As a result, the patient was started on a combination of propranalol and quinidine therapy, which was found to be reasonably effective in controlling the ventricular ectopy. After a 6-month trial on propranolol, however, the patient continued to complain about lethargy and depression. Therefore the decision was made to change medications and evaluate the patient's cardiovascular responses to exercise during an individually monitored exercise session.

Current medications

Atenolol (Tenormin), 50 mg/day

Quinidine, 300 mg 4 times a day

Discussion. Both propranolol and atenolol are beta blocking drugs, which act to significantly lower the resting and exercise heart rate and blood pressure. Therefore it is essential that the therapist be aware of the use of medications and follow adjustments in the dosage given to interpret exercise responses and design exercise programs appropriately. Awareness of the relative strength of the various beta blockers is important as well. We have found atenolol to be a potent beta blocker which in some patients results in significant exercise hypotension, even at mild levels of activity.

Summary

These cases demonstrate the importance of reviewing the medical record carefully and identifying the patient's current medical therapy. The medications listed often will give an indication of the cardiovascular abnormalities a patient has had such as arrhythmias, hypertension, congestive heart failure, or angina. Familiarity with the action, purpose, and side effects of the numerous cardiac drugs will help the therapist provide the most pertinent information to the physician. Finally, many cardiac drugs will alter the cardiovascular responses to exercise, and therefore their effects must be taken into consideration when one is evaluating and designing a treatment plan (see Chapter 4).

CLINICAL SUBSETS OF CORONARY ARTERY DISEASE

One of the major reasons for a thorough review of the medical record is to determine which clinical subset the patient is in because of its implications for evaluations and program planning. As I have mentioned in Chapter 2, the prognosis of the coronary patient is strongly influenced by the degree of left ventricular dysfunction and number of arteries diseased. There are several items in the medical record that should give the therapist some insight regarding the patient's clinical course.

In the acute patient who has had a myocardial infarction the description of the hospital course during the first 4 days after the myocardial infarction contained in the admitting note is of great value. Patients with a complicated early hospital course, as defined by the criteria in the boxed material, commonly have either poor left ventricular (LV) function as a result of a large infarction or multiple vessel disease. One should keep in mind that the absence of these complications does not rule out poor LV function or multivessel disease.

The 12-lead ECG may also be of some value in predicting poor LV function if it contains evidence of a large myocardial infarction or a ventricular aneurysm, or both. The degree of rise in the enzyme levels during the infarction also correlates with the amount of myocardial damage. Currently, there are several noninvasive methods available to evaluate LV function at rest, of which, two-dimensional echocardiography and radioisotope studies seem to be of the greatest value. The results of these studies should be carefully reviewed whenever they are available. The most definitive study is, of course, the cardiac catheterization, since it identifies the degree of disease in the coronary arteries, as well as documenting resting LV function. One should keep in mind that in order to appreciate the hemodynamics and functional consequences of the patient's disease, one should take the patient through a series of activities that are graduated in terms of the pa-

---

CRITERIA FOR A COMPLICATED POST– MYOCARDIAL INFARCTION HOSPITAL COURSE*

Ventricular tachycardia or fibrillation
Rapid supraventricular dysrhythmia
Second- or third-degree atrioventricular block
Persistent sinus tachycardia ($\geq$100 bpm)
Persistent hypotension (systolic blood pressure, 90 mm Hg)
Pulmonary edema
Cardiogenic shock
Persistent angina or extension of infarction

*McNeer, J.F., and others: Circulation **51**:410-415, 1975.

tient's physiological demand. This series of activities should include procedures such as the activities-of-daily-living (ADL) evaluation, monitored ambulation, low-level exercise testing, and eventually maximal exercise testing. Noninvasive evaluation of LV function during either the low-level exercise test or the maximal test, especially in suspected cases of poor LV function, can be most helpful.

INITIAL PHYSICAL THERAPY EVALUATION

The foundation for patient assessment and treatment is established through the initial evaluation process. At any stage of cardiac disease and treatment (acute, subacute, chronic, post–myocardial infarction, or pre– and post–bypass or valvular surgery) the patient's treatment program will be based on the evaluation findings. The evaluation process includes both the patient interview and a physical examination.

Patient interview

The patient interview is a dynamic interchange of information between the therapist and the patient. An interview session introduces the concept of cardiac rehabilitation to the patients and their families. It is also the mechanism to establish the therapist and patient relationship. Conversations centered around the subjects listed in the boxed material provide insight for the therapist regarding the patient's knowledge about his own disease, his perspective on how it affects his life, and what support mechanisms are available to him.

Understanding of the disease. The patient's understanding of cardiac disease is essential before participation in the rehabilitation process. Each person approaches the program with his or her personal biases regarding cardiac disease and the degree and progress of the disability. The patient's level of knowledge then affects the willingness and ability to participate. Additionally, assessment of the patient's educational level provides the therapist with the information needed to accurately educate and motivate the patient at the appropriate level.

Patient description of symptoms. The patient's description of the symptoms specifies familiar terminology for use in future communications. The terms each patient uses to describe cardiac symptoms (i.e., chest tightness, shortness of breath, discomfort, pain, burning, shoulder ache, or dizziness) are highly variable. For example, when a patient describes his or her symptoms as a fullness, the therapist should use the patient's description of the symptom when asking the patient about the symptom. Personal descriptions will aid the therapist during reassessment. An established base line allows judgment regarding the severity of symptoms if they reoccur.

Family. Family participation is integral to the success of the rehabilitation program. They are needed to both support the patient and participate in the educational experience. Education of the family helps them understand both

---

> **TOPICS FOR DISCUSSION IN A PATIENT INTERVIEW**
>
> Understanding of the disease
> Patient symptoms
> Family
> Vocation
> Psychological profile
> Risk-factor profile
> Leisure activities and exercise history
> Patient's goals

---

the disease process and the need for life style modification. Often a spouse can contribute to or detract from the patient's ability to cope with the patient's disease. Children also benefit from involvement because education can inform them and provide incentives for the prevention of coronary disease.

Vocation. Discussion concerning the specifics of the patient's vocational history aids in the assessment of the patient's functional capabilities. Important aspects to consider include both physical activity on the job and level of responsibility and stress. This information is valuable for setting goals and planning the patient's return to work.

Psychological profile. Consultation with the team member responsible for psychological care before or after the patient's interview helps to place your assessment of the patient in the proper prospective. The recommendations from the psychological assessment often indicate appropriate ways to approach the patient, as well as make suggestions for program modifications. Both the patient's ability to participate in the rehabilitation program and the patient's attitude toward education are closely linked to his or her psychological status, that is, denial, fear, depression.

Risk-factor profile. While interviewing the patient and discussing his or her history, one can obtain specifics such as the patient's family history of cardiac disease, smoking history, or social eating and drinking habits. This information is recorded, and a personal "risk-factor profile" is formed. Identifying individual problem areas is the key to focusing the patient's education and accomplishing modification of risk factors.

Leisure activities and exercise history. A list of the patient's leisure activities provides information necessary for individual program planning. Specific activities patients enjoy can be used to achieve increased function and performance. Early discussion of the patient's potential to return to vigorous leisure activities often has a positive effect on the patient's psychological status.

Patient's goals. Recognition of the patient's goals throughout the rehabilitative process is essential. When the program goals and patient goals are not synchronized, there will be less chance for the patient's compliance.

Physical examination

Physical examination of a cardiac patient by the physical therapist requires the skills of observation, palpation, and auscultation. Observation includes the analysis of musculoskeletal deficits such as posture, gait, muscle strength and tone, skin color and tone, and facial expression. Notation of the musculoskeletal deficits is necessary because these patients may require program adaptation and modifications based on their disability. Traditional walking or jogging programs may not be a possibility for a patient with a cerebrovascular accident or lower extremity amputation. Skin color, tone, and facial expression changes can be significant indications of circulatory responses to exercise or indicative of the patient's attitude and degree of discomfort or weariness. When observation has been completed, palpation is performed to collect further information. Palpation of the thorax, chest wall, head, neck, shoulder girdle, arms, and upper thoracic spine provides feedback on specifics about complaints of chest wall pain. During the period after myocardial infarction, many patients experience residual chest wall pain or musculoskeletal soreness. It is essential to determine the origin of that pain and distinguish it from angina. Palpation also focuses on circulation to the extremities. Many patients with coronary artery disease have accompanying peripheral vascular disease. It is therefore necessary to include palpation of femoral and peripheral pulses during the examination. Although the point of maximal impulse and some heart sounds can be palpated, heart sounds are primarily evaluated through auscultation. Auscultation of heart sounds is an art and a science (see Goldberger[18]). The additional information obtained from establishment of a base line and then detection of a change or continued stability of a patient's heart sounds may be critical to his program planning. The therapist should be able to identify normal heart sounds, rubs, murmurs, third heart sounds (gallops), and fourth heart sounds. Auscultation of breath sounds is found in Chapter 12.

The findings of the gross physical examination are continuously used as reference points for future evaluation and assessment of the patient and are essential to program development and revision throughout the patient's rehabilitation process.

Dynamic evaluation

After completion of chart review, patient interview, and gross evaluation there is a sufficient data base to initiate further patient evaluation including response to activity. The patient's inpatient (phase I) exercise program is based on the results of (1) a self-care evaluation and (2) monitored ambulation. A third exercise activity, low-level treadmill testing, is done before the patient's discharge. The exercise test results are the foundation for patient program planning and progression in phase II. The common objective for all evaluation procedures is the identification and interpretation of any abnormal or unsafe responses in heart rate, blood pressure, ECG, symptoms, or heart sounds that the patient exhibits during progressively increasing levels of activity.

Self-care evaluation

The self-care evaluation is performed for evaluation of the cardiac patient's response to activities of daily living. The evaluation is usually initiated 3 to 6 days after infarction and is optimally completed before the patient's transfer out of the coronary care unit. (Resting values are obtained in the supine, sitting, and standing positions.)

Patients are asked to perform several activities including tooth brushing, hair combing, dressing, ambulation, and a Valsalva maneuver. Heart rate, blood pressure, ECG changes, symptoms, and heart sound responses are recorded for each activity. This information is documented on a self-care evaluation form and subsequently placed in the patient's chart (Fig. 6-2).

Collection procedures. To perform a self-care evaluation, two trained persons are required. One person continuously observes the patient's ECG response, obtains sample ECG strips during each activity, and records the patient's responses on the evaluation form. The other person takes the patient's blood pressure and monitors clinical signs and symptoms both during the activity and continuously through observation and questioning. Heart sounds are auscultated supine at rest and immediately after ambulation.

The activities included in the self-care evaluation are known to cause mild increases in heart rate and blood pressure in various body positions. A study by Butler and others[7] demonstrated that the heart rate, blood pressure, and ECG changes that occur with self-care are strongly correlated to the responses of the patient during monitored ambulation activities.

Monitoring clinical responses to exercise

Heart rate. Heart rate is a simply obtained, yet extremely useful indicator of patient response to activity. It can be counted from the pulse or read from the ECG tracing. The heart rate is dependent on many factors, which include medication levels, ventricular function, and level of patient activity. The highest heart rates achieved clinically occur during upper extremity activities, such as hair combing and tooth brushing. However, these activities rarely cause heart rates in excess of 100. Most self-care activities require a minimal increase in oxygen consumption. Thus there should be a minimal change in the patient's heart rate with the activities listed.

SELF-CARE MONITOR

Department of Physical Therapy and Rehabilitation
Cardiac Rehabilitation Program

Patient name _____

Hospital No. _____

Risk factors: HBP _____ Family history _____ Overweight _____

                Smoking _____ Diabetes _____ Age _____

                Lack of exercise _____ Other _____

	HR	BP
Rest (supine)		
Sitting		
Standing		
ADL activity		
Ambulation		
Valsalva		

ECG strips

INTERPRETATION

Therapist _____ Date _____

Fig. 6-2. Self-care monitor form. This form serves to record data and can be used as an initial progress note.

Patients with large infarctions, continuing ischemia, or borderline heart failure may exhibit a sharp increase in the heart rate (20 to 40 bpm). Poor ventricular function dictates that the heart rate must rise rapidly to meet the demand for increased cardiac output. If a rapid heart rate is documented (greater than 100), the therapist immediately determines the significance of this response by noting the patient's blood pressure, symptoms, and heart sounds. A patient with poor ventricular function may also exhibit a flat, low blood pressure response (systolic less than 100), shortness of breath, and a third heart sound. A rapid heart rate response alone may have minimal significance except to indicate anemia or deconditioning. The combination of a heart rate greater than 100 with low blood pressure, shortness of breath, and a third heart sound indicates a severely limited cardiac reserve. Thus careful monitoring and a slower progression of the patient's activities are necessary. Discussion of the evaluation findings with the referring physician is mandatory.

Blood pressure. A major key to the clinical usefulness of the blood pressure response is to record accurate and interpretable blood pressures. Blood pressure recordings are most useful if obtained during an activity and recorded as such. Therapists can then use base-line or resting pressures and compare them to those taken during an activity and those recorded as the patient completes an activity. For example, a single resting blood pressure obtained sitting cannot be used as a base line for interpretation of upright activities. A blood pressure obtained only 15 seconds after a patient has stopped walking may have already fallen significantly and thus is of little value. Therefore, because of the dynamic nature of the blood pressure, it is taken frequently and accurately and recorded specifically.

The blood-pressure response to self-care activities and ambulation is generally unremarkable. Low levels of self-care activity should not evoke even moderate elevations in systolic or diastolic pressure. A 30 mm Hg rise in systolic pressure is uncommon. A fall in systolic pressure with an increase in heart rate or the development of symptoms may be quite ominous (see Chapter 5). Again a singular finding of a flat or falling systolic pressure is of little significance. Although, when found in combination with angina or shortness of breath, a fall in systolic pressure may indicate significant ischemia or poor ventricular function.

ECG changes. Physical therapists require knowledge of and ability to interpret the full spectrum of electrocardiogram changes. An excellent reference for learning basic ECG interpretation is by Dubins, *Rapid Interpretation of EKG's*.[10] Although arrhythmias and conduction defects can be identified and recorded using telemetry monitoring (see Chapter 9), ST-segment changes cannot be quantified. Telemetry units cannot be calibrated; therefore any ST-segment interpretation is at best subjective and limited.

The significance of ECG interpretation lies in its relation to the patient's clinical picture. Three factors of major importance to the ECG are (1) the patient's pharmacological regimen, (2) the severity and therefore the potential danger of the arrhythmia or conduction defect, and (3) the symptoms associated with an arrhythmia or conduction defect.

Antiarrhythmic medications. A description of the effects and side effects of antiarrhythmic medications is found in Chapter 4. Because some of these medications can cause arrhythmias or conduction defects, a clear identification and understanding of the type and effects of the medication the patient is taking is required (See Chapter 4). It is not unusual to find that patients well controlled on their antiarrhythmic medications at rest do not have that same control with activity.

Severity and potential danger of arrhythmias or conduction defects

Arrhythmia. A therapist involved in a cardiac rehabilitation program should be clinically competent in defining, recognizing, and determining the significance of all arrhythmias.

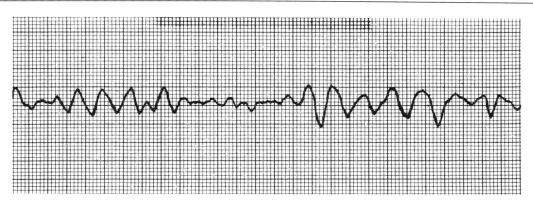

Fig. 6-3. ECG recording of ventricular fibrillation.

Categorization of arrhythmias from least dangerous to most dangerous is difficult because their severity is relative to the symptoms evoked and the frequency of the arrhythmia. Asymptomatic patients who exhibit arrhythmias are generally categorized as less serious, but this is not always true. Patients can be asymptomatic while in ventricular tachycardia, but this arrhythmia frequently deteriorates into fibrillation (Fig. 6-3), which is lethal.

Ventricular arrhythmias may be ranked from least serious to most serious in the following order:

Unifocal premature ventricular contraction (PVC) (Fig. 6-4)

Multifocal PVC's (Fig. 6-5)

Coupled PVC's (R-on-T PVC's) (Fig. 6-6)

Ventricular tachycardia (Fig. 6-7)

Ventricular fibrillation (Fig. 6-3)

Atrial arrhythmias without conduction block are generally less dangerous (lethal) than ventricular arrhythmias. Their primary effect is to reduce cardiac output by decreasing preload (see Chapter 3). Thus a true ranking is really not related to the arrhythmia as much as the symptoms it produces.

Premature atrial contractions (PAC's) (Fig. 6-8, *B*) or premature nodal contractions (PNC's) (Fig. 6-8, *A*)

Atrial fibrillation (Fig. 6-9)

Paroxysmal atrial tachycardia (PAT) (Fig. 6-10)

Atrial flutter (is a block) (Fig. 6-11)

Conduction defects. There are two categories of conduction defects. One category results in an interruption of the electrical transmission of an impulse from the atrioventricular node to the ventricular bundle branches. These are called "AV blocks." The other category involves the bundle of His and its branches. These are called "bundle-branch blocks."

AV blocks are categorized as first- (Fig. 6-12), second- (Fig. 6-13), and third-degree (Fig. 6-14) blocks. First-degree block is defined as a PR interval that exceeds 0.20 second (200 milliseconds). Second-degree block is characterized as having more than one P wave for each QRS. There are several types of second-degree block (i.e., Wenckebach, two-to-one block, three-to-one block, atrial flutter, etc.). Third-degree block is the most serious type of heart block and requires medical intervention. It is characterized by a complete dissociation between sinoatrial

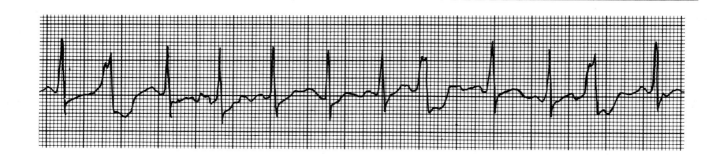

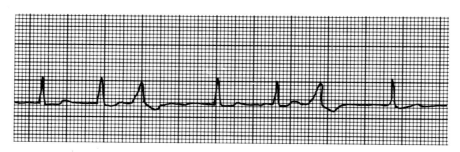

Fig. 6-4. Two examples of unifocal premature ventricular contractions (PVC's). Common characteristics of PVC's are that (1) they are early, (2) they have no conducted P wave, (3) they have a wide bizarre QRST, and (4) there is a complete compensatory pause.

node depolarization and ventricular depolarization.

Bundle-branch blocks (Fig. 6-15) are caused by a disruption in the normal conduction of an impulse through the right and left bundle branches of the heart's conductive system. The QRS duration is prolonged and exceeds 0.12 second (120 milliseconds). Some asynergy of ventricular contraction may occur because a bundle-branch block may create a decrease in cardiac output.

Symptoms. The most difficult patient responses to interpret are the patient's symptoms. The spectrum of symptoms are as varied and widespread as the patients in the program. The primary symptom, which the therapist learns to recognize, is angina.

The classic description of angina is a dull substernal ache or pain that is brought on by eating, exercise, or emotional upset. In my clinical experience, the best description of angina is as follows: "angina is any discomfort that occurs above the waist and is reproduced by ex-

ertional activites." Angina *must be differentiated* from other musculoskeletal or neurological discomforts. The therapist should understand and recognize the significance of the difference to reassure patients and inform the patient's physician.

Angina can be described by patients as a burning, tightness, pressure, indigestion, shortness of breath, aching, fullness, jaw pain, backache, toothache, shoulder pain, or arm pain. Patients can often be characterized by one of two responses; those who deny and those who exhibit hysteria. The denial group will continue to exercise and push themselves, yet do not want to discuss or reveal any of their symptoms. Hysterics complain about every ache and pain. Both roles can be difficult to detect and allow assessment of the patient's condition. The group using the denial mechanism can cause themselves serious harm before they will admit or discuss their symptoms. The hysterical reactors often have serious anginal symptoms, but

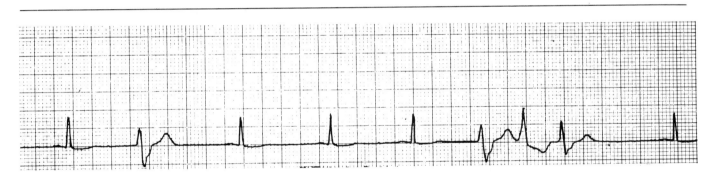

Fig. 6-5. Multifocal premature ventricular contractions arise from more than one focus. They are characterized by an electrocardiographic configuration that varies in form and direction.

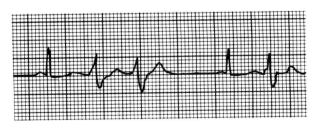

Fig. 6-6. Coupled premature ventricular contractions are two PVC's that occur in sequence with each other. They may be multifocal or unifocal. They are often seen before or during runs of ventricular tachycardia.

the symptoms are masked by a myriad of additional aches and pains. Differentiation of nonanginal discomforts from angina is not easy. Some guidelines and suggestions are listed in Table 6-2.

The content of these lists indicates that distinguishing angina from nonanginal discomforts should be fairly easy. This determination is clouded by the existence of two other types of angina; unstable angina and Prinzmetal's angina. Unstable, preinfarction angina occurs at any time, even at rest, may last longer than stable anginal episodes, and may be associated with chest wall soreness or a frozen shoulder. Prinzmetal's angina, angina caused by coronary vasospasm, has characteristics similar to unstable angina. It can also occur anytime and is improved only slightly by administration of nitroglycerin.

The therapist should also recognize and appropriately interpret symptoms of shortness of breath, dizziness, pallor, and general fatigue. Shortness of breath is common and may be equivalent to angina for some patients. They describe the symptom of shortness of breath to have all the characteristics of angina as described previously. Patients with poor ventricular function, borderline heart failure, or a combination of ischemia and poor ventricular function will often be limited by shortness of breath. It is important to distinguish between cardiogenic or respiratory induced shortness of breath. A patient's pulmonary function test (PFT) values will be the best indicators to aid differentiation. Abnormal PFT values may indicate that the shortness of breath is attributable to pulmonary dysfunction. Normal PFT values in a patient with no history of bronchospasm generally eliminates pulmonary dysfunction as a cause of shortness of breath. The patient's data base, including an enlarged heart on chest radiograph, poor blood pressure response to exercise, need for inotropic medications (glycoside derivatives), number and size of infarctions, or a combination of these variables should assist in the identification of a patient's shortness of breath as cardiogenic.

Dizziness and pallor are also associated with signs of failure and ischemia. Hypotension will cause dizziness and pallor. Although these symptoms are not common in cardiac patients, they should not be ignored. These symptoms should be added to all the other pieces of information in the patient's data base and interpreted appropriately.

Auscultation. The final clinical tool to be discussed is auscultation of heart sounds. Effective auscultation requires clinical experience under the tutelage of a knowledgeable clinician. A self-care evaluation starts with auscultation of the patient's heart sounds. Recognition of different heart sounds and murmurs is essential. The ability to auscultate does not have to be at a diagnostic level because a level of expertise that affords the therapist clinical recognition of heart sounds that have changed is sufficient. A change in heart sounds can indicate a change in heart function because of infarction, ischemia, failure, or inflammation. A complete review of heart sounds and

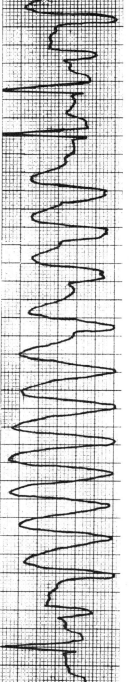

Fig. 6-7. Ventricular tachycardia. A run or string of PVC's in a row.

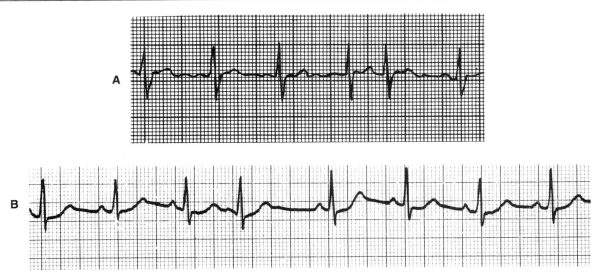

Fig. 6-8. A, Premature nodal contraction (PNC) is characterized by (1) being early, (2) having no P wave, inverted P wave, or a P wave after the QRS, and (3) having an incomplete pause. **B,** Premature atrial contraction (PAC) is characterized by (1) being early, (2) having a bizarre, abnormal P wave, and (3) having an incomplete pause.

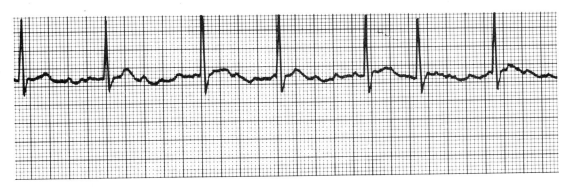

Fig. 6-9. Atrial fibrillation is characterized by irregular QRS intervals and multiple bizarre P waves.

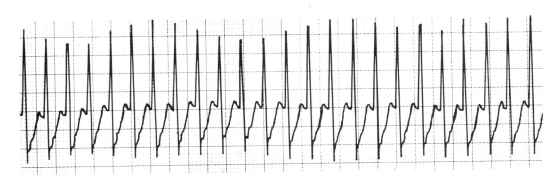

Fig. 6-10. Paroxysmal atrial tachycardia (PAT). Characterized by high heart rates, sudden onset, and relief by vagal stimulation.

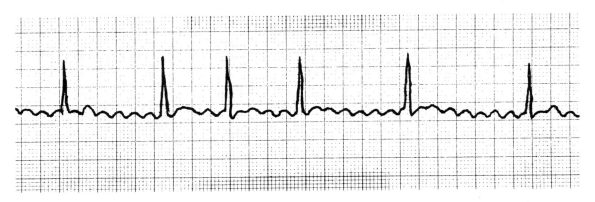

Fig. 6-11. Atrial flutter is characterized by (1) multiple P waves that occur in saw-tooth pattern, (2) atrial P wave rate of 300, and (3) usually more than one P wave to each QRS.

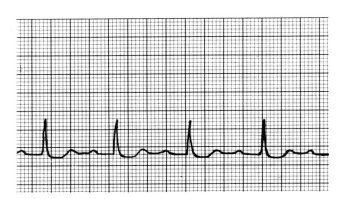

Fig. 6-12. First-degree atrioventricular (AV) block is characterized by a prolonged PR interval (0.20 m/sec).

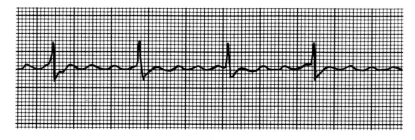

Fig. 6-13. Second-degree AV block is characterized by more than one P wave being required to generate a QRS.

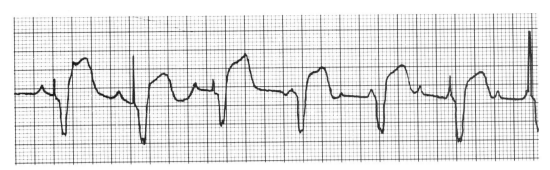

Fig. 6-14. Third-degree AV block is characterized by a complete disassociation of atrial (P wave) and ventricular (QRS) relationships. The P waves occur at their own rate and the QRS complexes occur at their own rate.

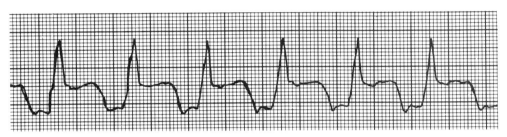

Fig. 6-15. Bundle branch block is characterized by a widening of the QRS duration to 0.12 m/sec or more.

Table 6-2. Differentiation of nonanginal discomforts from angina

Stable angina	Nonanginal discomfort (chest wall pain)
1. Relieved by nitroglycerin (30 seconds to 1 minute)	1. Nitroglycerin generally has no effect
2. Comes on at the same heart rate and blood pressure and is relieved by rest (lasts only a few minutes)	2. Occurs any time; lasts for hours
3. Not palpable	3. Muscle soreness, joint soreness, evoked by palpation
4. Associated with feelings of doom, cold sweats, shortness of breath	4. Minimal additional symptoms
5. Often seen with ST-segment depression	5. No ST-segment depression

causes of heart sounds will not be discussed here, but some common clinical examples are worth review.

Because of an increase in bypass surgery, we anticipate that patients will be enrolled in cardiac rehabilitation programs after surgery. It is common with patients early after bypass surgery (less than 6 weeks) to have pericarditis. Some will have audible rubs, and some will have only a rub sound after exercise. Patients with pericarditis should

not exercise vigorously. Occasionally, patients are referred to cardiac rehabilitation and subsequently develop a rub. This is a heart sound change the therapist can identify through auscultation of the patient's heart sounds.

Another example of a significant heart sound change is when a patient develops a third heart sound after exercise. Although a third heart sound may be auscultated in children and athletes, it is generally pathological when found in patients over 35 years of age. Third heart sounds correlate strongly with a decrease in ventricular compliance. Loss of compliance results from either a distended ventricle or large areas of ischemia or infarction. A combination of these changes produces the same loss. Patients who exhibit normal heart sounds at rest and develop a third heart sound are perhaps being exercised too strenuously. Their heart is literally being distended to its limits to compensate for the increased demands for cardiac output. Again, the presence of a third heart sound alone may have minimal significance, but as is often seen when this change occurs with shortness of breath, falling systolic blood pressure, or pronounced ST-segment depression, the patient's exercise should be terminated and a lower level of activity should be assumed during any future exercise sessions.

In this brief review, murmurs have been identified as a heart sound that requires recognition. The importance of documentation relates again to recognition rather than diagnosis. On some occasions, outpatients without a murmur will describe an episode of prolonged chest pain that they did not report to their physician. The therapist should auscultate this patient and obtain an ECG. The auscultation may reveal the development of a murmur. This information is vital and should be immediately communicated to the patient's physician. Consequently, the therapist's ability to recognize significant changes in a patient's heart sounds is a necessity.

Summary

Dynamic cardiac patient evaluation requires incorporation of good clinical skill (to obtain data) and rapid accurate interpretation of the data obtained. Self-care evaluation and monitored ambulation are performed to obtain guidelines for patient exercise programming and progression. The five dynamic clinical monitoring skills available to assist the therapist in patient evaluation and treatment are heart rate, blood pressure responses, ECG and heart sound changes, and symptoms.

Low-level exercise testing

Low-level exercise testing is usually the final procedure of the definitive evaluation in phase I. As discussed earlier, it provides the data base from which the hemodynamics and functional consequences of the patient's disease can be assessed. Furthermore, it provides the additional information needed to decide whether the patient is a candidate for exercise therapy (phase II) and, if so, what intensity of exercise appears to be indicated.

The low-level exercise test is a multistage procedure progressing from a work-load equivalent of 2 to 3 METs (metabolic equivalents) up to a work-load equivalent of no greater than 6 to 7 METs. There are numerous protocols for low-level testing in the literature. The key is to correlate the protocol with the purpose of the test and with the patient population to be evaluated. Table 6-3 defines the

Table 6-3. Low-level treadmill test protocol and estimated metabolic equivalent (MET) for each work load

Stage	Speed (mph)	% grade	Duration (min)	Estimated MET level
I	1.7	0	3	2.3
II	1.7	5	3	3.5
III	1.7	10	3	4.6
IV	2.5	12	3	6.8

From Schwartz, K.M., and others: Ann. Intern. Med. **94:**727-734, 1981.
Note: For a more debilitated deconditioned patient we sometimes precede stage I with a stage A of 1.3 mph, 0% grade for 3 minutes.

Table 6-4. Additional commonly utilized low-level treadmill test protocols

Stage	Speed (mph)	% grade	Time (min)	Metabolic equivalent
Lerman-Bruce Protocol				
I	1.2	0	3	2.1
II	1.2	3	3	2.3
III	1.2	6	3	3.0
IV	1.7	6	3	3.3
Modified Naughton Protocol				
I	2	3.5	3	3
II	2	7.0	3	4
III	2	10.5	3	5
IV	2	14.0	3	6
V	2	17.0	3	7
VI	3	12.5	3	8
VII	3	15.0	3	9
VIII	3	17.5	3	10

From Hassack, R.F., and Bruce, R.A.: Primary Cardiol., pp. 106-112, Feb. 1980, and from Starling, M.R., and others: Am. J. Cardiol. **46:**909, 1980.

various stages and corresponding estimated MET levels for the protocol we employ with our post–myocardial infarction and, when indicated, post–bypass surgery patient population. Two additional treadmill protocols for low-level testing are listed in Table 6-4. It is becoming increasingly more common to perform the low-level exercise test before hospital discharge for the post–myocardial infarction patient. The realization that the patient is likely to perform activities soon after discharge that are equivalent to the work loads performed on a low-level test has definitely influenced the physicians' thinking regarding the timing of the test. The precise timing of the test will depend on the hospital course of the patient and, generally, the uncomplicated post–myocardial infarction patient is tested as early as 7 to 10 days after the event. The interval for testing in the complicated patient will depend on the length of time required for stabilization, but generally these patients are tested within 2 to 3 weeks after the event. The safety of the procedure when performed within 1 to 3 weeks after the myocardial infarction has been borne out by the numerous reports in the literature. According to an editorial published in the June 1981 issue of the *Annals of Internal Medicine* there have been only two deaths related to low level testing and ''the concern about safety need not arise,'' provided that the test is designed to reproduce the physiological demands of the activities that the patient is likely to perform early after discharge.[34]

Purpose

The low-level exercise test has at least three major purposes:

1. To help identify the high-risk patient, i.e., the patient who demonstrates signs or symptoms of myocardial ischemia or poor left ventricular function at low work loads.
2. To evaluate the effectiveness of medical therapy designed to control hypertension, arrhythmias, and angina.
3. To provide the basis from which to make recommendations for activity and exercise therapy (phase II).

The ability to identify the high-risk patient by low-level testing is essential to the process of determining the candidacy of a given patient for early exercise therapy. Starling and others[35,36] reported that uncomplicated post–myocardial infarction patients, with the combination of exercise-induced ST-segment depression and inadequate blood pressure response (peak systolic blood pressure less than 140 mm Hg, or a 20 mm Hg or more drop from peak systolic pressure during exercise) on low-level testing, had a significantly greater evidence of cardiac death within 11 months than patients without ischemic treadmill abnormalities. Schwartz and others[32] found that 90% of patients with ischemic ECG changes or angina had multiple vessel disease compared to 55% of patients with no ischemic treadmill abnormalities. In addition, his group reported that exercise-induced ST-segment elevation predicted poor left ventricular function. The work of both Schwartz and Starling has been supported by Théroux[38] and Fuller[38] with others. A review of the data of 134 post–myocardial infarction patients tested in our laboratory within 7 to 10 days after the event revealed that the most prevalent ischemic treadmill abnormality was angina pectoris (Table 6-5). However, our data suggest that ST-segment depression of 2 mm or a hypoadaptive systolic blood pressure response (drop from peak exercise pressure of 10 or more mm Hg) are highly predictive of the high-risk subset of patients with triple vessel or left main coronary disease. The sensitivity, specificity, and predictive value of these two markers for severe coronary disease is summarized in Table 6-6. In essence, our findings possibly indicate that if the patient has less than 2 mm of ST-segment depression

Table 6-5. Prevalence of ischemic findings during low-level testing in 134 post–myocardial infarction patients

	N	%
Angina pectoris	29	22
ST-segment depression	23	17
Drop in systolic blood pressure of 10 mm Hg	13	10
Complex arrhythmias	1	1

Table 6-6. Significant ST-segment depression and exercise hypotension as predictors of severe coronary artery disease

Positive test	2 mm ST-segment depression or decrease in peak exercise systolic blood pressure of 10 mm Hg
"Significant" coronary disease	Triple vessel or left main disease
Sensitivity	62%
Specificity	90%
Predictive value of a negative test	88%
Predictive value of a positive test	67%

and an adequate blood pressure response he has a 88% chance of not having severe coronary disease, whereas two thirds of the time if a patient has either or both of the ischemic treadmill abnormalities discussed above, he will demonstrate triple vessel or left main disease by angiography.

CASE EXAMPLE E.B.

Consider the case example of Mr. E.B. who had a documented myocardial infarction and a hospital course complicated by congestive heart failure, persistent chest pain and sinus tachycardia, and complex ventricular arrhythmias. The complicated post–myocardial infarction hospital course suggests either a large myocardial infarction or severe coronary artery disease. After E.B.'s course in the hospital became stabilized, he underwent activities-of-daily-living evaluation and monitored ambulation without demonstrating any major cardiovascular abnormalities. Fourteen days after the myocardial infarction E.B. was referred for exercise testing before being referred for exercise therapy. His 12-lead ECG appears in Fig. 6-16. There is evidence of an anteroseptal myocardial infarction on the cardiogram but no suggestion of extensive myocardial damage. The heart rate and systolic and diastolic blood pressure responses to exercise are summarized on the graph in Fig. 6-17. Note the sharp drop in systolic blood pressure occurring after 2 minutes

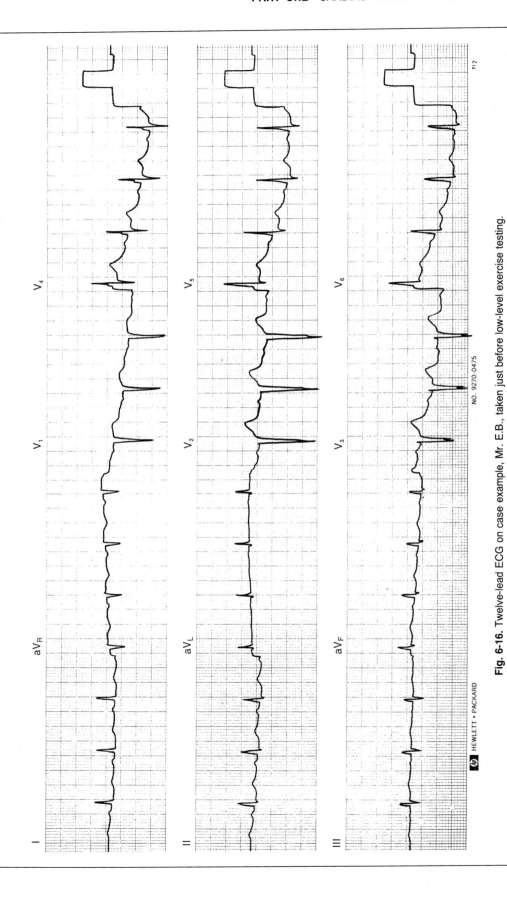

Fig. 6-16. Twelve-lead ECG on case example, Mr. E.B., taken just before low-level exercise testing.

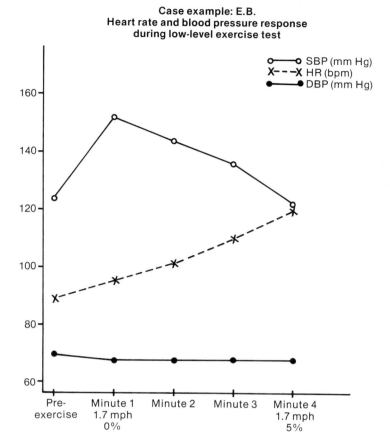

Fig. 6-17. Blood pressure and heart rate response of Mr. E.B. during low-level exercise testing.

of exercise at 1.7 mph, 0% grade at a heart rate of 104 bpm. Figs. 6-18 and 6-19 show the baseline ST-segment changes (preexercise standing) and the pronounced ST-segment changes occurring in multiple exercise leads at maximal exercise. Based on the prior discussion the findings on E.B.'s exercise test suggests that he has severe coronary disease and that he was not a candidate for rehabilitation until the degree of his coronary disease had been documented by angiography. In fact, E.B. was found to have 80% occlusion of the left main coronary artery and significant occlusions in the right coronary, the left anterior descending and the circumflex arteries. After bypass surgery, E.B. was referred to the cardiac rehabilitation program.

On the other hand, the absence of significant ischemic treadmill abnormalities usually clear the way for hospital discharge and referral for early outpatient rehabilitation.

CASE EXAMPLE J.T.

Ms. J.T. was a 44-year-old woman with a documented myocardial infarction and an uncomplicated course. The activities-of-living evaluation and monitored ambulation were unremarkable, and thus the patient was referred for low-level exercise testing 6 days after the myocardial infarction. The 12-lead ECG shown in Fig. 6-20 indicates that this patient had an anterior myocardial infarction and there are the corresponding T-wave abnormalities.

The graph of this patient's blood pressure response (Fig. 6-21) and the preexercise and maximal exercise testing ECG strips (Figs. 6-22 and 6-23) demonstrate appropriate cardiovascular responses to exercise. Because of the age of this patient, she did undergo coronary angiography, which documented single-vessel coronary disease (left anterior descending) and good left ventricular function as would be predicted from the post–myocardial infarction hospital course and the exercise test results. This patient was discharged from the hospital 7 days after the infarction and returned on day 9 after the infarction to begin outpatient cardiac rehabilitation.

The value of low-level exercise testing in providing the data base from which to design a individualized exercise prescription is discussed in detail in Chapter 7. Case examples are included to illustrate the exact method in which exercise prescriptions are formulated with these data at hand.

Contraindications and termination points

As mentioned earlier, low-level testing is a safe procedure. This is especially true when specific contraindications for testing are observed and appropriate end points for testing are enforced. Table 6-7 lists the contraindica-

Text continued on p. 90.

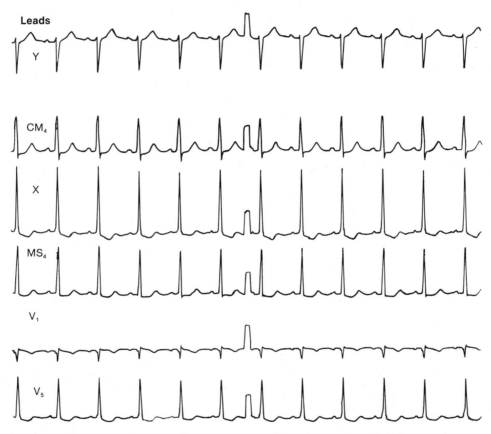

Fig. 6-18. Preexercise multiple-lead ECG tracing demonstrating ST depression in the X, MS$_4$, and V$_5$ leads.

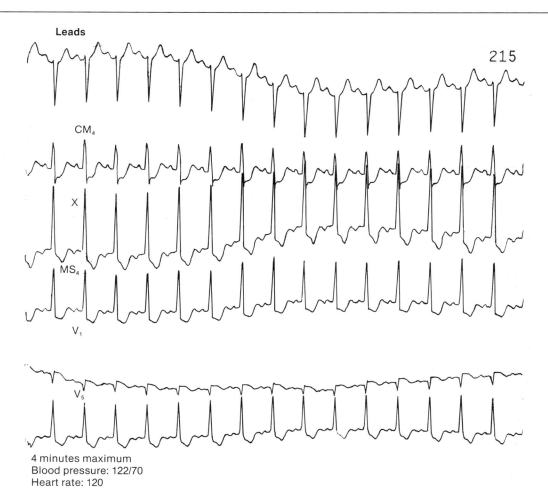

Leads

215

CM$_4$

X

MS$_4$

V$_1$

V$_5$

4 minutes maximum
Blood pressure: 122/70
Heart rate: 120

Fig. 6-19. Maximal exercise ECG tracing demonstrating pronounced net ST depression in four of the six leads and ST elevation in V$_1$.

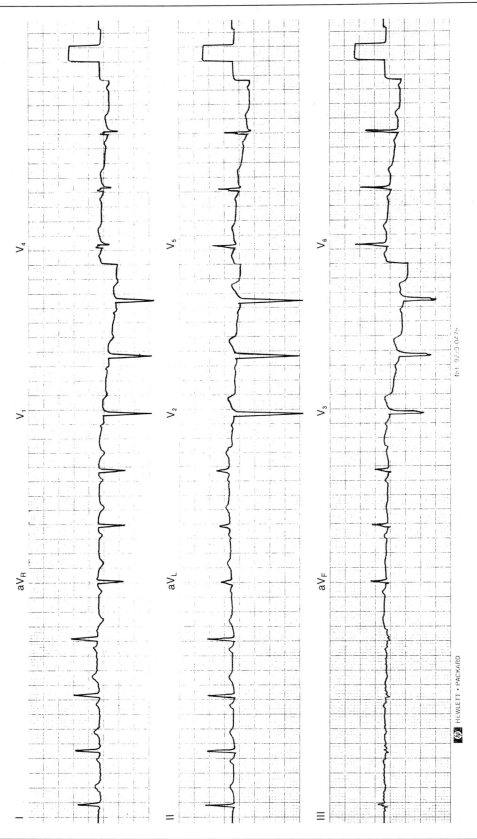

Fig. 6-20. Resting 12-lead ECG in case example, Ms. J.T., before exercise testing.

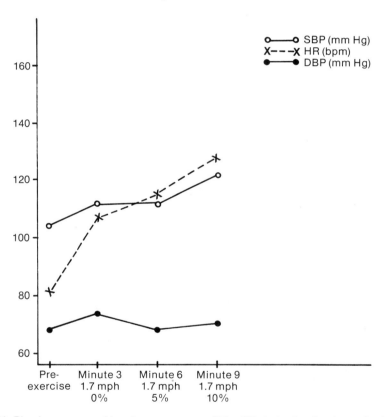

Case example: J.T.
Heart rate and blood pressure response
during low-level exercise test

Fig. 6-21. Blood pressure and heart rate response of Ms. J.T. during low-level exercise testing.

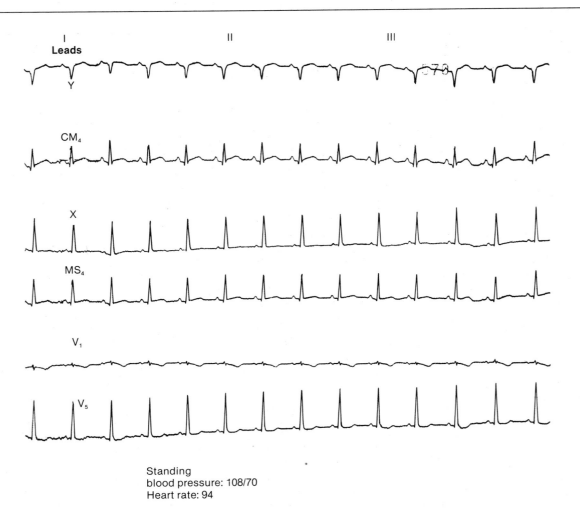

Standing
blood pressure: 108/70
Heart rate: 94

Fig. 6-22. Pre-exercise multiple-lead ECG tracings demonstrating essentially isoelectric ST segment.

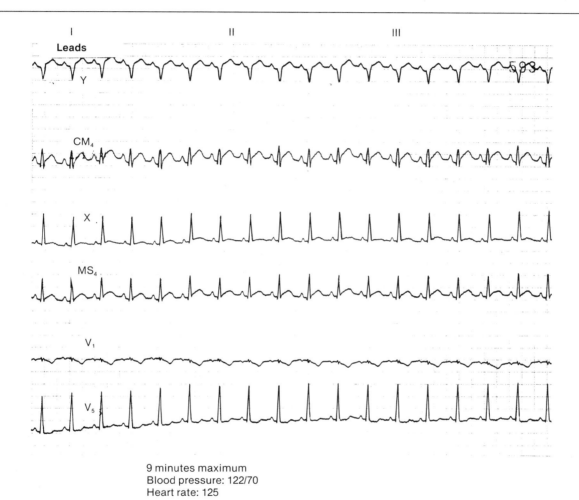

9 minutes maximum
Blood pressure: 122/70
Heart rate: 125

Fig. 6-23. ECG tracings of maximal exercise at a heart rate of 128 bpm documenting the absence of ischemic ST changes.

Table 6-7. Contraindications to low-level exercise testing

Patient less than 5 days after myocardial infarction or after coronary artery bypass graft surgery
Incomplete pretest data base
Acute congestive heart failure
Severe aortic stenosis
Recent episodes of chest pain suggestive of unstable angina
Hypotension (PB, 80/50)
Hypertension (BP, 170/100) at rest
Uncontrolled arrhythmias before exercise such as atrial fibrillation, frequent, or complex premature ventricular contractions

Table 6-8. End points for low-level treadmill tests

Achievement of heart rate equivalent to 75% to 80% of the age-predicted maximum valve (unless the patient is taking beta blockers)
Hypoadaptive systolic blood pressure response
Onset of symptoms consistent with mild angina pectoris
Two or more millimeters of ST-segment depression
Frequent multifocal premature ventricular contractions, (PVC), paired PVC's, ventricular tachycardia
Sustained supraventricular tachycardia
Fatigue
Patient request

Table 6-9. Low-level test end points (N = 134)

	N	%
Reached target heart rate	57	43
Fatigue	36	27
Angina	22	16
Hypotension	8	6
Hypertension	4	3
Leg pain, claudication	3	2
Dyspnea	3	2
Arrhythmias	1	1

tions for testing we utilize at our facilities. The end points for testing, like the test protocols, should be determined with the test objectives and patient population in mind. The criteria for terminating a low-level test are listed in Table 6-8. Our data (Table 6-9) indicate that 60% of the patients tested have their test terminated because they achieve their target heart rate or fatigue. Ischemic abnormalities (angina and hypotension) account for 22% of tests being terminated, and only 1% of the tests are stopped because of serious arrhythmias.

Summary

In summary, the low-level exercise test is a safe and extremely useful procedure, especially as a part of the definitive evaluation of the post–myocardial infarction patient. For this procedure to be as useful as possible, the therapist should consider all the available data including the total test time and maximum work load completed, the heart rate and blood pressure response, ECG changes, rhythm, exertional symptoms, reasons for terminating the test, and heart sounds before and after exercise. The therapist should carefully examine the test results (even if he is not directly involved in the procedure) to finalize his assessment of the patient and, if indicated, begin designing the treatment program.

MAXIMAL EXERCISE TESTING

In general, physical therapists that are involved with cardiac rehabilitation are not often directly involved with maximal exercise testing, though the therapist should be involved because this test is perhaps the most definitive evaluation for a patient before entry in a cardiac rehabilitation program. As the emphasis shifts from inpatient rehabilitation to outpatient rehabilitation, the importance of the data base provided by the maximal exercise test will become more evident. The objectives of the next section in this chapter is to provide an overview of the purposes

of maximal exercise testing, to illustrate how the test results influence treatment program planning, to provide examples of protocols used in testing, and to provide references, which include a more detailed discussion of the various subjects addressed.

It is not common to perform maximal exercise tests on the post–myocardial infarction patient and the post–coronary artery bypass surgery patient as early as 4 to 6 weeks after the event. In fact, the maximal test is usually done at the completion of the early outpatient phase of the exercise rehabilitation program, and it precedes the point in time in which the patient is cleared to return to work. The maximal exercise test, by definition, involves exercising a patient to a symptom-limited end point, which is most commonly severe leg fatigue or dyspnea. Heart rate, magnitude of exercise-induced ST-segment depression, and mild angina, unlike those produced by the low-level exercise test, are not used as test end points (see Appendix A, p. 99).

Purposes of maximal exercise testing
Diagnosing coronary artery disease

The fact that the majority of patients who are referred to exercise rehabilitation programs have known coronary

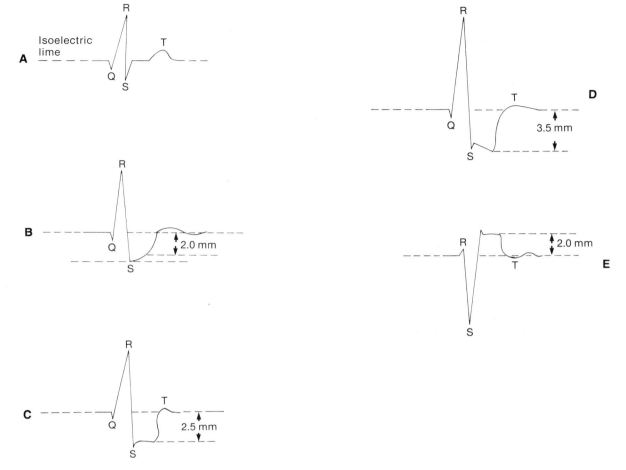

Fig. 6-24. A, Normal ST segment. **B,** Slowly upsloping ST-segment depression. **C,** Horizontal ST-segment depression. **D,** Downsloping ST-segment depression. **E,** Horizontal ST-segment depression.

artery disease does not diminish the importance of being knowledgeable of the diagnostic parameters of maximal exercise testing. Not only do the electrocardiographic and physiological ischemic indicators seen on exercise testing identify those that are likely to have coronary artery disease, but also these indicators are useful in predicting the severity of the disease. Furthermore, when exercise testing is done serially, as it is on most patients involved with long-term rehabilitation, changes in the ischemic indicators correlate with changes in the hemodynamics of the native coronary vessels or the bypass grafts.

There are a number of changes in the electrocardiogram induced by exercise that are predictive of myocardial ischemia, hence, coronary artery disease. ST-segment changes are the most commonly referred to electrocardiographic indicators of exercise-induced ischemia. The various types of alterations in the ST segment that potentially can occur during or after exercise as a result of myocardial ischemia

are illustrated in Fig. 6-24 and include a normal ST segment, a slowly upsloping ST-segment depression, a horizontal ST depression, a downsloping ST depression, and a horizontal ST elevation. The precise causes of the shift in the ST segments that are associated with ischemia are not clearly understood. Ellestad has proposed that the ischemic electrophysiological changes result from both hemodynamic and metabolic factors including elevated left ventricular end-diastolic pressures, incomplete relaxation of the myocardium, and potassium leak from the myocardial cells.[11]

Research has provided the clinician with some guidelines for understanding the value and limitations of exercise-induced ST-segment changes or shifts. In most exercise laboratories, the electrocardiographic criteria for ischemia involves a net change (when compared to the base-line preexercise tracing) of 1 mm or more of either horizontal or downsloping ST-segment depression or hori-

Table 6-10. Predictive accuracy of ST-segment changes related to prevalence of disease in the population being tested

Disease prevalence (%)	Predictive accuracy of ST depression	Predictive accuracy of no ST depression
5	50	99.7
10	68	99.4
20	83	98.7
30	90	97.5
50	95	95.0

zontal ST-segment or 1.5 to 2 mm of slow upsloping ST-segment depression.[11] However, the predictive accuracy of the above criteria for myocardial ischemia is not 100% and, in fact, is related directly to the prevalence of the disease in the population of patients being tested (Table 6-10). In other words, the predictive value of exercise-induced ST-segment changes is poor in a population of patients with low prevalence of coronary disease such as asymptomatic males less than 35 years of age[15] or premenopausal females.[8] On the other hand, in a population of older males or females with multiple risk factors or typical angina pectoris, or both, the predictive value of ST changes occurring with exercise for ischemia is very high. Furthermore, in a population of patients who previously had normal exercise electrocardiograms and develop ST changes with exercise on subsequent tests, there is a very high likelihood of progression of disease either in the native coronary arteries or in the bypass grafts.

One should keep in mind that exercise-induced ST-segment changes can result from a number of factors other than ischemia including (1) conduction abnormalities such as Wolff-Parkinson-White syndrome, left ventricular hypertrophy, and left and right bundle-branch block, (2) medications such as digitalis and diuretics, (3) valvular disorders such as mitral valve prolapse and aortic stenosis, (4) extreme base-line ST-segment abnormalities, and (5) electrolyte disturbances such as hypokalemia. Therefore, when any of the above conditions exist, the ST-segment changes must be interpreted cautiously.

On the other hand, the absence of ST-segment changes does not by itself rule out myocardial ischemia, especially in a population of patients with either a high prevalence of coronary disease or known ischemic heart disease. The predictive accuracy of a negative test (absence of electrocardiographic changes) depends on a number of factors such as (1) absence of physiological indicators for ischemia (i.e., hypotension, arrhythmias, angina), (2) achievement of a maximal heart rate that is equivalent to at least 85% of the age-predicted maximum, (3) the use of multi-

ple exercise electrocardiographic leads, and (4) the clarity and stability of the exercise and postexercise electrocardiographic tracing.

In addition to exercise-induced ST-segment changes, studies have indicated that there are a number of other electrocardiographic indicators of myocardial ischemia. Recently, R-wave amplitude changes with exercise have been reported to be a useful indicator of myocardial ischemia and left ventricular function, though there is some controversy in the literature. Theoretically, R-wave amplitude is directly related to left ventricular end-diastolic volume.[5] In the normal subject, R-wave amplitude decreases when the preexercise standing voltage is compared to the immediate postexercise value. It is assumed that this decrease in R-wave amplitude is attributable to the decrease in the left ventricular end-diastolic volume that occurs in the person with normal coronaries and normal left ventricular function. In the patient with coronary disease who becomes ischemic with exercise and whose left ventricular function deteriorates resulting in increased end-diastolic volumes, one would expect the R-wave amplitude to increase. In fact, there are studies indicating that R-wave amplitude changes increase the diagnostic value of exercise testing.[2,16] The problems with R-wave changes is that they can occur in patients with poor ventricular function without ischemia and in a small percentage of "normal" subjects, and therefore there are studies questioning their usefulness.[41] It seems the most reasonable approach for use of R-wave changes is to combine ST-segment changes with R-wave changes as done by Ellestad and others (Fig. 6-25).[12] According to Ellestad, if the net ST-segment changes are a "positive" 1 mm or more, once the R-wave changes have been taken into consideration, there is a stronger likelihood of coronary disease.

Exercise-induced septal Q-wave changes have been studied, and the results indicate that decreases in the amplitude of the Q wave (in lead CM_5) is highly predictive of disease in the left anterior descending artery.[27] Finally, although it is a rare finding, post-exercise inversion of the U wave is highly predictive of coronary disease even in the absence of ST-segment depression according to Gerson and others.[17]

As mentioned earlier, there are a number of physiological indicators of myocardial ischemia that can develop during exercise testing in conjunction with the various electrocardiographic changes or despite the absence of electrocardiographic changes such as ST-depression or R-wave amplitude changes. Blood pressure response to exercise is one physiological parameter that must be evaluated carefully throughout the test (see Chapter 5). Another hemodynamic indicator of compromised left ventricular function, usually associated with myocardial ischemia, is exercise bradycardia, also referred to as "chronotropic incompetence" (see Chapter 5). When the exercise bradycardia accompanies other electrocardiographic and hemo-

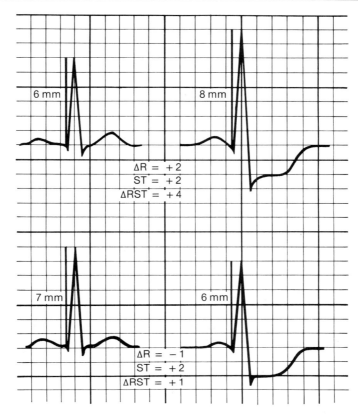

Fig. 6-25. Calculation of index (RST) in two cases with ST-segment depression and R wave increased and decreased. (From Bonoris. P.E., and others: Circulation **57**(5): 904-910, 1978.)

dynamic indicators of ischemia, the patients are more likely to have severe coronary disease.[3]

Exercise-induced ventricular arrhythmias· by themselves (in absence of electrocardiographic changes and other signs of myocardial ischemia) are not predictive of coronary disease. The combination of ST changes and exercise-induced arrhythmias is however predictive of more severe coronary disease.

The presence of angina discomfort during exercise testing without electrocardiographic changes has been shown to be as predictive as electrocardiographic changes alone.[42] The nature of the anginal discomfort can be quite variable, involving burning, pressure, tightness, tiredness in the chest, upper extremities, neck, jaw, or midscapular region. The common denominator, however, is that the discomfort becomes more intensive with increased heart rate and systolic blood pressure, and it is usually relieved within 5 minutes after exercise or after nitroglycerin administration.

It should be clear at this point that exercise-induced myocardial ischemia can be detected during and after testing by a variety of electrocardiographic and physiological indicators. It is obviously inappropriate to use the "tunnel-vision" approach of equating ischemia with ST changes alone.

Prognostic implications from exercise testing

Exercise testing provides a great deal of information regarding the prognosis of patients with known coronary disease. It is the most important functional assessment of the consequences of the degree of coronary disease and left ventricular dysfunction seen at the time of cardiac catheterization. For therapists involved with phase III cardiac rehabilitation candidates, the prognostic implication of exercise testing is important because it (1) identifies the priority for involvement in an ongoing program based on the likelihood of a future cardiac event (i.e., myocardial infarction, progression of angina, or sudden death), (2) provides part of the data base from which decisions can be made regarding the frequency of phase III visits, and (3) provides part of the data base from which decisions about the specific exercise program can be made.

As mentioned in Chapter 2, the two major determinants of prognosis for the patient with coronary disease are the number of diseased arteries and the degree of left ventricular dysfunction. There are several electrocardiographic and physiological indicators obtained from exercise testing that predict the likelihood of a future coronary event, since they relate directly to the degree of coronary disease and left ventricular impairment. A discussion of these prognostic variables follows.

The slope, magnitude, time of onset, and persistence of ST-segment abnormalities after exercise have been shown to be related to the severity of coronary disease and therefore the likelihood of future coronary events. Goldschlager and others[19] found downsloping ST depression (versus horizontal or slow upsloping ST depression) to be more commonly associated with multivessel or left main coronary disease. Patients who demonstrate significant ST-segment depression within the first 3 minutes of the test are at a much higher risk of a future coronary event.[13] In addition, the magnitude (number of millimeters of depression) of the ST change is predictive of future coronary events, especially when one compares ST changes occurring within the first 6 minutes of a Bruce or treadmill test. For example, according to Ellestad's data, a patient with 3 mm of ST-segment depression has an 82% chance of a future event compared to 50% likelihood of a future event for the patient with 1 mm at the same point on the test. However, patients with 1 to 2 mm ST depression at 5 minutes of the test have approximately a 35% likelihood of a future coronary event compared to a 42% likelihood in patients with 4 mm of ST depression at the same point on the test. From these data it appears that the time of onset is the more powerful prognostic variable. The onset of angina early in the test (within the first 3 minutes), in combination with early onset of ST depression, worsens the prognosis for the patient as well.[11] The persistence of the ST-segment depression after exercise appears to be a predictor of more severe coronary disease provided that 1 to 2 mm of horizontal or downsloping ST depression is used as end points for testing.[19] Goldschlager found that over 40% of patients whose ischemic ST depression resolved within 1 minute after exercise had normal coronaries or single-vessel disease. Ninety percent of patients whose ischemic ST depression persisted for 9 or more minutes had multivessel disease, however. One should note that the predictive value for postexercise persistence of ST-segment changes might differ in patients who are taken to a symptom-limited end point despite the magnitude of ST-segment depression.

McNeer and others[24] demonstrated that patients (not on beta adrenergic receptor–blocking agents) with impaired chronotropic reserve (low maximum heart rate) had a poor prognosis with a clear distinction between those with a maximum heart rate (1) equal to or greater than 160 bpm, (2) between 120 to 159 bpm, and (3) less than 120 bpm. Forty percent of patients with a maximum heart rate below 120 had died within 4 years of follow-up. Likewise, Irving and others[22] found patients with a limited inotropic reserve to have a poor prognosis. The annual rate of sudden death

was 97.9 per 1000 men if the maximal systolic pressure was less than 140 mm Hg, 25.3 if the response was between 140 and 155, and 6.6 if the systolic pressure was equal to or greater than 200 mm Hg.

Recently, the exercise capacity of the patient has also been shown to be an important prognostic indicator. McNeer and others[24] showed that patients able to perform through the third stage or longer on the Bruce test have a significantly better prognosis than those patients able to complete only stage I or II. In fact, patients able to complete only stage I had a 2-year survival rate less than 60%. Podrid[29] and Dagenais[9] both found that even in patients with 2 or more millimeters of ST depression the survival was closely correlated with exercise duration and patients able to enter the third or fourth stage of the Bruce test had an excellent prognosis.

Udall and Ellestad[40] have shown in the past that exercise-induced premature ventricular contractions have prognostic value in a population of patients with known coronary artery disease. Their results indicate that the annual incidence of a new coronary event (progression of angina, myocardial infarction, or death) was 1.7% in patients without premature ventricular contractions or ischemic ST changes, 6.4% in those with premature ventricular contractions alone, 9.5% in those with only ischemic ST changes, and 11.4% in those exhibiting both premature ventricular contractions and ischemic ST changes.

Exercise prescription and activity recommendations based on maximal-exercise test results

Exercise testing to a true symptom-limited end point (versus terminating a test at a predetermined end point such as 85% of the predicted maximal heart rate) allows for an objective measurement of the patient's physical work capacity. Each work load on a test, whether it be a treadmill or bicycle ergometer, has an oxygen requirement equivalent, and there are tables or nomograms from which the predicted values can be obtained (Fig. 6-26). Therefore by taking a patient to a symptom-limited end point one can predict their maximal oxygen-uptake capacity and compare their results to age- and sex-matched norms to assess the patient's degree of impairment. For clinical purposes, predicting the patient's maximal oxygen-uptake capacity may be useful. However, one must keep in mind that the majority of tables and nomograms that exist for oxygen-uptake work load equivalent are based on normal data and therefore there is a tendency to overestimate the cardiac patient's values by as much as 10% to 15%. As Adams and others[1] suggest, the prediction error is probably directly related to the severity of disease of the patient and the degree of ventricular dysfunction during exercise. Bruce[6] has published a nomogram for male cardiac patients from which the degree of impairment in maximal oxygen uptake can be calculated based on the treadmill test duration and the age of the patient. Once again, Bruce's

Functional class	Clinical status	O₂ requirements (ml O₂/kg/min)	Treadmill tests Bruce* (3-min stages) mph %gr	Treadmill tests Kattus⁺ (3-min stages) mph %gr	Treadmill tests Balke# % grade at 3.4 mph	Bicycle ergometer For 70 kg body weight kg/min
Normal and I	Physically active subject / Sedentary healthy / Diseased, recovered / Symptomatic patients	56.0			26	For 70 kg body weight
		52.5		mph %gr	24	
		49.0	mph %gr	4 22	22	kg/min
		45.5	4.2 16		20	1500
		42.0		4 18	18	1350
		38.5			16	1200
		35.0		4 14	14	1050
		31.5	3.4 14		12	900
		28.0		4 10	10	
II		24.5	2.5 12	3 10	8	750
		21.0			6	600
		17.5	1.7 10	2 10	4	450
		14.0			2	300
III		10.5				150
		7.0				
IV		3.5				

Fig. 6-26. Classification and oxygen requirements for various work loads on treadmill and bicycle ergometers. *gr*, Grade. (From Fortuin, N., and Weiss, J.L.: Circulation **56**(5): 699-712, 1977.)

nomogram is a useful clinical tool; however, the nomogram was developed from an undefined group of cardiac patients in terms of their ventricular function and the severity of their disease.

Another point to keep in mind when assessing maximal oxygen uptake from symptom-limited exercise testing is that both the protocol and the mode of exercise can be important variables. Studies have shown that normal sedentary subjects achieve a 10% to 15% higher value for maximal oxygen uptake on a treadmill protocol compared to bicycle ergometry testing.[20,26] Our unpublished results on cardiac patients indicate that a similar disparity in the actual measured maximal oxygen uptake obtained during treadmill and bicycle testing is evident in both the sedentary patient and the active patient using jogging as the primary mode of training. However, in the active cardiac patient using cycling as the primary mode of training, we found no significant difference in the measured maximal oxygen uptake obtained from the two testing modes. Based on a review of the literature and our results, it appears that part of the reason for the difference in maximal oxygen uptake values obtained on treadmill and bicycle testing is attributable to the local muscle fatigue (quadriceps) that

prevents a true maximal cardiovascular effort during bicycle testing of the untrained or noncyclist subject. Froelicher and others[14] compared maximal oxygen-uptake values obtained on three treadmill protocols in 15 normal subjects. Their results indicate that the highest oxygen-uptake values were obtained on the Taylor protocol (compared to the Bruce and Balke protocols), and the smallest coefficient of variation (a measure of reliability) was seen on the Taylor and Bruce tests.

In consideration of the above discussion, it would appear that ideally it is better to measure directly the cardiac patient's physical work capacity or maximal oxygen-uptake capacity by expired-gas collection and analysis. Our results indicate that the reliability of measured oxygen uptake in cardiac patients is equal to that of sex-matched inactive and active normals.[21]

The value of objective assessment of the patient's physical work capacity is at least threefold. First, the decision to allow a patient to return to work (especially a job involving relatively high levels of energy expenditures) cannot be appropriately made without knowing the patient's maximal capacity. As a guideline, the Committee on Exercise of the American Heart Association suggests that the vocational-setting work intensity during an 8-hour shift should fall within 25% to 40% range of the difference between the resting oxygen uptake and the maximal oxygen uptake. Similarly, the decision to clear the patient to perform activities of daily living and recreational activities should be based in part on the relationship between the energy demand of a given activity and the patient's maximal capacity. Finally, objective evaluation of the patient's work capacity will allow for evaluation of the effectiveness of exercise therapy, medications, and surgery when the results of future tests are compared.

The results of the maximal exercise test also provide the basis from which the intensity of the therapeutic aerobic exercise program is initially formulated. Studies indicate that the minimum aerobic training needed to stimulate improvement in the oxygen-consumption capacity of patients with coronary disease is a work-load equivalent to 60% of the person's maximal oxygen consumption (which corresponds to 70% of his maximal heart rate). The desired training threshold for each patient, in terms of the workload and heart-rate range, can be calculated from the results of the maximal-exercise test. In addition, the exercise test results provide guidelines for the therapist to determine whether it is appropriate to exercise the patient at the desired training threshold, that is, heart rates equivalent to 70% or greater of the patient's maximum heart rate achieved on the exercise test. In other words, does the patient develop significant hypotension or hypertension, arrhythmias, angina, and dyspnea at heart rates below 70% of maximum? Obviously, the current clinical status and medical history has a bearing as well on the establishment of the patient's recommended therapeutic intensity of exercise. Once the exercise prescription has been formulated, it is the responsibility of the therapist to evaluate the patient at the established therapeutic heart rate range, using the same skills needed for exercise testing, to determine the appropriateness of the initial exercise treatment plan (see Chapter 7).

Interpretation of maximal-exercise test results

The following is meant to be a guideline for obtainment of the key results from the maximal-exercise test whether it be from the standpoint of extracting the data from a test administered by the physician or by the therapist. Refer to Appendix B for an example of a test-result work sheet.

1. Demographic data
   Age, sex, activity level of patient (i.e., sedentary, mildly active, training).
   Current medication list including dose, frequency, and time of last dose taken before test.
   Time of test.
2. Protocol used (Appendix C)
   Sheffield, Bruce, Ellestad, Balke.
   Intermittent versus continuous, bicycle ergometer, or arm ergometer.
3. Minutes or maximum work load completed

4. Resting heart rate and blood pressure
   Note if significant changes occur in heart rate or blood pressure with position change, i.e., supine to sitting, sitting to standing.
5. Base-line ST-segment depression or elevation and slope
   Note if changes occur with position changes or breathing maneuvers (10-second breathholding and 30 seconds of hyperventilation).
6. R-wave amplitude in standing position
7. Maximum heart rate and percentage of age-predicted rate achieved
8. Maximum blood pressure achieved and pressure at peak work load if different
9. Interpretation of resting and exercise systolic and diastolic blood pressures
10. Major limiting factors of test or reason test was terminated (Appendix D)
11. Statement regarding presence or absence of anginal symptoms
    If symptoms noted, description of the location and nature of symptoms, time and heart rate at onset, and postexercise persistence should be given.
12. Summary of ST-segment changes
    To include time and heart rate at onset, maximum magnitude of ST changes, ST-segment slope, and time required for resolution of ST changes
13. Description of significant pre- and postexercise auscultatory findings
    Including heart sounds, lung sounds, and carotid or femoral bruits.
14. Description of arrhythmias
    Including the type(s) and frequency (range in terms of numbers per minute)
15. Assessment of physical work capacity
    To include predicted maximum oxygen consumption value and a comparison to age- and sex-matched norms.

Safety of maximal exercise testing

The rationale for performing maximal symptom-limited tests has been discussed earlier and should be evident at this point (Appendix E). How safe is it to perform maximal exercise tests? In 1970, Rochmis and Blackburn, in a survey of 170,000 exercise tests, reported a mortality of approximately 1 in 10,000 and a morbidity (prolonged chest pain or arrhythmias, requiring hospitalization) of 2.4 per 10,000.[31] Stuart and Ellestad[37] reported on a survey involving a half-million tests with a mortality of 0.5 per 10,000 and a complication rate of 9 per 10,000. Table 6-11 summarizes the major studies in the literature on safety of exercise testing.

Who should perform exercise tests? The Committee on Exercise Testing of the American Heart Association recently recommended that exercise testing be delegated to appropriately trained and competent nonphysician health

Table 6-11. Safety of exercise testing literature review

Author	Year	Number of tests	Complications
Rochmis and Blackburn[30]	1971	170,000 (73 centers)	1 death per 10,000 tests 2.4 morbid events per 10,000 (requiring hospitalization)
Stuart and Ellestad[37]	1980	444,396 treadmill tests 44,460 bike tests 25,592 master's tests 514,448 total (1375 centers)	0.5 deaths per 10,000 3.5 myocardial infarctions per 10,000 4.8 serious arrhythmias per 10,000 Total: 8.8 complications per 10,000
Scherer and Kaltenbach[31]	1979	1,065,923 total 353,638 "sports persons" 712,285 "coronary patients"	0 morbidity and mortality 0.24 deaths per 10,000 1.4 life-threatening complications per 10,000

Table 6-12. Exercise testing* at Ross-Loos Medical Center, 1980-1982

Total	Type of test
2426 (50%)	New diagnostic exercise tests (rule out coronary artery disease)
2151 (44%)	Known coronary artery disease (myocardial infarction, cardiac catheterization, coronary artery bypass graft)
305 (6%)	Other cardiac diagnoses (hypertension, arrhythmias, mitral valve prolapse, etc.)

*All tests were performed independently by physical therapists with an M.D. in the immediate vicinity but not present in the testing laboratory.

Table 6-13. Exercise testing* at Ross-Loos Medical Center, known coronary artery disease tests

Total	Type of patient
1386 (64%)	Status after myocardial infarction or coronary artery disease by angiography including 157 low-level exercise tests
765 (36%) 2151 (100%)	Status after coronary bypass surgery

*All tests were performed independently by physical therapists with an M.D. in the immediate vicinity but not present in the testing laboratory.

care professionals as long as there is a physician in the immediate vicinity. We recently reviewed the safety of stress testing done independently by properly trained physical therapists at our facilities in Los Angeles. We have performed 4882 tests between 1980 and 1982 without any deaths or myocardial infarctions. The complete summary of our data analysis is given in Tables 6-12 to 6-14.

SUMMARY

Patient evaluation is performed systematically throughout the cardiac rehabilitation program. To effectively evaluate a patient with coronary artery disease the therapist should be able to obtain useful clinical data and understand the relationships of that data to the basic sciences of exercise physiology, pathology, hemodynamics, and pathophysiology. As the patient moves into the program (phase I) to hospital discharge (phase II) to independent exercise (phase III), a matching evaluation is performed. Using the clinical monitoring tools of heart rate, blood pressure, ECG changes, symptoms, and heart sounds and the pa-

Table 6-14. Safety of exercise testing by physical therapists at Ross-Loos Medical Center

Years:	1980-1982
Number of tests:	4882
Complications:	
Mortality:	0%
Morbidity:	
Cardiac arrest:	0%
Other*:	5

*Other includes three patients with sustained ventricular tachycardia requiring hospitalization of one patient with cyanosis and confusion after the test and one patient with history of cerebrovascular accident 15 years previously and severe hypertension that developed a new cerebrovascular accident after the test.

tient's demographic information and medical status, the therapist can gain useful assessments of the patient's activity tolerance. Phase I begins with the self-care evaluation. Phase II begins with a low-level exercise test, and phase III can be initiated after maximal exercise testing and cardiac catheterization.

Each assessment will afford the therapist the clinical information necessary to develop a safe, yet effective, program of exercise and education.

We recommend that each exercise-testing laboratory develop specific policies and procedures that take into consideration the patient population to be tested, the expertise of the staff involved with performance of the tests, and the equipment utilized.

REFERENCES

 1. Adams, G.E., and others: Oxygen uptake in cardiac patients during treadmill testing, Cardiovasc. Pulmonary Technol. **2**:11, 1980.
 2. Berman, J.L., and others: Multiple-lead QRS changes with exercise testing, Circulation **63**:53, 1980.
 3. Blessey, R.L., and others: Aerobic capacity and cardiac catheterization results in 13 patients with exercise bradycardia, Med. Sci. Sports Exerc. **8**:50, 1976. (Abstract.)
 4. Bonoris, P.E., and others: Evaluation of R wave amplitude changes versus ST segment depression in stress testing, Circulation **57**:904, 1978.
 5. Brody, D.A.: A theoretical analysis of the intercavity blood mass influence on the heart lead relationship, Circ. Res. **4**:731, 1956.
 6. Bruce, R.A., and others: Maximal oxygen uptake and nomographic assessment of functional aerobic impairment in cardiovascular disease, Am. Heart J. **85**:846, 1973.
 7. Butler, S.M.: Phase one cardiac rehabilitation: the role of functional evaluation in patient progression, master's thesis, Atlanta, 1983, Emory University.
 8. Cumming, G.R., and others: Exercise electrocardiography in normal women, Br. Heart J. **35**:1055, 1973.
 9. Danegais, G.R., and others: Survival of patients with a strongly positive exercise electrocardiogram, Circulation **65**:452, 1982.
10. Dubin, D.: Rapid interpretation of EKG's, ed. 3, Tampa, 1974, Cover Publishing Co.
11. Ellestad, M.H.: Stress testing: principles and practice, ed. 2, Philadelphia, 1980, F.A. Davis Co.
12. Ellestad, M.H., and Wan, M.K.C.: Predictive implications of stress testing, Circulation **51**:363, 1975.
13. Ellestad, M.H., and others: Stress testing: clinical application and predictive capacity, Prog. Cardiovasc. Dis. **21**:431, 1979.
14. Froelicher, V.F., and others: The correlation of coronary angiography and the electrocardiographic response to maximal testing in 76 asymptomatic men, Circulation **48**:597, 1973.
15. Froelicher, V.F., and others: A comparison of three maximal treadmill exercise protocols, J. Appl. Physiol. **38**:720, 1974.
16. Fuller, C.M., and others: Early post–myocardial infarction treadmill stress testing: an accurate predictor of multivessel coronary disease and subsequent cardiac events, Ann. Intern. Med. **94**:734, 1981.
17. Gerson, M.C., and others: Exercise-induced U wave inversion as a marker of stenosis of the left anterior descending coronary artery, Circulation **60**:1014, 1979.
18. Goldberger, E.: Textbook of clinical cardiology, St. Louis, 1981, The C.V. Mosby Co.
19. Goldschlager, N., and others: Treadmill stress test indicators of presence and severity of coronary artery disease, Ann. Intern. Med. **85**:277, 1976.
20. Hermansen, H., and Salten, B.: Oxygen uptake during maximal treadmill and bicycle exercise, J. Appl. Physiol. **26**:31, 1969.
21. Ice, R., and others: The reliability of maximal oxygen uptake in trained and untrained normal and cardiac patients, Med. Sci. Sports Exerc. **14**:168, 1982. (Abstract.)
22. Irving, T.B., and others: Variations in and significance of systolic blood pressure during maximal exercise testing, Am. J. Cardiol. **39**:841, 1977.
23. Linhart, S.W., and others: Maximum treadmill exercise electrocardiography in female patients, Circulation **50**:1173, 1974.
24. McNeer, J.F., and others: The course of acute myocardial infarction: feasibility of early discharge of the uncomplicated patient, Circulation **51**:410, 1975.
25. McNeer, J.F., and others: The role of the exercise test in the evaluation of patients for ischemic heart disease, Circulation **57**:64, 1978.
26. Miyamura, M., and Honda, Y.: Oxygen intake and cardiac output during maximal treadmill and bicycle exercise, J. Appl. Physiol. **32**:185, 1972.
27. Morales-Ballejo, H., and others: Septal Q wave in exercise testing: angiographic correlation, Am. J. Cardiol. **48**:247, 1981.
28. Morris, S.N., and others: Incidence and significance of decreases in systolic blood pressure during graded treadmill exercise testing, Am. J. Cardiol. **41**:221, 1978.
29. Podrid, P.J., and others: Prognosis of medically treated patients with coronary artery disease with profound ST segment depression during exercise testing, N. Engl. J. Med. **306**:111, 1981.
30. Rochmis, P., and Blackburn, H.: Exercise tests: a survey of procedures, safety, and litigation experience in approximately 170,000 tests, J.A.M.A. **217**:1061, 1971.
31. Scherer, D., and Kaltenback, M.: Frequency of life-threatening complications associated with stress testing, Dtsch. Med. Wochenschr. **104**:1161, 1979.
32. Schwartz, K.M., and others: Limited exercise testing soon after myocardial infarction: correlation with early coronary and left ventricular angiography, Ann. Intern. Med. **94**:727, 1981.
33. Sheps, D.S., and others: Exercise-induced increase in diastolic pressure: indicator of severe coronary artery disease, Am. J. Cardiol. **45**:708, 1979.
34. Stange, J.M., and Lewis, R.P.: Early exercise test after MI, Ann. Intern. Med. **94**:814, 1981.
35. Starling, M.R., and others: Exercise testing early after myocardial infarction: predictive value for subsequent unstable angina and death, Am. J. Cardiol. **46**:909, 1980.
36. Starling, M.R., and others: Treadmill exercise tests pre-discharge and six weeks post-myocardial infarction to detect abnormalities of known prognostic value, Ann. Intern. Med. **94**:721, 1981.
37. Stuart, R.J., and Ellestad, M.H.: National survey of exercise stress testing facilities, Chest **77**:94, 1980.
38. Théroux, P., and others: Prognostic value of exercise testing soon after myocardial infarction, N. Engl. J. Med. **301**:341, 1979.
39. Thompson, P.D., and Deleman, M.H.: Hypotension accompanying the onset of exertional angina: a sign of severe compromise of left ventricular blood supply, Circulation **52**:28, 1975.
40. Udall, J.A., and Ellestad, M.H.: Predictive implications of ventricular premature complexes associated with treadmill stress testing, Circulation **56**:985, 1977.
41. Wagner, S., and others: Unreliability of exercise-induced R wave changes as indexes of coronary artery disease, Am. J. Cardiol. **44**:1241, 1979.
42. Werner, D.A., and others: The predictive value of chest pain as an indicator of coronary disease during exercise testing, Circulation **54**(Suppl. 2):10, 1976. (Abstract.)

APPENDIX A
Guidelines for maximal exercise testing

Definition

A maximal symptom-limited exercise test is an electrocardiographically monitored evaluation of a person's maximal oxygen consumption during dynamic work (exercise) utilizing large muscle groups. It begins with submaximal exertion, allows time for physiological adaptations, and has progressive increments in work loads until individually determined end points of fatigue are reached or limiting symptoms or signs occur.

Purpose

1. To establish the diagnosis and severity of coronary artery disease through exercise-induced ECG changes. This may occur as confirmation of clinically suspected coronary artery disease or detection of latent coronary artery disease in an asymptomatic individual.
2. Evaluate the functional cardiovascular capacity and reserve in response to exercise in patients with coronary artery disease for assessment of return to work or leisure activities and candidacy for exercise-training programs.
3. To evaluate prescribed therapy as an objective measure of medical or surgical intervention. This is particularly important in the assessment of the effect of a person's participation in an ongoing aerobic exercise program.

4. To serve as motivation and as stimulus to make needed changes in behavior or life-style (e.g., to stop smoking, alter diet, or adhere to an exercise program).

Indications for procedure

1. After myocardial infarction or coronary artery bypass graft surgery, 4 or more weeks after either event in uncomplicated patients, greater than 4 weeks in complicated patients.
2. Outpatient referral for admission to a cardiac rehabilitation program in a patient suspected of having coronary artery disease.
3. To distinguish angina from noncardiac chest pain.
4. Development of a change in the patient's medical status that requires reevaluation of cardiovascular status (onset of hypertension, inability to maintain habitual exercise program because of onset of dyspnea, excessive fatigue, or angina), or evaluation of a change in medications.
5. Ongoing periodic reevaluation of the patient's cardiac status and physical work capacity as part of a treatment program (i.e., exercise conditioning, surgery, etc.).
6. To assist in determining whether a coronary patient can return to a particular type of vocational or recreational activity.

APPENDIX B

TREADMILL TEST WORKSHEET

INSTITUTION: _____

Name _____ Patient No. _____ Date _____ Age _____
Sex _____ Weight _____ Height _____ Diagnosis _____
Reason for test _____ Protocol _____
12 Lead ECG Interp. _____
Time _____ Medications _____
Time last dose _____ Time last cigarette _____ Time last meal _____
Physician: _____ Activity Status: _____

TEST RESULTS

Minutes Completed _____ Limiting Factors _____
Resting Heart rate _____ Max. Heart rate _____ Resting BP _____ / _____
Max. BP _____ / _____ BP Response _____

Chest Pain _____

Summary ST Segment Changes _____

Heart Sounds _____ Arrhythmias _____

Physical Work Capacity _____

_____ Remarks/Recommendations _____

Interpreted by _____ M.D. _____ *Continued.*

TREADMILL TEST WORKSHEET—cont'd

STAGE	Workload	Time	HR	BP	Angina	Arrhy.	Y	ML	X
Supine Pre-Exercise		1							
Supine Pre-Exercise		2							
Breath-Holding		3							
Hyperventilation		3							
Sitting Pre-Exercise		4							
Standing Pre-Exercise		5							
		1							
		2							
		3							
		4							
		5							
		6							
		7							
		8							
		9							
		10							
		11							
		12							
		13							
		14							
		15							
Immed. Post-Exercise		0							
		1							
		2							
		3							
		4							
		5							
		6							
		7							
		8							
		9							

MS 4	ST changes		V L/m	Vo₂ L/min	Vo₂ ml/kg/m	O₂ Pulse	RQ
	V₁	V₅					

APPENDIX C
Exercise Test Protocols

Bruce Multistage Continuous Protocol

Stage	Speed (mph)	Grade (%)	Time (minutes)	Metabolic equivalents (work loads)
1	1.7	10	3	4-5
2	2.5	12	3	6-7
3	3.4	14	3	8-9
4	4.2	16	3	10-12
5	5.0	18	3	Greater than 14

Arm ergometry tests
1. Continuous protocol
   a. Initial work load not less than 150 kg.
   b. A total of 4 or 5 work loads, each with a duration of 2 minutes.
   c. Work load increments not less than 50 kg.
   d. Crank speed 50 to 60 rpm.
2. Intermittent protocol
   a. Initial work load not less than 150 kg.
   b. A total of 4 or 5 work loads each 3 minutes in duration followed by 3-minute recovery periods.
   c. Work-load increments not less than 50 kg.
   d. Crank speed 50 to 60 rpm.

Bicycle ergometry tests—intermittent protocol
1. Initial work load not less than 150 kg.
2. A total of 4 or 5 work loads, each 4 minutes long, followed by 4-minute recovery periods.
3. Seat height adjusted so that there is no more than 5 to 10 degrees of flexion in the knee at the lowest point in the pedal revolutions.
4. Work-load increments should be 20% to 25% of the difference between the initial work load and the estimated maximal work load.
5. Crank speed should be maintained at 50 to 60 rpm.

APPENDIX D
Criteria for termination of test
1. Patient's report of fatigue, which would make continued exertion uncomfortable.
2. Patient's report of dizziness.
3. Increasing premature ventricular contractions becoming multifocal.
4. Recurrent coupled premature ventricular contractions or ventricular tachycardia (three PVC's in a row).
5. Development of rapid atrial arrhythmias.
6. Level III angina (scale of I to IV).
7. A progressive fall in systolic blood pressure of 20 mm Hg or more in the presence of increased heart rate and work load, confirmed by second blood pressure taken within 20 seconds.
8. Extreme hypertensive response (systolic 250/diastolic 130).
9. Severe musculoskeletal pain as in leg claudication.
10. Uninterpretable electrocardiographic tracing.
11. Patient signs such as cold and clammy skin, ataxic gait, or other signs of vascular insufficiency.

APPENDIX E
Contraindications and precautions to exercise testing
1. Contraindications
   a. Overt congestive heart failure.
   b. Rapid intensifying or unstable angina.
   c. Recent acute myocardial infarction (less than 3 weeks).
   d. Dissecting aneurysm.
   e. Second- or third-degree heart block.
   f. Recurrent ventricular tachycardia.
   g. Rapid atrial arrhythmias.
   h. Acute myocarditis or pericarditis.
   i. Severe aortic stenosis.
   j. Recent pulmonary embolus.
   k. Acute infections or other active disease process.
2. Precautions (attending physician to be consulted before beginning of test)
   a. Repetitive or frequent ventricular ectopic activity at rest (more than 10 premature ventricular contractions per minute).
   b. Resting hypertension (systolic 180/diastolic 110).
   c. Severe cardiomegaly.
   d. Resting tachycardia of greater than 110 bpm or a recent change in cardiac symptoms.

7

RANDY ICE

Program planning and implementation

In 1978, Jan Kellerman, one of the early pioneers in the field of cardiac rehabilitation, gave the following definition of cardiac rehabilitation: "Rehabilitation of cardiac patients is the sum of activities required to insure the best possible physical, mental and social conditions so they may, on their own efforts, regain an active and productive life." The key phrase in this definition is "on their own efforts," which implies that for a cardiac patient to be rehabilitated the patient assumes control and direction of the program. In this chapter, the sequence for planning and implementing such a program in a team-oriented fashion will be presented for the inpatient (phase I), subacute patient (phase II), and stable long-term patient (phase III). A review of the goals of each of these phases is presented, as well as several case studies and supportive literature.

PHASE I—INPATIENT CARDIAC REHABILITATION

Phase I cardiac rehabilitation, the most recently developed programs, are undergoing rapid change. This has occurred because of a remarkable evolution in the overall care of both patients with acute myocardial infarction and those admitted for acute coronary insufficiency or coronary artery bypass graft surgery. These changes have created a noticeable reduction in the number of hospital days for these patients. Data now available for post–myocardial infarction patients classify these patients into complicated or uncomplicated categories within the first 4 days of hospital admission (see Chapter 6). Research studies have found that patients without complications during the first 4 days after infarction can be discharged from the hospital at 7 days without increasing their mortality during the next 6 months.[56] Uncomplicated patients therefore can be treated more aggressively, and they have progressed more rapidly in phase I than the complicated patients have. Complicated patients are often not referred for cardiac rehabilitation for fear that increased activity may provoke a catastrophic event (i.e., repeat infarction, cardiac arrest).

Work by our group with this type of patient at the Ross-Loos Medical Center in Los Angeles and the Presbyterian Intercommunity Hospital in Whittier, California, has indicated that the safety of progressive ambulation in the complicated patient is as good as with the uncomplicated patient provided that an individualized program is formulated and very close feedback with the referring physician is maintained. Quite often, day-to-day adjustments in antiarrhythmic, antihypertensive or antianginal medications will help to stabilize the patient much more rapidly and facilitate patient progress, as well as an earlier hospital discharge.

The rationale for many inpatient phase I programs has previously centered around the need to prevent the detrimental effects of bed rest.[90] Although that is still a goal, it is clear that most patients do not require extended periods of bed rest. Early mobilization and discharge has required phase I programs to assume alternate emphasis and rationale. With careful activity assessment (see Chapter 6), uncomplicated patients may be out of bed performing self-care activities and ward ambulation as early as the third day after the infarction. Complicated patients may be up as early as the fifth day after the infarction. Thus the goals and rationale for phase I are as follows:

1. Assessment of hemodynamic responses to self-care and progressive ambulation activities.
2. Determination of the effectiveness of the patient's medications in controlling abnormal physiological or electrocardiographic responses to activity.
3. Establishment of clinical data that contribute to the patient's prognosis and thus optimal medical management.
4. Early behavioral modification and risk factor reduction.
5. Family education.

These goals and the approach to patient evaluation discussed in detail in Chapter 6 encompass the treatment program for phase I. In other words, phase I patient treatment for myocardial infarction patients or patients after bypass

Table 7-1. Protocol for phase I cardiac rehabilitation program

Day	Protocol	Team member responsible
1	Coronary care unit	M.D.
2	(stabilization)	
3	↓	
4	Self-care evaluation	Physical therapist, nurse, or occupational therapist
5	Monitored ambulation	Physical therapist
6	↓	
7	Low-level exercise test	Physical therapist or physician
8	Discharge	Physician

ACTIVITY LEVELS

1. a. Complete bedrest
   b. Do own morning care: wash hands, face, brush teeth with arms supported
   c. Feed self, with arms supported
   d. Complete bed bath; male patients shaved by nurse
   e. Bedside commode
2. a. Complete bed bath; male patient may shave self; patient does own genital area
   b. Teaching materials given to patient
   c. Bedside commode
   d. Up in chair, at bedside with feet elevated, 20 to 30 minutes twice a day
   e. Flat, sitting, and standing blood pressure and apical pulse before moving to the chair on the first day
   f. Monitored self-care evaluation
3. a. In bed, patient bathes arms, chest, and genitals; nurse bathes back, legs, and feet.
   b. May walk to bathroom with help. Flat, sitting, and standing blood pressure and pulse before ambulation on the first day.
   c. Walk to chair and sit for 30 to 60 minutes three times a day
4. a. Same as level 3
   b. Up to bathroom as desired
   c. Up in room and chair three times a day for 30 to 60 minutes
   d. Monitored ambulation
5. a. Sponge-bathe self, sitting in bathroom (nurse bathes back)
   b. Up in room and chair as desired
   c. Continue progressive monitored ambulation
6. a. Sit down shower
   b. Walk in hall three times a day
7. Walk up and down one flight of stairs
8. Low-level treadmill test before discharge

surgery is simply evaluation of the patient's progress through ever-increasing levels of activity. In addition, emphasis is placed on education of the patient's family. The patient is included in these educational activities, but in the acute setting, denial, anxiety, and medications make cognitive learning a difficult and poorly accepted process for the patient.[17]

To facilitate the cardiac rehabilitation team's effectiveness, an overall protocol for patient progression in phase I is developed. Table 7-1 illustrates a protocol for cautious progression of a patient after a myocardial infarction (MI) or a coronary artery bypass graft surgery (CABG) through a phase I rehabilitation program. This protocol is based on recent literature indicating the safety and efficacy of early ambulation programs[9,19,28,37] as well as the prognostic value of early exercise testing before hospital discharge.[1,31,81,86] The protocol permits individualized treatment programs to be formulated based upon objective findings of evaluation. No blanket recommendations can be made for initial activity levels or speed of progression of each patient during phase I. Such recommendations would be overly optimistic for some patients and not progressive enough for others.

Phase I protocol

This protocol calls for a self-care evaluation as the first activity for the patient after myocardial or coronary artery bypass graft surgery (see Chapter 6). If no serious abnormalities are documented during the self-care evaluation, this level of activity is determined to be safe. The evaluator recommends to the referring physician that the patient perform these self-care activities as part of the daily routine.

We have developed an activity level chart to aid the referring physician to select an appropriate level of activity. The choice is based on the evaluation and treatment procedures performed by the cardiac rehabilitation team as well as the physician's medical assessment. These activity-level guidelines are illustrated in the boxed material. If the patient completes the self-care evaluation without significant cardiovascular problems, the recommendation is to clear the patient for activity level 4.

Monitored ambulation

Monitored ambulation refers to an individualized form of treatment where the patient participates in a walking program while being monitored one on one by a physical therapist. Initially, supine, sitting, and standing heart rates and blood pressures are recorded, and a resting single-lead electrocardiographic tracing is done. Heart and breath sounds may also be auscultated in selected patients (see

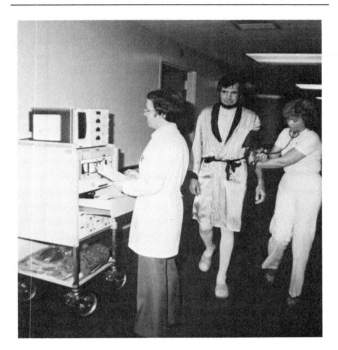

Fig. 7-1. Blood pressure and telemetry ECG are carefully monitored during ambulation. Blood pressures should be taken *while* walking, not afterwards.

Chapter 6). The patient is then ambulated under supervision by the therapist.

The initial distance walked is individualized for each patient. The total walk may vary from 10 to 20 feet for severely deconditioned and incapacitated patients and from 50 to 100 yards in the uncomplicated or less deconditioned patients. During the course of ambulation the physical therapist measures an ambulation blood pressure while a telemetry electrocardiogram is continuously being observed and recorded (Fig. 7-1). When ambulation is completed, the therapist evaluates the patient's hemodynamic and cardiovascular responses to determine whether activity progression is warranted (see Chapter 6).

During phase I, most patients begin with 2 to 5 minutes of continuous monitored ambulation and often progress to 15 to 30 minutes. The goal is to increase endurance at a relatively mild level of energy expenditure and document the cardiovascular responses at that level.

In most patients, this level of activity will provoke heart rates in the range of 80 to 125 beats per minute and systolic blood pressures of 90 to 150 mm Hg. If the patient is on drug therapy, which alters heart rate or blood pressure, values will be significantly lower. The overall rate pressure product during phase I will not usually exceed 20 $\times 10^3$ and is usually in the range of 7 to 15 $\times 10^3$. Thus, it is hoped that activity progression at low rate pressure products will not induce ischemic or other detrimental car-

diovascular responses and allow the patient to progress to higher levels of independent self-care and endurance. Abnormal responses at low rate pressure products is a signal that further medical intervention is necessary. Following are guidelines proposed as criteria for modifying or terminating monitored ambulation or the self-care evaluation during phase I:

1. Hypertensive blood pressure response (systolic greater than 180 mm Hg, diastolic blood pressure greater than 110 mm Hg).
2. Hypotensive systolic blood pressure response (greater than 10 to 15 mm Hg fall) (see Chapters 5 and 6).
3. Narrowing of the pulse pressure to less than 20 mm Hg between systolic and diastolic pressures.
4. Development of coupled premature ventricular contractions (PVC's) or a salvo of three or more PVC's in a row (ventricular tachycardia).
5. Greater than 10 PVC's per minute with ambulation.
6. PVC's with R-on-T phenomenon during exercise.
7. Level I/IV angina pectoris.
8. Onset of severe fatigue or dizziness.
9. 2 + /4 + dyspnea with ambulation.

When these signs or symptoms occur, the patient's physician is notified and appropriate documentation is made in the medical chart.

In keeping with McNeer's definition of complicated patients, the following criteria are proposed as contraindications to the initiation of phase I therapy:

1. Overt congestive heart failure.
2. Myocardial infarction or extension of infarction within the previous 2 days.
3. Second- or third-degree heart block, coupled with PVC's or ventricular tachycardia at rest.
4. Hypertensive resting blood pressure (systolic greater than 160 mm Hg, diastolic greater than 105 mm Hg).
5. Hypotensive resting blood pressure (systolic less than 80 mm Hg).
6. Greater than 10 to 15 PVC's per minute at rest, particularly if there is a variable coupling interval.
7. Severe aortic stenosis (gradient of $\geq$ 80 mm Hg).
8. Unstable angina pectoris with recent changes in symptoms (less than 24 hours).
9. Dissecting aortic aneurysm.
10. Uncontrolled metabolic diseases.
11. Psychosis or other unstable psychological condition.

Further medical management should precede phase I cardiac rehabilitation in these instances.

The deconditioning effects of bed rest are often cited as an indication that patients require inpatient cardiac rehabilitation.[90] However, with the shorter length of stay in coronary care units and earlier out-of-bed activities, the complications of excessive bed rest are rarely seen. Passive or active movement of the patient's extremities while in

```
10-60    18-108
11-66    19-114
12-72    20-120          Name _____ Dr. _____
13-78    21-126
14-84    22-132
15-90    23-138       INPATIENT EXERCISE LOG
16-96    24-144
17-102   25-150       TARGET HEART RATE _____
```

SPECIAL INSTRUCTION/PRECAUTIONS _____

_____

_____

Date	Rest. HR	Distance	Time	Peak HR	Symptoms or comments

Fig. 7-2. During the last few days of hospitalization, inpatients may ambulate independently utilizing this inpatient exercise log to record results.

bed can be better accomplished by the encouragement of self-care activities in and out of bed for active range of motion.

Quite frequently, the uncomplicated patients after myocardial infarction or coronary artery bypass graft perform their individualized ambulation activities on the ward several times each day. Instructions are given to capable patients to keep a record of their ambulation distance, time, and heart rate response as illustrated in Fig. 7-2. When the attending physician clears the patient for higher levels of activity, independent ambulation is done with the ward clerk monitoring the telemetry bed electrocardiograms. This monitoring method is more cost effective because the patient requires only one or two formal supervised and monitored ambulation sessions per day. The patient can then exercise an additional two to three times per day on his or her own. This independent ambulation improves the self-confidence of the patient and helps to psychologically prepare the patient for subsequent predischarge exercise testing.

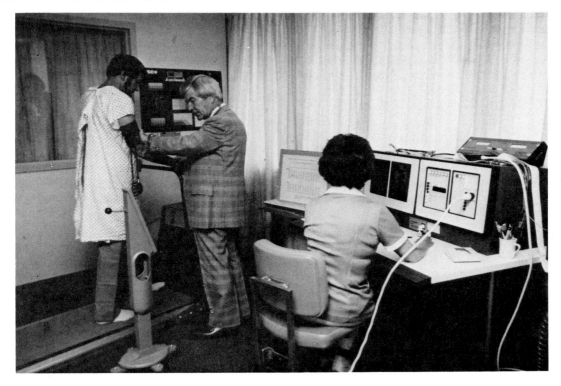

Fig. 7-3. Low-to-moderate level exercise testing before discharge gives valuable prognostic and therapeutic data.

Low to moderate level exercise testing

Before hospital discharge a properly completed multistage exercise test is essential for a number of reasons. First, several recent studies have documented the safety as well as prognostic value of such a test.[1,31,81,86] Since there are subsets of patients admitted with myocardial infarction or unstable angina who are at high risk of repeat infarction or of sudden death, particularly in the first few months after discharge, it is important that these high-risk patients be screened from those at lower risk. An exercise test done to a heart rate of 120 to 140 beats per minute depending on the patient is the best physiological evaluation tool currently available to uncover those patients at higher risk (see Chapter 6).

The low-level exercise test is important to perform on patients before hospital discharge because it gives the rehabilitation team information regarding the safety of recommending a patient resume home activities that require between 4 to 6 metabolic equivalents of exertion (i.e., driving, housework, sexual activity, etc.). High-risk persons will demonstrate a hypoadaptive blood pressure response,[75,87] 2 or more mm of ST-segment depression,[32,88,89] angina pectoris,[87] or complex ventricular arrhythmias with this type of predischarge exercise testing (see Chapters 5 and 6). With these test results the physician can accurately prescribe a return to these normal activities or recommend a lower functional level (Fig. 7-3).

The physical therapist can also use the test results to formulate the initial intensity of exercise training in the post–discharge phase II program. Finally, predischarge exercise testing also determines the effectiveness of medical therapy, particularly in complicated patients with angina, ventricular arrhythmias, or poor left ventricular function. Stein elicited angina in 29% of his post–myocardial infarction patients on early exercise testing, 55% of whom were not expected to have angina.[81] Severe arrhythmias were also seen in 31% of his patients, 60% of whom then required the addition of antiarrhythmic therapy. As a result of the testing, 47% of the population had their post–myocardial infarction medical therapy altered.[81]

Very little has been written on the value of this type of test for the postbypass patient[35,72]; however, we believe it to be an essential part of the overall patient evaluation before discharge. It helps to determine the patient's readiness for discharge and establish activity guidelines. Some centers have progressed to the use of symptom-limited maximal exercise testing for their postbypass patients before discharge.[72] The rationale is that with successful myocardial revascularization it is unlikely the patient will demonstrate abnormal responses to testing such as ST-segment depression or angina. However, it is expected that these patients will have blunted or hypoadaptive blood pressure response because of their anemia or temporary postoperative ventricular dysfunction. They will usually be very tachycardic with exertion, fatigue easily, and quite often demonstrate atrial irritability (i.e., premature atrial contractions, short runs of supraventricular tachycardia, etc.) during exercise.

A poor work capacity with angina and pronounced ST-segment changes (greater than 2 mm) is suggestive that other vessels are "at risk" or a zone of ischemia exists around an infarcted area. Additional drug therapy such as beta blocking agents and long-acting nitrates may be needed for these patients to exercise. These drugs should optimally be used in a phase II program after discharge where close monitoring is available. Surprisingly, very few arrhythmias have occurred during this low to moderate level exercise testing in the early post–myocardial infarction period.[6] This supports the safety of this predischarge exercise test.

At the Ross-Loos Medical Center in Los Angeles patients had low-level exercise tests a mean of 8 days after the myocardial infarction. Of these patients, 6% were found to have serious ventricular arrhythmias (greater than 10 premature ventricular contractions per minute, couplets, or ventricular tachycardia).[8] By identification of those complicated patients before discharge and elimination of them or modification of their program, the remaining patients were not prevented from progressing quickly and safely.

Case studies

The five case studies included in Appendices A through E (pp. 158 to 164) illustrate individualized protocol planning and its effective use. Included are a typical uncomplicated postbypass patient and a severely impaired patient with multiple complications after infarction.

PHASE II—OUTPATIENT CARDIAC REHABILITATION

The term "phase II" refers to that part of the cardiac rehabilitation program conducted on an outpatient basis immediately after hospitalization. It involves a closely supervised and carefully monitored exercise program with a structured basic education series. This program may include patients who have been recently discharged from the hospital, either after myocardial infarction or after coronary bypass surgery. Other patients who may be included in a phase II program are those with stable angina pectoris hypertrophic cardiomyopathy, or mitral valve prolapse with ventricular arrhythmias, or asymptomatic patients with latent coronary artery disease.

Following are purposes of phase II programs:
1. Increase exercise capacity and endurance in a safe and progressive manner.
2. Ensure the continuity of the exercise program with a transition to the home environment.

3. Assess the cardiovascular responses of mild to moderate external work loads and give feedback to the referring physician.
4. Teach the patient to apply techniques of self-monitoring to home activities.
5. Obtain monitored objective information on medication effectiveness in such areas as angina, blood pressure regulation, and arrhythmia control.
6. Relieve anxiety and depression.
7. Increase the patient's knowledge of the atherosclerotic disease process and how personal health habits affect it.

It is advantageous for patients to be referred to phase II immediately after hospital discharge. In addition to the medical reasons previously discussed, coronary patients are more easily influenced and educated at this time because of fear and anxiety about their health and longevity. As many studies have documented, coronary patients go through an adjustment period after a myocardial infarction consisting of initial denial or anger followed by depression.[17,82] Cardiac rehabilitation is the process that directs and supports physical, emotional, and psychological recovery. We believe it is a process that should begin in the hospital and continue without interruption.

Training program

Physical training of patients in phase II requires consideration of many variables. These variables include exercise intensity, duration, frequency and mode, age, sex, general musculoskeletal status of the patient, time since myocardial infarction or coronary bypass surgery, size of the infarction, subsequent complications such as development of angina pectoris or other signs of myocardial ischemia, and medications, as well as the patient's own goals. In addition, specific monitoring needs are identified in phase II to assist in individualizing the training programs. The five key monitoring techniques and tools are (1) heart rate, (2) blood pressure, (3) electrocardiogram, (4) heart sounds, and (5) signs and symptoms. An individualized approach to each patient utilizing these variables is required (see Chapter 6).

Identification of lower extremity problems before initiation of cardiovascular training may prevent the development of orthopaedic problems. These kinds of problems develop frequently in middle-aged and older people who embark on exercise programs. A brief musculoskeletal evaluation is necessary for identification of lower extremity problems such as arthritis, old orthopaedic injuries, and unusual biomechanical abnormalities (excessive pronation of the foot, genu valgum). Although in many cases these biomechanical abnormalities are of no consequence in a patient's everyday routine, under specific lower extremity training, they may develop into symptomatic orthopaedic problems that will interfere with the normal cardiovascular conditioning program.

The current literature supports a phase II training pro-

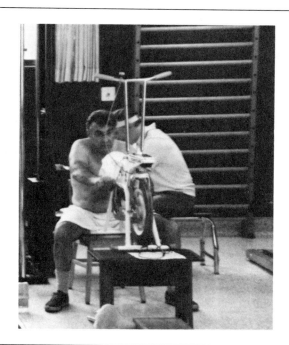

Fig. 7-4. Upper extremity ergometry may be done when a stationary bike is placed on a chair and stool.

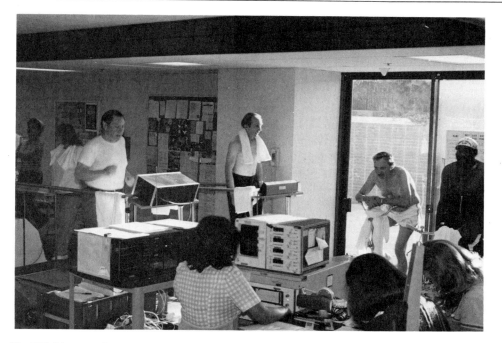

Fig. 7-5. Many cardiac patients will prefer treadmill exercise in phase II, though bicycle ergometers are necessary for those with lower extremity orthopaedic problems.

gram that is varied in nature and includes a combination of upper and lower extremity training.[30,92] Training of the lower extremities is specific to the lower extremities, and there is little cardiovascular carry-over to upper extremity work and vice versa.[14] Therefore, since a goal of physical conditioning is reduction of myocardial oxygen demand with arm or leg activities at any given level of submaximal work, it is essential to train both arms and legs (Fig. 7-4). Lower extremity aerobic exercise is accomplished with stationary equipment such as treadmills and bicycle ergometers (Fig. 7-5). Upper extremity training is done with arm ergometer units and rowing machines. Programs that employ this type of equipment can improve both endurance and physical work capacity of post–myocardial infarction and postbypass patients during phase II. A variety of programs that include oxygen-demanding cardiovascular exercises can be planned with this equipment; however, upper extremity training is not started until 3 to 4 weeks after surgery in postbypass patients. Chest soreness and bone healing precludes aggressive armwork for several weeks after bypass surgery.

Intensity of exercise

Before entering into phase II, outpatients are exercise tested. A low to moderate level test with a predetermined end point is appropriate for the early post–myocardial infarction and postbypass patient. The training intensity of exercise during phase II should be a percentage of the maximum heart rate achieved on this exercise test. The goal of physical training for the early post–myocardial infarction and postbypass patient is oriented toward an endurance gain, and so training levels are set at an intensity of work that will not interfere with the healing process or produce cardiovascular complications.

In our experience training post–myocardial infarction and postbypass patients, we noted that patients were able to tolerate training at 80% to 95% of the heart rate achieved during the low level test. Training at this level is not associated with any increased risk of reinfarction, congestive heart failure, or other morbidity or mortality.[6] The patients referred for a phase II program are monitored continuously by a telemetry electrocardiographic system throughout each exercise session. Occasionally, we have found that patients who demonstrate no arrhythmias or symptoms on a low to moderate level exercise test may exhibit one or more of these symptoms during the initial sessions in phase II. Again, close communication with the private physician and medical director is required to ensure medical stabilization of these patients.

Early post–myocardial infarction and postbypass patients can usually only tolerate 10 to 15 minutes of continuous low-intensity training. The emphasis during this initial 2 to 4 weeks is on increasing the peak interval time to 30 to 45 minutes of continuous exercise.

After the first 2 to 3 weeks of phase II, patients with good blood pressure responses, no ECG abnormalities, and no angina are progressed to an increased level of intensity by raising the target heart rate 10 beats per minute. For uncomplicated patients, the target heart rate during exercise may be raised 10 beats every 1 to 2 weeks. Complicated patients may have their target heart rate increased, or they may stay at the same level until the maximum exercise test is done. Increases in the intensity of training (target heart rate increases) are determined by careful review of the patient's monitored responses. If the patient exhibits angina, serious arrhythmias, poor blood pressure responses, symptoms of poor ventricular function, or mus-

culoskeletal difficulties, the intensity of exercise may remain unchanged or even be decreased. As these abnormalities resolve or decrease in severity, closely supervised work load increases are applied. Each time the target heart rate is raised to a higher level, close attention is paid to symptomatic and physiological adaptations to the higher training levels. Complicated patients who are limited by angina, have excessively hypertensive blood pressure responses, or develop ventricular arrhythmias require close monitoring. Oral and written communication regarding these medical problems are maintained with the patient's physician (see Chapter 9). Phase II is similar to phase I in its monitoring methods and examination of the effectiveness of medical management during the early recovery process.

Supervision and program progression

Progression to an independent exercise program is a goal during phase II. Promoting the ability to exercise only within the monitored hospital-based sessions fosters an attitude of dependency on the electronic hardware and supervisory personnel who conduct the exercise sessions. Ultimately, a cardiac rehabilitation program should attempt to develop an attitude of self-responsibility for medical care, including the physical exercise program. It has been our experience that patients improve more rapidly psychologically when they reach a state of illness adjustment that acknowledges their contribution to their health and a willingness to accept the responsibility for performing home exercise. During phase II, the patient usually progresses to 30 to 45 minutes of continuous lower extremity exercise and is encouraged to perform 10 to 15 minutes of continuous upper extremity exercise as well. With this combination the overall peak exercise period is approximately 45 to 60 minutes. A 5-minute warm-up and cool-down period precedes and terminates all training sessions. The frequency of exercise recommended is three times per week with the supervision and monitoring of the program. The patients assume personal responsibility for monitoring and the completion of additional exercise sessions at home. Home sessions begin in the first 1 to 2 weeks of phase II. The patients exercise for the same period of time and at similar training intensities as the sessions conducted at the hospital. The total number of exercise sessions recommended per week is five or six. The physical therapist can review problems the patient has during home exercise sessions when the patient comes in for monitored follow-up sessions. Medical intervention and program modifications are made at that time.

Monitoring of patients during phase II exercise employs continuous portable radiotelemetry electrocardiographic equipment (see Chapter 9) and continues for up to 6 weeks in uncomplicated patients and longer as necessary for more complicated patients. Continuous ECG monitoring of every exercise session does not last more than 8 to 12

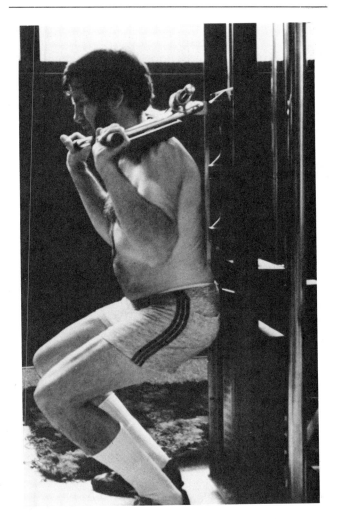

Fig. 7-6. This cardiac patient, who had coronary artery bypass surgery (CABG) 8 weeks before, is performing half-squats with 70 pounds.

weeks unless arrhythmias are consistently documented. Each patient "weans off" the monitor by decreasing to every other and then every third session. This process continues until "spot" checks are performed with paddle defibrillators. By the end of phase II, the majority of patients rely only on self-monitoring their heart rate.

In addition, we have found it of value to incorporate some form of "anaerobic" training into the second half of phase II. A weight training program individualized to each patient that emphasizes high repetitions and low weights is a safe and effective adjunct (Fig. 7-6). This type of training has proved valuable to help patients recover quickly from myocardial infarction or coronary bypass surgery. Weight training improves both peripheral muscle tone and strength. It adds to their self-confidence, and they are better able to perform daily activities. Most daily activities,

either around the home or at work, are not aerobic in nature and often require some degree of static effort. Examples of anaerobic activities include yard work, grocery shopping, and housework such as vacuuming, mopping, or window washing. Since these activities do require muscle strength, incorporating mild strength training into the phase II program is essential.

Selected patients who are candidates for weight training include myocardial infarction patients a minimum of 3 weeks after the event and surgical patients 3 to 4 weeks after the bypass. A multistation apparatus is used for three selected arm and leg exercises. Patients are instructed to avoid the Valsalva maneuver and to coordinate inhalation and exhalation with the concentric and eccentric phases of the exercise movements (Fig. 7-7). Usually two sets of a weight that can be handled easily for 10 to 12 repetitions is the starting point. The emphasis is initially on adding sets the first 2 to 3 weeks, and weight usually 5 to 10 pounds at a time is added the next 2 to 3 weeks. Continuous ECG monitoring is done during the initial anaerobic exercise sessions. In our experience the myocardial oxygen demand is lower during anaerobic training than during the aerobic portion of the training program as measured by lower rate pressure products. We have observed few ventricular arrhythmias and have had no complications during this type of "isotonic" exercise. As the patient is weaned off telemetry monitoring at the end of phase II, we encourage non–ECG monitored weight training with therapist supervision. Many patients who graduate from our phase II program continue with weight training either at home, in phase III, or at a local health club.

Safety in phase II

The early post–myocardial infarction and postbypass patient is at high risk of cardiovascular complications during the first 3 to 6 months after discharge from the hospital.[60] Statistics show that early exercise conditioning during this period and later is not associated with any higher risk of morbidity and mortality.[5,6,85] At the Ross-Loos Medical Center we studied 85 post–myocardial infarction patients who were entered into an early exercise training program immediately after hospital discharge. The patients were divided into complicated and uncomplicated groups based on McNeer's criteria (see Chapter 6). During 802 patient hours of early exercise training there were no adverse effects noted in either subgroup.[6] Since 1979 in the rehabilitation program at Presbyterian Intercommunity Hospital at Whittier, California, we have had over 10,000 hours of early exercise conditioning accumulated in phase II with no cardiovascular mortality and no cardiac arrest.

Basic patient education lecture series

Our phase II program offers a series of lectures conducted by several team members. These talks are designed to educate the cardiac patient about atherosclerosis, the

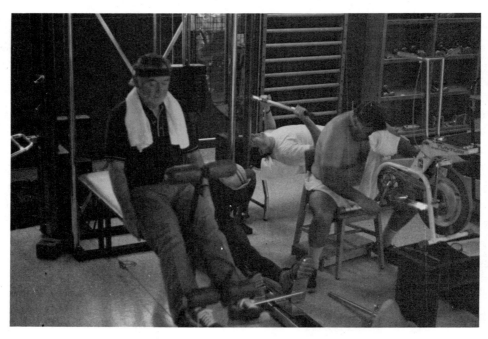

Fig. 7-7. The patient in the foreground is exhaling during concentric work with 40 pounds (knee extensions), whereas the other patient is inhaling during eccentric work with 50 pounds (bench press).

CARDIAC REHABILITATION PROGRAM
BASIC PATIENT EDUCATION SERIES

Time: 4:00 to 5:00 P.M.   *Place:* Santa Fe Springs Room

Date:	Lecture topic	Instructor
Jan. 5	Structure and function of the heart, coronary atherosclerosis, heart attack, angina pectoris, coronary bypass	Larry Cahalin, RPT
Jan. 7	The causes of atherosclerosis (risk factors and atherosclerosis)	Diane Tatman, RPT
Jan. 10	Cardiac medications: their purposes and side effects	Joyce Knopp, RN
Jan. 12	The therapeutic effects of exercise	Peggy Johnson, RPT
	Film: Quite an Accomplishment	
Jan. 14	Managing stress: film and discussion	Barbara Lane, MSW
Jan. 17	Diet, blood fats, and coronary artery disease	Karen Broxson, RD
Jan. 19	Sex and the heart patient*	Barbara Lane, MSW
Jan. 21	Shaking the salt habit: Relationship of diet and hypertension	Karen Broxson, RD
Jan. 24	*Film: Coping with Life on the Run*	Dr. George Sheehan
	Film: The Cardiac TransAmerica Express	Randy Ice, RPT
	*Please bring spouse or significant other to the January nineteenth talk on sex	

---

risk factors for heart disease, and the effects of exercise, diet, stress, and medications on this disease (see boxed material). Often, patients do not retain the educational information provided during phase I because they are not receptive to learning during their acute hospitalization. Learning is enhanced when the patient is out of the hos-

pital and living in a familiar environment. A variety of audiovisual aids (slides, movies, posters, etc.) are used to simplify concepts (atherogenesis, role of smoking, and diet in disease progression).

Individual conference sessions are also helpful. For example, fasting serum lipid panels are routinely obtained

LIPID PROFILE

Name: _____		Risk		Total Chol/HDL
Date: _____	Men:	$\frac{1}{2}$	Average	3.43
Initial _____ F/U _____			Average	4.97
Cholesterol _____		2X	Average	9.55
Triglycerides _____		3X	Average	23.39
HDL _____	Women:	$\frac{1}{2}$	Average	3.27
LDL _____			Average	4.44
VLDL _____		2X	Average	7.05
Total Chol/HDL _____		3X	Average	11.04

Fig. 7-8. This lipid profile form is used to give feedback to each patient on initial and serial lipid results.

(cholesterol, triglycerides, HDL, LDL, and VLDL cholesterol, and phenotype) on all patients 4 weeks after a myocardial infarction or surgery (Fig. 7-8). These lipids are reviewed individually with each patient and covered again during the dietitian's lecture. This serves as a base line for measuring the effects of the intervention program every 6 months thereafter (see Chapter 8). A written multiple-choice pretest was recently developed by our team to measure the level of knowledge and understanding of outpatients before starting the education series. The same test was given at the end of the 4-week lecture series for assessment of each patient's learning. Collection of data on the before and after tests over the last few years has been helpful in improving our teaching methods and determining the level of understanding and knowledge obtained by individual patients.

Termination of phase II

Because phase II is considered a recovery period as well as a physical conditioning time, the process usually takes a minimum of 6 to 8 weeks. Post–myocardial infarction and postbypass patients who make initial endurance gains by 6 to 8 weeks after the event are often anxious to pursue higher intensity exercise and other activities (bowling, golf, hiking, swimming, running, camping in the mountains, etc.). At this point, our protocol calls for a maximal symptom-limited exercise test. The patient is exercise tested through a symptom-limited end point (see Chapter 6). This test serves as a diagnostic procedure to further evaluate the extent of coronary artery disease in post–myocardial infarction patients and provides an objective measurement of physical work capacity. A maximal symptom-limited test will also indicate the effectiveness of revascu-

larization procedures and documents any symptomatic changes with exercise.

If the patient does exceptionally well on the maximal exercise test, the patient's physician may clear them to return to either full- or part-time work and the patient will have completed phase II. At the completion of phase II the patient is encouraged to continue a physical training program independently at home with further instructions from the physical therapist. Our patients are encouraged to continue cardiac rehabilitation participation in a phase III program.

Return to work after phase II

Literature regarding return-to-work statistics for post–myocardial infarction or postbypass patients participating in phase II cardiac rehabilitation programs is sparse. There are many variables that influence return to work after the onset of coronary artery disease. Many of these variables are completely unrelated to the degree of coronary disease or myocardial damage. Such factors as employment before myocardial infarction or bypass surgery, job satisfaction, employer attitudes, financial incentives, physician attitude, and other socioeconomic factors play a role in determining whether a post–myocardial infarction or postbypass patient will return to work. Cardiac rehabilitation promotes a positive attitude toward return to work for such patients. This attitude is instilled early in a phase II training program.

In our experience, 75% to 80% of rehabilitated patients will return to work within 8 to 10 weeks after myocardial infarction. In our rehabilitation program, of the 75% of the total postbypass patients who worked before surgery, 62% go back to work after surgery. In a control group of patients who did not undergo cardiac rehabilitation, the percentages before and after surgery were very similar; however, cardiac rehabilitation patients returned to work an average of almost 40 days sooner than nonrehabilitation patients.[85] Our work supports the concept that a cardiac rehabilitation environment fosters the concept of early return to work and may reduce the length of disability after bypass surgery. This finding is significant in light of the fact that many studies have lamented the clear-cut lack of improvement in return to work after coronary bypass surgery.[3,33,53]

Results of training

Exercise training begun early after myocardial infarction or bypass surgery is new and consequently there is little in the literature on its effects. Blessey and others[8] examined the effects of early exercise training in 85 post–myocardial infarction patients. These patients were subdivided into complicated and uncomplicated subsets based on McNeer's criteria. The exercise training was started between 7 and 14 days after myocardial infarction, and all patients had a low level exercise test before referral to the program. These patients were trained at 75% of their actual maximum heart rates as determined from their maximum exercise test, which were completed after their phase II program (approximately 6 to 8 weeks after the event).

Fifty-two of the uncomplicated patients had a better performance on both the predischarge low level test and post-training maximum exercise test when compared with 33 complicated patients. After training, both groups of patients demonstrated significantly better exercise capacity on maximum exercise testing when compared to age- and sex-matched controls.

During the phase II follow-up period, 9% of patients in each group demonstrated either resting or exercise hypertension or the new onset of angina. Complex ventricular arrhythmias were observed in a total of six patients, with five of these being in the complicated group. Follow-up of 802 patient hours of early exercise training revealed no cardiovascular morbidity or mortality in either subset. Thus it was concluded that selected patients, uncomplicated and complicated, could safely participate and respond favorably to early exercise training. Uncomplicated patients had a tendency to demonstrate a better exercise tolerance initially as well as after training, and they were less likely to have complex ventricular arrhythmias.[8] The case studies illustrate examples of post–myocardial infarction and postbypass patients that have progressed through a phase II training program and responded in a very favorable fashion.

PHASE III—OUTPATIENT CARDIAC REHABILITATION
Overview of phase III

A phase III cardiac rehabilitation program (also known as phase IV or "maintenance" in some facilities) is an ongoing, supervised, exercise conditioning program. It provides the coronary artery disease patient the opportunity to achieve a higher level of physical, mental, and sociological function. Typically, a phase III program provides incentives for the patient to continue a lifelong habit of exercise, risk factor reduction, and on-going education. These programs should also provide a mechanism for serial evaluation to assess progress and disease stability.

Typically, patients referred for phase III rehabilitation programs are post–myocardial infarction or postbypass surgery and are at least 4 to 6 weeks after the event. Patients with stable angina pectoris or patients who have abnormal exercise tests or who are asymptomatic and have a high risk for the development of symptomatic coronary disease are also referred to phase III. Many phase III programs are open ended without discharge criteria. The patient also assumes a greater financial burden in a phase III program after the initial 6 months to 1 year.

Although several nonrandomized studies have suggested a decreased morbidity and mortality for patients who participate in long-term cardiac rehabilitation,[38,39,45] randomized trials have not been as supportive.[68,78,93] Compliance with the prescribed program is a major problem in both types of study. This difficulty exists because of the nature of the life-style changes involved. Typically, the noncompliant cardiac rehabilitation patient is a habitual smoker, is a blue-collar worker, spends leisure time in sedentary activities, and works at a job that requires little energy expenditure.[62] Frequently with long-term rehabilitation programs, the participant rate may drop to as little as 30% to 40% after the first year and decrease at a rate of 10% per year thereafter (see Chapter 8). The reasons for this high drop-out rate may relate to psychological changes the patient is experiencing. Fear will motivate most patients for only a short period of time, and compliance with exercise, diet, nonsmoking, etc., will change as fear abates. Over the long run, compliance will come only with external and internal rewards for behavior modification. If the patient perceives his life-style change to be one of deprivation and giving up enjoyable life habits such as smoking, eating highly saturated fat foods, or a high-pressure job and if these needs are not replaced with habits that are equally or more rewarding, it is only a matter of time until the patient returns to his premorbid level of risk factors and life-style. The phase III program should provide ongoing rewards, feedback, and encouragement to help the patient adjust to this kind of problem and successfully adhere to the program.

Location of phase III program

To establish a phase III program, one has to examine the personnel available to staff a program, the geographic location, and the medical support systems available. The minimum equipment requirement for phase III include a radiotelemetry system with the capability to monitor patients exercising on a track, an outdoor exercise area preferably with lights, locker rooms with shower facilities,

---

CARDIAC REHABILITATION PROGRAM
ADVANCED LECTURE SERIES
JANUARY AND FEBRUARY 1983

Time: 6:00 PM   *Location:* Hacienda Heights Room
Date: *Lecture topic:*   *Speaker:*
Jan. 3   Cardiopulmonary "Heartsaver" course (open to all)   Rehab. faculty
                             Note: On this night, we will have "Dance For Your
                             Heart." All rehab. members and spouses will par-
                             ticipate in an aerobic dance session led by Sarah
                             Shea. I will personally sponsor all participants for
                             1¢ per minute of dancing.
Jan. 10   *Videocassette and discussion:* "Treatment of Obes-   Karen Broxson, RD
                             ity"
Jan. 17   *Film: Stress and the "Hot Reactor"*   John Camp, MD
Jan. 24   *Film: Heart Attacks*   Randy Ice, RPT
Jan. 31   *Guest speaker:* The U.S.C. Lipid-Lowering Study   Miguel Sanmarco, MD
Feb. 7   *Discussion:* Coping with illness   Barbara Lane, MSW
Feb. 21   *Lecture:* Oh my aching back! Prevention and treat-   Randy Ice, RPT
                             ment of low back pain
Feb. 28   *Lecture:* A survey of home exercise devices: their   Sarah Shea and Randy Ice, RPT
                             cost and effectiveness

AEROBIC DANCING

For the month of January, we will have aerobic dancing offered *every* Monday as part of the American Heart Association's Dance For
Heart program. The idea is to get sponsors to pay you for dancing aerobically for 1 to 4 hours (it's your choice). All participants will
be expected to dance on January 3, while the other dates are optional. Aerobic dancing will be on February 14 and 28.
Remember on February 12 the Fourth Annual Walk/Jog/Run/Wheel For your Heart 5 or 10 km.

---

and an educational room with facilities for audiovisual aids such as slides, movie projectors, or videocassette systems (see Chapter 9).

Since the patient has achieved a higher level of fitness by phase III and requires less supervision and monitoring, a greater variety of exercise modalities and procedures can be carried out. For this reason, phase III programs can be established at either a hospital facility or a community facility such as a YMCA, health club, or college. Hospital-based facilities have the advantage of greater continuity for patients progressing from phase I through phase III. They also provide complete medical support systems for any emergencies that occur. Unfortunately, many hospitals lack both space and varied exercise equipment. Another disadvantage is that hospitals are considered a place where "sick people" go. Community-based facilities have the advantage of being geographically closer to patients' homes and usually have adequate equipment and space. Their disadvantages lies in less medical support and a breakup of the continuity in phases I, II, and III. Competitive environments, which may cause patients to exceed safe exercise limits, often exist in these facilities.

Purpose of phase III

The designated purpose of the phase III program is to improve the physical fitness and endurance level in coro-

nary patients as well as produce long-term reductions in coronary risk factors (see Chapter 8). In addition, the program should improve the patient's knowledge of his or her disease process and role in health maintenance. Because most patients ready for and referred to phase III programs are working, the program is usually conducted in the evening between the hours of 4:30 and 9:00 PM. This scheduling encourages the patient to continue working as a productive contributing member of society while providing an ongoing individualized training program to evaluate his or her progress and disease stability. Coronary artery disease is a progressive disease process. Despite maximum medical therapy, the disease may jeopardize the patients' lives and may produce unstable symptoms. By being seen on a regular basis in a phase III program patients have an ongoing weekly or monthly evaluation, which may detect changes in the course of the disease.

We also incorporate an advanced educational series that continues to build on the knowledge of inpatient education lectures presented during phase II. They provide continued information on new therapeutic or diagnostic techniques in coronary disease, ongoing dietary management, cooking workshops, psychological intervention to reduce stress and adjust to illness, and motivational talks from inspirational speakers (see boxed material).

A major objective of cardiac rehabilitation is to enhance

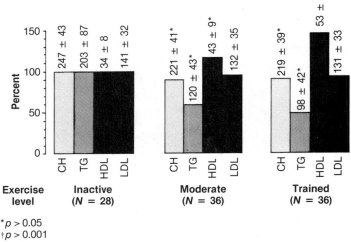

Fig. 7-9. *Inactive,* no exercise. *Moderate,* 1 to 2 hours of exercise per week. *Trained,* 5 to 6 hours of exercise per week. Mean follow-up time, 36 months (unpublished data). *HDL,* High-density lipoproteins; *LDL,* low-density lipoproteins; *CH,* carbohydrates; *TG,* triglycerides.

the patient's quality of life. Indeed, phase III programs through group interaction, peer support, and comraderie helps contribute to this improved quality of life. We have also found that if the program can be oriented toward the production of research articles patients are more likely to comply because they feel as though they are contributing to a body of knowledge that will benefit others, including their family members and children.

Training program

Patients referred into the phase III program must undergo an evaluation procedure not unlike phase II; that is, the patient is interviewed and goals are established. A chart review to obtain the clinical medical history and pertinent laboratory data must be taken (see Chapter 6). We require all our patients to have a lipoprotein profile including total serum cholesterol, total serum triglycerides, HDL cholesterol, LDL cholesterol, VLDL cholesterol, and phenotype before beginning the exercise program. A maximal symptom-limited exercise test is required. The results of that test are used to determine initial levels of physical work and establish initial training target heart rates and monitoring needs. Establishing a training intensity includes development of a target heart rate range. This range of target heart rate training intensity should be high enough to produce cardiac (central) improvements. This is a level of exercise that is at least 60% of the total chronotropic reserve; that is, the target heart rate should be at least 60% of the difference between a resting and maximal heart rate.[92] (Resting heart rate minus maximum heart rate times 60% plus the resting heart rate)—this formula is referred to as Karvonen's formula.

This is only a rough guideline, however, because many other clinical variables should be considered. These vari-

ables include angina, drop in systolic blood pressure or ST-segment depression of greater than 3 to 4 mm, medications, severe dyspnea, fatigue, musculoskeletal limitations, and the patient's goals.

In phase III, emphasizing distance goals and not speed is of primary importance.[44] It is our impression that not enough emphasis is placed in cardiac rehabilitation on encouraging the patient to train for longer periods of time, particularly those patients with greater degrees of lipid or carbohydrate metabolism abnormalities. Research we have done on coronary patients who either ran or bicycled more than 5 to 6 hours per week demonstrated consistently higher HDL cholesterol levels as compared to men who exercised only 1 to 2 hours per week. The latter subset also demonstrated higher HDL cholesterol than patients who did no training at all (Fig. 7-9).

Many patients may not desire to train at high intensities and desire only the level of training that is minimum required to maintain fitness. This may be achieved with low to moderate levels of exercise training by emphasizing increasing the duration of exercise. Thus the mode, intensity, frequency, and duration of each patient's program is individualized to the capabilities and interests of that patient. It is the physical therapist's responsibility to direct the progress of the patients from week to week. It may include telemetry monitoring, particularly in the first several weeks for new patients or only periodically for patients who have graduated from the phase II program. All patients are oriented to proper clothing and, in particular, are given instructions in proper footwear. The patient will often progress from walking to jogging or running and needs good footwear to prevent orthopaedic injuries. Our sessions are conducted on a track either at the hospital or at a local community school site. The therapist works with each patient individually and helps the patient achieve a desired level of training intensity and gradually increases the duration from 30 minutes to 45 to 60 minutes per session.

Advanced lecture series

Immediately after the phase III exercise session, the group education session is conducted by any of a number of cardiac rehabilitation team members. The dietitian may discuss weight-loss programs, diets, or the polyunsaturated versus saturated fat controversy. The social worker or psychologist may discuss stress and its management and coping with illness or family adjustments. Current advances in diagnostic or therapeutic cardiology are often presented by an invited speaker. Individual case study presentation of patients who have shown excellent improvement serve to give the patient a "pat on the back" and motivate newer patients to persevere in their own rehabilitation efforts.

A basic CPR course (usually the heart-saver course) is taught every 6 to 12 months so that all patients and family members are certified in basic life support. This is done not only out of concern over the patient's risk of sudden death, but because these patients are educated about the causes of coronary artery disease and its risk factors and can respond to other emergency situations in an appropriate fashion.

In summary, we have found these advanced patient education lectures to be very valuable in maintaining a viable active and interesting phase III program. To help to enhance overall compliance, rewards are given out to the patients and inspirational guest speakers.

Phase III compliance programming

Several years ago we started week-end activity programs (jogging and cycling clubs) as one mechanism of facilitating patient compliance and to assist in a achievement of maximum fitness levels in an environment of social comraderie and support. The SCOR Cardiac Cyclists Club and SCOR Jogging Club have now been in existence for 9 and 7 years respectively. Cardiac patients, spouses, and family members are in each club and participate in week-end endurance-building activities.

The cycling club began in 1974 with a flat 15-mile bike ride on Saturday morning with four or five selected patients from our phase III program. The club now has over 60 cardiac patients, many of whom complete 100-mile (century) rides routinely. More recently, several ambitious patients in the cycling club decided to bicycle across the United States. The Cardiac Transamerica Relay Ride was a 24-hour per day nonstop bicycle relay ride that left Los Angeles on June 5, 1982, and set a United States Cycling Federation Relay Ride record of 12 days, 1 hour, and 50 minutes and arrived in Central Park in New York City on June 17, 1982. Fourteen men with coronary artery disease made the trip to demonstrate the benefits of cardiac reha-

bilitation and the value of an anticoronary life-style. In this ride, each patient rode 1 to 2 hours at their own pace each day. There were no cardiovascular complications during the 3000-mile trip, and none were anticipated. The actual physical exercise of 1 to 2 hours of bicycling each day was less than most of what these patients do on their own in training sessions with the club and at home. Environmental factors of heat, altitude, and hills were the only variables that imposed additional demands on these patients, but even these factors were well tolerated by all the riders.

Collectively, the SCOR Cardiac Cyclists Club has ridden over 400,000 miles. Only two cardiac events have occurred during exercise in the last 8 years.[42] A 59-year-old postbypass patient sustained a myocardial infraction while cycling. He had continued to smoke cigarettes and had a very complicated course with multiple cardiac arrests. He survived this event and was found to have occluded all his bypass grafts. Despite this, he eventually recovered sufficiently to rejoin the cycling club. The other incident was a 56-year-old man who had an extensive anterior wall myocardial infarction 17 years before his sudden death while cycling. His ventricular function was fair at best with a resting ejection fraction of 31%. Yet, despite this, he rode with the club for over 7 years and made dramatic improvements in his stamina and endurance.

These two case examples serve to illustrate an important factor to remember in long-term cardiac rehabilitation. Despite the medical and surgical interventions currently available coronary artery disease is an enigma, and episodic recurrent events are sometimes unpredictable. Their temporal relationship to exercise may imply a slightly greater risk of training but are probably offset by the long-term protective effects observed in multiple nonrandomized uncontrolled rehabilitation studies[39,45,77] (see Chapter 8).

The SCOR Jogging Club has undergone a similar metamorphosis with over 75 patients now participating in Saturday morning training sessions at various locations around Los Angeles (Fig. 7-10). Ten patients have trained to a level of successfully completing a marathon. One man with triple-vessel disease has completed over 85 marathons in the last 5 years. Many patients are routinely participating in week-end 5 and 10 km runs in a noncompetitive fashion. Family participation is strongly encouraged in these clubs, and both spouses and children often train with these patients on weekend outings.

To achieve these levels of fitness, patients in phase III begin by either walking on the track or perhaps on a treadmill indoors and progress to walk-jogging and later to continuous jogging as they can tolerate it. When the physical therapist observes the patient is stable, requires infrequent monitoring, and has developed a basic fitness that is compatible with these weekend activities, the patient is encouraged to join the jogging or biking club. This is usually at least 2 months after starting the phase III program.

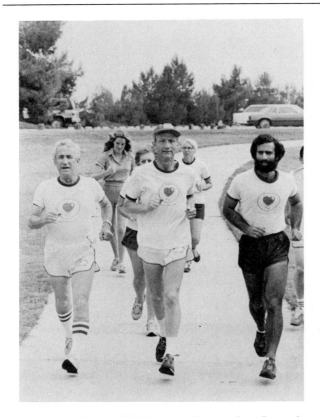

Fig. 7-10. Ray Blessey, R.P.T., runs with several cardiac patients, their spouses and family members on a typical Saturday morning SCOR Jogging Club meeting.

The overall accomplishments of the patients in both of these groups (1) provides good public relations for the patient's hospital and cardiac rehabilitation program and (2) serves as very positive feedback for new patients. The tremendous life-style changes and fitness improvements that these patients have demonstrated over relatively short periods of time are inspirational and motivational for patients and staff of the program.

Reevaluation in phase III

Patients who participate in phase III programs for greater than 6 months need periodic assessment of their disease stability. We have a protocol for doing this, which is standardized but flexible enough to meet specific patient requirements. For example, for assessment of lipid changes, particularly HDL cholesterol, sufficient training time is necessary. A lipid profile is routinely repeated after 3 months in the program and every 6 months thereafter. These results are always sent to the referring physician and are individually reviewed by the therapist or dietitian with the patient. If the patient's lipid values are worse, and the

change appears to be the result of an improper diet, individual counseling is done with the team dietitian. If all dietary and training modes of intervention have failed to improve lipid values, the referring physician will be contacted and alternative therapy (drugs, medication changes) will be discussed.

In terms of monitoring disease stability we recommend two follow-up procedures: (1) periodic ECG monitoring during exercise and (2) all patients being instructed to record hospital and home exercise sessions in a monthly diary (Fig. 7-11). These serial exercise sheets are turned into the physical therapist at the end of each month. A review of these diaries by the physical therapist may uncover subtle changes in performance or the presence of new symptoms. Either finding can indicate disease progression and need for repeat assessments.

We attempt to monitor electrocardiographically all phase III patients at least once every 4 to 8 weeks during an exercise session. Although some patients will tell you when they feel arrhythmias in their pulse, some patients will not feel them or perhaps do not regularly take their pulse. Routine monitoring during moderate to high intensity exercise, particularly in the cool-down phase, may help to detect asymptomatic ventricular arrhythmias or ST-segment changes. Blood pressure responses to exercise are also an important factor to follow (see Chapters 5 and 6).

We repeat a maximum symptom-limited exercise test every 6 months to 1 year on patients enrolled in phase III. This is the best noninvasive means of measuring functional improvement (increased time or increased maximal oxygen uptake) and coronary disease stability. A decrease in exercise tolerance, an increase in ST-segment abnormalities, abnormal blood pressure responses, and the appearence of ventricular arrhythmias or angina may be indicative of worsening coronary disease. Communication of these findings to the patient's referring practitioner often results in medication changes or further evaluative and therapeutic procedures to prevent any cardiac event. The frequency of this testing is every 3 to 6 months in new, particularly complicated patients, or every 12 months in uncomplicated apparently stable patients. An important point to emphasize is that coronary patients demonstrate training changes that develop more slowly than healthy subjects of the same age. Thus testing may not show improvement if it is done over too short of a testing interval (less than 3 months). Likewise, it is not unusual to see compliant, well-motivated patients continue to improve objectively with testing over a 3- to 5-year period from the time of their initial training program.[41,44,45] The following case studies illustrate the type of long-term program changes associated with a successful phase III program.

```
                        S.C.O.R.
        (Specialized Coronary Outpatient Rehabilitation) ─────────────────
                      Exercise Diary


Prescription:  Distance_____mile(s)

Time:_____minutes    Physical fitness stage:_____

Target heart rate:_____bpm    Weight (end of month):_____
```

Day	Rest. HR	Exercise mode	Distance (peak)	Time (peak)	Work load	W-U HR	Peak HR	C-D HR	Symptoms or remarks
1									
2									
3									
4									
5									
6									
7									
8									
9									
10									
11									
12									
13									
14									
15									
16									
17									
18									
19									
20									

Fig. 7-11. All exercise sessions, both at the hospital and at home, are logged on this exercise diary form. The physical therapist reviews it at the end of each month, makes comments, and gives a copy back to the patient.

Continued.

Day	Rest. HR	Exercise mode	Distance (peak)	Time (peak)	Work load	W–U HR	Peak HR	C–D HR	Symptoms or remarks
21									
22									
23									
24									
25									
26									
27									
28									
29									
30									
31									

MONTHLY SUMMARY

Average resting heart rate =
Average peak heart rate =
Total days exercise =
Average peak interval = _____ miles
Average peak duration =
Total monthly mileage =

DEFINITIONS

Level of angina
L_1 mild discomfort
L_2 moderately painful
L_3 severe pain
L_4 intolerable

SOB—Shortness of breath
PVC—Premature ventricular
      contraction

Recommendations: _____

_____

_____

_____

Fig. 7-11, cont'd. Exercise diary.

CASE STUDIES
MR. F.D.

The following case study illustrates long-term training changes that can occur in a well-motivated man with single-vessel coronary artery disease and angina pectoris. Both peripheral and central training adaptations have accounted for the tremendous improvement in symptoms this man achieved.

Patient: Mr. F.D.

Age: 48 (at onset of symptoms in early 1977)

Medical history: Beginning in January 1977, Mr. F.D. noticed the onset of substernal chest pain while walking uphill to his office in downtown Los Angeles. It was relieved by rest or with nitroglycerin. He saw his family doctor who referred him to a cardiologist at the Ross-Loos Medical Center for evaluation. His risk-factor profile at the time included the following:

> Pipe smoker for many years, overweight (6 feet tall; 193 pounds), inactive sedentary life-style, family history of coronary disease with a father who died at age 54 from a myocardial infarction, serum lipids were unknown, and there was no history of hypertension or diabetes. He worked as a construction inspector for the City of Los Angeles, which he considered as a very stressful occupation.

He underwent a symptom-limited treadmill exercise test to confirm the diagnosis of angina pectoris and define noninvasively the extent of coronary artery disease.

Treadmill test results (Jan. 24, 1977)
Completed 6 minutes of Bruce Protocol
Test stopped by moderate angina pectoris (level 2 + /4)
Resting heart rate: 56
Maximal heart rate: 119
Resting blood pressure: 128/84
Maximal blood pressure: 160/80
Maximal rate-pressure product (RPP): 19×10^3
RPP at onset of angina: 14×10^3
RPP at onset of ST-segment changes: (not measured)
1.5 mm ST-segment depression at maximal RPP
No arrhythmias
Fair symptom-limited physical work capacity

The cardiologist subsequently started the patient on Inderal (propranolol) 20 mg q.i.d. and Nitrobid (nitroglycerin) 2.5 mg b.i.d. A cardiac catheterization was done on Feb. 14, 1977 revealing:

Ventriculogram: Normal left ventricular contractility with an ejection fraction of 70%
Coronary angiogram:
Left anterior descending artery: 90% obstruction distal to the first septal perforator and first diagonal
Circumflex artery: intimal irregularities
Right coronary artery: intimal irregularities

Because of continuing angina symptoms, Inderal was increased to 40 mg q.i.d. and subsequently to 60 mg q.i.d. The latter dosage caused the patient to feel dizzy, and the dosage was decreased back to 40 mg q.i.d. and Nitrobid was increased to 5 mg b.i.d. To assess the effectiveness of this medical regime, his treadmill test was repeated.

Treadmill test results (June 1977)
Completed 5 minutes
Test stopped by severe angina (level 3 + /4)

Resting heart rate: 45
Maximal heart rate: 90
Resting blood pressure: 100/60
Maximal blood pressure: 114/72
Maximal RPP: 10.3×10^3
RPP at onset angina: 7.0×10^3
1.5 mm ST-segment depression at maximal RPP
Decreased symptom-limited performance with increased symptoms at lower RPP's.

After this test, Nitrobid was increased to 5 mg t.i.d. The patient was not exercising in any systematic fashion and underwent another exerise test in August 1977 with the same results.

As discussed in Chapter 6, in some patients increasing left ventricular dilation may offset myocardial oxygen demand decreases achieved by beta blockade of heart rate and blood pressure. This patient's Inderal was subsequently reduced to 20 mg q.i.d., and his cardiologist referred him to begin an exercise program with the SCOR Cardiac Cycling Club. The goals of his phase III cardiac rehabilitation program were to (1) improve physical work capacity and endurance, (2) decrease anginal symptoms with exertion, and (3) reduce risk actors through patient education and life-style changes.

He began a home bicycling program with instructions on how to train, the frequency of exercise, at what intensity to train, and how to deal with exertional angina. The emphasis was on increasing the duration of bicycling time at a mild (level 1/4) exertional angina threshold. Within 2 months, Mr. F.D. was cycling outdoors 4 to 15 miles on a 10-speed bike. Nitroglycerin was required to relieve his angina bout 50% to 60% of the time during these exercise sessions.

Subsequently, the patient's Inderal was reduced from 40 mg q.i.d. to 20 mg q.i.d., then to 10 mg q.i.d. A routine follow-up exercise test revealed:

Treadmill test results (Nov. 1977):
Completed 7.5 minutes
Test stopped by severe angina (level 3 + /4)
Resting heart rate: 58
Maximal heart rate: 125
Resting blood pressure: 114/72
Maximal blood pressure: 154/68, dropping to 148/64 the last minute of exercise
Maximal RPP: 19.2×10^3
RPP at onset angina: 15.4×10^3
RPP at onset ST-segment changes: 15.4×10^3
2.0 mm ST-segment depression at maximal RPP
Improved symptom-limited performance

Over the next 6 months, Mr. F.D. continued cycling, began riding longer distances of 20 to 35 miles on Saturday morning outings with the cycling club, and began a formal phase III hospital-based rehabilitation program for periodic monitoring and educational lectures. He rapidly progressed from 95 to 400 miles per month of bicycling and completed a 100-mile "century" ride in one day in May 1978. In August 1978, his Inderal was reduced to 5 mg q.i.d. and then discontinued in January 1979. Nitrobid was continued a while longer and also discontinued in late 1979. Table 7-2 illustrates the continuing improvement Mr. F.D. has made from May 1978 to June 1982 as a result of his continued excellent compliance to endurance exercise and life-style changes.

Table 7-2. Improvement in cardiac capacities over a 4-year period

	May 78	Nov. 78	June 79	Dec. 79	Sept. 80	Sept. 81	June 82
Treadmill time	9.0	10.5	10.5	10.5	10.5	10.5	10.33
Limiting factor	L_3AP	L_3AP	L_2 and fatigue	L_2 and fatigue	Fatigue	Fatigue	Fatigue
Resting heart rate	51	46	44	53	50	46	53
Maximal heart rate	135	141	160	170	170	170	168
Resting blood pressure	108/62	112/74	112/80	104/68	106/76	124/76	122/72
Maximal blood pressure	152/62	170/70	190/90	176/70	204/74	200/92	192/78
Maximal rate pressure product ($\times 10^3$)	20.8	22.5	30.4	28.1	34.6	34.0	32.3
Rate pressure product at angina pectoris ($\times 10^3$)	20.2	21.8	23.2	22.7	AP after exercise only	No AP	AP after exercise only
Rate pressure product at ST ($\times 10^3$)	14.2	19.5	16.8	N.A.	23.7	26.8	24.1
Maximal ST depression (mm) (CM$_4$ lead)	2.5	3.0	5.0	5.0	4.5	3.0	2.5
Medications	Inderal 5 mg q.i.d. Nitrobid 6.5 mg b.i.d.	Same	Nitrobid 6.5 mg b.i.d.	None	None	None	None

L, Level; AP, angina pectoris; N.A., not applicable.

As Mr. F.D.'s symptoms have abated over the years, he has expanded his recreational pursuits into other areas. He has become an avid cross-country skier with minimal symptoms in cold weather and at altitudes up to 8000 feet. He continues long-distance cycling and has completed two "double centuries" in 1 day. In the summer of 1980, he took a 4-week cycling trip through England, Scotland, and Ireland with myself and two other cardiac patients from the SCOR Cardiac Cycling Club.

Mr. F.D. had a decrease in angina symptoms at progressively higher rate pressure products until he became completely asymptomatic during the tests. The ST-segment depression initially became more prominent as he was able to exercise at higher rate-pressure produces; however, their magnitude has decreased in the last 2 years. The onset of ST changes has also been occurring at progressively higher rate-pressure products. Concurrently the patient's medications (beta blockade and vasodilator therapy) was tapered off. It is planned that yearly exercise tests will be continued to assess his stability and freedom from angina symptoms. Certainly, the quality of his life is infinitely better in terms of the great many vigorous leisure activities he is now capable of participating in.

MR. D.D.

The following patient demonstrates an uncomplicated phase I post–coronary artery bypass surgery program. Very clear-cut goals, set by the patient, helped to speed his recovery and allow for early hospital discharge.

Patient: Mr. D.D.

Age: 57

Medical history: This 57-year-old man noted the onset of substernal chest pains occurring after running or hiking in the mountains. He had previously been an active jogger before the onset of the symptoms; however, he had cut back considerably on the amount of running he had done in the last 3 to 4 years. During the time that he was jogging, he would do 2 to 4 miles, 2 to 3 days each week. The patient saw his private physician, who referred him to a cardiologist, who subsequently did a Bruce Treadmill Test (see Chapter 6). This test showed abnormalities of both angina and ischemic ST changes with greater than 1 mm of depression during exercise. The patient subsequently was catheterized on September 20, 1980.

Results

Ventriculogram
  Normal contractility, ejection fraction 60%
Coronary angiogram
  Right coronary artery: proximal 70% obstruction
  Left anterior descending artery: proximal 70% obstruction
  Circumflex artery: 30% stenosis midportion
On October 7, 1980, the patient had coronary artery bypass graft surgery with independent grafts to the left anterior descending, right coronary artery, and diagonal. The patient had an uncomplicated postoperative course except for a temporary right bundle branch block.

Phase I cardiac rehabilitation

The patient's cardiologist referred Mr. D.D. for inpatient cardiac rehabilitation on October 10, 1980, 3 days postoperatively. His medical history was reviewed by a thorough chart review, and it was noted at that time that his hemoglobin was 12.0 and his hematocrit was 40.

After completion of a normal self-care evaluation, the patient began monitored ambulation sessions and on his initial session was able to ambulate 200 yards in 5 minutes with no ectopy, no symptoms, and no ST changes.

Oct. 10, 1980
  Resting heart rate: 102
  Peak heart rate: 114
  Resting blood pressure: 112/80
  Peak blood pressure: 120/62
Oct. 11, 1980: monitored ambulation 200 to 300 yards, 10 minutes, no symptoms, no ectopy
  Resting heart rate: 96
  Peak heart rate: 120
  Resting blood pressure: 108/76
  Peak blood pressure: 124/70
Oct. 12, 1980: monitored ambulation 300 to 400 yards, 9 minutes, no symptoms
  Resting heart rate: 96
  Peak heart rate: 120
  Resting blood pressure: 112/70
  Peak blood pressure: 120/70
Oct. 13, 1980: Mr. D.D. underwent a low-level treadmill test utilizing the modified protocol described in Chapter 6.

Results

Time completed: 11 minutes (Sheffield)
Limiting factor: reached target heart rate
  Resting heart rate: 98
  Peak heart rate: 155
  Resting blood pressure: 142/70
  Peak blood pressure: 148/70
Flat systolic blood-pressure response
  No angina
  No ST changes
  No arrhythmias
On October 13, 1980, the patient was discharged home, being 6 days after coronary artery bypass graft surgery. His medications were Fergon (ferrous gluconate), one tablet three times daily.

Phase II cardiac rehabilitation

The patient returned on October 16, 1980, for an initial interview with the rehabilitation team. The physical therapy assessment was that this was a 57-year-old man who was strongly motivated to improve his physical condition and was 9 days after bypass with an uncomplicated course. The low-level treadmill test suggested good revascularization results with the flat blood pressure response probably secondary to mild anemia. The patient's goals, upon entering phase II were to (1) return to work by 2 months after the operation and (2) build up to 5 miles of continuous jogging as soon as possible

Phase II exercise program

On October 15, 1980, the patient began phase II as an outpatient. He was started on stationary ergometry, utilizing 62.5 watts for 15 minutes.
  Resting heart rate: 108
  Peak heart rate: 132
  Resting blood pressure: 92/70
  Peak blood pressure: 132/60
  No ST changes, no ectopy
In addition, the patient was instructed in walking at home, which he began with three fourths of a mile, four times a day.

On October 22, 1980, patient performed 40 minutes at peak exercise at 87.5 watts.
  Resting heart rate: 102
  Peak heart rate: 150
  Resting blood pressure: 100/70
  Peak blood pressure: 138/66
On October 24, 1980, the patient came to phase II. His resting heart rate was 92, and it was noted that he had frequent premature atrial contractions at rest on the radiotelemetry system. He performed his usual bicycle ergometry workout of 87.5 to 100 watts.

At a peak heart rate of 144, the patient developed multiple premature atrial contractions and a burst of supraventricular tachycardia immediately after exercise at a rate of 160 to 170 beats per minute. This resolved spontaneously during the postexercise period. Cardiac examination revealed an S_4 heart sound with no S_3 and no pericardial friction rub, nor any paradoxical pulse. The program cardiologist then examined the patient and found again no obvious signs or symptoms of pericarditis, and the cause of the supraventricular tachycardia remained unknown. The physician subsequently digitalized the patient and recommended continuing telemetry exercise sessions.

Oct. 29, 1980: 40 minutes at 100 watts, peak heart rate 144, no ectopy
Nov. 3, 1980: 40 minutes at 112 watts, peak heart rate 150
Nov. 14, 1980: 40 minutes at 3.5 mph 7% grade, peak heart rate 144 (resting heart rate 66)
Nov. 24, 1980: 40 minutes at 3.5 mph 10% grade, peak heart rate 150; began arm ergometry at 50 watts for 8 minutes, peak heart rate 126
Dec. 12, 1980: 40 minutes at 3.5 mph per 11% grade, peak heart rate 140; 10 minutes at 62.5 watts for arm ergometry, peak heart rate 120
Dec. 19, 1980: 40 minutes at 3.5 mph per 13% grade, peak heart rate 144; arm ergometry 10 minutes at 62.5 watts, peak heart rate 120

Home program

The patient was now walk-jogging 2 to 4 miles at a peak heart rate of 138 to 144 and progressed from 4 miles in 57 minutes to 4 miles in 45 to 50 minutes by the end of November. On November 13, 1980, the patient returned to work part time as a workman compensation adjuster for the state of California and on December 12, 1980, returned to work full time

Phase III cardiac rehabilitation

Dec. 22, 1980: Initial phase III visit with 4-mile peak jog, 38 minutes, peak heart rate 150, no ectopy

Jan. 12, 1980: 4-mile peak jog, 36 minutes, peak heart rate 144

Jan. 26, 1980: 5-mile peak jog, 42½ minutes, peak heart rate 150

January monthly exercise log summary
Number of workouts: 27
Average resting heart rate: 66
Average peak heart rate: 144
Total miles: 155
Average peak: 5.1
Average peak time: 55 minutes

The patient subsequently joined the SCOR Jogging Club and began training on Saturdays with this group. He continued to gradually increase his distances on up to 8 to 12 miles and in March 1981 was taken off his Lanoxin (digoxin) without recurrence of supraventricular arrhythmias. Through the course of the next year, Mr. D.D. continued to attend phase III, one or two times per month, while working full time and running at home. With the help of several other members in the SCOR Jogging Club, Mr. D.D. began to increase his mileage with the idea in mind of training for a full marathon. He did complete the Los Alamitos Marathon in March 1982 in 4 hours and 15 minutes and was extremely proud of his accomplishment.

The patient continues with his long-distance running program and maintains an excellent level of risk factor reduction, having improved his cholesterol/high-density lipoprotein ratio to 3.9 and maintaining a nonsmoking status and a normotensive blood pressure.

MR. P.P.

The following case study illustrates a complicated acute myocardial infarction, which subsequently demonstrated the importance of recognizing the effects of a myocardial infarction on all aspects of heart function.

Patient: Mr. P.P.

Age: 72

Medical history: The patient was feeling well until January 9, 1980, when at work he developed a severe pressure-like discomfort in the retrosternal area associated with nausea. After going home from work and having the pain persist, the patient called the paramedics to his house and he was transferred to the Presbyterian Intercommunity Hospital emergency room. According to the patient's wife, he lost consciousness for 2 to 3 minutes and was found by the paramedics to have occasional premature ventricular contractions. He was admitted to the coronary care unit and suddenly went into ventricular tachycardia at a rate of 140 per minute, with a stable blood pressure of 120/80. This was treated with lidocaine given intravenously. The electrocardiogram revealed an acute inferoposterior myocardial infarction with first-degree atrioventricular block and left atrial enlargement. Myocardial enzyme changes were positive for myocardial damage.

Risk factors

1. Previous cigarette smoker, one pack per day for 30 years; quit cigarettes in 1968 and subsequently smoked a few pipefuls of tobacco or cigars daily
2. *Hypertension:* 22-year history of high blood pressure
3. *Lipids* on January 14, 1981: *cholesterol* 197; *triglycerides* 100; *HDL* 55; *LDL* 128; *cholesterol/HDL ratio* 3.9
4. *Diabetes:* negative
5. *Sedentary life-style:* positive
6. *Obesity:* negative, height 5'10", weight 155 pounds
7. *Stress:* mild levels of stress associated with part-time work as a salesperson for a hardware store
8. *Diet:* extremely high in saturated fats, cholesterol, and caffeine

Hospital course

Jan. 9, 1981: Potassium 3.1; therefore it was believed that hypokalemia secondary to diuretic used for hypertension may have contributed to his arrhythmia.

Jan. 12, 1981: The patient was weaned off lidocaine and developed coarse rhonchi and wheezing in both lungs, believed to be acute bronchitis.

Jan. 13, 1981: Cardiac rehabilitation ordered. The patient was transferred from the coronary care unit to the telemetry ward.

Monitored self-care evaluation

Chest wall exam: negative
Resting heart rate: 92
Resting blood pressure: 108/62
Peak heart rate:
  104 (during dressing and ambulation)
  108 (during hygiene and grooming)
Peak blood pressure: 110/60 throughout all self-care activities, except for 140/60 during Valsalva maneuver. There were no arrhythmias and no ST changes. An S_4 heart sound was auscultated at rest and after ambulation.

Self-care evaluation summary and recommendations

The patient was asymptomatic without ST-segment changes or arrhythmias. However, the blood pressure failed to rise with increasing heart rate.

Plan: Increase current activity levels; closely monitor HR, BP, ECG and symptoms, breath and heart sounds.

Jan. 14, 1981: initial monitored ambulation session
  Resting heart rate: 90
  Resting blood pressure: 110/74
  Peak heart rate: 110
  Sitting: 102/66
  Standing: 102/64
  Peak blood pressure: 100-110/70

Patient ambulated 50 yards initially and then 75 yards after a 5-minute rest period with no ectopic beats.

Jan. 15, 1981: monitored ambulation
  Resting heart rate: 94
  Peak heart rate: 111
  Resting blood pressure: 114/70
  Peak blood pressure: 136/76

Patient ambulated 100 yards with 5 minutes of rest and then 200 yards with occasional premature arterial and ventricular contractions being noticed.

Jan. 16, 1981
  Resting heart rate: 90
  Peak heart rate: 112
  Resting blood pressure: 116/80
  Peak blood pressure: 110/70

Patient ambulated 200 yards, 5 minutes rest, then 300 yards, with occasional premature atrial and ventricular contractions being noticed.

Jan. 17, 1981: Patient noticed the onset of slight precordial chest pain lasting approximately 30 minutes and subsiding without medications. Repeat electrocardiogram revealed extension of an inferior wall infarction with deeper Q waves in leads 2, 3, and aV_L with hyperacute ST changes in the same leads, as well as reciprocal ST-segment depression in leads 1 and aV_L. The patient was returned to bed rest. He was started on lidocaine and then weaned off on January 20, 1981, and put on Pronestyl (procaine amide) and Inderal (propranolol).

A self-care evaluation was again ordered and completed on January 23, 1981.

Results
  Resting heart rate: 84
  Peak heart rate: 102
  Resting blood pressure: 100/62
  During hygiene and grooming, peak blood pressure: 102/70

It was noted that the patient had a progressive drop in blood pressure to 82/58 while dressing upper extremities and 80/52 during Valsalva maneuver, returning to 102/66 1 minute after activity. No ST-segment changes were seen. Occasional premature atrial contractions were noticed.

Jan. 23, 1981: monitored ambulation restarted
  Resting heart rate: 89
  Peak heart rate: 105
  Resting blood pressure: 112/72
  Peak blood pressure: 118/78

Patient ambulated 100 yards without chest discomfort, had one premature atrial contraction with ambulation, and was mildly short of breath.

Jan. 24, 1981: monitored ambulation
  Resting heart rate: 88
  Peak heart rate: 96
  Resting blood pressure: 114/68
  Peak blood pressure: 92/60

Patient ambulated 100 yards, with 5 minutes of rest and then 200 yards. This hypotensive response was a definite new finding.

Jan. 29, 1981: monitored ambulation
  Resting heart rate: 89
  Peak heart rate: 102
  Resting blood pressure: 102/70
  Peak blood pressure: 90-96/60

Patient ambulated 200 and then 400 yards with no ST changes; however, multiple premature ventricular contractions with short runs of trigeminy and occasional coupled premature ventricular contractions were noticed.

Because of the possibility the arrhythmias represented an ischemic response, the patient's beta blockade dose was increased, nitrates increased, and Pronestyl increased to 750 mg every 6 hours. Later in the day, the patient had several long runs of ventricular tachycardia, which required lidocaine, given intravenously.

Jan. 28, 1981: Because of multiple arrhythmias and an abnormal blood pressure response, the patient underwent a low-level treadmill test.

Results
  Time completed: 8.5 minutes
  Limiting factor: stopped because of a 30 mm Hg fall in systolic blood pressure during the last 2 minutes of exercise.
  Resting heart rate: 80
  Peak heart rate: 108
  Resting blood pressure: 110/70
  Peak blood pressure: 112/80 (minute 6)

Blood pressure fell to 84/60 by minute 8.5. During recovery, the patient again developed ventricular tachycardia with a rate of 140. This lasted for 3 minutes and required lidocaine, given intravenously for conversion to sinus rhythm. The patient was asymptomatic before, during, and after exercise. No significant ST changes were seen. The test was interpreted as being abnormal, with a falling blood pressure and ventricular arrhythmias suggestive of ischemic left ventricular dysfunction. The patient may have had extensive, severe, three-vessel coronary artery disease.

Jan. 30, 1981: cardiac catheterization
  Ventriculogram:
    Akinesis of the inferior wall of the left ventricle because of moderate-sized inferior infarction
    Left ventricular end-diastolic pressure 8
    Ejection fraction 43%
  Coronary angiogram:
    Right coronary artery: proximal 100% obstruction (distal to the first diagonal)
    Left anterior descending artery: 40% obstruction
    Circumflex artery: 30% obstruction proximally with an additional 30% obstruction distal to the first marginal artery

Jan. 31, 1981: monitored ambulation (reordered)

Patient again demonstrated, while walking at a very slow pace, a decrease in blood pressure from 120/70 to 94/60 with a heart rate rise from 80 to 96. No ventricular ectopic beats were observed.

The patient had a short episode of ventricular tachycardia that occurred while at rest in the afternoon and resolved spontaneously. It was believed that the recurring ventricular tachycardia was caused by a reentry mechanism in peri-infarction tissue. The exertional hypotension in the face of a moderate-sized inferior infarction with apparently good perfusion through the left coronary system indicated a myocardial depressant effect of the patient's antiarrhythmics and beta blocking medications. Subsequently, Isordil (isosorbide dinitrate) and Lopressor (metoprolol tartrate) were decreased, however, Pronestyl (procaine amide) was increased to one gram every 6 hours.

Feb. 1, 1981: monitored ambulation

The patient continued to show 15 to 20 mm decrease in blood pressure with a 12 to 20 beat per minute increase in heart rate over resting levels. Occasional premature atrial and ventricular contractions were observed.

Feb. 4, 1981:

Because of the persistent arrhythmias and poor blood pressure response, it was decided to do an exercise radionuclide wall-motion study. The patient exercised on a supine bicycle ergometer in three stages, at 3 minutes per stage, and at 200, 300, and 400 kgm (kilogram meters). The test was terminated by the patient because of leg fatigue.

Results

Resting heart rate: 72
Maximum heart rate: 90
(Blunted heart rate because of beta blocking medications)
Resting blood pressure; 112/70
Peak blood pressure: 80/50

A fourth heart sound was auscultated before exercise and an S₃ developed after exercise. There were no arrhythmias and no significant ST-segment changes.

Wall-motion results

Heart rate	Left ventricular ejection fraction	Right ventricular ejection fraction
72	45%	21%
83	54%	—
88	65%	—
90	64%	26%

The right ventricle was dilated with inferior wall akinesis, and the remaining portion of the right ventricle was severely hypokinetic.

An interpretation of this study revealed that left ventricular function was mildly impaired at rest and improved with exercise, while the right ventricle was greatly dilated and demonstrated a very poor ejection fraction at rest and with exercise. It was postulated that this patient's limitation in cardiac reserve was not attributable to left ventricular dysfunction but rather to right ventricular dysfunction and a very large akinetic segment (or possibly aneurysm). Diastolic tamponade of the left ventricle caused by the dilated right ventricle during exercise was also considered as an explanation. Lopressor (metoprolol tartrate) was discontinued and Dyazide (triamterene and hydrochlorothiazide) was added to decrease the right ventricular preload.

Feb. 5, 1981: monitored ambulation
Resting heart rate: 92
Peak heart rate: 110
Resting blood pressure: 89/70
Peak blood pressure: 130/70

Occasional premature ventricular contractions were noticed, and an adaptive blood pressure response was observed with ambulation of 100 yards.

Feb. 6, 1981: monitored ambulation
Resting heart rate: 88
Peak heart rate: 120 to 132
Resting blood pressure: 102/70
Peak blood pressure: 134/70

One premature ventricular contraction with ambulation of 300 yards

Feb. 7, 1981: Patient discharged home on Pronestyl (procaine amide), 1000 mg q.i.d.; Isordil Tembids (isosorbide dinitrate) 40 mg b.i.d.; and Aldactazide (spironolactone and hydrochlorothiazide), one tablet b.i.d., with K-Lyte for potassium supplementation. With a normal blood-pressure response and no significant arrhythmias, it was believed that the patient was safe to perform self-care and home activities to a heart rate of 130.

This case clearly demonstrates three aspects of Phase I cardiac rehabilitation. First, the monitoring activities (self-care and am-

bulation) when completed accurately and interpreted appropriately correlated well with the patient's ventricular performance. This patient's hypotension, tachycardia, and heart sounds, repeatedly described a person with poor ventricular function. Second, these data were used by the patient's physician to make decisions about further diagnostic tests and medication changes. Finally, the monitored ambulation was used to make appropriate discharge decisions.

Phase II cardiac rehabilitation

Feb. 9, 1981: The patient was interviewed by the entire cardiac rehabilitation team for entry into the phase II program. The physical therapy assessment was that this was a 72-year-old man with a very complicated hospital course with recurrent ventricular arrhythmias and low blood pressure response to activity because of severe right ventricular decompensation during exercise. The patient had been quite depressed at times in the hospital because of the multiple complications and setbacks; however, he was very well motivated to improve his physical capacity and to return to work.

Goals

1. Improve physical work capacity and endurance.
2. Reduce risk factors.
3. Educate the patient regarding coronary artery disease, risk factors, diet, exercise, etc.
4. Return to work as soon as possible.

Plan

1. Begin phase II, three times a week, for outpatient exercise program with arm and leg ergometry. Add weight training in 4 weeks.
2. Basic education lecture series.
3. Schedule for maximal exercise test in 4 weeks.

Feb. 11, 1981: initial phase II session
Resting heart rate: 90
Peak heart rate: 120
Resting blood pressure: 92/62
Peak blood pressure: 100/60

Fifteen minutes of lower extremity ergometry with 50 watts, 5 minutes of upper extremity ergometry with 30 watts, no arrhythmias, moderate dyspnea

Feb. 23, 1981:
Resting heart rate: 84
Resting blood pressure: 106/76
Peak heart rate: 114
Peak blood pressure: 120/70

25 minutes of lower extremity ergometry at 50 watts, 10 minutes of upper extremity ergometry at 37½ watts, no ectopy

March 11, 1981:
Resting heart rate: 84
Peak heart rate: 114
Resting blood pressure: 110/60
Peak blood pressure: 120/74

35 minutes of lower extremity ergometry at 62½ watts, 10 minutes of upper extremity ergometry at 55 watts; only occasional premature atrial contractions were noticed.

March 25, 1981:
Resting heart rate: 78
Peak heart rate: 114
Resting blood pressure: 104/60
Peak blood pressure: 120/62

35 minutes of lower extremity ergometry at 68 watts, 10 minutes of upper extremity ergometry at 62½ watts, no ectopic beats

April 3, 1981: Maximum treadmill test results

Completed 9.2 minutes of Sheffield Protocol

    Limiting factor: Dyspnea

    Resting heart rate: 76

    Resting blood pressure: 146/92

    Peak heart rate: 136

    Peak blood pressure: 92/70

    No angina

    S_4 before and after exercise

    No arrhythmias, no ST-segment changes

    Fair physical work capacity for 72-year-old man

The patient began a home program of walking, upon entering into phase II, consisting of one-half mile, twice a day, for 15 minutes each time to similiar heart rates seen in monitored exercise sessions. By the end of February, he had increased this to 2 miles in 43 minutes and in March and April increased this to 3 to 4 miles in 60 to 70 minutes, at a peak heart rate of 120. The patient elected to retire from work at this point, and in mid-May was transferred to our phase III program.

Phase III

On May 18, 1981, the patient began in the phase III program with a large group exercise class. Because of a lack of arrhythmias in late April and early May, he had been weaned off the continuous telemetry monitoring but was monitored the first two initial sessions in phase III as a routine check.

May 18, 1981: initial phase III program

    Resting heart rate: 78

    Peak heart rate: 114

    Resting blood pressure: 120/90

    Peak blood pressure: 130/68

Patient completed 3 miles in 47 minutes of a fast walk, no arrhythmias.

The patient continued weekly phase III visits for the next 6 months, while continuing to exercise at home 5 or 6 days a week. During this time, he gradually built his endurance up to 3 miles in 50 minutes with a peak heart rate of 108 to 114 beats per minute while his resting heart rate had dropped to 72. At this point the patient was interested in beginning a walk-jogging program. Since the patient had been in the program 9 months, it was elected to repeat his maximum treadmill test first.

Nov. 25, 1981: maximum treadmill test results

    Completed 12.2 minutes of Sheffield Protocol

    Resting heart rate: 76

    Peak heart rate: 136

    Resting blood pressure: 146/92

    Peak blood pressure 126/80, 104/64

    Blunted blood pressure response with 16 mm Hg fall in last 6 minutes

    Occasional premature ventricular contractions throughout

    No ST-segment changes; R-wave amplitude increased 8 mm

    Mildly impaired physical working capacity (PWC) for 72-year-old man

    Functional aerobic impairment (FAI): 2%

    Three-minute improvement since last test of April 1981

Nov. 30, 1981: The patient began short-distance jogging, reducing his 3-mile time from 50 to 45 minutes, while maintaining the peak heart rate of 114 to 120 with an appropriate albeit blunted blood pressure response. The patient continues to feel well and participates in all of his premorbid recreational activities, including golf, bowling, and hiking, and continues to maintain his walk-jogging program. It is planned that yearly treadmill tests will be performed to assess the stability of the patient's disease and to document any further improvement in his physical work capacity.

To summarize, this 72-year-old man demonstrates how a carefully prescribed and supervised cardiac rehabilitation program can significantly improve physical performance and assist to determine the appropriate medications despite multiple complications and severe ventricular dysfunction.

Mr. G.F.

The following case study illustrates the difficulties that may be encountered with an extremely complicated myocardial infarction. Although this is clearly a "high-risk" patient, a carefully monitored program allowed this completely bedridden patient to ultimately become quite vigorous.

Patient: Mr. G.F.

Age: 63

Medical history: This 63-year-old man was well until January 5, 1980. While walking after lunch in Newport Beach, he experienced the onset of retrosternal pain. This persisted on and off all afternoon, and he went to a local emergency room at 11 PM. An ECG was normal, and he was given Mylanta and Dalmane (flurazepam) and sent home. The pain continued and the patient had a more severe episode at 1 AM associated with pronounced diaphoresis. Early that morning (January 6) his wife drove him to Presbyterian Intercommunity Hospital where he was admitted.

Risk factors

1. Negative family history
2. Cigarette smoking: one-third pack per day for 30 years, quit before myocardial infarction
3. *Lipids: cholesterol* 189; *triglycerides* 118; *HDL* 33; *cholesterol/HDL* ratio 5.9 (see Chapter 6)
4. *Obesity:* admission weight 220 pounds, height 6 feet
5. Sedentary
6. Negative for hypertension and diabetes
7. *Stress:* worked as president of local bank

On admission, he had evidence of an acute anterolateral wall myocardial infarction with chest pain. He developed congestive heart failure with cardiomegaly and pulmonary vascular congestion on chest radiograph and inspiratory rales bilaterally. He was medically controlled with morphine and Lasix (furosemide) initially until January 8, when he developed atrial fibrillation and Lanoxin (digoxin) was added. Atrial fibrillation continued intermittently through January 11, but his chest radiograph showed improvement, and Nitropaste, Isordil, and Dyazide were added. He was allowed by his physician to be up in a chair and walk around in his coronary care unit room by January 12. On January 14, he had increasing premature ventricular contractions requiring lidocaine given intravenously but was transferred from the CCU to a telemetry ward the same day. On January 15, the intravenous tubing was removed, and the physician ordered "increased activity."

On January 16, the patient had a cardiac arrest requiring defibrillation several times, and he was returned to the CCU where a Swan-Ganz catheter was inserted, the patient was intubated, and lidocaine started intravenously with additional diuretic added because of basilar rales. He was weaned off lidocaine on January 20 and started on Norpace (disopyramide phosphate); however, he fibrillated again on the same day. The chest radiograph showed an increase in pulmonary congestion and more Lasix was given. Oral Pronestyl and quinidine were added.

Enzyme changes:	*1/6/80*	*1/7/80*	*1/8/80*	*1/12/80*	*1/17/80*
Creatine phosphokinase	895	1670	535	80	320
Creatine phosphokinase Isoenzymes	MM-75% MB-25%	MM-77% MB-23%	MM-93% MB-7%	—	MM-93% MB-7%

On January 20, it was believed that the patient was in impending cardiogenic shock and intra-aortic balloon counterpulsation was started. A cardiac catheterization was done because of these multiple complications.

Coronary angiogram
  Left anterior descending artery: 99% occluded from first to fourth septal perforators (pattern suggested recanalization)
  Circumflex artery: marginal branch irregularity
  Right coronary artery: normal
Ventriculogram
  Left ventricular end-diastolic pressure: 12 mm Hg, 24 mm Hg after angiography, normal (0 to 12)
  Pulmonary artery pressure: 38/20 mm Hg (mean 27), normal (25/10)
  Aortic blood pressure: 132/68 mm Hg (mean 96)
  Stroke volume: 107 ml
  Heart rate: 84
  Cardiac index: 2.4 L/min/M$_2$
  Ejection fraction: 24%

On January 23, the intra-aortic balloon was removed. The patient was encouraged to sit at bedside, but multiple attempts at this and standing were unsuccessful because of severe hypotension (BP 50/0). Various arrhythmias continued despite high doses of Pronestyl, quinidine, Norpace, Inderal, and intravenous lidocaine. (Inderal was discontinued January 30.)

In early February, the Pronestyl was increased to 875 mg q4h and Anturane (sulfinpyrazone) 100 mg twice a day added. Intravenously given lidocaine was discontinued on February 6; however, on February 13 an asymptomatic episode of prolonged ventricular tachycardia occurred. Mr. G.F. was transferred to a telemetry bed on February 20; however, his congestive heart failure persisted, basilar rales were present, and more Dyazide was given. By early March, the patient could sit at bedside for only a few minutes because of hypotension and was very light headed.

Phase I cardiac rehabilitation

On March 12, cardiac rehabilitation was ordered for Mr. G.F.

After 2 months in the hospital with multiple complications, this patient was totally incapacitated, severely depressed, and dependent on nursing care for all his self-care needs. The goals of phase I cardiac rehabilitation for this patient were as follows:
1. Reduce orthostatic hypotension and increase sitting and standing tolerance.
2. Increase self-care capabilities.
3. Progress to short-distance ambulation and improve blood pressure response.

4. Decrease depression; improve self-confidence.
5. Prepare patient for hospital discharge and phase II cardiac rehabilitation immediately after discharge

Phase I program (self-care evaluation, physical therapy evaluation, interview)
1. Sitting out of bed four times a day to tolerance, with blood pressure heart rate and telemetry ECG recorded continuously while up.
2. Lower extremities resistive exercises while sitting
3. Monitored ambulation twice a day (10 to 20 feet)
4. Bicycle ergometry twice a day (less than 5 minutes)

Initial session
  Resting heart rate: 78
  Peak heart rate: 84
  Resting blood pressure: 56/38 (sitting) after 5 minutes of sitting with active toe raises
  Standing blood pressure: 50/28
  Walk 50 feet, with blood pressure 48/20 while ambulating
By March 21:
  Resting heart rate: 78
  Peak heart rate: 88
  Resting blood pressure: 90/60 but 82/50 with walking 200 feet, repeated four times
By March 23:
  96/60 but 84/50 with walking 1000 to 1400 feet; also riding ergometer at 25 watts for 5 minutes
By March 31:
  Discharged home
  Able to walk 1700 feet with assist
  Blood pressure: 85/50
  Infrequent hypotensive episodes
  Discharge medications: Lanoxin, Pronestyl, quinidine, Norpace, Anturane, Isordil, and Coumadin (warfarin)

A low-level treadmill test was not attempted. The results of the monitored ambulation indicated that further work loads would not be tolerated.

Phase II goals

Although this patient was able to walk a few hundred feet and perform most self-care activities at the time of discharge, his physician did not believe that a low-level treadmill test was indicated. The goals for this patient were based on the knowledge of his ventricular function from catheterization and the following physiological detrimental effects of bed rest:
1. Decrease exercise-induced hypotension
2. Increase walking distance initially and then speed and intensity if indicated
3. Increase upper extremity strength and endurance
4. Increase self-confidence

Unknown at the time of hospital discharge was the degree and cause of this patient's functional limitations. The limitations could have been a result of peri-infarction ischemia, the myocardial depressant effects of multiple antiarrhythmic drugs, prolonged bed rest with muscle atrophy and deconditioning (the patient lost 40 pounds in the hospital) or infarcted myocardium.

Phase II program (three-times-a-week outpatient program)
1. Monitored ambulation, with increases in distance as physiological responses and tolerance warrant.

2. Bicycle ergometry emphasizing low resistance and increasing time and endurance.
3. Add arm ergometry when capable.

Program progress

March 2, 1980: first phase II session
Walked 2000 feet in 15 minutes; on ergometer at 37 watts
Resting blood pressure: 84/60
Resting heart rate: 72
Peak heart rate: 90
Peak blood pressure: 86/50
May 5, 1980
Walking 1 mile in 25 minutes
Resting blood pressure: 76-84/42
Peak blood pressure: 96-106/60
20 minutes at 50 watts with lower extremity ergometry
June 9, 1980
Walking 3 miles in 56 minutes
Resting blood pressure: 84/50-60
Peak blood pressure: 88-96/40
Started arm ergometry for 10 minutes at 30 watts (taken off Norpace, and Pronestyl was decreased)
June 20, 1980: low-level exercise test: 4-minute Sheffield Protocol stopped secondary to blood-pressure drop

Resting heart rate: 82
Maximal heart rate: 100
Resting blood pressure: 90/50
Maximal blood pressure: 90/50, which fell to 80/36 last minute of exercise
Negative for angina, ST changes or arrhythmias
S_4 before exercise
Pronestyl and quinidine dosages decreased again
July 2, 1980: Resting gated blood pool study with first-pass angiogram results: "diffuse hypokinesis of the left ventricle with the apex and inferior wall almost akinetic."
July 9, 1980
Walking 3 miles in 46 minutes
Peak heart rate: 96
Resting blood pressure: 80/50
Peak blood pressure: 102/40, doing 15 minutes at 50 watts with arm ergometry
Aug. 9, 1980
Began walk-jogging 3 miles in 46 minutes
Peak heart rate: 102-108
Resting blood pressure: 90/52
Peak blood pressure: 102/44
Jogged 100 feet, alternated with walking 900 feet

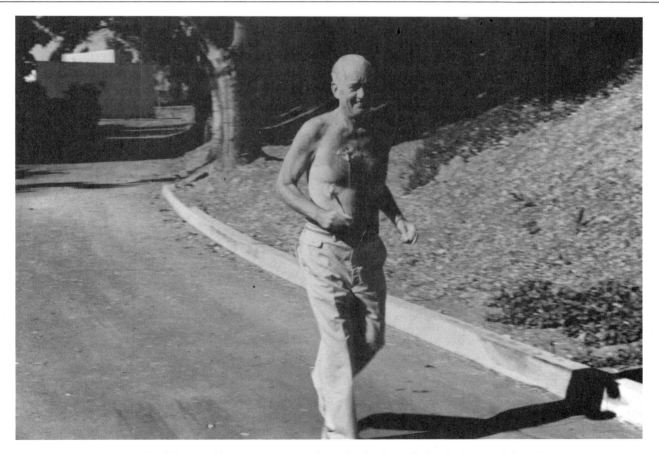

Fig. 7-12. Mr. G.F. was able to progress to walk-jogging in phase III despite his poor left ventricular function on angiography. His resting and exercise blood pressures gradually became adaptive over a 12-month period.

Sept. 9, 1980
Walk-jogging 3 miles in 45 minutes
Peak heart rate: 102/114
200-foot jog, 500-foot walk
Resting blood pressure: 94/60
Peak blood pressure: 110/60

Sept. 29, 1980: started phase III program (one time a week in phase III, 2 times a week in phase II); arm ergometry increased to 15 minutes at 60 to 65 watts (Fig. 7-12).

Because of the history of multiple cardiac arrests and changing antiarrhythmic therapy, continuous ECG monitoring in phase II was continued for many months. Only occasional premature ventricular contractions were observed.

In December 1980, the patient's physician cleared Mr. G.F. to return to work. He desired to work part-time and did so on January 5, 1981.

Phase III program

With return to work, phase II was completed and Mr. G.F. was seen once a week for continued endurance building and periodic monitoring.

Jan. 5, 1981
Walk-jog for 3 miles in 43 minutes
Resting heart rate: 72
Peak heart rate: 114
Resting blood pressure: 102/66
Peak blood pressure: 130/68
No arrhythmias
Fig. 7-12

Feb. 12, 1981: Mr. G.F. participated in the Presbyterian Intercommunity Hospital "Walk-Jog-Run for Your Heart" 5 and 10 km. Exactly 1 year earlier, he had watched the race from a wheelchair while still an inpatient. He completed the 5 km in 40 minutes winning a first-place award for coming closest to his predicted time!

Mr. G.F. continues to participate in phase III on a weekly basis, walk-jogging 3 miles in 37 to 39 minutes with appropriate cardiovascular responses. All antiarrhythmics have been eliminated except quinidine. He exercises two to three times a week on his own, continues to work 20 hours a week, fishes at high altitudes, and travels around the country to see relatives from time to time.

MR. E.R.

This case study is another example of the long-term training effects that may be seen in patients who comply with a vigorous aerobic exercise program. Despite severe triple vessel coronary artery disease and angina, this patient was able to alleviate his symptoms through the conditioning program, improve his physical work capacity by nearly 50% over an 8-year period, and demonstrate some apparent degree of regression of his coronary atheroma.

Patient: Mr. E.R.

Age: 61 (at time of entry into rehabilitation program)

Medical history: This 61-year-old man first began to note the onset of substernal chest pressure in 1959 at 48 years of age. He began a limited walking program on his own, gradually progressing up to 2 miles per day. His angina symptoms improved with this self-prescribed exercise program until 1972 when they be-

came more frequent and more severe. He saw his private physician, who referred the patient for a bicycle ergometry test. This was done in July 1972.

Results:

Completed: 800 kgm (kilogram meters)
Limited by fatigue and falling blood pressure
Resting heart rate: 62
Peak heart rate: 145
Resting blood pressure: 140/70
Peak blood pressure: 160/60 (falling to 120/50 at peak heart rate)
Patient experienced level 1 angina pectoris during the third and fourth work loads, which was not limiting
No arrhythmias
4 mm of flat ST-segment depression noted in V_5 lead at peak rate
Physical work capacity: fair to good in a mildly active 61-year-old man
Resting electrocardiogram: normal

The patient was then subsequently referred for catheterization because of the hypoadaptive blood pressure response along with pronounced ischemic ST changes and angina symptoms.

Cardiac catheterization (July 13, 1972)

Ventriculogram
Normal contractility of the left ventricle
Left ventricular end-diastolic pressure: 12 mm Hg
Stroke index: 65 ml/m²
Cardiac index: 4.7 l/min/m²
Ejection fraction: 78%

Coronary angiogram
Left anterior descending artery: 95% obstruction proximal to first septal perforator with an additional long narrow segment of 70% to 85% obstruction between the first and second septal perforators with good distal runoff
Circumflex artery: 95% occlusion, just proximal to the marginal branch with rapid filling of the marginal and distal circumflex arteries
Right coronary artery: 75% obstruction, 2 cm from the origin with excellent distal runoff

Risk factors

1. Positive family history of coronary disease: patient's brother died of a myocardial infarction at 55 years of age
2. Negative for smoking
3. Positive for hypertension: systolic blood pressures found to be 140 to 160 mm Hg
4. Lipids: only one cholesterol was available in 1972, that being 215 mg/dl
5. No history of diabetes
6. Body weight: at the onset of the patient's angina in 1959, he weighed 145 pounds, height 5' 9"
7. Stress/type A personality: patient worked as a shoe salesman for many years under a considerable amount of stress in the patient's estimation.

Phase III rehabilitation program

After the patient's initial catheterization in July 1972 he began exercising on his own again and returned to walking up to 4 miles per day and bicycling a stationary ergometer 6 miles per day. His physician subsequently referred him to a phase III program in April 1973.

Initial evaluation revealed a well-motivated 61-year-old man who experienced mild to moderate anginal symptoms with walking. He had severe triple-vessel coronary artery disease with normal ventricular function; however, he developed a severely ischemic ventricle at heart rates above 120 beats per minute with a hypoadaptive blood pressure on objective testing.

Goals:
1. Reduce angina pectoris symptoms
2. Improve physical work capacity and endurance
3. Reduce risk factors
4. Patient education on the value of exercise and risk-factor reduction in reducing the risk of coronary atherosclerosis progression

Mr. E.R. began phase III and was monitored while performing his usual level of exercise, that is, 4 miles of walking to a peak heart rate of 96. He would experience level 1 angina with an appropriate blood pressure response and no arrhythmias. During bicycle ergometry he would train up to a heart rate of 114 or 120, also with level 1 angina but an appropriate blood pressure response (probably secondary to warm-up).

Over the course of the next year, the patient maintained this level of exercise and found his anginal symptoms progressively decreasing to the point where he required very infrequent nitroglycerin use. No other cardiac medications were required.

In September 1973, the patient again underwent repeated cardiac catheterization.

Results (Sept. 1973)

Ventriculogram
  Normal contractility
  Ejection fraction: 63%
  Left ventricular end-diastolic pressure: 18 mm Hg
Coronary angiogram
  Unchanged except for the circumflex artery, where a new 60% proximal obstruction was observed

Despite the progression of the patient's coronary artery disease, it was elected to continue to treat him medically because of the symptomatic improvement he had experienced in the previous year from his exercise conditioning program. In addition, objective exercise testing revealed an improved physical work capacity (900 kgm) with very mild angina symptoms in the fourth work load only.

Over the next 7 years, as seen in Fig. 7-13, the patient maintained a very high level of compliance to an exercise conditioning program. He consistently averaged between 5 to 7 days per week of training during this time with very infrequent interruption. In 1977, he became virtually asymptomatic and began to jog, and by 1978 he was jogging continuously 5 miles. In addition to his early-morning jogging program, the patient would exercise again in the late afternoon, riding a stationary bicycle, progressing up to 10 miles in 45 minutes. Fig. 7-14 reveals that over this 7-year period, the patient was able to train to higher heart rates, ultimately training at pulse rates of 120 to 138 beats per minute with no angina symptoms. Fig. 7-15 reveals that Mr. E.R. averaged, through a combination of cycling and walk-jogging, between 1 to 2 hours of exercise per day throughout this 7-year period.

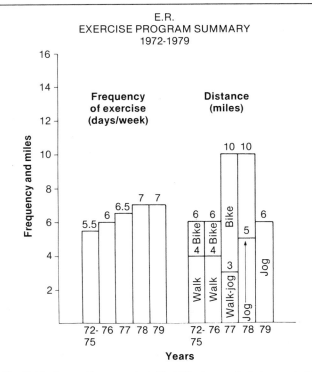

Fig. 7-13. Over a 7-year period, Mr. E.R. demonstrated remarkable consistency in his adherence to an aerobic conditioning program. He attended phase III weekly during the entire time.

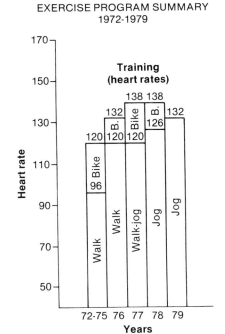

Fig. 7-14. As his angina symptoms abated, Mr. E.R. was able to train at higher heart rates, eventually being able to jog continuously at a heart rate of 132 to 138 beats per minute without symptoms.

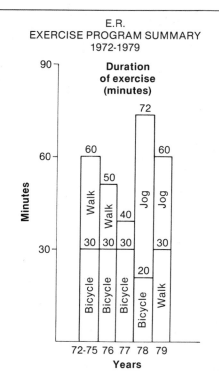

Fig. 7-15. Mr. E.R. enjoyed exercising and usually rode a stationary bike 20 to 30 minutes in the afternoon after walk-jogging or jogging 40 to 70 minutes in the morning.

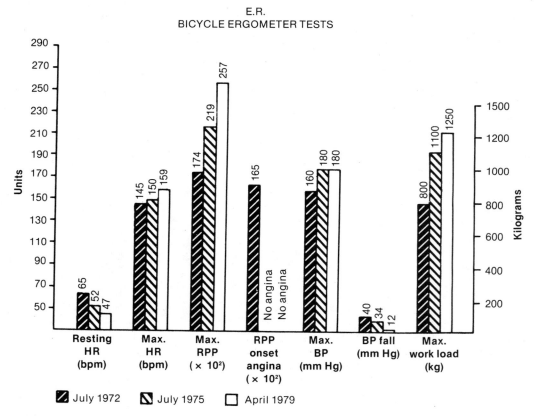

Fig. 7-16. This graph demonstrates the tremendous central and peripheral changes Mr. E.R. developed over a 7-year period.

Mr. E.R. was seen in phase III on a weekly basis and monitored periodically with radiotelemetry ECG and blood-pressure measurements while jogging for 7 years. Frequently with an appropriate warm-up interval, even at these higher heart rates, it was found that the patient's blood pressure was always adaptive and only infrequent premature ventricular contractions were observed. In 1977, the patient joined the SCOR Jogging Club as a result of his new-found jogging abilities and did his Saturday morning training sessions with this group. Between 1977 and 1980 the patient participated in a number of local 10 km runs, enjoying the friendship and comraderie of doing these physical activities with other cardiac runners.

During this 7-year period of time, bicycle ergometry testing demonstrated rather dramatic physiological changes despite his severe coronary disease and advancing age. His resting pulse rate dropped progressively into the mid-40s, while his maximal chronotropic reserve also increased to 159 beats per minute by 1979 (Fig. 7-16). Consequently, the patient's maximal rate pressure product improved dramatically from 174×10^2 in 1973 to 257×10^2 by April 1979. From 1974 on, no anginal symptoms were experienced during the patient's yearly exercise tests. Interestingly, the degree of hypoadaptive blood pressure response became progressively less over this time, and by April 1979 the patient experienced a rather small drop of 12 mm Hg from 180 to 168 at the peak of exercise at 1250 kgm. Only occasional premature ventricular contractions were observed during all these tests, and the degree of ST-segment depression remained stable at 4 to 6 mm in the V_5 lead. Thus this patient demonstrated a 50% improvement in his work capacity over a 7-year period of time with complete resolution of angina symptoms and an ability to exercise at a progressively higher rate pressure product.

In May 1979, because of the tremendous improvement this patient had experienced with medical management, it was believed that another cardiac catheterization was warranted to examine the stability of the patient's severe coronary obstructions.

Results (May 1979)

Ventriculogram
  Normal contractility
  Ejection fraction: 65%
Coronary angiogram
  Left anterior descending artery: unchanged with a proximal 95% obstruction
  Circumflex artery: 60% obstruction proximal with apparent regression of the second lesion from 95% to 70% (Figs. 7-17 and 7-18)
  Right coronary artery: apparent regression from 75% in 1973 to 30% to 40% in 1979

Thus this patient showed regression of coronary atherosclerosis in two of his three major arteries with symptomatic relief of the angina pectoris. Excellent adherence to exercise conditioning and risk-factor modifications may have accounted for these findings. The lipids in 1979 were observed to be the following:

  Cholesterol: 151
  Triglycerides: 54
  HDL: 51
  LDL: 109
  Cholesterol/HDL ratio: 3.0

The patient had lost a total of 15 pounds over this 7-year period of time, being 130 pounds in 1979. His percent body fat had

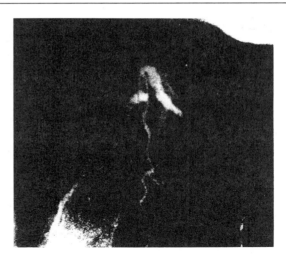

Fig. 7-17. In 1972, the left coronary injection (left anterior oblique view) revealed a proximal 95% LAD (left anterior descending artery) lesion and a midcircumflex lesion of 95%.

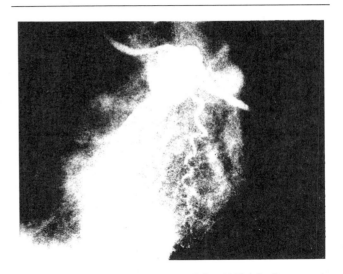

Fig. 7-18. Although the angulation of the 1980 injection appears slightly different, it was believed that definite regression to 70% obstruction in the circumflex had occurred.

decreased from 19% in 1973 to a very lean 13% in 1979. Blood pressures were well controlled with exercise, weight loss, and sodium restriction, averaging 120 to 130 mm Hg systolic pressure.

Again, because of these findings, it was elected to continue to treat the patient medically, and he became somewhat of a celebrity in the program because he was the most dramatic example of regression seen in the program to that point in time (approximately 5% of middle-aged patients in our long-term phase III program were found to have some degree of regression on repeat coronary angiograms).

The patient had elected to retire from his job as a shoe salesman in 1972 and often took 2- to 3-week vacations on trips around the world, in which he would continue to exercise either by running around the deck of a ship or running up and down the stairs of a hotel where he was staying.

On January 20, 1980, the patient died during his sleep. He apparently suffered a fatal arrhythmia while sleeping. A subsequent autopsy revealed no evidence of acute myocardial infarction or coronary thrombosis with stable coronary atherosclerotic lesions, as described at angiography in 1979. Patchy fibrosis of the myocardium was observed, however. This patient experienced a rhythm death during sleep of unknown cause. Many theories have been advanced trying to explain these occurrences, including myocardial ischemia, low-potassium or low-magnesium levels within the myocardium, inadequate intake of linoleic acid in the diet, and so on.

In any case, we can certainly say that this man experienced a greatly improved quality of life over the 21-year history of his coronary disease and may well have extended his life as a result of his compliance to the overall cardiac rehabilitation program. His dedication, compliance, and tremendous improvement served as an inspiration for other patients to adhere to life-style changes.

REFERENCES

1. Akhras, F., and others: Early exercise testing and coronary angiography after uncomplicated myocardial infarction, Br. Med. J. **284:**1293, 1982.
2. Barndt, R., Jr., and others: Regression and progression of early femoral atherosclerosis in treated hyperlipoproteinemia patients, Ann. Intern. Med. **86:**109, 1977.
3. Barnes, G.K., and others: Changes in working status of patients following coronary bypass surgery, J.A.M.A. **238:**1259, 1977.
4. Bemis, C.E., and others: Progression of coronary artery disease: a clinical anteriographic study, Circulation **47:**55, 1973.
5. Blessey, R., and others: Therapeutic effects and safety of exercising coronary patients at their angina threshold, Med. Sci. Sports Exerc. **11:**110, 1979. (Abstract.)
6. Blessey, R., and others: Early exercise training in complicated and uncomplicated post-myocardial infarction patients, Med. Sci. Sports Exerc. **12:**100, 1980. (Abstract.)
7. Blessey, R., and others: Angiographic, clinical and exercise data in marathoning coronary patients, Med. Sci. Sports Exerc. **13:**131, 1981. (Abstract.)
8. Blessey, R., and others: Post–myocardial infarction hospital course and response to early exercise training, Med. Sci. Sports Exerc. **114:**155, 1982. (Abstract.)
9. Bloch, A., and others: Early mobilization after myocardial infarction: a controlled study, Am. J. Cardiol. **34:**152, 1974.
10. Block, T.A., and others: Improvement in exercise performance after unsuccessful myocardial revascularization, Am. J. Cardiol. **40:**673, 1977.
11. Brown, C.A., and others: Prospective study of medical and urgent surgical therapy in randomizable patients with unstable angina pectoris: results of in-hospital and chronic mortality and morbidity, Am. Heart J. **102:**959, 1981.
12. Bruce, R.A., and others: Difference in cardiac function with prolonged physical training for cardiac rehabilitation, Am. J. Cardiol. **40:**597, 1977.
13. Clausen, J.P.: Circulatory adjustments to dynamic exercise and effect of physical training in normal subjects and in patients with coronary artery disease, Prog. Cardiovasc. Dis. **18:**459, 1976.
14. Clausen, J.P., and others: The effects of training on the heart rate during arm and leg exercise, Scand. J. Clin. Lab. Invest. **26:**295, 1970.
15. Clement, D.B., and others: A survey of overuse running injuries, Phys. Sports Med. **9:**47, 1981.
16. Conn, E.H., and others: Exercise responses before and after physical conditioning in patients with severely depressed left ventricular functions, Am. J. Cardiol. **49:**296, 1982.
17. Cook, R.: Psychological responses to myocardial infarction, Heart Lung **2:**62, 1973.
18. Cookey, J.D., and others: Exercise training and plasma catecholamines in patients with ischemic heart disease, Am. J. Cardiol. **42:**372, 1978.
19. De Busk, R.F., and others: Exercise training soon after myocardial infarction, Am. J. Cardiol. **44:**1223, 1979.
20. Detry, J.M., and others: Effects of physical training on exertional ST-segment depression in coronary heart disease, Circulation **44:**390, 1971.
21. Detry, J.M., and others: Increased arteriovenous oxygen difference after physical training in coronary heart disease, Circulation **4:**109, 1971.
22. DeWood, M.A., and others: Medical and surgical management of myocardial infarction, Am. J. Cardiol. **44:**1356, 1979.
23. Dion, W.F., and others: Medical problems and physiologic responses during supervised inpatient cardiac rehabilitation: the patient after coronary bypass grafting, Heart Lung **11:**248, 1982.
24. Ehsani, A.A., and others: Effects of 12 months of intense exercise training on ischemic ST-segment depression in patients with coronary artery disease, Circulation **64:**1116, 1981.
25. Eikelans, D.W., and others: High density lipoprotein-cholesterol in survivors of myocardial infarction, J.A.M.A. **242:**2185, 1979.
26. Erdman, R.A.M.: Psychological evaluation of an existing cardiac program: a randomized clinical trial in patients with myocardial infarction. In II World Congress on Cardiac Rehabilitation: Abstracts of free communications, Jerusalem, p. 124, 1982.
27. Felig, P., and others: Fuel homeostasis in exercise, N. Engl. J. Med. **293:**1078, 1975.
28. Ferguson, R.J., and others: Changes in exercise coronary sinus blood flow with training in patients with angina pectoris, Circulation **58:**41, 1978.
29. Freedman, B., and others: Pathophysiology of coronary artery spasm, Circulation **66:**705, 1982.
30. Froelicher, V.F.: Does exercise conditioning delay progression of myocardial ischemia in coronary atherosclerotic disease? Cardiovasc. Clin. **8:**11, 1977.
31. Fuller, C.M., and others: Early post–myocardial infarction treadmill stress testing: an accurate prediction of multivessel coronary disease and subsequent cardiac events, Ann. Intern. Med. **94:**734, 1981.
32. Goldman, S., and others: Marked depth of ST-segment depression during treadmill exercise testing: indicator of severe coronary disease, Circulation **61:**572, 1980.
33. Hammermeister, K.E., and others: Effect of surgical vs medical therapy on return to work in patients with coronary disease, Am. J. Cardiol. **44:**105, 1979.
34. Harri, M.N.E.: Physical training under the influence of beta blockade in rats, III. Effects in muscular metabolism, Eur. J. Applied Physiol. **45:**25, 1980.
35. Hartman, C.W., and others: The safety and value of exercise testing soon after coronary artery bypass surgery, J. Cardiac Rehabil. **1:**142, 1981.
36. Haskell, J.H.: Physical activity after myocardial infarction, Am. J. Cardiol. **33:**776, 1974.
37. Hayes, M.J., and others: Comparison of mobilization after two and nine days in uncomplicated myocardial infarction, Br. Med. J. **3:**10, 1974.
38. Hellerstein, H.K.: Effects of an active physical reconditioning intervention program on the clinical course of coronary artery disease, Med. Cardiovasc. **10:**461, 1969.

39. Hellerstein, H.K., and others: The influence of active conditioning upon subjects with coronary disease, Can. Med. Assoc. J. **96**:901, 1967.
40. Hoffman, W.E.: The effect of propranolol on change in HDL level in cardiac patients involved in exercise training, Med. Sci. Sports Exerc. **14**:124, 1982. (Abstract.)
41. Ice, R., and others: Descriptive data on marathon runners with severe coronary artery disease: results from cardiac catheterization, exercise tests and serum lipids, Med. Sci. Sports Exerc. **10**:35, 1978. (Abstract.)
42. Ice, R., and others: The safety and effectiveness of long distance bicycling in the treatment of coronary artery disease, Proceedings of the First International Conference on Sports Cardiology, Rome, 1978, Aulo Gaggi (publisher).
43. Kallio, V., and others: Reduction in sudden deaths by a multifactorial intervention program after acute myocardial infarction, Lancet **2**:1091, 1979.
44. Kavanaugh, T., and others: Characteristics of post-coronary marathon runners, Ann. N.Y. Acad. Sci. **301**:455, 1978.
45. Kavanaugh, T., and others: Prognostic indices for patients with ischemic heart disease enrolled in an exercise-centered rehabilitation program, Am. J. Cardiol. **44**:1230, 1979.
46. Kellerman, J.: In Proceedings of the International Conference on Sports Cardiology, Rome, 1978, Aulo Gaggi (publisher).
47. Kimbiris, D., and others: Devolutionary pattern of coronary atherosclerosis in patients with angina pectoris, Am. J. Cardiol. **33**:7, 1974.
48. Jensen, D., and others: Improvement in ventricular function during exercise following cardiac rehabilitation, Am. J. Cardiol. **46**:770, 1980.
49. Lee, A., and others: Long-term effects of physical training on coronary patients with impaired ventricular function, Circulation **60**:1519, 1979.
50. Lehtonen, A.: The effects of exercise on high density (HDL) lipoprotein apoproteins, Acta Physiol. Scand. **106**:487, 1979.
51. Lie, J.T., and others: Aortocoronary bypass saphenous vein graft atherosclerosis: anatomic study of 99 vein grafts from normal and hyperlipoproteinemic patients up to 75 months postoperatively, Am. J. Cardiol. **40**:906, 1977.
52. Lindberg, H.A., and others: Totally asymptomatic myocardial infarction: an estimate of its incidence in the living population, Arch. Intern. Med. **106**:628, 1960.
53. Logue, B., and others: A practical approach to coronary artery disease with special reference to coronary artery bypass surgery, Curr. Probl. Cardiol. **1**:5, 1976.
54. López, S.A., and others: Effect of exercise and physical fitness on serum lipids and lipoproteins, Atherosclerosis **20**:1, 1974.
55. McNeer, J.F., and others: The course of acute myocardial infarction: feasibility of early discharge of the uncomplicated patient, Circulation **51**:410, 1975.
56. McNeer, J.F., and others: Hospital discharge one week after acute myocardial infarction, N. Engl. J. Med. **298**:229, 1978.
57. Miller, N.E., and others: The Tromsø Heart study: high density lipoproteins and coronary artery disease: a prospective case control study, Lancet **1**:965, 1977.
58. Mitchell, J.H.: Exercise testing in the treatment of coronary heart disease, Adv. Intern. Med. **20**:249, 1975.
59. Morganroth, J., and others: Echocardiographic detection of coronary artery disease, Am. J. Cardiol. **46**:1178, 1980.
60. Moss, A.J., and others: Cardiac deaths in the first six months after myocardial infarction: potential for mortality reduction in the early post-hospital periods, Am. J. Cardiol. **39**:816, 1977.
61. Oldridge, N., and others: Noncompliance in an exercise rehabilitation program for men who have suffered a myocardial infarction, Can. Med. Assoc. J. **118**:361, 1978.
62. Oldridge, N., and others: Compliance in exercise rehabilitation, Phys. Sports Med. **7**:94, 1979.
63. Oscai, L.B.: The role of exercise and weight control, Exerc. Sport Sci. Rev. **1**:103, 1973.
64. Oscai, L.B, and others: Normalization of serum triglycerides and lipoprotein electrophoretic patterns by exercise, Am. J. Cardiol. **30**:775, 1972.
65. Palac, R.T., and others: Risk factors related to progressive narrowing in aortocoronary vein grafts studied 1 and 5 years after surgery, Circulation **66**(suppl. 1):1, 1982.
66. Patterson, D.H., and others: Effects of physical training on cardiovascular function following myocardial infarction, J. Appl. Physiol. **47**:482, 1979.
67. Rahimtoola, S.H.: A consensus on coronary bypass surgery, Arch. Intern. Med. **94**:272, 1981.
68. Rechnitzer, P.A.: The effects of training: reinfarction and death—an interim report, Med. Sci. Sports Exerc. **11**:382, 1979.
69. Rechnitzer, P.A., and others: The effect of exercise prescription in the recurrence rate of myocardial infarction in men, Am. J. Cardiol. **47**:419, 1981. (Abstract.)
70. Redwood, D.R., and others: Circulatory and symptomatic effects of physical training in patients with coronary artery disease and angina pectoris, N. Engl. J. Med. **286**:959, 1972.
71. Rigo, P., and others: Hemodynamic and prognostic findings in patients with transmural and nontransmural infarction, Circulation **51**:1064, 1975.
72. Rod, J.L., and others: Symptom-limited graded exercise testing soon after myocardial revascularization surgery, J. Cardiac Rehabil. **2**:199, 1982.
73. Russell, R.O., and others: Unstable angina pectoris study group: unstable angina pectoris: national cooperative study group to compare surgical and medical therapy. II. In-hospital experience and initial follow-up results in patients with one, two, or three vessel disease, Am. J. Cardiol. **42**:839, 1978.
74. Sable, D.L., and others: Attenuation of exercise conditioning by beta-adrenergic blockade, Circulation **65**:679, 1982.
75. Sanmarco, M.E., and others: Atherosclerosis: its progression and regression, Primary Cardiology, p. 51, July/Aug. 1978.
76. Sanmarco, M.E., and others: Abnormal blood pressure response and marked ischemic ST-segment depression as predictors of severe coronary artery disease, Circulation **61**:572, 1980.
77. Selvester, R., and others: Exercise training and coronary artery disease progression, Ann. N.Y. Acad. Sci. **301**:495, 1978.
78. Shaw, L.W.: Effects of a prescribed supervised exercise program on mortality and cardiovascular morbidity in patients after myocardial infarction: The National Heart Disease Project, Am. J. Cardiol. **48**(1):39, 1981.
79. Sim, D.N., and others: Investigation of the physiologic basis for increased exercise threshold for angina pectoris after physical conditioning, J. Clin. Invest. **54**:763, 1974.
80. Stamford, B.A., and others: Task specific changes in maximal oxygen uptake resulting from arm versus leg training, Ergonomics **21**:1, 1978.
81. Stein, R.A., and others: Clinical value of early exercise testing after myocardial infarction, Arch. Intern. Med. **140**:1179, 1980.
82. Stern, M.J.: Psychosocial adaptation following an acute myocardial infarction, J. Chronic Dis. **29**:513, 1976.
83. Streja, D., and others: Moderate exercise and high density lipoprotein-cholesterol, J.A.M.A. **242**:2190, 1979.
84. Szklo, M., and others: Survival of patients with nontransmural myocardial infarction: a population-based study, Am. J. Cardiol. **42**:648, 1978.
85. Tatman, D., and others: Exercise conditioning and early return to work after coronary bypass surgery, Med. Sci. Sports Exerc. **113**:133, 1981. (Abstract)

86. Théroux, P., and others: Prognostic value of exercise testing soon after myocardial infarction, N. Engl. J. Med. **301:**341, 1979.

87. Thompson, P.D., and Keleman, M.H.: Hypotension accompanying the onset of exertional angina, Circulation **52:**28, 1975.

88. Weiner, D.A., and others: ST segment changes post-infarction: predictive value for multi-vessel coronary disease and left ventricular aneurysm, Circulation **58:**887, 1978.

89. Weiner, D.A., and others: Identification of patients with left main and three vessel coronary disease with clinical and exercise test variables, Am. J. Cardiol. **46:**21, 1980.

90. Wenger, N.K.: Rehabilitation of the patient with acute myocardial infarction: early ambulation and patient education. In Pollack, M.L., and Schmidt, D.H., editors: Heart disease and rehabilitation, Boston, 1979, Houghton Mifflin Co.

91. Wenger, N.K.: Research related to rehabilitation, Circulation **60:**1636, 1979.

92. Wenger, N.K., and others: Cardiac conditioning after myocardial infarction: an early intervention program, Cardiovasc. Rehabil. Q. **2:**17, 1971.

93. Wilhelmsen, L., and others: A controlled trial of physical training myocardial infarction, Prev. Med. **4:**491, 1975.

94. Williams, R.S., and others: Physical conditioning augments the fibrinolytic response to venous occlusion in healthy adults, N. Engl. J. Med. **302:**987, 1980.

95. Wilmore, J., and others: Validity of skinfold and girth measurements for predicting alterations in body composition, J. Appl. Physiol. **29:**313, 1970.

96. Young, D.T., and others: A prospective controlled study of in-hospital myocardial infarction rehabilitation, J. Cardiac Rehabil. **2:**32, 1982.

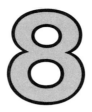

RAYMOND L. BLESSEY

The beneficial effects of aerobic exercise for patients with coronary artery disease

It has been emphasized in several of the preceding chapters that coronary disease is a multifactorial disease. It follows therefore that the treatment of coronary disease should be multifaceted including life-style modification aimed at risk-factor reduction, diet, medication, and exercise therapy. It is inappropriate to think of any of the previously mentioned treatment approaches by itself as the panacea for coronary disease.

The value of exercise for coronary patients is often questioned, and the skeptics continue to state that there is no "definitive proof" that exercise is beneficial to the coronary patient in terms of prolonging life or "preventing" a repeat myocardial infarction. This negative view of the value of exercise for coronary patients stems from a limited perspective and, in fact, is poorly founded. The "definitive" lack of proof is not available for a number of reasons including the following: (1) It is virtually impossible to design and implement a study that "proves" that exercise therapy significantly reduces coronary death rate and repeat infarction rate because of the large number of subjects needed, and (2) previous attempts at proving or disproving the protective effect of exercise have often used less than adequate exercise intensity and duration and have not properly handled the problem with "crossover" in the treatment and control groups. Furthermore, the skeptic's view of exercise for coronary patients is short sighted in that the benefits of properly designed exercise programs are not limited to reduction in mortality and morbidity and, as mentioned earlier, treatment of the coronary patient should be multifaceted.

Our view regarding the benefits of aerobic exercise for the coronary patient is that there is more than adequate evidence clinically and in the literature to support it as one of several essential treatment modalities for the coronary patient. The key to achieving beneficial results is the de-

sign and implementation of an aerobic exercise program that is appropriate in terms of the intensity, duration, and frequency (refer to Chapter 7). On the next page there is a list of the ranges of exercise intensity, duration, and frequency and the various modes of exercise we have utilized with our patients in the last 10 years.

This chapter is designed to discuss the various beneficial effects of aerobic exercise for coronary patients who have been well documented. In addition, there will be some discussion regarding the need to study further the effects of chronic exercise in certain specific areas.

AEROBIC EXERCISE AND RISK-FACTOR REDUCTION

Several major factors that are associated with an increased risk for the development of coronary disease and the progression (worsening) of the disease can be modified by consistent aerobic exercise programs.

Serum lipid levels and exercise

The beneficial effect of aerobic exercise on serum lipids in normals have been well documented.[35,84] There have also been similar studies involving patients with known coronary disease. Hartung and others demonstrated that a 3-month training program utilizing an intensity of 70% to 85% of the patient's maximal heart rate, a frequency of three times per week, and a duration of 30 minutes per session was adequate to significantly increase the serum high-density-lipoprotein cholesterol (HDL-C).[36] There was a significant correlation ($r = .79$, $p < .05$) between the change in HDL-C and improvement in estimated maximal oxygen consumption based on treadmill test duration. In Hartung's study there was no major change in the total cholesterol, low-density cholesterol (LDL-C), or the triglyceride values after training. Streja, using a similar ex-

Table 8-1. Summary of training effects on serum lipids in coronary patients

Author/year	n	Training average duration (months)	% change in total cholesterol	% change in HDL cholesterol	% change in LDL cholesterol	% change in triglycerides
Streja, 1979	32	3	+4.7*	+9.7*	+6.6	−8.0
Hartung, 1981	18	3	−2.0	+15*	−5.7	−8.1
Erkelens, 1979	18	6	−5.0	+14.0*	—	−6.0
Oschrin, 1982	17	6	−3.0	+11.0*	−3.0	−34*

*$p = \leq .05$

SUMMARY OF AEROBIC EXERCISE PROGRAMS UTILIZED FOR CORONARY PATIENTS

EXERCISE MODE:
Walking, jogging, cycling, aerobic dancing, cross-country skiing, roller skating, rope jumping, trampoline, jogging, swimming, arm cranking, rowing, circuit weight training

EXERCISE INTENSITY:
65% to 95% of patient's maximum heart rate

EXERCISE DURATION:
30 to 60 minutes

FREQUENCY:
3 to 6 days per week

---

ercise program, also documented significant increases in the HDL-C values after training. Unfortunately, his patients also demonstrated increased total cholesterol values ($p < .05$) as well.[78]

Both Oschrin[59] and Erkelens[24] documented increased HDL-C values after 6 months' training of 11% to 14% above pretraining values. The major difference in the results of these two studies was that Oschrin also reported triglyceride values that were 34% lower after training ($p < .05$). The higher training intensity (mean of 83% of maximum heart rate) and greater frequency of training (mean of 5.1 days per week) in our patients and thus greater total caloric expenditure, probably is responsible for the different findings in the posttraining triglyceride values. The findings from all four of these studies are summarized in Table 8-1.

We have also investigated the relationship between various levels of aerobic exercise and HDL values in patients with documented coronary disease. Our study involved 98 male patients divided into three groups: (1) inactive pa-

tients, (2) patients performing up to 96 minutes of aerobic exercise per week, and (3) patients performing more than 120 minutes of aerobic exercise per week.[29] Both exercising groups demonstrated significant decreases in serum triglyceride values and increases in high-density lipoprotein values. However, although there was a trend for a greater magnitude of change in the patients performing a greater duration of exercise, the difference between the two subgroups pre- and posttraining values ($n = 10$ in each group) were not statistically significant.

In summary, there is consistent evidence that aerobic exercise can result in significantly increased serum HDL cholesterol values and significantly decreased serum triglycerides after 3 to 6 months of training in coronary patients. The data on the effects of exercise on serum total cholesterol and LDL cholesterol do not indicate any consistent beneficial effect of aerobic exercise on these lipids. There are epidemiological and angiographic studies indicating that higher HDL values and lower triglyceride values are associated with a decreased likelihood of progression of coronary disease.[55,71] Additional studies are needed to investigate whether the magnitude of the changes that occur in serum lipids in exercising coronary patients are likely to affect the probability of progression of disease.

Aerobic exercise and hypertension

The literature indicates that consistent long-term aerobic exercise can result in at least a 10 to 20 mm Hg decrease in both the resting and exercise (at a given submaximal work load) blood pressure of hypertensive subjects.[9,11,13,67] Boyer and Kasch's study[11] was especially impressive, since it involved 23 hypertensive men whose resting blood pressure did not respond to medical therapy alone. However, after 6 months of aerobic exercise combined with medical therapy, these investigators reported a mean decrease in resting systolic and diastolic blood pressures of 14 and 12 mm Hg respectively. It is important to note that the improved blood pressures in these men were not associated with a significant decrease in body weight or sodium intake. Krotkiewski also reported significant decreases in the blood pressures of obese hypertensive subjects after phys-

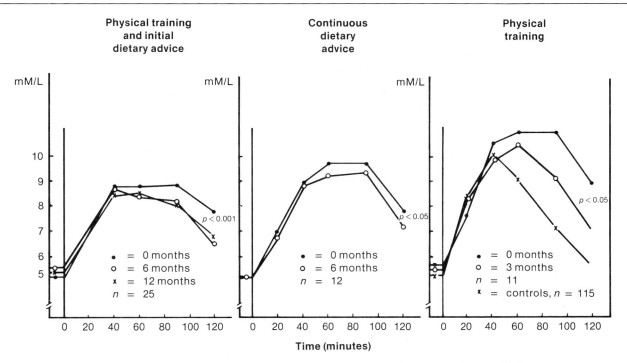

Fig. 8-1. Oral glucose tolerance test results in middle-aged men with chemical diabetes. Notice that physical training by itself and in combination with dietary advice had significantly improved glucose tolerance test results. (From Saltin, B., and others: Diabetes **28** (Suppl. 1):30-32, 1979.)

ical training that were not associated with decreases in body weight or body fat.[48] In fact, the greatest reduction in both the systolic and diastolic blood pressures in those obese subjects occurred in the group of patients with the least change in body weight and body fat.

What are the mechanisms through which aerobic exercise modifies systolic and diastolic blood pressure? This is an area that definitely requires further study. Björntorp has concluded from his work and his review of the literature that the major mechanism through which physical training mediates its antihypertensive effect is through a decrease in the sympathetic nervous system activity.[2] Hartley and others work[34] supports this theoretical explanation.

We have noted a sharp reduction in the blood pressures of our hypertensive coronary patients involved with chronic physical training. The changes in these patients are not unlike those reported in the hypertensive patients discussed above. A recent study at Duke University Medical Center of 125 cardiac rehabilitation participants with hypertension supports our clinical impression.[54] After training, the mean diastolic blood pressure decreased from 98 to 80 mm Hg and 73% of these patients achieved a diastolic pressure below 90. In this study, unlike those cited earlier, the decreased blood pressures were associated with decreased weight loss and sodium intake.

How important is the control of hypertension in the pre-

vention of cardiovascular mortality and morbidity? This was the focus of the Hypertension Detection and Follow-up Program Study involving 10,940 participants.[85] The conclusion of this 5-year randomized prospective trial was that effective management of hypertension has great potential for reducing mortality for the large numbers of individuals with elevated blood pressure, even those with mild hypertension. In addition, there are data from the Mayo Clinic indicating that effective treatment of hypertension improves the survival of patients with known coronary disease.[16] The survival rates at 1, 5, and 10 years for 300 patients (with angina pectoris or who had a myocardial infarction) treated for hypertension was 91%, 82%, and 74% and in the untreated patients 76%, 65%, and 41% respectively. Based on this data and that of the Hypertension Detection and Follow-up Study, hypertension is a major prognostic variable, and thus therapy aimed at modifying the degree of hypertension is definitely in the patients's best interest.

Aerobic exercise and glucose intolerance

The Framingham data suggest that diabetes is a powerful risk factor in that diabetic men and women have two to three times the risk of developing coronary disease compared to their nondiabetic counterparts.[41] Furthermore, the diabetic patient has a higher risk of more rapid progression of coronary disease,[68] multiple myocardial infarctions,[18] and a higher mortality from coronary disease[47] compared to the nondiabetic patient. Thus the goal of modifying the risk factor of glucose intolerance by exercise and other therapies appears to be indicated for the patient with known coronary disease, as well as the patient with multiple-risk factors for the disease.

Glucose intolerance has been shown to be associated with obesity and a sedentary life-style.[17,53] Thus physical training would have a positive effect on the tendency toward glucose intolerance, and, in fact, studies have shown that the serum insulin levels are reduced during oral glucose tolerance tests in obese men after training.[4] More importantly, Saltin and other's studies of subjects with documented chemical diabetes demonstrated that after 3 to 6 months of aerobic exercise, the glucose tolerance tests of these subjects were normalized[70] (Fig. 8-1). Ruderman and others suggested that the improvement in glucose disappearance rate found in the intravenous glucose tolerance tests of adult-onset diabetics after training was attributable to either an enhanced sensitivity to endogenous insulin or a decreased or diminished "anti-insulin" factor.[68]

In those coronary patients who perform regular aerobic exercise, we have frequently noticed a decreased need for insulin or oral medication. Björntorp and other's study of post–myocardial infarction patients on a regular training program supports our clinical findings in that they noted lower serum insulin levels after a glucose challenge in the trained patients presumably because of an increased insulin sensitivity at the cellular level.[3] These improved results were associated with significantly decreased serum triglycerides and body fat levels.

In summary, aerobic exercise has been shown to be effective in altering several of the major risk factors for coronary disease, including low serum HDL-cholesterol level, hypertriglyceridemia, hyperglycemia, and arterial hypertension. More significantly, several of these risk factors have also been shown to be related to the risk of progression of coronary disease[63] and coronary artery bypass graft occlusion.[60]

AEROBIC EXERCISE AND IMPROVEMENT IN PHYSICAL WORK CAPACITY OF PATIENTS WITH KNOWN CORONARY DISEASE

In the 1950s, exercise therapy was used primarily to help the coronary patient to overcome the detrimental effects of prolonged bed rest. In the early and mid 1960s, several of the more "aggressive" centers began to use exercise therapy for the purpose of conditioning the coronary patient with the overall aim of returning the patient to a more active life-style. Formal studies documenting the beneficial effects of physical training for coronary patients began appearing in the literature in the early mid-1960s.[1,37,57,80] Frick and Katila reporting on seven coronary patients exercised for 1 to 2 months three times per

week concluded that after training (1) the stroke volume was improved during exercise, (2) the heart volume was unchanged, (3) the arterial blood lactate levels during exercise were reduced, (4) the exercise tolerance was improved, and (5) there was some evidence suggestive of increased coronary flow.[26] These same authors cautioned, however, that there is a "need for proper selection of patients and close medical supervision during training." Since the early 1960s, when it became clear that coronary patients are capable of responding appropriately to exercise training, clinicians and researchers have continued to ask two major questions. What degree of improvement in maximal aerobic capacity is reasonable to expect in the coronary patient? What are the mechanisms through which coronary patients improve their aerobic capacity? Not surprisingly, these two questions are closely related. Based on a review of the literature and some 10 years of clinical experience, it is my opinion that the major variable that determines the coronary patient's adaptations to training, that is, the degree of improvement in maximal oxygen uptake and the specific cardiovascular adaptation accounting for the change in the maximal volume of oxygen $Vo_{2 \, max}$, is the training stimulus, that is, training intensity, duration, frequency, and period of time the program is carried out (see Chapter 7). To a lesser extent, the degree of coronary disease and left ventricular dysfunction and the use of beta-adrenergic blocking agents such as propranolol, atenolol, and timolol may influence the coronary patient's responses to chronic training.

Detry and other's results are representative of most of the earlier studies on the hemodynamic consequences of physical training in coronary patients.[19] After 12 patients (six with angina, six after myocardial infarction without symptoms) underwent exercise training for 45 minutes three times per week for 3 months, Detry and others reported a 22.5% improvement in $Vo_{2 \, max}$. The exercise intensity used in this study was not specified. The results of this study indicated that the classic posttraining bradycardia at rest and at a given submaximal work load was attributable to peripheral changes, that is, increased arteriovenous differences, and not related to changes in left ventricular function, that is, increased stroke volume or ejection fraction. Many clinicians continue to believe that the only mechanism through which coronary patients improve their aerobic capacity is the increased extraction of oxygen by the trained skeletal muscle. However, in the late 1970s, there were several studies published that challenged the conclusions of Detry and others. Patterson and others studied two groups of coronary patients randomly assigned to either a low-intensity or a high-intensity exercise program.[61] The high-intensity group exercised for 30 to 45 minutes at work loads equivalent to 65% to 80% of their $Vo_{2 \, max}$. As expected, the high-intensity group showed the classic changes in aerobic capacity over the course of the 1-year study. More importantly, however, the high-intensity group demonstrated improvements (10% increase in stroke volume) in ventricular function that did not appear until the last 6 months of training. Patterson's results suggest that in order to stimulate central cardiac adaptations to exercise training in coronary patients it is important to evaluate the patients over a longer period than 2 to 3 months as most of the previous studies had done. Shortly after Patterson published his results, Jensen and others, using radionuclide ventriculography, reported improvements in exercise left ventricular ejection fractions in a subset of coronary patients trained for 3 to 9 months (mean of 6 months) at an intensity equivalent to 65% to 85% of maximal oxygen uptake.[38] A randomized study using a larger patient population and similar techniques for evaluating posttraining ventricular function changes is currently underway by Jensen and Froelicher's group.[27] Hagberg and others documented impressive changes in left ventricular function after training in a group of coronary patients as well.[31] Once again, the training program was carried out over a period of 12 months, with the last 6 months of training consisting of exercise sessions 50 to 60 minutes in duration at 70% to 90% of $VO_{2\ max}$, four to six times per week. These patients had a mean increase in their aerobic capacity of 39% and demonstrated significant increases in stroke volume at both a given submaximal work load and the same relative work load (i.e., same percent of $VO_{2\ max}$). Those authors appropriately concluded that these results demonstrated that "if training is continued and progressively increased in intensity, duration and frequency, some patients with coronary artery disease can, over 12 months, have improved cardiac function as reflected in an increase in stroke volume and stroke work." These studies support the earlier statement that training stimulus is in fact the key variable in determining the cardiac patient's adaptations to chronic aerobic exercise.

What about the influence of the degree of coronary disease and left ventricular dysfunction on the patient's ability to respond to training? Neither Patterson[61] nor Jensen[38] were able to correlate the degree of improvement in aerobic capacity or left ventricular function to the clinical status of the patient. We have reported on a group of patients with relatively poor ventricular function (resting ejection fraction less than 40%) who trained over a period of 12 to 42 months and demonstrated the classic training responses and no evidence of deterioration in ventricular function.[50] Our data and those of Letac[51] indicate that poor left ventricular function does not necessarily prevent the patient from responding appropriately to an individualized exercise training program. We have also reported on a subset of patients with good ventricular function but with severe coronary disease (three with severe double-vessel, five with triple-vessel disease) who have trained for and completed numerous marathon (26.2-mile) runs.[7] Several of these patients had limiting exertional angina before initiating their training program. Thus it has been our observation that severe coronary disease and angina does not necessarily prevent patients from training to high levels of fitness. The combination of poor ventricular function and multiple coronary artery lesions has neither been closely examined nor is it likely to be in the future because of the aggressive use of surgery in these patients. It is possible that this subset of patients would be limited in their ability to respond to training.

The effect of beta blockers on the coronary patients' ability to improve their aerobic capacity has been studied.[52,58,62] It is difficult, however, to draw any general conclusions because of the variety in the training programs utilized, the individual patient's sensitivity to the drug, and the variety in doses used. Both Obin[58] and Pratt's[62] results suggest that certain coronary patients on beta blockers can significantly increase their aerobic capacity. In fact, Pratt reported that a group of patients receiving 120 to 240 mg of propranolol per day were able to increase their $VO_{2\ max}$ by 46% 3 months after training compared to a group of clinically matched patients not receiving propranolol who demonstrated a 27% improvement in their aerobic capacity. Pratt's data may be somewhat misleading because of the self-selected nature of the patient population.

In summary, it is clear from the literature that coronary patients can significantly improve their aerobic capacity. The degree of improvement that occurs appears to be primarily related to the training stimulus and perhaps secondarily related to the clinical status and medical therapy of the patient. In addition, it is evident from the literature that coronary patients continue to improve their aerobic capacity over extended periods of time (years) provided that an adequate training stimulus is utilized. The specific type of cardiovascular adaptations that occur in coronary patients may vary, again, dependent on the training stimulus and the duration of the exercise program. The key point, however, is that no matter what specific physiological adaptations take place in the trained coronary patient, an increased aerobic capacity means a greater reserve for both recreational and occupational activities and therefore the potential for a greater quality of life.

EXERCISE TRAINING AND IMPROVEMENT OF ISCHEMIC SYMPTOMS

A relatively high percentage of patients referred to our centers for rehabilitation have stable exertional angina pectoris despite medical or surgical intervention. In fact, we are seeing increasing numbers of postbypass patients who have had a return of their exertional angina. In addition, we see a significant number of patients with the combination of coronary artery and peripheral artery disease who are primarily limited by their claudication symptoms. This next section of the chapter is a discussion of the therapeutic effects of aerobic exercise for patients with effort angina and claudication symptoms.

Exercise training and angina patients

In the early 1970s, we had a patient enter our outpatient cardiac rehabilitation program with the primary diagnosis of angina pectoris. At the time this gentleman was 64 years of age and had sought medical attention because of exertional symptoms of chest pressure that were becoming progressive in nature. The patient was limited to walking slowly with his dog two or three blocks at a time because of his symptoms. He underwent exercise testing and angiography at another facility. On his exercise test, he demonstrated both symptoms and electrocardiographic changes consistent with myocardial ischemia at a relatively low work load and myocardial oxygen demand. Fortunately, on his ventriculogram he had evidence of normal left ventricular function at rest with an ejection fraction of 75%. His left ventricular end-diastolic volume and pressures were both elevated, however, being 149 m/m^2 and 18 mm Hg, respectively. The results of his angiography were not quite so encouraging. His angiogram findings were as follows:

Left main artery: no significant lesions

Left anterior descending artery (LAD): 90% occlusion proximally; 95% occlusion distal to the first septal perforator and diagonal; diffuse distal disease extending throughout the course of the LAD. 95% occlusion in the proximal portion of the diagonal artery.

Circumflex artery: 90% occlusion of the midportion, distal to the take-off of the main marginal artery.

Right coronary artery (RCA): 50% to 60% lesions proximally; complete (100%) obstruction of the distal RCA.

In summary, this patient had triple-vessel coronary disease, and he was told by the surgeons that he was not a candidate for bypass surgery because both the LAD and RCA had distal lesions and were therefore not suitable "targets." Furthermore, he was not a candidate for beta receptor–blocking agents because of an inherent resting and exercise bradycardia. In essence, he was told to go home, take it easy, use nitroglycerin as needed, and not to make any long-range plans. Despite this advice from an outside facility, he did enter our rehabilitation program shortly after his angiogram. Using an individualized exercise program initially involving walking the patient up to his angina threshold, this patient began to make improvements in his exercise capacity. In fact, within 4 months after initiating exercise therapy, he began a walk-jog program and was eventually able to progress to a continuous jog. Provided that the patient warmed up sufficiently and jogged at a reasonable pace, he was eventually asymptomatic with exercise. He went on to participate in numerous 10-kilometer runs and half-marathon runs. In addition, he completed over 20 marathon runs during his 9-year involvement with our program. The dramatic changes in the exertional symptoms of this patient and many others like him raise several questions in the minds of clinicians.

What are the mechanisms that allow patients with exertional angina to significantly improve their exercise capacity? Furthermore, what allows certain subsets of these initially symptomatic patients to eventually exercise to considerably higher levels of exertion and not perceive angina? (See Chapter 5.)

We examined the exercise test data on the previously referred-to patient and 17 others with documented coronary disease who were either on no medication or the same medication throughout the course of a 20-month training program.[6] This particular group of patients was exercised at their angina threshold for 60 to 300 minutes per week. Nearly half (44%) of the patients after training demonstrated higher rate-pressure products (RPP) at the onset of angina and 56% had higher maximal RPP on their maximal exercise tests. Several of the patients demonstrated higher maximal RPP after training because they were asymptomatic. Unfortunately, there were more questions than answers raised by this study. We were unable to predict which patients were more likely to improve their angina threshold or become asymptomatic based on their angiography, training program, or initial exercise test results. In addition, the specific mechanisms leading to improvement of symptoms were not studied.

There is considerable controversy in the literature regarding the adaptations that occur in the symptomatic coronary patient after training. The earlier studies explained the beneficial effects of physical training on exertional angina in terms of the relationship between the RPP (indicator of myocardial oxygen demand) and a given external work load[14,28,80]; that is, after training, angina patients were able to exercise at a higher work load before reporting angina because of the lower RPP at comparable pretraining work loads. Therefore it was concluded that the patient's symptoms improved at a given workload because of a lower level of myocardial oxygen demand and not because of any change in myocardial oxygen delivery. The more recent work of Clausen and others made it evident that not all patient's symptomatic improvement could be explained by the RPP changes at a given work load.[15] They noted that after training a subset of patients exercised to significantly higher RPP's before reporting angina. They speculated that an improvement in myocardial oxygen supply caused by increased vascularization or increased content of oxidative enzymes in myocardial muscle cells might have explained these changes. These authors also cautioned that using the RPP alone as an indicator of myocardial oxygen demand (MVO$_2$) may be misleading. RPP does not take into account the left ventricular end-diastolic volume, which is another determinant of MVO$_2$. Both Sim and Neill[76] and Redwood and others[65] have concluded after studying symptomatic coronary patients that after training the improved symptoms could be explained by increased myocardial oxygen supply. Other mechanisms that have been considered in explaining the adaptation to exercise training in angina patients include (1) a higher threshold for perception of exertional angina, (2) improved left ventricular function with decreased exercise end-diastolic volumes, and (3) enhanced mechanical efficiency.[20] In addition, Ehsani and others have shown prolonged high level exercise training results in a reduction in myocardial ischemia (as indicated by ECG changes) at the same or higher RPP's.[21] This raises the point again that perhaps some disparity in the mechanism through which the patient with effort angina improves is related to the training stimulus and the length of the training program. Finally, Rizi and others have speculated that transient coronary spasm superimposed on a high-grade arterial obstruction was responsible for ''walk-through'' angina in a patient they studied.[66] This raises the question about the influence of changes in the coronary vasomotor tone on posttraining symptoms. Up to now there have been no studies dealing with this phenomena.

Does exercise training angina patients with the lower extremities (trained limbs) influence their angina threshold during performance of upper extremity exercise (untrained limbs)? This was the basis for Thompson and other's recent study involving a total of 15 patients— four trained with the arms, seven trained with the legs, and four as controls.[79] The exercise training program was 8 weeks in duration. In summary, they reported that the posttraining angina threshold (absolute work load) was enhanced primarily because of a lower rate-pressure product at a given work load. These authors also concluded that it is not necessary therefore to use upper extremity exercise as part of the total exercise rehabilitation program to improve the upper extremity angina threshold. Our clinical impression goes along with their findings regarding the carry-over effect between trained and untrained limbs or extremities; however, using more aggressive exercise programs of longer duration, we have noticed a greater degree of symptomatic improvement specific to the trained muscle group, not explained entirely by a decreased rate-pressure product and therefore have used upper extremity exercise training in addition to lower extremity training when indicated. Additional studies involving larger patient populations and longer training programs are needed for further investigation.

Exercise therapy in the treatment of peripheral vascular disease

Claudication pain manifested as burning or numbness in the feet or pain in the ''calf'' (gastrocnemius and soleus muscles) or, in some cases, as hip discomfort can be more limiting to the coronary patient than angina pectoris. Claudication symptoms are ischemic in nature, that is, attributable to an imbalance between oxygen supply and demand and, as a result, precipitated by exertion and relieved promptly by rest. Patients with these symptoms tend to want to avoid exertion and therefore are somewhat difficult to motivate to exercise regularly. However, these patients often respond favorably to exercise therapy in a relatively short period of time. According to the Framingham statistics, approximately one fourth of coronary artery disease patients suffer from claudication.[40] Approximately 5% to 10% of all the coronary patients referred to our centers report claudication symptoms.

Foley was probably the first to document a beneficial effect of exercise training for patients with advanced peripheral vascular disease in the lower extremities.[25] Since that time, there have been other reports on the favorable responses to exercise training in patients with claudication symptoms; however, the explanations for the symptomatic improvement in these patients remains controversial. Zetterquist, after studying nine patients with claudication who were treated with a combination of a daily walking program and isotonic exercise for three to four months, reported a 73% increase in the walking tolerance of his study population. He used venous occlusion plethysmography to evaluate arterial inflow capacity and, basing his views on the posttraining results, did not see any evidence of improved regional arterial circulation despite considerable clinical improvement. He concluded that the major mechanism for improvement was more efficient distribution of blood flow to the exercising muscle. Finally, he speculated that increased concentration of the oxidative enzymes and increased mechanical efficiency may have accounted for some of the increased functional capacity. Larsen and Larsen reported that a subset of patients with claudication did demonstrate significant improvement in calf-muscle blood flow during exercise.[49] Their findings have been supported by Skinner and Strandness.[77] Saltin, after reviewing the literature, concluded that the reasons for improved walking tolerance in these patients include any and possibly all of the following: (1) improved mechanical efficiency, thereby lowering the oxygen demand during walking, (2) enhanced anaerobic energy yield, and (3) increased oxygen supply to the working muscle.[69] Finally, the literature does not support the hypothesis that severe proximal stenosis or resting claudication symptoms prohibit patients from responding favorably to exercise therapy.[22,39]

The recent reports of Hall suggest that exercise training by itself may not be the ideal therapy for claudication patients.[32,33] He has documented improved muscle blood flow using Doppler studies (arm/ankle index) in patients treated with the combination of high complex carbohydrate, high-fiber, low-fat diet, and exercise training. The improvement in walking time and maximum metabolic equivalent level was associated with a decrease in the serum cholesterol and triglycerides of 28% and 32%. Earlier investigators have reported increased blood flow both at rest and during reactive hyperemia in patients treated with the combination of exercise training and vitamin E.[23]

Summary

In summary, aerobic exercise is effective in improving the exercise capacity of patients with exertional angina. This improvement in angina threshold appears to be attributable to a number of factors. First, after training, the myocardial oxygen demand at a given exercise level (as measured by the heart rate and systolic blood pressure) is lower, and therefore the likelihood of an imbalance between MVo_2 demand and supply is reduced. Furthermore, there appears to be a subset of patients who, after training, are able to achieve higher rate-pressure products with little or no symptoms, apparently as a result of better oxygen supply to the myocardium.

The coronary patient who is limited by symptoms of peripheral vascular disease also often dramatically improves his exercise tolerance after training. The mechanisms that allow these patients to improve after training include more efficient distribution of cardiac output to the working muscle, improved oxygen extraction of the trained muscle, and improved blood supply to the previously ischemic muscle as a result of improved collateral circulation.

EXERCISE AND CORONARY MORTALITY AND MORBIDITY: DOES EXERCISE PROVIDE A PROTECTIVE EFFECT?

The preceding sections in this chapter dealt with the discussion of the documented benefits of chronic aerobic exercise in risk-factor reduction, improvement in maximal aerobic capacity, and relief or improvement in symptoms of exertional angina and claudication. As was mentioned earlier, there has not been, as yet, definitive proof through a randomized prospective trial that exercise significantly influences the mortality and morbidity of coronary patients. Following are several of the major reasons why the previous studies have not reported a significant protective effect of exercise:

1. Need for large randomized sample groups because of the relatively low mortality and morbidity and because of the various subsets of coronary patients
2. High drop-out rates in exercising groups
3. Improper handling of crossover in the control and treatment groups
4. Use of low-intensity and short-duration exercise programs.
5. Treatment of a multifaceted disease with a single intervention, i.e., exercise

After one reviews the above, it becomes apparent that there are both inherent problems with the disease (i.e., multifaceted, relatively low mortality and morbidity, and various subsets of patients) and problems with study design that have clouded the results of previous trials. Table 8-2 summarizes the results of the major studies that have previously examined the value of exercise in reducing coronary morbidity (reinfarction) and mortality (attributable to all causes and cardiac death specifically). A careful review of this table reveals that there has been a consistent trend toward a lower recurrence rate (reinfarction or death) in the exercise groups with the exception of Kentala's data.[46] However, the differences in the recurrence rates between the treatment and control groups, more often than not, have not been found to be statistically significant. Once again, some of the reasons for the lack of statistically significant differences relate to those points previously listed.

The National Exercise and Heart Disease Project was the most recent randomized controlled trial attempted in this country.[56] Further discussion of this project is warranted because it is the largest randomized trial of its kind completed in the United States. This trial was originally designed to randomize some 4000 participants in order to provide a sufficient number of treatment and nontreatment subjects from which statistically significant results could be found. However, because of a lack of funding, only 651 men between 30 and 64 years of age and with a previous documented myocardial infarction were randomized into either the exercise or the nonexercise group.[75] The number of actual randomized subjects is equivalent to 16% of the desired number, and thus the study had limited probability of demonstrating statistically significant differences between the two randomized groups.

The exercise program for the treatment group appeared to barely meet the "minimum" intensity recommendations of most authorities in the field. During the first 8 weeks of the study, the subjects exercised three times per week for 24 minutes; 4 minutes at six different exercise stations, that is, treadmill, bicycle, arm ergometer, and shoulder wheel. Thereafter the participants completed 15 minutes of continuous aerobic exercise followed by 25 minutes of "games" three times per week. It is assumed that the relatively mild exercise program was implemented by the investigators to minimize the problem with subject dropout.

The study also had problems with crossover between the two groups. By the end of 2 years, 23% of the exercising group reported that they had discontinued regular exercise, and 31% of the nonexercising group stated that they were exercising regularly. However, in analysis of the data, because this crossover was ignored, it obviously biased the data against the positive effects of exercise.

Despite the problem of a less than aggressive exercise program and crossover, there were some encouraging findings from the study. The mortality in the exercise group (4.3%) was 37% lower than that in the nonexercise group (6.1%). This difference was not statistically significant because of the relatively small group size; however, if this difference had been seen in a study population of 1400, the lower death rate would have been significant. In addition, the exercise group had a death rate from cardiovascular causes of 1.9% versus 4.3% in the nonexercise group. Furthermore, of the nine deaths related directly to

Table 8-2. Summary of major studies on exercise and coronary mortality and morbidity (1968-1978)

Authors	Follow-up period (years)	Number of exercise groups	Exercise group			Control group		
			Recurrence and mortality (%/year)	Mortality (%/year)	Cardiac mortality (9%/year)	Recurrence and mortality (%/year)	Mortality (%/year)	Cardiac mortality (%/year)
Bruce (1974)	Up to 4.0	195	10.3	3.1	—	—	11.2	—
Gottheiner (1968)	5.0	1103	—	0.88	0.72	—	4.8	—
Kavanagh and others (1975)	2.0	31	2.3	2.3	2.3	5.0	—	—
Kentala (1972)	2.0	77	9.7	7.1	5.8	8.6	6.8	6.2
Rechnitzer and others (1972)	7.0	68	5.0	3.6	—	14.3	9.0	—
Sanne (1972)	1.9	158	6.6	3.8	2.9	12.5	8.8	3.3
Wilhelmsen and others (1975)	4.0	158	8.4	4.4	3.6	10.0	5.6	5.3

recurrent myocardial infarction, eight occurred in the control group and one in the treatment group ($p < .05$). Also of note was that men with a peak systolic blood pressure of 140 mm Hg or greater in the final stage of their exercise test at entry who were in the exercise group had a statistically significant ($p < .05$) lower death rate than their counterparts in the control group. There were no statistically significant differences in the two groups in morbidity though the exercise group had 31% less events.

Summary

In summary, despite a number of design problems and relatively small sample size, the data from The National Exercise and Heart Disease Project are somewhat encouraging in regard to the protective effects of exercise on mortality and morbidity. At the very least, the data from this study suggests that the protective effect may be more significant in certain subsets of post–myocardial infarction patients. It is unfortunate that this project was unable to randomize an adequate number of subjects, since it is unlikely that the funding agencies will support similar projects in the future.

Dr. Terence Kavanagh, director of the largest cardiac rehabilitation program in the world, published data on the influence of exercise compliance on the prognosis in men with a previous myocardial infarction.[45] Although this was not a randomized trial, the data are very impressive and warrant further discussion at this point. Kavanagh's study involved a consecutive series of 610 men referred to the Toronto Rehabilitation Center after a documented myocardial infarction. These men were followed for a mean of 36 months to assess which were the most important prognostic indicators of cardiac events (death, reinfarction). The goal of the exercise program was to complete 3 miles in 30 to 36 minutes, five times per week. Of the study sub-

jects 505 were exercising three times per week and 78 of the remaining 105 men were following through twice per week.

During the follow-up period, there were 23 cardiac deaths and 21 recurrent myocardial infarctions. Risk ratios were calculated for the various factors believed to influence prognosis. Patients with an elevated cholesterol value (≥ 270 mg/dl) had a risk ratio of 1.98. In other words, patients with elevated cholesterol levels had nearly twice the risk of a future coronary event compared to those with a lower value. Cigarette smokers had a risk ratio of 1.93. Exercise noncompliance, on the other hand, had a risk ratio of 22.6, meaning that those who did not continue to comply with the exercise program had nearly 23 times the chance of suffering a second coronary event.

In fact, exercise noncompliance was the major prognostic factor, even more important that the presence of more than 2 mm of ST-segment depression on the initial exercise test, age, hypertension ($\geq 150/110$), persistent angina, evidence of ventricular aneurysm, or enlarged heart on the radiograph. Once again, these data very definitely indicate that exercise compliance dramatically lowers the probability of repeat coronary events.

If one interprets the data from The National Exercise and Heart Disease Project and The Toronto Rehabilitation Center as evidence that exercise training decreases the probability of future coronary events in post–myocardial infarction patients, then the question becomes through which mechanism or mechanisms does exercise provide its protective effect? Following are several mechanisms through which exercise may theoretically influence the prognosis of the coronary patient:

1. Alteration of the normal rate of progression of coronary atherosclerosis through risk-factor reduction and other mechanisms.

2. Improvement in the myocardial oxygen supply and demand balance partly as a result of increased collateral circulation or increased size of the lumen of the coronary vessels.
3. Decreased tendency to form coronary thrombi because of increased fibrolytic activity.
4. Decreased coronary vasomotor tone resulting in decreased tendency toward coronary spasm.

Does risk factor reduction influence the progression of atherosclerosis as suggested above? Barndt and others have demonstrated that reduction of serum cholesterol and triglycerides and blood pressure in hyperlipidemic patients can result in regression of early femoral atherosclerosis over a 13-month period of follow-up.[10] Blankenhorn, after analyzing the data further on these patients with early femoral lesions, reported that the percent change in atherosclerosis was highly correlated with the serum triglyceride level in the type IV hyperlipidemic patients[5]; that is, the lower the serum triglyceride level, the greater the degree of regression in these patients. The earlier studies on atherosclerotic changes in the coronary arteries are somewhat conflicting partly because of the failure either to control some of the major risk factors or aggressively to attempt risk-factor reduction. Furthermore, these studies have involved subjects with clinical manifestations of the disease and therefore more advanced degree of atherosclerosis. It is possible that factors such as ulceration, hemorrhage, calcification, and thrombosis may influence the course of the disease as much as if not more than the major risk factors such as smoking and hypertension. However, Sanmarco and others have reported on 38 men with advanced coronary atherosclerosis studied with serial angiography. They found that changes in coronary lesions are directly related to the risk factors of cigarette smoking and serum HDL cholesterol levels, as well as the age of the patient at the onset of his clinical manifestation of coronary disease.[71] Sanmarco stated, after reviewing his data, that "a program consisting of diet modification, regular exercise, cessation of cigarette smoking, and control of blood pressure and hyperlipidemia will at least stabilize the disease process in some patients and offers the greatest chance of reducing cardiovascular morbidity and mortality.[72] Selvester and others' data suggest that both cigarette smoking and exercise training are related to progression in coronary lesions.[74] In those patients who were nonsmokers and complied with high levels of exercise training, 20% of their vessels demonstrated progression (worsening) of disease over a course of 18 months, whereas nonsmokers who were inactive demonstrated progression in 30% of their vessels. The more recent work by Raichlen cited earlier supports the concept that progression of coronary disease is related to blood pressure, cigarette smoking, control of diabetes, and exercise habits.[63] Thus it appears that risk-factor reduction through exercise and other intervention is worthwhile and may help to stabilize coronary disease.

Thus far, the other "mechanisms" listed previously have not been studied. Specifically, no studies are available on the influence of exercise training on the size of the coronary vessels or on vasomotor tone. In addition, the studies on exercise training and collateralization have been inconclusive. Williams and others have reported that regular aerobic exercise over a 10-week period in healthy adults 25 to 69 years of age can enhance fibrinolysis in response to thrombotic stimuli.[83] They concluded that the augmented fibrinolytic response to venous occlusion "could be an important mechanism in the beneficial effect of habitual physical activity on the risk of cardiovascular disease." Further study is needed to see if the coronary patient demonstrates a similar tendency toward enhanced fibrinolysis and what influence it has on future coronary events.

PSYCHOLOGICAL EFFECTS OF EXERCISE TRAINING

Kavanagh and others have studied the effects of exercise training on depression in coronary patients after myocardial infarction and have noted reduced depression scores after training.[43] The control group in this study did not demonstrate a similar trend. Furthermore, in a group of coronary long-distance runners, posttraining depression scores and psychological profiles were dramatically improved.[44] Based on our and others' observations much of the postevent (myocardial infarction, surgery, or onset of angina) depression seen in coronary patients is a result of fear over loss of life and, just as important, loss of ability to "safely" participate in various recreational and everyday activities. Once the coronary patient realizes that through a program of exercise rehabilitation he or she can become (in most cases) more active than he or she was before the event, much of the depression and fear is overcome.

Finally, Blumenthal and others have published a preliminary report on the effects of chronic exercise (jogging) on type A behavior as assessed by the Jenkins Activity Survey in 10 healthy adults.[8] These authors reported a significant reduction in the survey scores after training. Coronary patients at both our centers in Los Angeles are currently participating in a study under the direction of Dr. Alan Abbott, designed to investigate whether exercise and rehabilitation efforts in general influence type A behavior as assessed by both the Jenkins Activity Survey and a structured interview.

As was mentioned earlier, no single intervention by itself should be considered the panacea for coronary disease, since its clinical course appears to be influenced by multiple factors. Exercise therapy is, however, a very essential component of rehabilitation and therapy for the coronary patient. Its potential benefits include improvement in aerobic and physical work capacity, risk-factor reduction, improvement or relief of effort, angina and claudication discomfort, and reduction in postevent depression. In addition, there is evidence to suggest that exercise training can influence the progression of coronary disease and the likelihood of future coronary events. To be truly effective, a therapeutic exercise training program must be designed to include an adequate intensity, duration, and frequency and the program must be ongoing. Finally, a great deal of effort and creativity must be expended on the therapist's part to ensure the highest possible exercise-compliance rate of his or her patient population.

REFERENCES

1. Barry, A.J., and others: Effects of physical training in patients who have had myocardial infarctions, Am. J. Cardiol. **17**:1, 1966.
2. Björntorp, P.: Hypertension and exercise, Circulation **4**(suppl. III):56-59, 1982.
3. Björntorp, P., and others: Effects of physical training on the glucose tolerance, plasma insulin and lipids and on body composition in men after myocardial infarction, Acta Med. Scand. **192**:439, 1972.
4. Björntorp, P., and others: Physical training in human hyperplastic obesity: IV. Effects on the hormonal states, Metabolism **26**:319, 1977.
5. Blankenhorn, D.H.: The rate of atherosclerosis change during treatment of hyperlipoproteinemia, Circulation **57**:355, 1977.
6. Blessey, R., and others: Therapeutic effects and safety of exercising coronary patients at their angina threshold, Med. Sci. Sports Exerc. **11**:110, 1979. (Abstract.)
7. Blessey, R., and others: Angiographic, clinical and exercise test data in marathoning coronary patients, Med. Sci. Sports Exerc. **13**:131, 1981. (Abstract.)
8. Blumenthal, J.A., and others: Effects of exercise on the type A (coronary prone) behavior pattern, Psychosom. Med. **42**:289, 1980.
9. Bonanno, J., and others: Effects of physical training on coronary risk factors, Am. J. Cardiol. **33**:760, 1974.
10. Barndt, R., Jr., and others: Regression and progression of early femoral atherosclerosis in treated hyperlipoproteinemic patients, Ann. Intern. Med. **86**:139, 1977.
11. Boyer, J.L., and Kasch, F.W.: Exercise therapy in hypertensive men, J.A.M.A. **211**:1668, 1970.
12. Bruce, R.A.: The benefits of physical training for patients with coronary heart disease. In Ingelfinger, F.J., and others, editors: Controversy in internal medicine, II, Philadelphia, 1974, W.B. Saunders Co.
13. Choquette, G., and Ferguson, R.J.: Blood pressure reduction in borderline hypertension following physical training, Can. Med. Assoc. J. **108**:699, 1973.
14. Clausen, J.P., and others: Physical training in the management of coronary artery disease, Circulation **40**:143, 1969.
15. Clausen, J.P., and others: Heart rate and arterial blood pressure during exercise in patients with angina pectoris, Circulation **53**:436, 1976.
16. Conolly, D.C.: Treatment of hypertension improves survival in patients with coronary heart disease. Circulation **64**(suppl. IV):300, 1981. (Abstract.)
17. Cooper, K.H., and others: Physical fitness levels versus selected coronary risk factors, J.A.M.A. **236**:166, 1978.
18. Dash, E., and others: Cardiomyopathic syndrome due to coronary disease. II. Increased prevalence in patients with diabetes mellitus: a matched pair analysis, Br. Heart J. **39**:740, 1977.
19. Detry, J.M., and others: Increased arteriovenous oxygen difference after physical training in coronary heart disease, Circulation **44**:109, 1971.
20. Dressendorfer, R.H., and others: Therapeutic effects of exercise training in angina patients. In Cohen, L.S., and others, editors: Physical conditioning and cardiovascular rehabilitation, New York, 1981, John Wiley & Sons.
21. Ehsani, A.A., and others: Effect of 12 months of intense exercise training on ischemic ST segment depression in patients with coronary artery disease, Circulation **46**:1116, 1981.
22. Ekroth, R., and others: Physical training of patients with intermittent claudication: indications, methods and results, Surgery **84**:640, 1978.
23. Erickson, B., and others: Maximal flow capacity before and after training. In Larsen, M.A., and Malmborg, R.O., editors: Coronary heart disease and physical fitness, Baltimore, 1971, University Park Press.
24. Erkelens, D.W., and others: High density lipoprotein cholesterol in survivors of myocardial infarction, J.A.M.A. **242**:2185, 1979.
25. Foley, W.T.: Treatment of gangrene of the foot and legs by walking, Circulation **15**:689, 1957.
26. Frick, M.H., and Katila, M.: Hemodynamic consequences of physical training after myocardial infarction, Circulation **37**:192, 1968.
27. Froelicher, V., and others: Cardiac rehabilitation: evidence for improvement in myocardial perfusion and function, Arch. Phys. Med. **61**:517, 1980.
28. Frick, M.H., and others: The mechanism of bradycardia evoked by physical training, Cardiologia **51**:46, 1967.
29. Goeransson, C., and Peppy, M.: Effects exercise on lipids and lipoproteins of men with coronary artery disease, masters's thesis, Los Angeles, 1979, University of Southern California, School of Physical Therapy.
30. Gottheiner, V.: Long-range strenuous sports training for cardiac reconditioning and rehabilitation, Am. J. Cardiol. **22**:426-435, 1968.
31. Hagberg, J.M., and others: Effects of 12 months of intense exercise training on stroke volume in patients with coronary artery disease, Circulation **67**:1194, 1983.
32. Hall, J.A., and others: Effects of diet and exercise on peripheral vascular disease, Physician Sports Med. **10**:90-101, 1982.
33. Hall, J.A., and others: Effects of an intensive short-term diet and exercise program on patients with peripheral vascular disease, Med. Sci. Sports Exerc. **14**:179, 1982. (Abstract.)
34. Hartley, L.H., and others: Multiple hormonal responses to graded exercise in relation to physical training, J. Appl. Physiol. **33**:602, 1972.
35. Hartung, H., and others: Relation of diet to high density lipoprotein cholesterol in middle-age marathon runners, joggers and inactive men, N. Engl. J. Med. **302**:357, 1980.
36. Hartung, G.H., and others: Effect of exercise training on plasma high density lipoprotein cholesterol in coronary disease patients, Am. Heart J. **101**:181, 1981.
37. Hellerstein, H.K., and others: Reconditioning of the coronary patient: preliminary report. In Likoff, W., and Moyer, J.H., editors: Coronary heart disease, New York, 1963, Grune & Stratton, Inc.
38. Jensen, D., and others: Improvement in ventricular function during exercise studied with radionuclide ventriculography after cardiac rehabilitation, Am. J. Cardiol. **46**:770, 1980.
39. Jonason, T., and others: Effect of physical training on different categories of patients with intermittent claudication, Acta Med. Scand. **206**:253, 1979.
40. Kannel, W.B., and others: Intermittent claudication: incidence in the Framingham Study, Circulation **41**:875, 1970.
41. Kannel, W.B., and McGee, D.L.: Diabetes and cardiovascular risk factors: the Framingham Study, Circulation **59**:8, 1979.
42. Kavanagh, T.; Intervention studies in Canada: primary and secondary intervention. In Pollack, M.L., and Schmidt, D.H., editors: Heart disease and rehabilitation, Boston, 1979, Houghton Mifflin Co.
43. Kavanagh, T., and others: Depression after myocardial infarction, Can. Med. Assoc. J. **113**:23, 1975.

44. Kavanagh, T., and others: Depression following myocardial infarction: the effects of distance running, Ann. N.Y. Acad. Sci. **301**:1029, 1978.

45. Kavanagh, T., and others: Prognostic indexes for patients with ischemic heart disease enrolled in an exercise-centered rehabilitation program, Am. J. Cardiol. **44**:1230, 1979.

46. Kentala, E.: Physical fitness and probability of physical rehabilitation after myocardial infarction in men of working age, Ann. Clin. Res. **9**(Suppl.):1, 1972.

47. Kessler, I.I.: Mortality experience of diabetic patients: a 26-year follow-up study, Am. J. Med. **51**:715, 1971.

48. Krotkiewski, M., and others: Effects of long-term physical training on body fat, metabolism, and blood pressure in obesity, Metabolism **21**:650, 1979.

49. Larsen, M.A., and Larsen, O.A.: Effect of training on the circulation in ischemic muscle tissue: observations of calf muscle blood flow in patients with intermittent claudication. In Larsen, M.A., and Malmborg, R.O., editors: Coronary heart disease and physical fitness, Baltimore, 1971, University Park Press.

50. Lee, A.P., and others: Long-term effects of physical training on coronary patients with impaired ventricular function, Circulation **60**:1519, 1979.

51. Letac, B., and others: A study of left ventricular function in coronary patients before and after physical training, Circulation **56**:375, 1977.

52. Malmborg, R., and others: The effect of beta blockade and/or physical training in patients with angina pectoris, Curr. Ther. Res. **16**:171, 1974.

53. Mann, G.U., and others: Exercise to prevent coronary heart disease: an experimental study of the effects of training on risk factors for coronary disease in man, Am. J. Med. **46**:12, 1969.

54. Mau, H.S., and Wagner, E.D.: Cardiac rehabilitation effects on exercise and diet on blood pressure, Circulation **64**(Suppl. IV):275, 1981. (Abstract.)

55. Miller, H., and others: Tromsø heart study: HDL and coronary artery disease: a prospective case control study, Lancet **2**:965, 1977.

56. Naughton, J.: The National Exercise and Heart Disease Project: the pre-randomized exercise program, Cardiology **63**:352, 1978.

57. Naughton, J., and Balke, B.: Effect of physical training on work capacity in post–myocardial infarction patients, J. Sports Med. **4**:185, 1964.

58. Obina, R., and others: Effect of a conditioning program on patients taking propranolol for angina pectoris, Cardiology **64**:365, 1979.

59. Oschrin, A., and others: Effects of aerobic exercise training on lipids and lipoproteins in coronary artery disease patients, Proceedings of the Ninth International Congress of the World Confederation of Physical Therapy, Stockholm, Sweden, Part I, p. 28, May 1982, Legitimerade Sjukgymnastears Ikssorbune.

60. Palac, R.T., and others: Risk factors related to progressive narrowing in aortocoronary vein grafts studies 1 and 5 years after surgery, Circulation **66**(Suppl. I):40, 1982.

61. Patterson, D.H., and others: Effects of physical training on cardiovascular function following myocardial infarction, J. Appl. Physiol. **47**:482, 1979.

62. Pratt, C.M., and others: Demonstration of training effect during chronic beta-adrenergic blockage in patients with coronary artery disease, Circulation **64**:1125, 1981.

63. Raichlen, J.S., and others: Risk factors and angiographic progression of coronary artery disease, Circulation **66**(Suppl. II):283, 1982. (Abstract.)

64. Rechnitzer, P.A., and others: Long-term follow-up study of survival and recurrence rate following myocardial infarction in exercising and control subjects, Circulation **43**:853, 1972.

65. Redwood, D.R., and others: Circulatory and symptomatic effects of physical training in patients with coronary artery disease and angina pectoris, N. Engl. J. Med. **286**:959, 1972.

66. Rizi, H.R., and others: Walk-through angina phenomenon demonstrated by graded exercise radionuclide ventriculography: possible coronary spasm mechanisms, Am. Heart J. **102**:292, 1982.

67. Roman, O., and others: Physical training program in arterial hypertension: a long-term prospective follow-up, Cardiology **67**:230, 1981.

68. Ruderman, N.B., and others: The effect of physical training on glucose tolerance and plasma lipids in maturity-onset diabetes, Diabetes **28**:89, 1979.

69. Saltin, B.: Physical training in patients with intermittent claudication. In Cohen, L.S., and others, editors: Physical conditioning and cardiovascular rehabilitation, New York, 1981, John Wiley & Sons, Inc.

70. Saltin, B., and others: Physical training and glucose tolerance in middle-aged men with chemical diabetes, Diabetes **28**:30, 1979.

71. Sanmarco, M.E., and others: Smoking and high density lipoproteins and coronary change in two and three vessel disease, Am. J. Cardiol. **41**:423, 1978. (Abstract.)

72. Sanmarco, M.E., and Blankenhorn, D.H.: Atherosclerosis: its progression and regression, Primary Cardiol., p. 51, July-Aug. 1978.

73. Sanne, H.: Preventive effect of physical training after a myocardial infarction. In Tibblin G., and others, editors: Preventive cardiology, New York, 1972, John Wiley & Sons, Inc.

74. Selvester, R., and others: Effects of exercise training on progression of documented atherosclerosis in men, Ann. N.Y. Acad. Sci. **301**:495, 1977.

75. Shaw, L.W.: Effects of a prescribed supervised exercise program on mortality and cardiovascular morbidity in patients after a myocardial infarction, Am. J. Cardiol. **48**:39, 1981.

76. Sim, D.N., and Neill, W.A.: Investigation of the physiological basis for increased exercise threshold for angina pectoris after physical conditioning, J. Clin. Invest. **54**:763, 1974.

77. Skinner, J.S., and Strandness, D.E., Jr.: Exercise and intermittent claudication. II. Effect of physical training, Circulation **36**:23-27, 1967.

78. Streja, D., and Mymin, O.: Moderate exercise and high density lipoprotein cholesterol, J.A.M.A. **242**:2190, 1979.

79. Thompson, P.D., and others: Effect of exercise training on the untrained limb: exercise performance of men with angina pectoris, Am. J. Cardiol. **48**:844, 1981.

80. Varnauskas, E., and others: Haemodynamic effects of physical training in coronary patients, Lancet **2**:8, 1966.

81. Waller, B.F., and Roberts, W.C.: Acceleration of coronary atherosclerosis in diabetes mellitus only with onset of diabetes less than 30 years of age: necropsy analysis of 275 diabetic patients (1100 arteries) aged 1 to 87 years and 242 aged-matched control subjects, Circulation **64**(Suppl. IV):80, 1981.

82. Wilhelmsen, L., and others: A controlled trial of physical training after myocardial infarction: effects on risk factors, nonfatal reinfarction, and death, Prev. Med. **4**:491, 1975.

83. Williams, R.S., and others: Physical conditioning augments the fibrinolytic response to venous occlusion in healthy adults, N. Engl. J. Med. **302**:987, 1980.

84. Wood, P., and others: Plasma lipoprotein distribution in male and female runners, Ann. N.Y. Acad. Sci. **301**:748, 1978.

85. Five year findings of the hypertension detection and follow-up program: I. Reduction in mortality of persons with high blood pressure, including mild hypertension, J.A.M.A. **242**:2562, 1979.

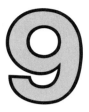

SCOT IRWIN

Administrative considerations

To initiate and maintain a cardiac rehabilitation (phases I to III), one must complete certain administrative details. These details include six broad areas: physician support, clinical knowledge and skills of the rehabilitation team members, communication procedures, space, equipment, and reimbursement. Clinical knowledge and skills for physical therapists have been discussed in the previous chapters. Each of the other areas are subject to the hospital or clinical environment and thus require adaptation to those environments.

PHYSICIAN SUPPORT

Each program needs a medical director. This is preferably one or more board-certified cardiologists. The medical director should have a well-established rapport with the facility administrator and potential referring physicians. The medical director has three major roles: referral, reinforcement of the philosophy, and supervision.

As a source of referral, the medical director should consider each of his patients as appropriate candidates for the program. The director should encourage other physicians to refer to the program by developing and distributing criteria and methods for admitting patients to the program. A director may quickly increase the referrals to the program through one-to-one discussions with potential referring physicians. These discussions should include careful orientation to the program, methods of referral, candidates, communication mechanisms, referring physician role, and program structure and goals. A sample written orientation guide is included as Appendix A of this chapter. With this orientation, an order for cardiac rehabilitation becomes all inclusive. In other words, the referring physician does not and should not have to order each step of the program. However, they should be consulted before exercise tests and an additional referral for testing may be required.

Referral to the program can be facilitated by making the referral mechanisms simple. Phase I referral can be enhanced by use of a check-off sheet in the coronary care unit (Fig. 9-1). Phase II and III referral is accomplished by use of a form that can be easily completed and returned. An example is shown in Fig. 9-2.

A medical director should emulate and constantly reinforce the program philosophy. A medical director who has few or no risk factors and actively participates in the exercise program will make the program go and grow. The opposite approach is also true. If the medical director even suggests to patients that smoking, overeating, or not exercising is all right, the team efforts at risk factor modification will not succeed.

Reinforcement of the program philosophy is another major responsibility of the medical director. As director, involvement in patient and team educational activities is essential. In my clinical experience, the cardiac rehabilitation programs that are most effective and have the greatest longevity are those programs with active, on-site, physician participation.

The third task of the medical director is to assist with supervision of the program. This task includes approving protocols, advising team members on patient medical problems, and making medication changes as necessary.

The following protocols need to be developed and approved by the medical director: resuscitation procedures (Appendix B, Fig. 9-3), consent forms, treadmill and program (Appendices C and D), exercise testing guidelines and protocols (Appendix E, Table 9-1), and all cardiac rehabilitation policies and procedures. All these protocols are commonly a part of most programs except the resuscitation procedures. The resuscitation procedures are critical to patient safety. In my opinion, a program that does not allow defibrillation by the team members involved in the exercise program is assuming an inordinate risk and liability. To work in a cardiac program that did not support resuscitation procedures like those found in Fig. 9-3 is not safe. At some time, despite all the assessments, monitor-

CCU to Step-down transfer orders

1. Transfer to Step-down Unit:

2. Diagnosis: Condition

3. Telemetry: yes   no

4. Diet: A. Regular   No added salt   Sanka

           B. Sodium restricted to   grams

           C. "Prudent"

           D. Other

5. TED hose: yes   no

6. IV:

7. Initiate cardiac rehabilitation: yes   no

8. Medications:

    A. NTG 1/150 gr. PRN angina

    B. Sedation

    C. Sleep

    D. Noncardiac analgesic

    E. Anticoagulant

    F. Antiarrhythmic

    G. Laxative

    H. Digoxin

    I. Propranolol (Inderal)

    J. Diuretic

    K. Other

9. Lab: A. PPT   q

         B. PT   q

         C. Other

Fig. 9-1. Sample transfer order sheet used to facilitate referral to cardiac rehabilitation (phase I).

```
            CARDIAC REHABILITATION REFERRAL FORM

        Department of Physical Therapy and Rehabilitation

The following person has applied for entry into the

Cardiac Rehabilitation Program:

Mr.
Mrs.
Miss _____   Address: _____
Telephone
number:   H _____   B _____   Age: _____   Sex: __ M or __ F

Participation in this program requires referral by the attending physician.

If you wish the above person to enter the program, please complete the fol-

lowing information.   Thank you.


I am referring the above-named person for participation in the Cardiac

Rehabilitation Program.

Diagnosis: _____

           _____


Major symptoms: _____

               _____


Medication: _____

            _____

            _____

            _____


            Signed _____ M.D.

Periodic progress reports will be sent to the referring physician.
```

Fig. 9-2. Outpatient referral form.

CARDIOPULMONARY RESUSCITATION FLOW SHEET

(See CPR procedures)

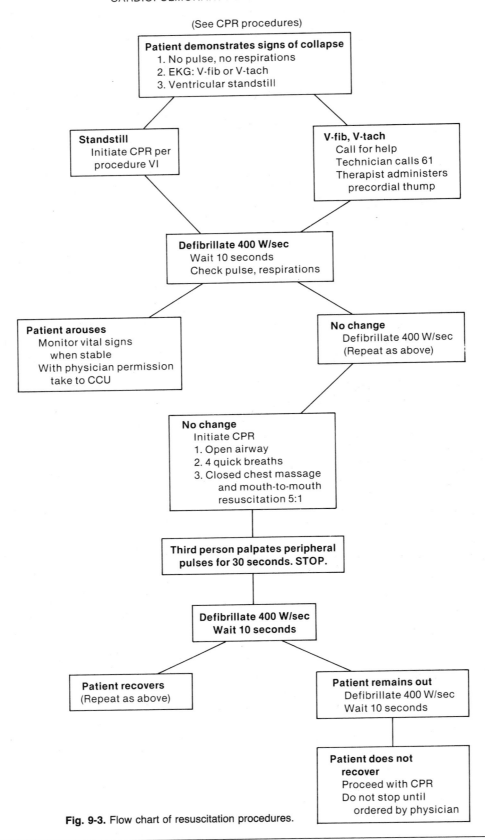

Patient demonstrates signs of collapse
1. No pulse, no respirations
2. EKG: V-fib or V-tach
3. Ventricular standstill

Standstill
   Initiate CPR per
   procedure VI

V-fib, V-tach
   Call for help
   Technician calls 61
   Therapist administers
      precordial thump

Defibrillate 400 W/sec
   Wait 10 seconds
   Check pulse, respirations

Patient arouses
   Monitor vital signs
      when stable
   With physician permission
      take to CCU

No change
   Defibrillate 400 W/sec
   (Repeat as above)

No change
   Initiate CPR
   1. Open airway
   2. 4 quick breaths
   3. Closed chest massage
      and mouth-to-mouth
      resuscitation 5:1

Third person palpates peripheral pulses for 30 seconds. STOP.

Defibrillate 400 W/sec
Wait 10 seconds

Patient recovers
   (Repeat as above)

Patient remains out
   Defibrillate 400 W/sec
   Wait 10 seconds

Patient does not recover
   Proceed with CPR
   Do not stop until
      ordered by physician

Fig. 9-3. Flow chart of resuscitation procedures.

Table 9-1. Treadmill protocols		
Maximal Bruce Multistage Protocol		
	Speed (mph)	*Grade (%)*
Stage I	1.7	10
Stage II	2.5	12
Stage III	3.4	14
Stage IV	4.2	16
Stage V	5.0	18
Stage VI	5.5	20
Stage VII	6.0	22
Low-level protocol—submaximal		
	Speed (mph)	*Grade (%)*
Stage I	1.7	0
Stage II	1.7	5
Stage III	1.7	10
Stage IV	2.0	12
Stage V	2.5	12

ing, and careful program design, a patient will go into ventricular tachycardia or ventricular fibrillation and require immediate resuscitation.

A second supervisory task of the medical director is to be familiar with all the program participants' medical histories and problems. The medical director can then answer team member questions about medical disorders (i.e., gout, pericarditis, arthritis, and diabetes) and their effects on disease progression, exercise tolerance, and exercise prescription.

Perhaps the most important task of the medical director is to respond to the team members' objective findings by making medication adjustments as needed. For example, a patient 3 weeks into phase II develops serious ventricular arrhythmias, and this information is communicated to the medical director. If there is no response to this new development, team member morale will fall and the program effectiveness will be impaired. A strong medical director will make the appropriate medication changes or explain to the team members why medical intervention is not necessary.

Physician support is essential, and the key to support comes from the program's medical director. The director's required duties include being a referral source, medical advisor, and a program supervisor.

CLINICAL KNOWLEDGE AND SKILLS OF THE TEAM

Several texts could be written describing the knowledge and skills required of each potential member of a cardiac rehabilitation team. That is not the intent of this section. If the philosophy of a cardiac program is the same as the one described in the first chapter of this text, the following knowledge and skills are needed.

Team members with knowledge in the following areas

are preferred: dietary content and food preparation, metabolism of cholesterol, medication interaction (effects and side effects), psychological manifestations of heart disease, community resources (financial, vocational) available to patients and their families, exercise training (methods and effects), and medical care.

Each team member should be knowledgeable in educational methods. Each should also be trained and certified in cardiopulmonary resuscitation.

COMMUNICATION PROCEDURES

There are three simple, but essential, communication procedures that will enhance the program's effectiveness and ensure safety. These procedures include physician contact, progress notes, and patient diaries.

A system for immediate physician contact is essential. As the previous chapters have demonstrated, patient complications can occur at any point in the patient's program (see Chapters 5 to 7). These complications are rarely life threatening or serious enough to require emergency procedures, but they may require medical intervention. Often, a simple change in frequency or dosage of a patient's medication will remedy a potentially serious complication. The therapist needs to have a direct line to the patient's physician or the program's medical director. Several physicians may be required, and a priority order of contact should be established in a written policy and procedure.

Written progress reports about the patient's program progression and current exercise assessment should be sent to the patient's physician at least monthly (phases II and III). A sample progress report is presented in Fig. 9-4. Daily reports are required in phase I as part of the patient's inpatient medical record. We have found that it is effective and convenient to generate progress reports before a patient's appointment with the referring physician. We then have the patient carry the report to the physician's office. In addition, we encourage the patients to take their exercise diaries (Fig. 9-5) with them when they visit their physician. A combination of monthly progress reports and exercise diaries ensures frequent written documentation of the patient's progress. This data sheet is also used for documentation to third-party reimbursement agencies.

The patient exercise diary is a crucial written communication for the physician, physical therapist, and patient (Fig. 9-5). These diaries help to constantly update the therapist about the patient's home exercise sessions. Careful review of the diaries can help identify patient compliance, current exercise intensity, and new signs or symptoms. Our therapists are encouraged to constantly check the patient diaries before each supervised session and to use the data from the diaries to assess patient progression.

A combination of physician contact, progress notes, and patient diaries are keys to good communication within the program. Without these communication procedures, pa-

CARDIAC REHABILITATION OUT-PATIENT PROGRESS REPORT

Name: _____ Plan established _____

Diagnosis: _____

Report period from _____ to _____

Current medications _____

General information _____

EXERCISE:

a. Dates attended: _____
b. Frequency: Home _____/week   Hospital _____/week _____/month
c. Max. HR: _____
d. Avg. rest. HR _____ Avg. exer. HR _____
e. Mode: Walk _____   Intensity: _____ mph _____ grade
          Walk-jog _____   _____ miles
          Jog _____   _____ minutes
          Stationary bicycle _____ Intensity: _____ miles
          Arm bicycle _____   _____ minutes
                                                  _____ resistance

f. Arrhythmias: None _____ Other _____
g. Avg. rest. BP: _____ Avg. peak BP with exercise:_____
h. BP response: Adaptive _____ Hypertensive _____ Hypotensive _____

i. Symptoms: Angina level _____ Leg pain _____ Dyspnea _____

   Other _____

EDUCATION:

Complete _____ Ongoing _____ Needs all sessions _____

ADHERENCE TO PROGRAM:

Poor _____ Fair _____ Good _____ Next report _____

COMMENTS (indicate major changes):

Signed _____ RPT   Date _____

Fig. 9-4. Sample progress report form.

Name:_____ Month:_____ Hospital:_____ Medications:_____

_____

S.C.O.R.
(Specialized Coronary Outpatient Rehabilitation) _____
Exercise Diary

Prescription: Distance_____mile(s)

Time:_____minutes   Physical fitness stage:_____

Target heart rate:_____bpm   Weight (end of month):_____

Day	Rest. HR	Exercise mode	Distance (peak)	Time (peak)	Work load	W-U HR	Peak HR	C-D HR	Symptoms or remarks
1									
2									
3									
4									
5									
6									
7									
8									
9									
10									
11									
12									
13									
14									
15									
16									
17									
18									
19									
20									

Fig. 9-5. Patient exercise diary and data recording sheet.

Continued.

Day	Rest. HR	Exercise mode	Distance (peak)	Time (peak)	Work load	W–U HR	Peak HR	C–D HR	Symptoms or remarks
21									
22									
23									
24									
25									
26									
27									
28									
29									
30									
31									

MONTHLY SUMMARY

Average resting heart rate =
Average peak heart rate =
Total days exercise =
Average peak interval =_____ miles
Average peak duration =
Total monthly mileage =

DEFINITIONS

Level of angina
L_1 mild discomfort
L_2 moderately painful
L_3 severe pain
L_4 intolerable
SOB—Shortness of breath
PVC—Premature ventricular
      contraction

Recommendations: _____

_____

_____

_____

Fig. 9-5, cont'd. Patient exercise diary and data recording sheet.

tient compliance, physician referral, and therapist assessments will be less than optimal.

SPACE

There are two major space requirements: an area for the exercise program (phases II and III) and an area for the educational sessions (phases I to III).

The educational area is best situated near the coronary care unit. An area large enough to accommodate the pa-

tients, their families, and audiovisual aids will suffice.

The space requirements for a cardiac rehabilitation program are often dependent on climate. Dry, temperate climates require less space because much of the exercise training can be conducted outdoors. Most regions are not fortunate enough to have that kind of climate, and space requirements can be a major block to development and implementation of a program.

The exercise program space is best situated within a

Table 9-2. Equipment list

Equipment	Approximate cost
Radiotelemetry monitoring unit	$6000 per channel
Treadmill	$5000-8000 each
Bicycle ergometer	$750-1000
Exercise bikes	$300-500
Arm ergometer/Rowing ergometer	$600-800
Defibrillator (400 W/sec)	$2000+
Crash cart and medications	$500+
Mobil standing-mercury sphygmomanom-eters	$200 per each
Stethoscopes	$40+ per each
Miscellaneous	Widely variable
Data board	
File cabinets	

gymnasium, but this is rarely available at a hospital. Space requirements for the exercise program should allow for sufficient equipment to have group exercise training sessions. Our facility has four treadmills, two bicycle ergometers, and an arm-crank ergometer. This allows for seven patients to be treated simultaneously. The space is 30 by 15 feet.

EQUIPMENT

Table 9-2 gives a brief description and approximate cost for the majority of equipment needed to conduct a cardiac rehabilitation program. Each piece of equipment has specific requirements that will make it useful to the program. These requirements and some helpful hints about purchases are found below.

Radiotelemetry monitoring units

Radiotelemetry monitoring units should have an oscilloscope, strip chart recorder, and transmitters. The strip chart recorder should have memory capabilities so that arrhythmias observed on the oscilloscope can be recorded on the strip chart. Group exercise sessions require at least enough telemetry channels to allow each patient to be monitored. These units will be the program's greatest equipment expense. Before including these units in your budget, check your hospital or clinic for outdated telemetry systems. Over the last few years, technological improvements have caused coronary care units to replace their telemetry systems. The old systems are usually quite adequate and will allay the expense of purchasing additional telemetry units.

Treadmills

Treadmills should be calibratable. They are more useful if they have the capability for fine speed and grade adjustments.

There are some details about treadmill purchases that it pays to watch out for. These details include but are not limited to ensuring that the treadmills have (1) acceptable leakage currents, (2) adequate power sources, and (3) acceptable ceiling height.

Bicycle ergometers and exercise bicycles

Bicycle ergometers should have work-load indicators that are easily observed and calibrated. They should be durable and have as comfortable seats as possible.

Exercise bicycles are simply stationary bicycles with resistance capabilities. Measurable work loads cannot be obtained, and they are generally less durable. These bicycles are adequate for patient use at home but rarely withstand the stresses of a busy outpatient cardiac program.

Emergency equipment (crash cart—defibrillator)

The key requirement for emergency equipment is that it is mobile. The defibrillator should have enough extension cord to be able to reach any part of the exercise area. Battery-powered defibrillator units are available, but in my experience they are not so reliable and tend to produce inadequate power outputs.

REIMBURSEMENT

Before developing a program, it is helpful to discuss reimbursement with the major third-party agencies. Each state has its own guidelines for reimbursement of cardiac rehabilitation programs. If guidelines or procedures for reimbursement are not established in your state, then help develop them.

In my experience, all major third-party reimbursement agencies will pay for cardiac rehabilitation except Federal Employees Blue Cross–Blue Shield. Medicare reimbursement is limited to 12 weeks of outpatient care, and billing should be labeled as cardiac rehabilitation. Medicare will not pay for physical therapy for cardiac patients if the clinic or hospital has a separate cardiac rehabilitation unit.

SUMMARY

To facilitate cardiac rehabilitation program development, several administrative procedures need to be established and controlled. This chapter is an endeavor to delineate some key administrative considerations and to highlight some potential problems. It may be helpful to identify one team member to coordinate these administrative procedures. Such a member should be responsible for physician support, clinical knowledge and skills of the team members, and communication mechanisms.

APPENDIX A
Cardiac Rehabilitation Program (Department of Physical Therapy and Rehabilitation)

The Cardiac Rehabilitation Program consists of two phases; inpatient (after infarction, etc.) and outpatient. The following is a general description of the program, along with other information of importance to physicians interested in entering their patients into the program.

Inpatient phase

A patient may enter the rehabilitation program only on his or her physician's referral. Optimally, this should coincide with the patient's transfer from the coronary care unit (CCU) to the step-down unit. Other patients not having suffered an acute myocardial infarction but who are otherwise candidates, (i.e., coronary prone, postbypass, etc.) for the program may be referred at an appropriate time in their hospital course or as outpatients. The new transfer orders (CCU to step-down) have a check-off space for cardiac rehabilitation. Other inpatients may enter the program by ordering "cardiac rehabilitation" on the hospital chart order sheet.

Upon transfer to the step-down unit and initiation of rehabilitation, the patient is visited by the nurse coordinator, who will introduce the patient to the inpatient educational program, discuss rehabilitation objectives, and explain the patient notebook used in the program. The inpatient educational program is 4 days in length and repeats every 4 days Tuesday through Friday. Patients may enter this phase on any week day.

While the patient is in the inpatient program, the following evaluative procedures constitute important "base-line" data on which each patient's program is individualized.

1. Self-care monitor. This monitor is a comprehensive evaluation of the patient's cardiac responses to normal daily activities. It includes monitoring heart rate, blood pressure, ECG, symptoms, and heart sound changes while the patient is supine, sitting, standing, dressing, grooming, ambulating, and performing a Valsalva maneuver. A full interpretation of this evaluation and recommendations will be placed in the medical chart. The physician and therapist can use these data and evaluation before allowing the patient to begin ambulating activities.

2. Based on the self-care monitoring results, the patient will begin supervised ambulation in the hall. Supervision may consist in observing the heart rate and blood pressure and ECG monitoring as is indicated by the self-care evaluation. The patient will be progressed according to his ability.

3. If the patient is to progress to the cardiac rehabilitation program as an outpatient, a low-level treadmill test is required. This is an important data base for developing low-level exercise training and as a final screening evaluation before discharge from the hospital. The protocol for this test is as follows:

Stage	Speed (mph)	Grade (%)	Time (min)	Metabolic equivalents
1	1.7	0	3	1-2
2	1.7	5	3	2-3
3	1.7	10	3	4

There are several predetermined termination points:
   a. Attaining a heart rate of 130
   b. Onset of angina
   c. Inappropriate hypotensive or hypertensive blood pressure response
   d. Coupled or tripled premature ventricular contractions
   e. Multifocal premature ventricular contractions
   f. Eight premature ventricular contractions per minute during exercise
   g. Completion of all three stages of the protocol

Outpatient phase

4. After the patient's discharge, he will be scheduled for an outpatient supervised low-level exercise program. The goals of this aspect of the program are to gradually and safely progress the patient's activity tolerance and give the physician objective feedback as to the effects of their medical regimen. For example, routine monitoring will allow the physical therapist to give the physician input regarding arrhythmia control or ventricular function. A referral from the physician and consent from the patient are required to enter this phase of the program.

5. Upon approval of the referring physician, approximately 6 to 8 weeks after the infarction, the patient will be scheduled for a maximal exercise test. The report of this test will be sent to the referring physician. The referring physician will also be sent monthly progress notes as to the patient's progression in the program.

6. After the maximal treadmill test, the patient's exercise program will be revised according to the results of the test. A progress note indicating this revision will be sent to the referring physician. Continuation with the program is subject to the referring physician's approval. The patient's educational program will continue as an outpatient with expansion of the inpatient sessions.

APPENDIX B
Cardiopulmonary resuscitation procedures
Cardiac Rehabilitation Program (Department of Physical Therapy and Rehabilitation

All personnel involved in the exercise training portion of the cardiac rehabilitation program shall be trained and certified in basic life support by the American Heart Association.

Patient demonstrates abnormal cardiopulmonary distress requiring emergency procedures (Fig. 9-3).

Assumptions
1. Witnessed arrest not on monitor
2. Defibrillator immediately available, turned on and functional
3. Physician not immediately available but on call

I. Definition of cardiac emergency
  a. Sustained ventricular tachycardia with hypotension
  b. Ventricular fibrillation
  c. Asystole
  d. Severe bradycardia
  e. Other (i.e., pulmonary emergency)
II. Standard precautions
  a. Defibrillator available and operational
  b. Full crash-cart equipment available
  c. All patients referred to the program by a qualified physician
  d. All patients have had a recent thorough cardiac examination, as well as treadmill testing

Procedures
Patient collapses
III. Call for help. Call for cardiologist on call and call code 7C, dial #61, and report "cardiac arrest."
IV. a. Shake and shout
  b. Check pulse and respirations; if no pulse, proceed to a precordial thump
  c. Check pulse; if no pulse, defibrillate at 400 W/sec.
V. Wait 10 seconds. Check pulse and respirations carefully. If still no response, defibrillate again.
VI. Initiate cardiopulmonary resuscitation per American Heart Association Guidelines.
  a. Open airway
  b. Four quick breaths
  c. Begin closed-chest massage and mouth-to-mouth resuscitation. Team 5:1 when a third rescuer enters, one should feel for peripheral pulses, preferably femoral artery. If the peripheral pulse is palpable, maintain CPR for 30 seconds. Discontinue CPR unless instructed otherwise.
VII. Defibrillate at 400 W/sec and recharge.
  Wait 10 seconds and review vital signs as in (V).

Patient remains in state of emergency
VIII. Defibrillate at 400 W/sec.
  Wait 10 seconds and review vital signs as in (V).
  If no recovery, resume CPR as in (VI) until directed to discontinue by a physician.
  Remember: Do not stop until requested to do so by a physician

APPENDIX C
Specialized Coronary Outpatient Rehabilitation Treadmill Consent Form

Name of patient _____
Date and time of patient's signature _____

I hereby authorize the Center to carry out the prescribed exercise stress testing and graded, monitored exercise indicated for me as the preliminary steps in a comprehensive cardiac rehabilitation program.

It is understood that I voluntarily enter into this program at the recommendation of my own physician and that the Center accepts me for the program only on my physician's recommendation and prescription.

In becoming a participant in this program, I agree to cooperate with the personnel at the Center and accept their recommendations pertaining to the amount of exercising prescribed. I further agree not to exceed these recommendations, and if I do so, it will be at my own risk.

I hereby consent to engage voluntarily in exercise stress testing to determine the state of my heart and circulation. The information thus obtained will help the physicians in prescribing an exercise program of activities in which I may engage.

The nature and purpose of the proposed testing and the procedures involved have been explained to me. There exists the rare possibility of a serious complication occurring during the tests and procedures. The risks, hazards, and possible complications have been explained to me. These may include occasional induction of chest discomfort or pain, decrease in blood pressure, fainting, disorders of heart rhythm, and very rarely a heart attack or even death. Every effort will be made to minimize these by the preliminary examination and by continuous observation during stress testing and monitored exercise by the physician or therapist. Emergency equipment and trained personnel are available to deal with unusual situations that may arise. However, I understand more detailed information is available if I wish to discuss it.

Should any complications arise, I consent to whatever is necessary to correct the complication, including cessation of the program as it pertains to me.

The information that is obtained will be sent to my personal physician and will not be released to any other person without my expressed written consent. The information, however, may be used for a statistical or scientific purpose.

I certify that I have read all the foregoing consent form and that I fully understand its contents.

Signed: _____ Date: _____
      Patient
      _____ Date: _____
      Witness

APPENDIX D
Informed Consent for Outpatient Cardiac Rehabilitation Program (Department of Physical Therapy and Rehabilitation)
Purpose of the outpatient cardiac rehabilitation program

The present cardiac rehabilitation program is designed to improve your physical exercise capacity and to reduce your level of physical impairment because of your heart condition. This program utilizes a form of physical exercise known as "aerobic" or "endurance" training, which has beneficial effects on cardiovascular performance. The program is expanding and will ultimately include additional areas such as nutritional and weight control education, vocational rehabilitation, psychological counseling, and other appropriate rehabilitative modalities.

Based on an "initial intake graded exercise test" you will begin at an appropriate level of physical exercise and then progress to more intense levels under skilled professional supervision. During the earlier stages of the program, especially if you are convalescing from a heart attack, you should attend three exercise sessions a week to closely supervise and evaluate your progress. In the later stages, as you become more familiar with the concept of aerobic training, heart rate response, and other important aspects of rehabilitative sessions, you will continue your exercise program at home on your own according to carefully planned exercise prescriptions. The graded exercise test at the end of convalescence and periodically throughout the year is the cornerstone of appraisal of "cardiovascular fitness."

Your doctor will receive periodic updates on your progress so that he may objectively prescribe medications and advise you regarding work, general daily activities, etc.

Possible risks

All possible precautions will be taken to avoid any complications of exercise. Strict adherence to your "exercise prescription" is essential to minimize any risks. We want you to understand, however, that a small possibility still exists of your developing an abnormal blood pressure, dizziness or even fainting, or an irritable heart beat during exercise. Close monitoring (telemetry) and supervision generally precludes these complications leading to a serious event; however, a rare heart attack or heart arrest can occur in such a program. Emergency equipment and trained personnel are available to deal with any situation that might arise.

Advantages

This program can benefit you in many ways, among which the most important are as follows:
1. To give you a carefully supervised progression of activity during your convalescence with important objective data feedback to your physician.
2. To maximize your cardiovascular exercise capacity as well as your overall physical conditioning.
3. To provide you with a sound basis to maintain your level of cardiovascular conditioning over the years.
4. To provide educational sessions and material regarding cardiovascular risk factors (diet, smoking, weight, etc.).
5. In some instances, to possibly reduce the quantity or types of medications.

Inquiries

All questions about the rehabilitation program are welcome. If you have doubts or questions, please discuss them with us.

Consent to participate

Entry into this program requires your physician's referral. Participation in the rehabilitation program is voluntary. You are free to withdraw, if you so desire, at any point in the program.

I have read this form and understand the rehabilitation program in which I will participate. I realize that there is a remote possibility of a complication occurring during the exercise sessions, including heart attack and cardiac arrest, but I believe the benefits far exceed any risks. I consent to participate in this rehabilitation program.

_____ Date: _____
Signature
_____
Witness

APPENDIX E
Maximal symptom-limited exercise test protocol
Definition

A maximal symptom-limited exercise test is an electrocardiographically monitored evaluation of a person's maximal oxygen consumption during dynamic work (exercise) utilizing large muscle groups. It begins with submaximal exertion, allows time for physiological adaptations, and has progressive increments in work loads until individually determined end points of fatigue are reached or limiting symptoms or signs occur.

Purpose

1. To establish the diagnosis or severity of coronary artery disease by observation of exercise-induced ECG changes. This may occur as confirmation of clinically suspected coronary artery disease or detection of latent coronary artery disease in asymptomatic persons.
2. Evaluate the functional cardiovascular capacity and reserve in response to exercise in patients with coronary artery disease for assessment of return to work or leisure activities and candidacy for exercise training programs.
3. To evaluate prescribed therapy as an objective measure of efficacy of medical or surgical intervention. This is particularly important in the assessment of the effect of a person's participation in an ongoing aerobic exercise program.
4. To serve as motivation and a stimulus to make needed changes in behavior or life-style (e.g., to stop smoking, alter diet, or adhere to an exercise program).

Indications for procedure

1. Surgery after a myocardial infarction or after coronary artery bypass graft; 4 or more weeks after either event in uncomplicated patients; greater than 4 weeks in complicated patients.
2. Outpatient referral for admission to a cardiac rehabilitation program in a patient suspected of having coronary artery disease.
3. Distinguishing angina from noncardiac chest pain.
4. Development of a change in the patient's medical status that requires reevaluation of cardiovascular status (onset of hypertension, inability to maintain habitual exercise program because of onset of dyspnea, excessive fatigue, or angina), or evaluation of a change in medications.
5. Ongoing periodic reevaluation of the patient's cardiac status and physical work capacity as part of a treatment program (i.e., exercise conditioning, surgery, etc.).
6. Assistance in determining whether a coronary patient can return to a particular type of vocational or recreational activity.

Personnel required for the procedure

1. Cardiac technician trained in the recognition of ECG arrhythmias.
2. Exercise tester, either physician or designated physical therapist or nurse, who is responsible for the actual conduction and preliminary interpretation of the test. This person is also responsible for supervision of the technician assisting in the test.
3. Physician who will assume overall responsibility for the conduction supervision and interpretation of the evaluation. The physician will be in the immediate vicinity of the test area during the test, though he may designate responsibility for the conduction of the test to a specific staff member.

PROCEDURES FOR CONDUCTING A MAXIMAL SYMPTOM-LIMITED EXERCISE TEST
Equipment and supplies required

1. Disposable ECG electrodes.
2. Conduction gel.
3. Treadmill and treadmill speed- and grade-control unit.
4. Alcohol swabs, razor, extrafine sandpaper for skin preparation.
5. Stethoscope.
6. Standing blood pressure apparatus.
7. ECG recorder with oscilloscope.
8. Defibrillator and crash cart.
9. Stretcher.
10. Linens: sheets, towels, pillow cases.
11. Patient's medical chart.
12. Treadmill data collection worksheet for maximal test.
13. Treadmill consent form.
14. ECG paper.

Preparation of patient

1. The purpose and potential hazards of the test are explained to the patient and a consent form is signed (if necessary).
2. Before the test, a 12-lead ECG is performed on all patients and read before testing.
3. Preliminary information (name and dose of medications, patient's age, height, and weight) is obtained and recorded.
4. The patient is instructed to report any chest discomfort, dizziness, leg cramps, or any other unusual or discomforting sensations.
5. The patient is instructed to describe any angina in terms of levels:
   Level 1. Very mild sensation or initial perception of discomfort
   Level 2. Moderately uncomfortable sensation of greater intensity
   Level 3. Severe, chest discomfort
   Level 4. Intolerable chest pain

6. The exercise tester or technician demonstrates how to walk on the treadmill including getting on the treadmill and instructions not to grip the handrails during the test. (If balance support is necessary, the patient may rest two fully extended fingers on the handrail.)
7. Electrode placement. The patient is monitored simultaneously by a lead system using these leads: Y, X, CM_4, MS_4, V_1, and V_5.
8. Women being tested should be wearing a bra to minimize interference on the ECG.
9. Emergency equipment. A defibrillator is in the room at all times and remains turned on throughout the test. A completely equipped crash cart is also present.

*STANDARD EVALUATIVE PROCEDURES
FOR PRETESTING, TESTING, AND POSTTESTING
(COMMON TO ALL PROTOCOLS INCLUDING LOW-
LEVEL TESTING)*

1. Preliminary information (name and dose of medications, patient's age, height and weight, etc.) is obtained and recorded on the raw data sheet.
2. Preexercise procedures
   a. Heart rate, heart sounds, blood pressure, and symptoms are evaluated and recorded in the supine position for 2 consecutive minutes.
   b. *Special considerations:* Nonambulatory patients will not undergo supine positioning before or after exercise. Heart rate and blood pressure are measured and recorded after 1 minute of sitting.
   When expired, air measurements are to be performed with either the arm or leg ergometry tests; the patient will remain seated at rest for 3 minutes while gas collection and analysis is performed.
   c. 10-second breath-holding and 30 seconds of hyperventilation are performed by the patient in the sitting position with continuous ECG recording during both maneuvers.
   d. Heart rate and blood pressure are measured and recorded immediately after 1 minute of standing.
   Special considerations:
   a. The attending measurements are not included in the arm and leg ergometry protocols.
   b. When expired air measurements are to be performed, the patient will remain standing for 3 minutes while base-line measurements are performed.
3. Exercise procedures
   a. Heart rate and blood pressure measurements are taken during each minute of exercise and recorded.
   b. The time of onset of angina is recorded, as are changes in the severity of discomfort on a minute-by-minute basis. Recording of the angina levels is to continue after exercise until pain subsides completely.

c. Continuous recording of ECG is with a paper speed of 10 mm/sec, except for last 10 seconds of each minute at 25 mm/sec, carried out for documentation of the type and frequency of arrhythmias and the frequency of ectopic beats is recorded.
4. After exercise
   a. Immediately after exercise the treadmill speed and grade or the ergometer work load is reduced over a 30 to 60-second period.
   b. Heart rate and blood pressure are recorded every minute after exercise.
   c. Postexercise monitoring continues until the heart rate is within 15 to 25 bpm of the resting rate, the systolic blood pressure is within 20 mm Hg, arrhythmias have stabilized, the patient is asymptomatic, and the net ST-segment depression or elevation is less than 1 mm above or below base-line measurements.
   d. When expired air collection is performed, gas sampling will continue for 5 minutes after exercise.
   e. In the intermittent ergometry tests, postexercise heart rate, blood pressure, and angina levels are recorded for the duration of the recovery intervals on a minute-to-minute basis.
   f. When expired air collection is performed as part of the intermittent tests, sampling will be discontinued at the end of each work load and resumed 1 minute before the beginning of the following work load.

TEST CONDUCTION

1. *Test protocol:* Bruce Multistage Continuous Protocol

Stage	Speed (mph)	Grade (%)	Time (min)	Metabolic equivalents
1	1.7	10	3	4-5
2	2.5	12	3	6-7
3	3.4	14	3	8-9
4	4.2	16	3	10-12
5	5.0	18	3	greater than 14

2. Continuous ECG monitoring is done and heart rate, blood pressure, and 10-second ECG strip recording are taken each minute of the test.
3. Upon reaching the designated end point of the test, one conducts a "cool-down" stage during which the treadmill speed and grade is reduced. (This may last up to 30 seconds.) At this point, the treadmill is turned off, and the patient is instructed to march in place on the treadmill while the heart rate, blood pressure, and continuous ECG are recorded for an additional 30 seconds. Thus the total time standing after exercise is 1 minute.
4. The patient then lies down, and the exercise tester again auscultates the chest for cardiac gallop rhythms, murmurs, etc.

5. Minute-by-minute heart rate, blood pressure, and ECG recordings are taken until values approximate resting pretest values. (Heart rate is within 15 bpm of resting value.) At this point, the patient is questioned regarding symptoms and is disconnected from the equipment and released if asymptomatic.
6. Continued monitoring is required if the patient demonstrates evidence of continuing ischemia or angina (persistent ST-segment depression or elevation), unstable arrhythmias, or unusual signs or symptoms.

ERGOMETRY TESTS
Arm ergometry tests

1. Continuous protocol
   a. Initial work load not less than 150 kg.
   b. A total of four or five work loads, each with a duration of 2 minutes.
   c. Work-load increments not less than 50 kg.
   d. Crank speed 50 to 60 rpm.
2. Intermittent protocol
   a. Initial work-load not less than 150 kg.
   b. A total of four or five work loads each 3 minutes in duration followed by 3-minute recovery periods.
   c. Work-load increments not less than 50 kg.
   d. Crank speed 50 to 60 rpm.

Bicycle ergometry tests

1. Intermittent protocol
   a. Initial work load not less than 150 kg.
   b. A total of four or five work loads, each 4 minutes long, followed by 4-minute recovery periods.
   c. Seat height adjusted so that there is no more than 5 to 10 degrees of flexion in the knee at the lowest point in the pedal revolutions.
   d. Work-load increments should be 20% to 25% of the difference between the initial work load and the estimated maximal work load.
   e. Crank speed should be maintained at 50 to 60 rpm.
2. Care of equipment
   a. Dispose of all used electrodes, alcohol swabs, and packages.
   b. Change sheets and pillow cases on gurney.
   c. Turn off defibrillator.
   d. Return ECG leads, blood pressure cuffs, and stethoscopes to proper place.
   e. Turn off all equipment.
   f. Check to assure that there are adequate supplies of electrodes, swabs, and ECG paper; replace as necessary.
3. Charting
   a. Immediately upon completion of the test, the exercise tester should enter a preliminary interpretation of test into the chart, which includes the following:
      (1) Date of test
      (2) Type of test

   (3) Minutes completed and limiting factor(s)
   (4) Resting heart rate and maximal heart rate achieved
   (5) Resting and maximal blood pressure values; comment whether hypoadaptive, normoadaptive or hypertensive
   (6) Angina: level I to IV during or after exercise
   (7) Additional symptoms, e.g. nausea, ataxia, dizziness
   (8) Arrhythmias: comment on any arrhythmias, e.g , supraventricular versus ventricular, number, type (multifocal, parasystolic, etc.), frequency, and when they occurred
   (9) Auscultation findings: presence or absence of S_4, S_3, murmurs
   (10) Positive ($+$), negative ($-$), or indeterminate for ischemia and degree of ST-segment change (or R-wave amplitude change)
   (11) Maximal or submaximal test and assessment of physical working capacity and functional aerobic impairment (FAI)
   (12) Recommendations for additional monitoring or follow-up tests
   b. A formal interpretation of the test is made after a complete review of data and is reviewed and signed by the physician. This interpretation should be entered into the chart, along with sample ECG strips taken from the test.

SPECIAL OBSERVATIONS, ASSESSMENTS, PRECAUTIONS
Criteria for termination of test

1. Patient's report of fatigue that would make continued exertion uncomfortable:
   a. Patient's report of dizziness
   b. Increasing premature ventricular contractions (PVC) becoming multifocal
   c. Coupled PVC's or ventricular tachycardia (three PVC's in a row)
   d. Development of rapid atrial arrhythmias
   e. Level III angina (scale of I to IV)
   f. A progressive fall in systolic blood pressure of 20 mm Hg or more in the presence of increased heart rate and work load
   g. Extreme hypertensive response (systolic 240/diastolic 130)
   h. Severe musculoskeletal pain as in leg claudication
   i. Uninterpretable ECG tracing
   j. Patient signs such as cold and clammy skin, ataxic gait, or other signs of vascular insufficiency
2. If patient becomes moderately uncomfortable, from any cause.

Contraindications and precautions to exercise testing

1. Contraindications.
   a. Overt congestive heart failure
   b. Rapidly intensifying or unstable angina
   c. Recent acute myocardial infarction (less than 3 weeks)
   d. Dissecting aneurysm
   e. Second- or third-degree heart block
   f. Recurrent ventricular tachycardia
   g. Rapid atrial arrhythmias
   h. Acute myocarditis or pericarditis
   i. Severe aortic stenosis
   j. Recent pulmonary embolus
   k. Acute infections or other active disease process
2. Precautions (attending physician to be consulted before beginning of test).
   a. Repetitive or frequent ventricular ectopic activity at rest (more than 10 PVC's/min)
   b. Resting hypertension (systolic 180/diastolic 110)
   c. Severe cardiomegaly
   d. Resting tachycardia of greater than 110 bpm or a recent change in cardiac symptoms

PART TWO

PULMONARY PHYSICAL THERAPY AND REHABILITATION

10

THOMAS H. SHAFFER
MARLA R. WOLFSON
JOAN H. GAULT

Respiratory physiology

The main function of the respiratory system is the exchange of gases such that arterial blood oxygen, carbon dioxide, and pH levels remain within specific limits throughout many different plysiological conditions. There are five fundamental processes involved in the maintenance of homeostasis, as follows:

1. Ventilation and distribution of gas volumes
2. Gas exchange and transport
3. Circulation of blood through the lungs
4. Mechanical interaction of respiratory forces that initiate breathing (respiratory muscles) and those that resist the flow of air (lung compliance and airway resistance)
5. Control and organization of respiratory movements

To appreciate the coordinated and integrated function of the entire respiratory system, it is essential to understand the functions of each of the five fundamental processes. We have attempted to analyze and present each fundamental process on an individual basis. We also discuss the integration and function of each of these processes with respect to the entire system.

Knowledge of respiratory physiology is paramount for proper diagnosis and effective treatment of pulmonary disease. With this in mind, we have presented basic scientific principles as viewed from the perspective of the physical therapist. The processes involved during normal respiration are described in detail in the following sections to establish a scientific basis for therapeutic interventions required for the patient with pulmonary disease.

VENTILATION AND DISTRIBUTION
Functional anatomy of the respiratory system

On gross inspection, each lung is cone shaped and covered by visceral pleura. The right lung is slightly larger than the left and is divided by the oblique and horizontal fissures into the upper, middle, and lower lobes. The left lung has two lobes, upper and lower, separated by an oblique fissure. The lobes are further subdivided into bron-chopulmonary segments, each receiving a segmental bronchus and artery, and giving rise to a vein (Fig. 10-1).

The airways, pleura, and connective tissue of the lung are vascularized by the systemic circulation through the bronchial arteries. The bronchial veins bypass the pulmonary circulation and join the pulmonary veins to return blood to the heart. Alveoli are perfused by the pulmonary circulation.

The lungs and airways are innervated through the pulmonary plexus. Located at the root of each lung, this plexus is formed from branches of the sympathetic trunk and vagus nerve. Recently, a nonadrenergic, noncholinergic inhibitory nerve fiber has been identified in the airway smooth muscle. Sympathetic stimulation causes bronchodilatation and marginal vasoconstriction, whereas parasympathetic stimulation produces bronchoconstriction and indirect vasodilatation.

The respiratory system is conceptually divided into two major divisions: (1) a *conducting portion,* which includes the nose, pharynx, larynx, trachea, bronchi, and bronchioles, and (2) a *respiratory portion,* consisting of the terminal portion of the bronchial tree and alveoli, the site of gas exchange (Fig. 10-2). The transitional zone, separating the conducting and respiratory portions, consists of the respiratory bronchioles.

In the conducting zone, air moves by bulk flow under the pressure gradients created by the respiratory muscles and the elastic recoil of the lung. The total cross-sectional area of the airways increases rapidly at the respiratory zone. Forward velocity of air flow therefore decreases, and the gases readily move by diffusion through the alveoli into the pulmonary capillaries. This is one example of the numerous histological (Fig. 10-3) and morphological alterations occurring throughout the respiratory system that provide for optimal ventilation and gas exchange.

Inspired air enters the body through the nose or mouth. Because of its architecture, large mucosal surface area, and fibrillae, the nose serves to filter, humidify, and warm

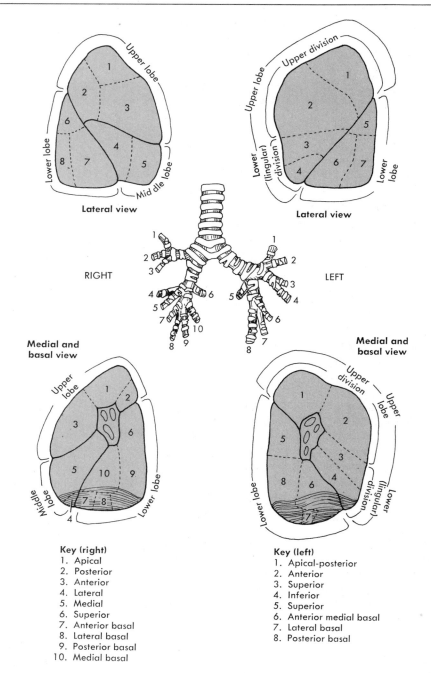

Key (right)
1. Apical
2. Posterior
3. Anterior
4. Lateral
5. Medial
6. Superior
7. Anterior basal
8. Lateral basal
9. Posterior basal
10. Medial basal

Key (left)
1. Apical-posterior
2. Anterior
3. Superior
4. Inferior
5. Superior
6. Anterior medial basal
7. Lateral basal
8. Posterior basal

Fig. 10-1. Bronchopulmonary tree (From Fishman, A.P.: Assessment of pulmonary function, New York, 1980, McGraw-Hill Book Co.)

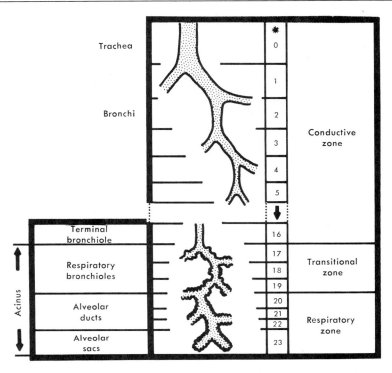

Fig. 10-2. Airway branching (Z-generation). (From Fishman, A.P.: Assessment of pulmonary function, New York, 1980, McGraw Hill Book Co.)

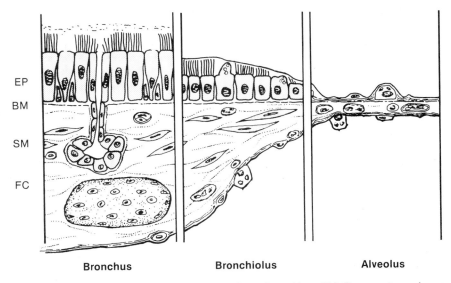

Fig. 10-3. Histological modification accompanying airway branching. *BM,* Basement membrane; *EP,* epithelial layer; *FC,* fibrous coating containing cartilage; *SM,* smooth muscle.

or cool the air to body temperature. This process protects the remainder of the respiratory system from damage caused by dry gases or harmful debris. The gas then passes through the pharynx where skeletal muscles contract during swallowing to prevent aspiration of food or liquid into the nose. The pharynx is essential for articulated speech and allows interaction between the sense of smell and taste; however, aside from serving as a conduit, it does not participate in respiration. Next, air travels through the larynx in which the epiglottis acts as a valve to prevent food stuffs from entering the trachea. The larynx, lined by a mucous membrane, is formed by cartilages that are connected by ligaments and moved by skeletal muscles. The most caudal cartilage, the cricoid, is of particular importance in ventilation. It is located at the upper end of the trachea and is the only complete cartilaginous ring around the trachea; as such, it protects the trachea from dynamic compression during forced inspiration or expiration.

The trachea is generally considered to be the differentiating structure between the upper and lower airways. It is continuous with the larynx and is lined by a pseudostratified ciliated columnar epithelium containing goblet cells and seromucinous glands. The latter structures produce a sol-gel mucus blanket in which the cilia are embedded. As the cilia beat, this mucous blanket is set into motion and carries unfiltered debris toward the pharynx. This process of mucociliary transport is one of the major defense mechanisms in the lung.

The trachea is formed by 16 to 20 horseshoe-shaped cartilaginous rings connected by smooth muscle that is interlaced with elastic fibers. The cartilage rings support the anterior and lateral walls of the trachea. The posterior wall consists of the tracheal muscle, a thin sheath of smooth muscle, whose horizontal fibers bridge the opened ends of the cartilaginous rings. The trachea divides at the carina into the right and left main bronchi, which in turn branch in an irregular dichotomous pattern forming the lobar and segmental bronchi.

The left main bronchus branches at a more acute angle and is longer than the right main bronchus, which is more directly in line with the trachea. This relationship predisposes to aspiration of material into the right rather than the left lung. Bronchial walls consist of irregular plates of cartilage joined by circular bands of smooth muscle. The walls are lined with a continuation of the tracheal epithelium. With further bronchial divisions, the cartilaginous plates become scant and smooth muscle and elastic fibers become prominent with respect to lumen diameter. Cartilage and glands disappear and goblet cells decrease in number at the level of the bronchiole. In addition, the pseudostratified epithelium is replaced by a simpler ciliated cuboid cell epithelium. The bronchioles proximal to the emergence of alveoli are the terminal bronchioles. The transitional zone is demarcated by the appearance of alveoli in the walls of the respiratory bronchioles. The

smooth muscle begins to spiral in the terminal bronchiole thereby providing the supportive function served by cartilage in the more proximal airways. Smooth muscle thins and cilia gradually disappear so that by the final division, the respiratory bronchiole wall consists of a few strands of muscle and elastic fiber and is lined by a simple cuboid epithelium. Alveolar macrophages are found at this level and provide another defense mechanism by ingesting small unfiltered particles.

Alveolar ducts, completely lined with alveoli, are formed by the branching of the respiratory bronchioles (Fig. 10-2). This division demarcates the respiratory zone of the lung where gas exchange occurs. The discontinuous wall of the alveolar duct is composed of elastic and sparse smooth muscle fibers. The lining is further reduced to a low cuboid epithelium. The alveolar duct gives rise to the alveolar sphincter, the final presence of smooth muscle, and terminates as simple alveoli and alveolar sacs that contain two or more alveoli.

Alveoli (Fig. 10-4) are small evaginations of the respiratory bronchioles, alveolar ducts, and alveolar sacs. Because adjacent alveoli share a common wall, their shape and dimensions vary depending on the arrangement of adjoining alveoli and on lung volume. This phenomenon is called ''interdependence,'' wherein an increase in volume in one alveolus will tend to increase the volume in the adjacent alveoli. A similar mechanism increases the lumen diameter of distal airways that are surrounded by and tethered to the alveoli. Furthermore, adjacent alveoli communicate through channels called ''pores of Kohn'' and with bronchioles through channels called ''Lambert's canals.'' All these alveolar and airway architectural features contribute to the stability and uniformity of lung expansion.

The thin alveolar lining is particularly suited for gas exchange (Fig. 10-5). It consists of two types of cells: (1) type I alveolar cells, which are large flat cells composing most of the internal alveolar surface and (2) type II alveolar cells, which are less numerous, are ovoid, and are involved in the synthesis of surfactant, a substance that facilitates alveolar stability.

Definition of ventilation and volumes

Ventilation is the cyclic process of inspiration and expiration whereby optimal levels of oxygen and carbon dioxide are maintained in the alveoli and arterial blood. Total ventilation $(\dot{V}_E)$ is the volume of air expired each minute. It is the product of the volume of gas moved in and out of the alveoli (V_A) and airways with each breaths (V_D), the tidal volume (V_T), and the number of breaths taken each minute, the respiratory rate (f). Therefore:

$$\dot{V}_E = V_T \cdot f$$

where $V_T = V_A + V_D$.

The volume of alveolar gas (V_A) in the tidal volume represents the volume of fresh gas entering the respiratory

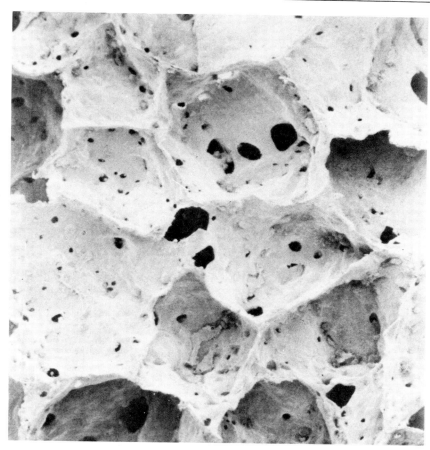

Fig. 10-4. Horse lung. Cut edges of interalveolar septa surround alveoli seen *en face*. Pores and alveolar epithelial cells are visible on the surfaces of the interalveolar septa, and pulmonary alveolar macrophages are seen in the alveoli. (Field width, 250 μm.) (From American Lung Association: In defense of the lung, New York, 1974, The Association.)

zone with each breath. Alveolar ventilation, $\dot{V}_A = V_A \cdot f$, is extremely important because it represents the amount of fresh air available for gas exchange per minute. Hyperventilation is defined as an increase in alveolar ventilation that decreases carbon dioxide levels below the normal limits ($Pco_2 = 40$ mm Hg), that is hypocapnia. Hypoventilation, in contrast, is defined as an increase in carbon dioxide (hypercapnia) levels caused by a decrease in alveolar ventilation. The oxygen tension of alveolar air is increased by hyperventilation and decreased by hypoventilation.

Therefore total ventilation is the combined volume of gases moving through the conducting and respiratory zones of the lung each minute. It is described as:

$$\dot{V}_E = \dot{V}_D + \dot{V}_A$$

where E is exhaled air, D is lead space, and A is alveolar air.

The terms used in the discussion of the dynamic process of ventilation are best understood with consideration of static lung volumes and lung capacities (Fig. 10-6). Although these values are essentially anatomic measurements, alterations in lung volumes or capacities may reflect the effects of cardiopulmonary disease. In general, lung volumes are subdivisions that do not overlap. Capacities include two or more primary volumes.

There are four primary lung volumes: (1) tidal volume, (2) inspiratory reserve volume, (3) expiratory reserve volume, and (4) residual volume. Tidal volume (V_T) is the volume of gas inspired or expired during each respiratory cycle. It reflects the depth of breathing and comprises the volume entering the alveoli (V_A) and the volume remaining in the airways (V_D). These values, when coupled with the respiratory frequency, are used to describe ventilation.

Reserve volumes represent the maximal volumes of gas

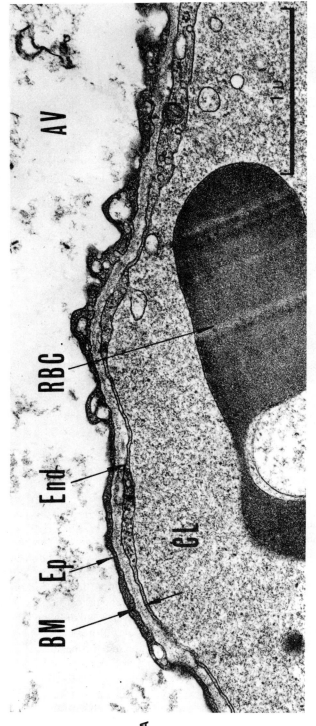

Fig. 10-5. A, Electron micrograph of the lung, showing the alveolocapillary region of the left lower lobe of a healthy 35-year-old man. **B,** Electron micrograph of the healthy human lung (specimen from the left lower lobe of a 74-year-old man), showing alveolocapillary structures with large epithelial (type B, type II) cell containing cytoplasmic lamellar bodies. *AV,* Alveolar space; *BM,* basement membrane; *CL,* capillary lumen; *C,* collagen; *End,* endothelial cytoplasm; *End Ret,* endoplasmic reticulum; *Ep* (in **A**), epithelial cytoplasm, type II; *Ep* (in **B**), epithelial cytoplasm; *Ep II,* cytoplasm of alveolar epithelial cell, type II; *Ep Nu,* epithelial nucleus; *Ep II Nu,* nucleus of alveolar epithelial cell, type II; *Lam,* lamellar body; *RBC,* red blood cell. **(A,** Courtesy A.E. Vatter, Department of Pathology, Webb-Waring Institute, University of Colorado Medical Center, Denver, Colo. **B,** Courtesy Robert L. Hawley, Mercy Institute of Biomedical Research, Denver, Colo.)

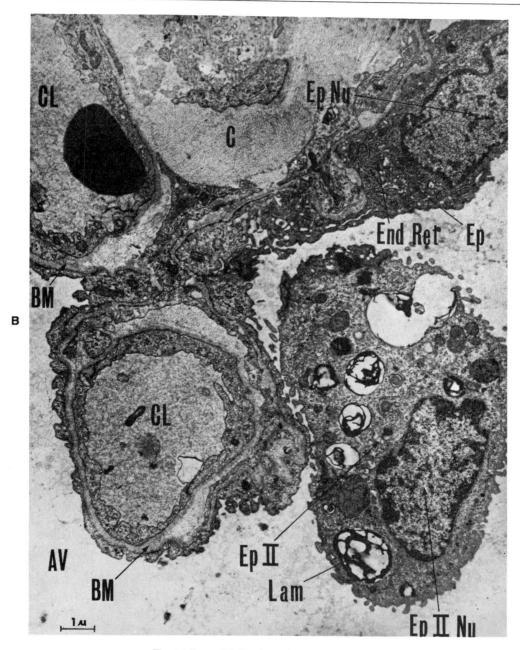

Fig. 10-5, cont'd. For legend see opposite page.

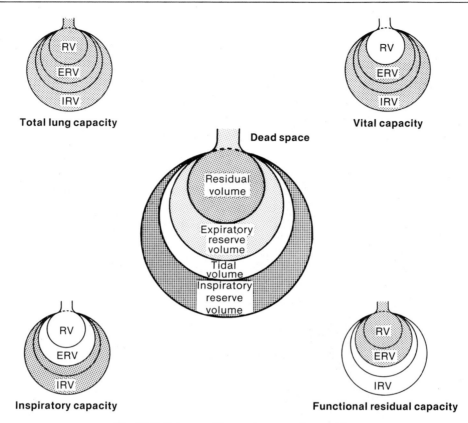

Fig. 10-6. Scheme of lung volumes and capacities.

that can be moved above or below a normal tidal volume. These values reflect the balance between lung and chest wall elasticity, respiratory muscle strength, and thoracic mobility. *Inspiratory reserve volume* (IRV) is the maximum volume of gas that can be inspired from the peak of a tidal volume. *Expiratory reserve volume* (ERV) is the maximum volume of gas that can be expired after a normal tidal expiration. Therefore reserve volumes are associated with the ability to increase or decrease the tidal volume. Normal lungs do not collapse at the end of the greatest expiration. The volume of gas remaining is called the *residual volume* (RV).

These four volumes can be combined to form four capacities: (1) total lung capacity, (2) vital capacity, (3) inspiratory capacity, and (4) functional residual capacity. *Total lung capacity* (TLC) is the amount of gas in the respiratory system after a maximal inspiration. It is the sum of all four lung volumes. *Vital capacity* (VC) is the maximal volume of gas that can be expelled from the lungs after a maximal inspiration. As such, the vital capacity is the sum of IRV + TV + ERV. *Inspiratory capacity* (IC) is the maximal volume of gas that can be inspired from the resting end-expiration level; therefore it is the sum of TV + IRV. *Functional residual capacity* is the volume of

gas in the lungs when the respiratory system is at rest, that is, the volume in the lung at the end of a normal expiration. The size of the FRC is determined by the balance of two opposing forces: (1) inward elastic recoil of the lung tending to collapse the lung and (2) outward elastic recoil of the chest wall tending to expand the lung. Functional residual capacity is the volume of gas above which a normal tidal volume oscillates. A normal FRC avails optimal lung mechanics and alveolar surface area for efficient ventilation and gas exchange.

Definition of dead space

Dead space (V_D) refers to the volume within the respiratory system that does not participate in gas exchange. It is composed of several components. *Anatomic dead space* is the volume of gas contained in the conducting airways. *Alveolar dead space* refers to the volume of gas in areas of "wasted ventilation," that is, in alveoli that are *ventilated* but poorly or underperfused. The total volume of gas that is not involved in gas exchange is called the *physiological dead space*. It is the sum of the anatomical and alveolar dead space. In a normal person, the physiological dead space should be equal to the anatomical dead space. For this reason, some investigators refer to physiological dead space as *pathological* dead space.

Several factors can modify the dead-space volume. Anatomical dead space increases as a function of airway size. Because of the interdependence of the alveoli and airways, anatomical dead space increases as a function of lung volume. Similarly, dead space increases as a function of body height, bronchodilator drugs, diseases such as emphysema, and oversized artificial airways. In contrast, anatomical dead space is decreased by reduction of the size of the airways, as occurs with bronchoconstriction or a tracheostomy.

Distribution of gas

Inspired air is not distributed uniformly throughout the lungs. One obvious explanation for this non-uniform distribution is the difference in size between the right and left lungs. Topographical differences in ventilation also occur within each lung. Because of intrapleural pressure gradients caused by gravitational, chest-wall, and lung forces, the alveoli in dependent portions of the lung are smaller and more compliant than alveoli within less dependent segments. Therefore, when breathing is around a normal functional residual capacity, the dependent alveoli receive three times more inspired air than the independent alveoli do. For example, apical ventilation exceeds basilar ventilation with the subject sitting or standing. In the supine position, the posterior portion of the lung is better ventilated than the anterior portion. Similar ventilation inequalities exist in the lateral and Trendelenburg positions.

This relationship changes if breathing occurs at very high or low lung volumes. At high volumes, all alveoli become less compliant; therefore the volume changes tend to be similar. However, at low lung volumes, airways in the dependent portion close, and distribution of air to the dependent areas is prevented.

The distribution of gas is further altered by local factors in disease. Regional airway obstruction, abnormal lung or chest wall compliance, or respiratory muscle weakness may significantly increase the nonuniformity of air distribution in the lung. However, collateral ventilation between adjacent alveoli through the pores of Kohn, or between alveoli and respiratory bronchioles through Lambert's canals, may help ventilate lung regions behind occluded airways.

Testing and evaluation

Lung volumes and ventilation. Lung volumes are measured by spirometry, inert gas dilution, nitrogen washout, and body plethysmography techniques. Because lung volumes are essentially anatomical measurements, they do not directly evaluate pulmonary function. However, changes in lung volumes are associated with respiratory pathological conditions. For this reason these tests offer valuable information to assist in the diagnosis and management of patients with cardiopulmonary disease.

Spirometry is a traditional technique used to measure lung volumes and specific ventilatory capacities. As originally described in the mid-1800s by Hutchinson, the spirometer records changes in lung volumes from movement of a lightweight bell that is inverted over a water bath. The patient's breathing through a mouthpiece causes the bell to rise or fall. The change in volume is recorded on a variable-speed rotating drum of graph paper by corresponding movements of a pen (Figs. 10-7 and 10-8). Recent modifications of this system enable rapid collection of data by a computer. Tidal volume and expiratory and inspiratory reserve volumes are measured when one performs particular respiratory maneuvers from which inspiratory and vital capacity can be determined. Because the lung cannot be emptied by maximal expiration, other techniques must be employed to measure residual volume, functional residual capacity, and total lung capacity. Typically, the functional residual capacity is determined and residual volume is calculated. Once residual volume is calculated, one deduces the total lung capacity by adding the vital capacity and residual volume.

Closed-circuit helium dilution is commonly used to determine residual volume and functional residual capacity. This technique is based on the facts that (1) helium is an inert gas that is insoluble in blood and not found in the lungs and (2) consumed oxygen is replaced and carbon dioxide is removed from the spirometer and therefore the total volume of the system is constant. The patient breathes through a spirometer containing a known concentration of helium (C_1). After several minutes the concentration of helium in the lung and in the spirometer equilibrates (C_2). The final helium concentration (C_2) reflects dilution of the initial helium volume (V_1) by the volume of gas in the lungs (V_2). Therefore the unknown value (V_2) can be calculated:

$$C_1 \times V_1 = C_2 (V_1 + V_2)$$

or

$$V_2 = V_1 \left(\frac{C_1}{C_2} - 1 \right)$$

Body plethysmography utilizes Boyle's law ($PV = K$) in the determination of lung volume (Fig. 10-9). Basically, a patient sits in an airtight booth and breathes against a mouthpiece that is occluded at the lung volume to be measured. According to Boyle's law, pressure and volume change inversely in the lung as a result of respiratory efforts. Because the "body box" is sealed, opposite pressure and volume changes occur in the box. By measuring the pressure inside the box and the volume change in the box, one can calculate the lung volume as follows:

$$P_1 V = P_2 (V - \Delta V)$$

or

$$V = \Delta V \frac{P_2}{P_2 - 1}$$

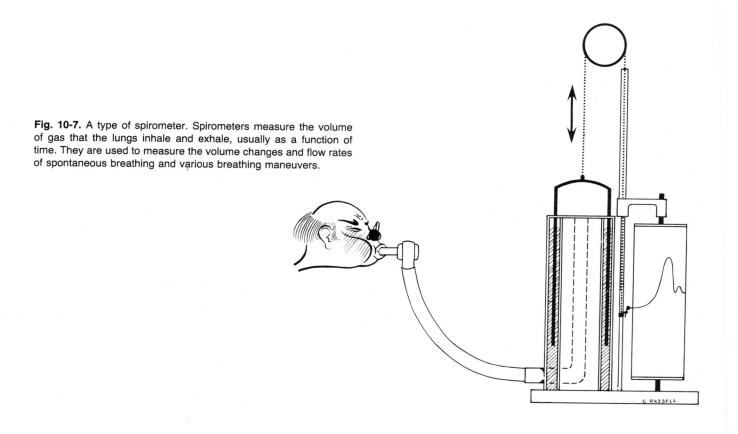

Fig. 10-7. A type of spirometer. Spirometers measure the volume of gas that the lungs inhale and exhale, usually as a function of time. They are used to measure the volume changes and flow rates of spontaneous breathing and various breathing maneuvers.

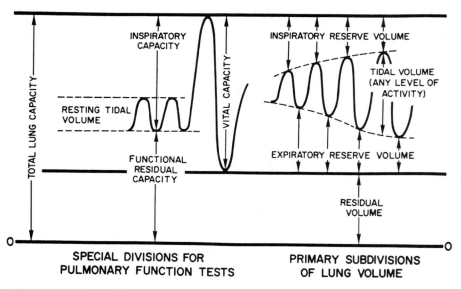

Fig. 10-8. Subdivisions of the lung volume. (Modified from Pappenheimer, J.R., and others: Fed. Proc. **9:**602, 1950.)

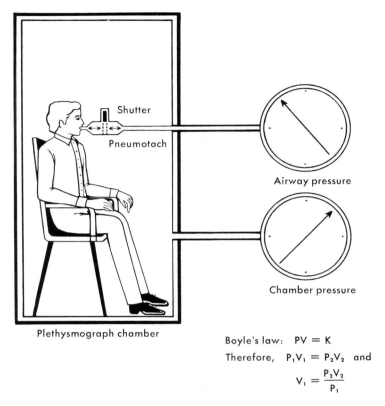

Boyle's law: PV = K

Therefore, $P_1V_1 = P_2V_2$ and

$$V_1 = \frac{P_2V_2}{P_1}$$

Fig. 10-9. Body plethysmography. (From Spearman, C., and Sheldon, R.: Egan's fundamentals of respiratory therapy, ed. 4, St. Louis, 1982, The C.V. Mosby Co.)

where P_1 is end-inspiratory pressure; P_2 is end-expiratory pressure; ΔV is change in volume of box; and V is unknown lung volume.

Ventilatory capacity is most commonly evaluated by the forced vital capacity (FVC). The maximal voluntary ventilation (MVV) test requires that the patient breathe as deeply and rapidly as possible for 15 seconds. This test is often too fatiguing for patients, and comparable diagnostic information is readily gained from the forced vital capacity. However, assessment of respiratory muscle endurance is best made on the basis of tests such as the MVV.

The forced expiratory volume at 1 second (FEV_1) is the volume of gas forcibly expired in 1 second after maximal inspiration. It is recorded by a spirometer when the patient exhales as hard, as much, and as fast as possible from maximal lung volume. The change in volume occurring in the first second and the total volume exhaled (FVC) can be directly measured (Fig. 10-10) from the curve on the spirometer graph. The FVC is a measurement of the maximal volume output of the respiratory system. As such, the FVC reflects the integrity of all the components involved with pulmonary mechanics. The FEV_1 provides information about airway resistance and the elastic recoil of the

lungs. In addition, the ratio of FEV_1/FVC varies in the presence of a pathological condition. Therefore this test can help distinguish between obstructive and restrictive lung disease. In restrictive disease, the total lung capacity and the forced vital capacity are decreased. However, because the elastic recoil of the lungs may be increased in restrictive disease, the FEV_1/FVC ratio may also increase. In contrast, increased airway resistance associated with obstructive lung disease decreases the FEV_1. The total lung capacity and functional residual capacity are typically increased as a function of airtrapping distal to the occluded airways. Therefore in obstructive lung disease the FEV_1/FVC ratio is decreased.

Ventilation is commonly determined by measurement of the total volume of expired gas over a given duration. Typically the patient breathes through a mouthpiece for about 3 minutes, and the expired gas is shunted into a collecting bag. The total ventilation ($\dot{V}_E$) is determined when the total volume of gas is divided by the duration of the collecting period. Alternatively, minute ventilation can be determined by calculation of the tidal volume, wherein the total volume (V) is divided by the total number of breaths (n) and multiplied by the number of breaths per minute (f). Therefore:

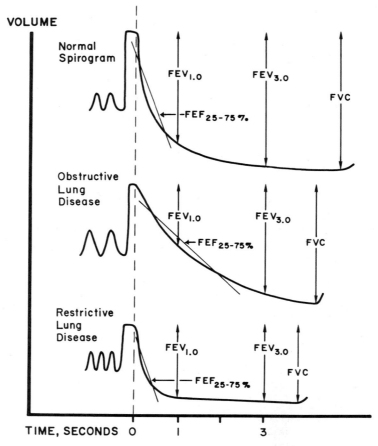

Fig. 10-10. Spirometric recording of forced expiratory volume (FEV) and forced vital capacity (FVC): normal, obstructive, and restrictive lung disease. (From Slonim, N.B., and Hamilton, L.H.: Respiratory physiology, ed. 4, St. Louis, 1981, The C.V. Mosby Co.)

$$\dot{V}_E = V_T \times f$$

or

$$\frac{V}{n} \times f = V_E$$

Alveolar ventilation is calculated in two ways: (1) by subtraction of dead-space volume from the tidal volume and (2) on the basis of CO_2 elimination by the lungs. Determination of dead space is discussed later. The second method measures alveolar ventilation from the concentration of CO_2 in expired gas. CO_2 is derived solely from alveolar air, since gas exchange does not occur in the conducting airways.

Inadequate alveolar ventilation is associated with faulty pulmonary mechanics and neural control and results in abnormal blood gas tensions.

Distribution of gases. Several techniques are employed to assess the distribution of inspired air. The three most commonly discussed tests are (1) single-breath nitrogen test, (2) multibreath nitrogen test, and (3) use of radioactive gases.

The single-breath nitrogen test involves plotting of the changing concentrations of nitrogen (N_2) in the expired gas after a maximal inspiration of 100% oxygen. As seen in Fig. 10-11, four phases are described. Phases 1 and 2 reflect gas expired from the dead space. Phase 3, the plateau phase, represents alveolar gas. In patients, the slope of phase 3 is steep, reflecting varying concentrations of nitrogen in the expired gas. This steep slope usually indicates that either the inspired oxygen was unevenly distributed or there are regional variations in the emptying rate of the alveoli. The abrupt rise in nitrogen concentration, phase 4, marks the onset of the "closing volume," the volume at which dependent airways close.

The multibreath nitrogen test records the nitrogen concentration at the end of each breath while the patient

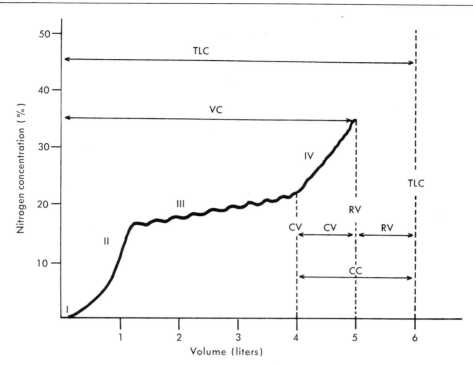

Fig. 10-11. Single-breath nitrogen test of uneven ventilation. (From Spearman, C., and Sheldon, R.: Egan's fundamentals of respiratory therapy, ed. 4, St. Louis, 1982, The C.V. Mosby Co.)

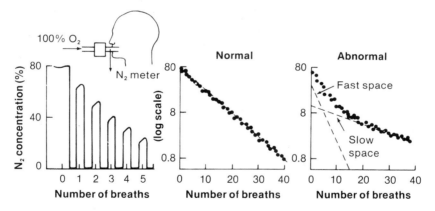

Fig. 10-12. Multibreath nitrogen washout test for determination of uneven ventilation. (From West, J.B.: Respiratory physiology, ed. 2, Baltimore, Md., 1979, The Williams & Wilkins Co.)

breathes 100% oxygen. A normal lung empties uniformly so that the nitrogen concentration decreases by the same proportion on each breath. In patients with lung disease, gross inequalities in ventilation dilute some alveoli before others; therefore a variable pattern of nitrogen-concentration decrease occurs (Fig. 10-12).

Radionuclide tracers are used to demonstrate regional differences in ventilation. A volume of radioactive xenon is inspired from a spirometer and is carried to alveoli. A radioactivity counter detects the gas and records the distribution through the lung.

Gross inequalities in ventilation are associated with many pulmonary diseases. Abnormalities in lung compliance, resistance, and collateral ventilation of alveoli obstructed by airway disease are associated with emptying and filling defects.

Dead space. Each component of respiratory dead space can be evaluated. Specific tests include (1) Fowler's single-breath nitrogen technique, which measures anatomical dead space, and (2) use of the Bohr equation to calculate physiological dead space. Total dead-space volume is estimated to be 1 ml for each pound of body weight.

The Fowler technique measures anatomical dead space through nitrogen concentration analysis of expired air after a single inspiration of 100% oxygen. The inspired gas enters the alveoli, and the last part of this tidal volume stays in the conducting airways (anatomic dead space). Nitrogen concentration begins to rise as the airways are cleared and alveolar gas is expired. The recorded volume to this point represents anatomical dead space.

The Bohr equation is used to calculate physiological dead space. This method requires analysis of the carbon dioxide (CO_2) in a collected volume of expired gas and of the CO_2 in the very end of the expired tidal volume. It is assumed that all the expired CO_2 is from the alveolar gas. Therefore:

$$V_D = \left(\frac{F_{ACO_2} - F_{ECO_2}}{F_{ACO_2}} \right) \cdot V_T$$

In the normal lung, measurements derived from the Fowler technique and the Bohr equation should be equal. A difference reflects alveolar dead space.

In the normal population, variations in lung volumes and ventilatory capacity are associated with age, position, body proportions, obesity, and cooperation. Once these factors are considered, values that deviate from normal standards are usually indicative of a pulmonary disease. The aforementioned tests aid in the differential diagnosis and therapeutic recommendations in the presence of abnormal findings. For example, body plethysmography measures thoracic gas volume, whereas spirometry and gas dilution measures only ventilated lung volume. Disparity between thoracic gas volume and ventilated lung volume indicate gas that is trapped by airway obstruction. Furthermore, reversible airway obstruction, associated with asthma, is demonstrated by improved FEV_1 and FVC values after administration of a bronchodilator.

MECHANICS OF BREATHING

The mechanics of breathing deals with the respiratory muscle forces required to overcome the elastic recoil of the lungs and thorax as well as frictional resistance to air flow through hundreds of thousands of conducting airways. The energy for ventilating the lungs is supplied by active contraction of the respiratory muscles, which are discussed in a subsequent chapter. This section discusses the elastic and nonelastic forces that resist movement of the lung and chest wall. We begin our discussion of pulmonary mechanics by considering the elastic nature of the lung.

Elastic behavior of the respiratory system

Elasticity is the property of matter such that if we disturb a system by stretching or expanding it the system will

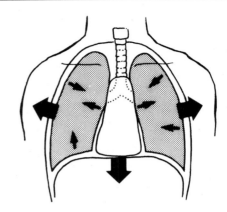

Fig. 10-13. Balance of elastic forces in the lung at rest.

return to its original position when all external forces are removed. Like a spring, the tissues of the lungs and thorax stretch during inspiration, and when the force of contraction (respiratory muscular effort) is removed, the tissues return to their resting position. The resting position or lung volume is established by the balance of elastic forces. Under these conditions, the elastic force of the lung tissues (Fig. 10-13) exactly equals those of the chest wall and diaphragm. This occurs at the end of every normal expiration when the respiratory muscles are relaxed, and the volume remaining in the lungs is the functional residual capacity (FRC).

The visceral pleura of the lung is separated from the parietal pleura of the chest wall by a thin film of fluid. In a normal person at the end of expiration, the mean pleural pressure is 3 to 5 cm H_2O below atmospheric pressure. This pressure results from the equal and opposite retractive forces of the lungs and chest wall. Since there is no air movement at the end of expiration, gas throughout the lungs is in equilibrium with atmospheric air.

During inspiration, the inspiratory muscles contract expanding the chest wall and lowering the diaphragm. Since the lungs tend to pull inward, this expansion results in a further reduction of pleural pressure. Therefore the more the chest wall is expanded during inspiration, the more subatmospheric is the resultant pleural pressure.

Lung compliance. If pressure is sequentially decreased (more subatmospheric) around the outside of an excised lung, as shown in Fig. 10-14, the lung volume increases. When the pressure is removed from the lung, it deflates along a pressure-volume curve that is different from that during inflation. The difference between the inflation and deflation levels of the pressure-volume curve is called "hysteresis." The elastic behavior of the lungs is characterized by the pressure-volume curve. More specifically, the ratio of change in lung volume to change in distending pressure defines the compliance of the lungs. Although the

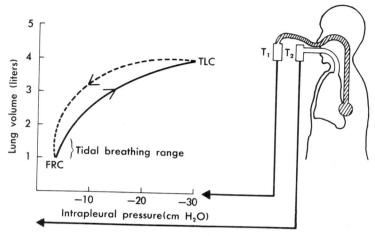

Fig. 10-14. Measurement of the pressure-volume curve of excised lung. (From Ruppel, G.: Manual of pulmonary function testing, ed. 3, St. Louis, 1982, The C.V. Mosby Co.)

pressure-volume relationship of the lung is not linear over the entire range, the compliance or slope ($\Delta V/\Delta P$) is linear over the normal range of tidal volumes beginning at functional residual capacity. Thus, for a given change in intrathoracic pressure, tidal volume will increase in proportion to lung compliance. As lung compliance is decreased, the lungs are stiffer and more difficult to expand. When lung compliance is increased, the lung becomes easier to distend, that is, more compliant.

Lung compliance and pressure-volume relationships are attributable to the interdependence of elastic tissue elements and alveolar surface tension. Tissue elasticity is dependent on elastin and collagen content of the lung. A typical value for lung compliance in a young healthy adult would be 0.2 L/cm H_2O. This value is dependent on the size of the lung (mass of elastic tissue). As may be expected, compliance of the lung increases with development as the tissue mass of the lung increases.

In pulmonary fibrosis, collagen content is increased, and lung compliance is reduced; in emphysema, elastin content is decreased (destruction of alveolar walls) and lung compliance is increased as compared to normal (Fig. 10-15).

The surface-active material (surfactant) lining the alveoli of the lung has significant physiological function. Surfactant lowers surface tension inside the alveoli, thereby contributing to lung stability by reducing the pressure necessary to expand the alveoli. Alveolar type II cells (Fig. 10-16) contain osmophilic lamellated bodies that are associated with the transformation of surfactant. Impaired surface activity, as occurs in some premature infants, typically results in lungs that are stiff (low compliance) and prone to collapse (atelectasis).

Chest-wall compliance. Like the lung, the chest wall is elastic. If air is introduced into the pleural cavity, the lungs will collapse inward and the chest wall will expand outward (Fig. 10-17). As previously discussed, there is a balance of elastic forces at rest (end of expiration) such that the lungs maintain a stable functional residual capacity (FRC) volume. In certain pathological conditions this balance of forces becomes disturbed. For example, as a result of destroyed elastic tissue in emphysema, the inward pull of the lungs is less than normal (increased compliance); therefore the chest wall is pulled out and the FRC is increased. In contrast, pulmonary fibrosis results in a greater elastic recoil than normal (decreased compliance), thereby pulling the chest wall inward and decreasing the FRC (Fig. 10-15).

Chest-wall compliance and pressure-volume relationships are attributable to the elastic-tissue properties of the rib cage and diaphragm. A normal value for chest wall compliance in a healthy young adult would be 0.2 L/cm H_2O, approximately the same as lung compliance. Chest-wall compliance may be decreased in kyphoscoliosis, skeletal muscle disorders, and abdominal disorders.

Nonelastic behavior of the respiratory system

Nonelastic properties of the respiratory system characterize its resistance to motion. Because motion involves friction or loss of energy, whenever two surfaces are in contact, resistance to breathing occurs in any moving part of the respiratory system. These resistances would include frictional resistance to air flow, tissue resistance, and inertial forces. Lung resistance results predominantly (80%) from frictional resistance to air flow. Tissue resistance

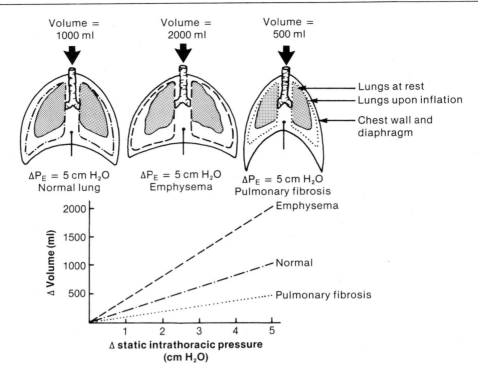

Fig. 10-15. Lung compliance changes associated with disease. (From Cherniack, R.M., and others: Respiration in health and disease, ed. 2, Philadelphia, 1972, W.B. Saunders Co.)

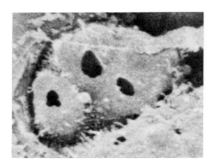

Fig. 10-16. Electron micrograph (10,000×) of type II alveolar epithelial cell demonstrating presence of osmophilic lamellated bodies (LB). (From West, J.B.: Respiratory physiology, ed. 2, Baltimore, Md., 1979, The Williams & Wilkins Co.)

(19%) and inertia (1%) also influence lung resistance, but under normal conditions have a relatively small effect. Airflow through the airways requires a driving pressure generated by changes in alveolar pressure. When alveolar pressure is less than atmospheric pressure (during spontaneous inspiration), air flows into the lungs; when alveolar pressure is greater than atmospheric pressure, air flows out

of the lungs. By definition, resistance to air flow (R_A) is equal to the pressure difference between alveolar and atmospheric pressure (ΔP) divided by air flow ($\dot{V}$); therefore:

$$R_A = \frac{\Delta P}{\dot{V}}$$

Under normal tidal-volume breathing conditions, there is a linear relationship between airflow and driving pressure. As shown in Fig. 10-18, the slope of the flow-pressure curve changes as the airways narrow indicating that the patient with airway obstruction has a greater resistance to air flow. Normal airway resistance in a young adult is approximately 1.0 cm H_2O/L/sec.

About 80% of the total resistance to air flow occurs in large airways to about the fourth to fifth generation of bronchial branching. Thus the finding that resistance to airflow is elevated in a patient usually indicates large-airway disease. Because the smaller airways contribute a small proportion of total airway resistance, they have been designated as the "silent zone" of the lung in which airway obstruction can occur without easy detection.

Mechanical factors influencing airway resistance. The dimensions (length and cross-sectional area) of airways are greatly influenced by lung volume. Small bronchi, bronchioles, and respiratory bronchioles have attachments to lung parenchyma so that with increases in volume, these

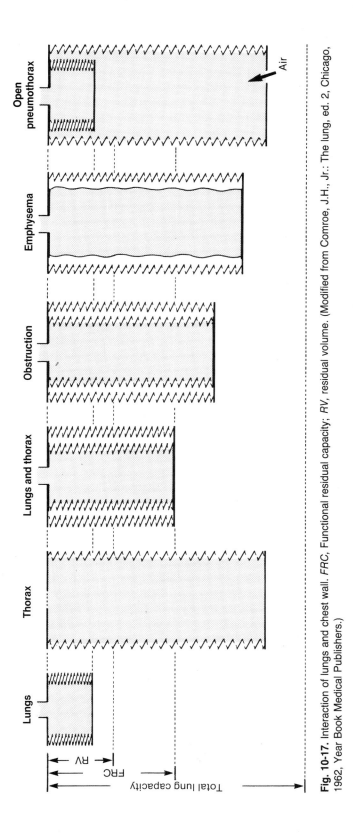

Fig. 10-17. Interaction of lungs and chest wall. *FRC*, Functional residual capacity; *RV*, residual volume. (Modified from Comroe, J.H., Jr.: The lung, ed. 2, Chicago, 1962, Year Book Medical Publishers.)

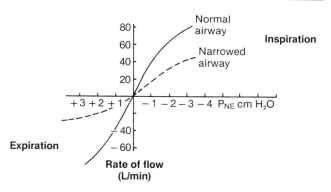

Fig. 10-18. Flow pressure curves for normal and narrowed airways. (From Cherniack, R.M., and others: Respiration in health and disease, ed. 2, Philadelphia, 1972, W.B. Saunders Co.)

airways are stretched. Like lung tissue, the airways are elastic. At high lung volumes, the pressure on the outer surface of the airway becomes more subatmospheric and transmural pressure (difference in inside and outside pressure of the airway) becomes greater. These pressure differences cause the airways to increase in cross-sectional area and decrease the resistance to airflow (Fig. 10-19).

During a forced expiration, dynamic compression of the airway can occur with a resulting increased resistance to airflow. Since smaller airways are more compressible than larger airways (no supporting cartilage in bronchiolar walls and beyond), smaller airways are more likely to collapse when the pressure outside the airway is greater than that inside (forced expiration) (Fig. 10-20). Further effort by the respiratory muscles produces no further increase in airflow. The increase in driving force is offset by dynamic compression of the airways. Patients with lung disease who have abnormal elastic and nonelastic properties of the lungs exhibit expiratory flow limitation at much lower levels of transmural pressure and lower lung volumes than that seen in normal subjects.

Neural control of airway resistance. The cross-sectional area of airways is also under control of airway smooth muscle tone, which results from constant parasympathetic impulses. Stimulation of parasympathetic cholinergic nerves causes contraction of airway smooth muscle with an increase in airway resistance, whereas sympathetic adrenergic stimulation causes relaxation with a decrease in airway resistance. Smooth muscle in large airways has a more dense innervation than in small airways. Stimulation of vagal bronchioconstrictor fibers narrows the bronchioles, increases airway resistance, and decreases anatomical dead space, but enlarges the alveoli because of gas trapping.

Airway obstruction. Airway obstruction refers to a reduction in relative cross-sectional area of an airway resulting in an increase in airway resistance. The degree or se-

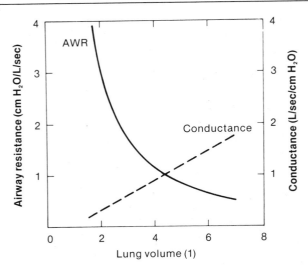

Fig. 10-19. Airway resistance and conductance as a function of lung volume. (From West, J.B.: Respiratory physiology, ed. 2, Baltimore, Md., 1979, The Williams & Wilkins Co.)

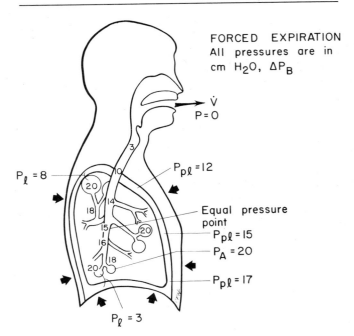

Fig. 10-20. Dynamic compression of the airways during forced expiration. (From Slonim, N.B., and Hamilton, L.H.: Respiratory physiology, ed. 4, St. Louis, 1981, The C.V. Mosby Co.)

verity of obstruction is also dependent on how diffusely the airways are involved. Finally, airway obstruction can be either partial or complete. Partial obstruction acts as a check valve by increasing resistance to air flow, impairing drainage of secretions, and reducing alveolar emptying to a greater degree during expiration. In complete airway obstruction there is no airflow or drainage of secretions.

Testing and evaluation

The mechanical properties of the lung play an important role in understanding lung volume as well as establishing the respiratory muscle force requirements for sustaining adequate alveolar ventilation. Like other pulmonary tests, the determination of lung mechanical properties is an important practical application of respiratory physiology for diagnosis and management of patients with lung disease.

Lung compliance. Lung compliance is a measure of the elastic properties of the lung and is defined as the change in lung volume per change in pressure across the lung.

To determine lung compliance, one first needs to measure intrapleural pressure. Clinically, as well as experimentally, intrapleural pressure has been estimated by intraesophageal measurements. This determination is accomplished when one has a subject swallow a small latex balloon attached to a catheter and pressure transducers. In addition, lung volume changes are determined by either spirometry or pneumotachography.

When lung compliance is measured during breathholding procedures (a subject breathes into or out of a spirometer in steps of 500 ml), this is termed "quasi-static." Thus the change in spirometer volume to the change in

esophageal pressure is an estimate of static lung compliance. It is also possible to measure lung compliance during quiet breathing. As shown in Fig. 10-21, there are two points in the respiratory cycle when airflow is zero: the end of inspiration and the end of expiration. Under these conditions all intrapleural pressure effort is associated with lung elastic forces. The change in tidal volume between these points per change in intrapleural (esophageal) pressure is a measure of dynamic lung compliance.

Lung resistance. Lung resistance is a measure of the nonelastic properties of lung and, by definition, requires a dynamic measurement. Like compliance evaluations, intrapleural pressure measurements are required. In addition, simultaneous measurements of tidal volume and air flow are necessary (Fig. 10-21). As shown, intrapleural pressure reflects the forces required to overcome both elastic and nonelastic forces. The pressure required to overcome the elastic forces is represented by the dashed lines, whereas the additional pressure (that between 1 and 1′, 2 and 2′, etc., on the intrapleural pressure trace) is necessary to overcome tissue and airway resistance. Lung resistance (tissue and airway resistance) can therefore be determined at a specific point in the respiratory cycle (e.g., at point 1) as the change in pressure ($P_1 - P_{1'}$) divided by the airflow at that instance in time.

To measure airway resistance directly, we need to know alveolar pressure, since by definition this is the pressure

A spontaneous breath

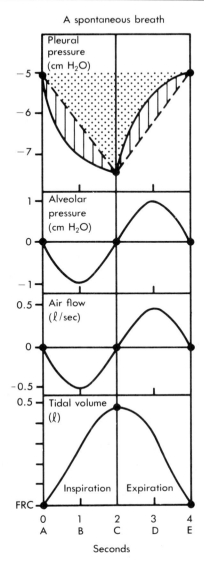

Fig. 10-21. Dynamic pressure: flow, volume recordings during quiet breathing. (From Moser, K., and Spragg, R.G.: Respiratory emergencies, ed. 2, St. Louis, 1982, The C.V. Mosby Co.)

difference between the alveoli and the mouth per unit of airflow. Alveolar pressure measurements (Fig. 10-21) require the use of a body plethysmograph (previously discussed in the measurement of functional residual capacity).

GAS EXCHANGE AND TRANSPORT

Respiratory gas exchange takes place in the alveoli. Oxygen enters the blood from the alveolar air; carbon dioxide enters the alveolar air from the blood. There are several hundred million alveoli, which provide an enormous surface area (about the size of a tennis court) for such gas exchange. Blood flows through the walls of these alveoli

in wide, short capillaries. It is as if a bubble of air were encased in a film of blood. The air and blood are separated by the thinnest of tissue barriers (less than 0.5 μm in width). These features make for rapid gas transfer between the air and blood.

Respiratory exchange ratio

The volumes of oxygen and carbon dioxide that are exchanged depend on the metabolic activity of the tissues. During strenuous exercise the oxygen uptake by the blood may be 10 times the resting uptake. The volume of carbon dioxide that must be expired is correspondingly increased. Indeed there is a relationship between the oxygen uptake and the carbon dioxide output that depends on the type of fuel (glucose, amino acids, or fatty acids) being utilized in energy production. This relationship is known as the respiratory exchange ratio *(R):*

$$R = \frac{CO_2 \text{ output}}{O_2 \text{ uptake}}$$

The body uses a mixture of fuels; the exchange ratio is normally 0.8. When measured under basal conditions the ratio is termed the respiratory quotient (RQ).

Determinants of gas exchange

Gas exchange takes place in the alveolus by a process of diffusion. Diffusion is the random movement of molecules down their concentration gradient. The term "partial pressure" can be substituted for "concentration" when speaking of gas mixtures because the contribution of each gas to the total pressure of a gas mixture is directly proportional to the concentration of that gas in the mixture (Dalton's law). If the fractional concentration (F) of oxygen in a dry gas mixture is 21%, the partial pressure exerted by the oxygen is 21% of the total pressure. The total pressure of ambient (atmospheric) air is the barometric pressure. At sea level this is one atmosphere, or 760 mm Hg. It is the barometric pressure that determines the total pressure of the air in the respiratory passages and the alveoli when the respiratory system is at rest.

Alveolar air is a mixture of nitrogen, oxygen, carbon dioxide, and water vapor (Fig. 10-22). The concentrations and consequently the partial pressures of these gases in the alveolar air differ considerably from their concentrations in the ambient air. In ambient air the water-vapor content (humidity) is variable. As the inspired air moves through the respiratory passages into the alveoli, it becomes fully saturated with water, and it is warmed to body temperature (37° C). Such air has a water vapor pressure of 47 mm Hg. The concentration of oxygen in the alveoli (about 14%) is much less than in ambient air (21%). Although the oxygen supply to the alveolus is periodically renewed during inspiration, oxygen is constantly removed from the alveolar air by the blood. The average partial pressure of oxygen in alveolar air (P_{AO_2}) at sea level is about 100 mm

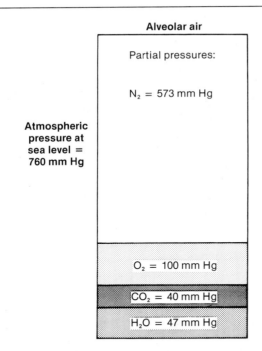

Fig. 10-22. Composition of alveolar air.

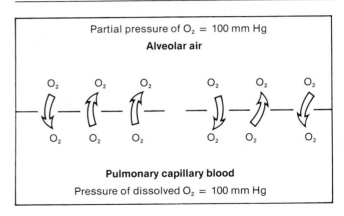

Fig. 10-23. Partial pressures of oxygen at an air-blood interface when the system is in equilibrium.

Hg. There is a negligible amount of carbon dioxide in ambient air and significant amounts (about 5.6%) in alveolar air because carbon dioxide is constantly being added to the alveolar air by the blood. During normal breathing the average partial pressure of alveolar carbon dioxide (P_{ACO_2}) is 40 mm Hg. If the carbon dioxide production by the tissues remains constant, a decrease in alveolar ventilation will result in an accumulation of carbon dioxide in the alveolus with an increase in its partial pressure. This is termed "hypoventilation." Conversely, an increase in alveolar ventilation will produce a decreased alveolar partial pressure of carbon dioxide.

When a liquid is exposed to a gas mixture, as pulmonary capillary blood is to alveolar air, the molecules of each gas diffuse between air and liquid until the pressure of the dissolved molecules equals the partial pressure of that gas in the gas mixture (Fig. 10-23). When equilibrium is achieved in the alveolus, the gas tensions in the end pulmonary capillary blood are the same as the partial pressures of the gases in the alveolar air.

Diffusion of respiratory gases

The diffusion pathway between air and red cells consists of both tissue and blood (Fig. 10-24). The tissue barrier, which is extremely thin, is made up of the surfactant lining the alveolus, the alveolar epithelium, the interstitial tissue, and the capillary endothelium. The blood barrier is made up of the plasma and the red cell membrane. Oxygen dif-

fuses from alveolar air through the tissue and plasma into the red blood cell where it combines with hemoglobin. The red blood cell also plays an important part in the handling of carbon dioxide. In the pulmonary capillary carbon dioxide diffuses out of the red blood cell through the plasma and the tissue barrier into the alveolar air.

The rate of diffusion of a gas through a tissue barrier is dependent on several physical factors: the surface area (A) available for gas exchange; the thickness (T) of the tissue; partial pressure gradient across the tissue ($P_1 - P_2$); and the diffusing constant (D) for the gas. The relationship of these factors is described in Fick's law:

$$\dot{V}_{gas} \propto \frac{A}{T} D (P_1 - P_2)$$

The alveolar surface area ranges from 50 to 100 square meters. However, for this surface to be available for gas exchange, blood must be flowing through the capillaries. This is not always the case even in normal persons, and not all the pulmonary capillaries are open all the time. In disease states alveolar walls may be destroyed (as in emphysema) or blood flow may be blocked by emboli.

Normally, the tissue barrier is extremely thin, but in disease states, such as pulmonary fibrosis, the interstitial tissues may be thickened. This widens the tissue barrier.

In addition to the direction of the partial pressure gradient being opposite (from air to blood for oxygen; from blood to air for carbon dioxide), the gradient for oxygen (100 to 40 mm Hg) is about 15 times that for carbon dioxide (44 to 40 mm Hg) (Fig. 10-25). Because carbon dioxide is more soluble than oxygen, the diffusing constant (D) for carbon dioxide is about 20 times that for oxygen. The net result of these two factors (partial pressure gradient and D) is that carbon dioxide diffuses across the tissue barrier more easily and faster than oxygen.

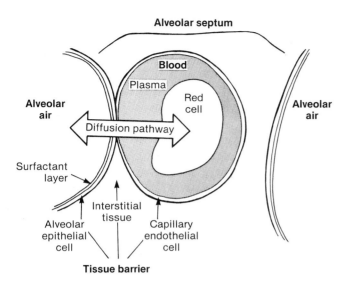

Fig. 10-24. Diffusion pathway for respiratory gases between alveolar air and pulmonary capillary blood.

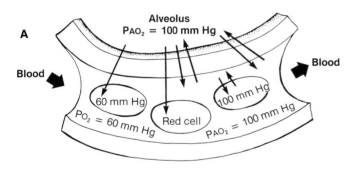

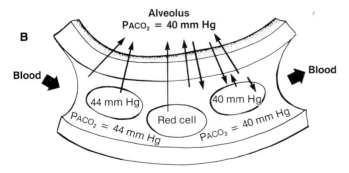

Fig. 10-25. A, Diffusion of O_2 from alveolar air into pulmonary capillary blood. B, Diffusion of CO_2 out of pulmonary capillary blood into alveolar air.

At the end of the diffusion pathway oxygen enters the red blood cell and combines with hemoglobin. This chemical reaction influences the rate of transfer of oxygen from air to blood. A reduction in the volume of blood flowing through the capillary, a reduction in the red cell mass (anemia), or the presence of abnormal hemoglobin molecules, which do not readily combine with oxygen, will reduce the volume of oxygen taken up by the blood.

The normal transit time for blood through a pulmonary capillary is less than 1 second. The rate of diffusion for both oxygen and carbon dioxide is so rapid that equilibrium occurs in less than a fourth of that time. Even when the velocity of blood flow is increased, as occurs during exercise, there is ample time for equilibrium to be achieved. Only in disease states where the tissues are greatly thickened or the partial-pressure gradients are drastically reduced is equilibration incomplete between air and blood.

Transport of gases

After the diffusion of oxygen from the alveolar air into the blood, oxygen is transported by the blood to the tissue capillaries. Here it diffuses out of the capillaries to the cells, which utilize it in the production of energy (ATP). The metabolic activity of the cells results in the production of carbon dioxide, which diffuses out of the cells into the tissue capillaries and is carried by the blood to the lungs, where it diffuses into the alveolar air and is expired.

As oxygen diffuses into the pulmonary blood, it is present as the dissolved gas. It quickly diffuses into the red blood cell where it combines with hemoglobin to form oxyhemoglobin. It is in this form that all but about 1% to 2% of the oxygen is transported by the blood.

The red blood cell is an ideal transport mechanism for oxygen. Its biconcave shape gives it a large surface area; it is flexible and slips easily through narrow capillaries. Within the cell, the hemoglobin molecules are densely packed. Also contained within the red blood cell are enzymes and agents, such as DPG (diphosphoglyceride), which aid in the rapid unloading of oxygen in the tissues.

Oxygen forms in a reversible chemical combination with hemoglobin (oxyhemoglobin). When the hemoglobin is 100% saturated with oxygen, each molecule is capable of combining with four molecules of oxygen, or 1 gram of hemoglobin can combine with 1.34 ml of oxygen (the oxygen capacity). It is the partial pressure of the dissolved oxygen molecules in the blood that primarily determines the volume of oxygen that combines with hemoglobin (percent hemoglobin saturation). The relationship is shown in the oxyhemoglobin dissociation curve (Fig. 10-26). As the partial pressure of dissolved oxygen (Po_2) increases, the percent saturation of hemoglobin increases. At the usual Pao_2 of arterial blood (100 mm Hg) the hemoglobin is about 97% saturated. Full saturation is achieved when the Pao_2 is in the range of 250 to 300 mm Hg.

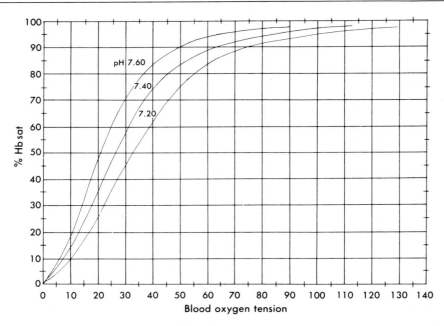

Fig. 10-26. Oxyhemoglobin dissociation curve for whole blood. (From Spearman, C., and Sheldon, R.: Egan's fundamentals of respiratory therapy, ed. 4, St. Louis, 1982, The C.V. Mosby Co.)

The relationship of P_{O_2} to percent hemoglobin saturation produces an S shaped curve. "Loading" of oxygen on the hemoglobin occurs in the flat portion of the curve. Despite variations of several millimeters of mercury in the "loading" pressures, the hemoglobin usually is about 96% to 97% saturated. At the lower partial pressures of oxygen that are found in the tissue capillaries (30 to 80 mm Hg), the curve is very steep. This is the "unloading" portion. Small decreases in the P_{O_2} will release relatively large volumes of oxygen. Hemoglobin unloads about 25% of its oxygen in the tissue capillaries. When a tissue is metabolically active, more oxygen is released or "extracted" from the hemoglobin.

An active tissue also produces more CO_2 and becomes acidotic, and the temperature of the tissue is raised. All these conditions increase the amount of O_2 released at any given P_{O_2}. The oxyhemoglobin dissociation curve is said to be "shifted to the right."

The volume of oxygen delivered to the tissues depends not only on the oxygen content of the blood, but also on the cardiac output. When the oxygen content is reduced because of decreased oxygen tensions and reduced oxygen saturation, a peripheral chemoreceptor reflex increases the heart rate and cardiac output and thus the oxygen supply to the tissues is maintained.

The transport of carbon dioxide from the tissues to the lungs is by way of the blood and also involves the red blood cell. Carbon dioxide diffuses out of the tissue into the plasma and then into the red blood cell. Here it is processed (Fig. 10-27): CO_2, in the presence of the enzyme carbonic anhydrase, is rapidly hydrated to H_2CO_3. This latter compound quickly dissociates into H^+ and HCO_3^-. The bicarbonate ion then diffuses out of the red blood cell into the plasma. The hydrogen ion that remains within the red blood cell is buffered by the hemoglobin. (Hemoglobin that has lost its oxygen is a better buffer than oxyhemoglobin.) About 65% of the carbon dioxide produced by the tissues is handled in this fashion, thus transported back to the lungs as bicarbonate.

Another 25% of the carbon dioxide entering the capillary combines with hemoglobin to form a carbamino compound. About 10% of the carbon dioxide remains as dissolved gas. It is the dissolved gas that produces the carbon dioxide tension of the blood.

Within the pulmonary capillaries the processes are reversed: CO_2 diffuses from the capillary blood into the alveolar air, and the chemical process within the red cell is reversed (Fig. 10-28). H^+ is released from the hemoglobin and HCO_3^- diffuses into the red cell from the plasma. These combine to form H_2CO_3, which is rapidly dehydrated to $CO_2 + H_2O$ and the CO_2 diffuses out. The CO_2 dissociates from the hemoglobin. It is the partial pressure of CO_2 within the alveolar air that determines the final tension of CO_2 in the arterial blood. It is this tension that is determined by the alveolar ventilation.

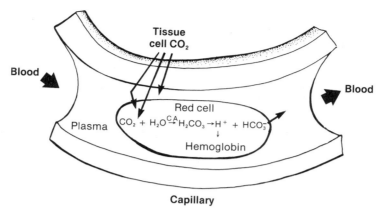

Fig. 10-27. Diffusion of CO_2 from tissue cell into tissue capillary blood. The major pathway for handling CO_2: the processing of CO_2 in the red cell in the presence of carbonic anhydrase (CA).

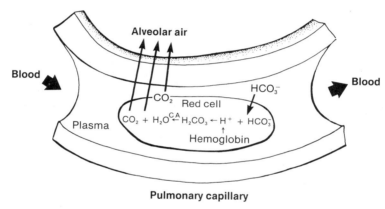

Fig. 10-28. Diffusion of CO_2 out of pulmonary capillary blood into alveolar air. Reversal of reactions seen in Fig. 10-31.

Testing and evaluation

The diffusing capability of the lung is known as the diffusing capacity ($D_{L\ gas}$). It is the measurement of the volume of a gas that diffuses into the blood per minute per millimeter of mercury as a partial pressure gradient. It differs for each gas, depending on the diffusing constant for the gas.

$$D_L = \text{ml of gas/min/mm Hg}$$

Clinically, carbon monoxide (CO) is used as the standard test gas. The patient breathes a very dilute mixture of known carbon monoxide concentration from a spirometer, holds his breath for 10 seconds, and then expels the mixture, and the carbon monoxide concentration in the expired air is measured.

$$D_{L_{CO}} = \frac{\text{vol of CO taken up by the blood/min}}{P_{ACO} - P_{aCO}}$$

where A is the alveoli and a is the artery. Since CO combines 250 times more readily with hemoglobin than O_2 does, no significant partial pressure builds up in the blood and the P_{aCO} is zero. The diffusion of CO is not limited by the blood flow but is purely a measure of the adequacy of the tissue component of the diffusion pathway.

The normal value for $D_{L_{CO}}$ is 25 ml/min/mm Hg. In exercise the $D_{L_{CO}}$ may be doubled as blood flow increases and capillaries are opened; in disease states, loss of surface area or thickening of the tissues may reduce the capacity to 4 to 5 ml.

PULMONARY CIRCULATION

Blood flow through the alveolar capillaries is an integral part of gas exchange. The pulmonary circulation carries the entire output of the right heart through the lungs to the left heart (Fig. 10-29). The pulmonary blood vessels are

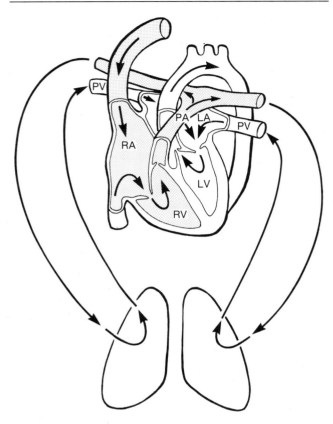

Fig. 10-29. The pulmonary circulation. *Shaded area,* Flow of unoxygenated blood. *RA,* Right atrium; *RV,* right ventricle; *PA,* pulmonary artery; *PV,* pulmonary vein; *LA,* left atrium; *LV,* left ventricle.

short and wide compared to their systemic counterparts. Their walls, which contain far less smooth muscle than systemic vessels, are thin and compliant. Mixed venous blood flows from the right ventricle through the pulmonary artery and its branches into the pulmonary capillaries, which lie in the alveolar septa. The short, wide, intersecting capillaries maximize the exposure of the blood to the alveolar air. Finally, oxygenated blood is collected by the pulmonary veins and emptied into the left atrium. The veins are distensible and demonstrate the capacity to store an extra 300 to 500 ml of blood. This occurs with a change in body position, wherein blood is shifted out of veins in the lower extremities with a change from standing to supine position.

At rest, some of the pulmonary capillaries are closed. When the cardiac output increases, as in exercise, closed capillaries are opened (recruitment) and those that were already open are distended. This increases the volume of blood exposed to alveolar air and increases the surface area available for gas exchange.

Vascular mechanics

Resistance to blood flow through the short wide vessels is only about one tenth of that found in the systemic vessels. The differential pressure (between pulmonary artery pressure and left atrial pressure) needed to drive blood across the circuit is proportionately decreased (average, 15 mm Hg). When cardiac output increases, the compliant pulmonary vessels distend and resistance to blood flow actually drops.

Indeed, there are very few situations in which pulmonary vascular resistance increases. Changes in the dimensions of the vessels during both deep inspiration and deep expiration cause increases in resistance. At high lung volumes the alveolar vessels are stretched and narrowed; at very low lung volumes the extra-alveolar vessels (small pulmonary arteries) narrow because of the elastic recoil of their walls, which are no longer pulled open by the lung parenchyma.

Active vasoconstriction will increase pulmonary resistance. Such vasoconstriction is produced chiefly by low alveolar oxygen tensions but also by high carbon dioxide tensions and acidosis. The response of the pulmonary vessels to the altered respiratory gases is in direct contrast to the response of systemic arterioles, which dilate when exposed to low interstitial oxygen tensions and high carbon dioxide tensions. When the alveolar gas changes are localized, blood is shunted away from these areas to alveoli that are better ventilated. However, when the vasoconstriction is generalized, the total pulmonary vascular resistance is increased. Pulmonary artery pressure rises (pulmonary hypertension), and so the work of the right ventricle is increased. In some cases right heart failure (cor pulmonale) develops.

Under normal circumstances sympathetic stimulation to the pulmonary vessels does not cause significant vasoconstriction. However, humoral substances, such as histamine, can cause vasoconstriction.

Blood flow is not evenly distributed to all alveoli. Flow through the pulmonary capillaries depends on the relationship of alveolar air pressures to capillary hydrostatic pressures. Although the alveolar air pressures are essentially the same in all alveoli, the capillary pressures are varied. In an upright person the effect of gravity lowers the hydrostatic pressure of the blood as it rises above the level of the pulmonary artery and augments the pressures in vessels below the level of the pulmonary artery. The zones of West (Fig. 10-30) describe the pressure-flow relationships. In zone I at the apex of the lung, there is no blood flow through the alveolar capillaries. Alveolar air pressures are greater than capillary hydrostatic pressures; the capillaries are compressed. By far the largest portion of the lung is zone II. Pulmonary arteriole pressures are greater than alveolar air pressures, but pressure at the venous end of the capillaries are less than air pressures. Blood flow is deter-

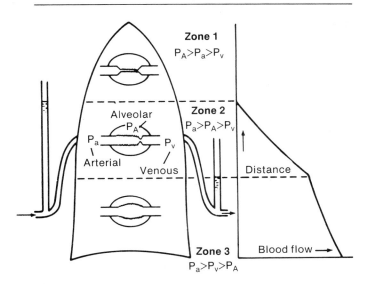

Fig. 10-30. Zones of West. (From West, J.B.: Respiratory physiology, ed. 2, Baltimore, Md., 1979, The Williams & Wilkins Co.)

Table 10-1. Starling forces

Pressure (mm Hg)	Promoting	
	Filtration	Reabsorption
Capillary hydrostatic	10	
Capillary osmotic		25
Interstitial tissue	−4	
Interstitial osmotic	15	
TOTAL	29	25

mined by the pressure difference between the pulmonary arterioles and alveolar air. With advancement toward the more dependent portions of the lung, the intracapillary pressures increase, and flow increases. In zone III, or the dependent portion of the lung, venous hydrostatic pressures exceed alveolar air pressures. Capillaries are wide open, and flow is unrestricted. In the normal lung, blood flow increases tenfold from apex to base in the upright person. In zone IV, in which high interstitial pressures compress the pulmonary vessels to reduce flow, there have been cases of interstitial edema but not under normal conditions.

The pulmonary capillaries are more permeable to plasma proteins than systemic capillaries are. The protein content of the pulmonary interstitial tissue is 10 to 20 times that of systemic tissues. The Starling forces are altered (Table 10-1). Filtration occurs along the entire length of the alveolar capillary. In normal persons the alveolar epithelium is quite impermeable to small solutes. The filtered fluid is carried out of the lung by the lymphatics. The lymphatics can handle up to 10 times the normal volume of lymph. When the rate of filtration increases, fluid accumulates in the interstitial tissue (pulmonary edema) and ultimately enters the alveoli.

Matching of blood and gas

For ideal gas exchange, equal volumes of fresh air entering the alveoli should come into contact with equal volumes of blood flowing through the alveolar capillaries. In other words alveolar ventilation ($\dot{V}_A$) should match the pulmonary blood blow ($\dot{Q}$). The relationship of the two flows

is the ventilation/perfusion ratio, or the $\dot{V}/\dot{Q}$ ratio. In the ideal matching of equal volumes of gas and blood, the ratio would be 1. However, when one is considering the lungs as a whole, the ratio is less than one. A normal alveolar ventilation of 4 L/min is usually matched with a 5 L/min cardiac output, which would give a $\dot{V}/\dot{Q}$ ratio of 4/5, or 0.8.

Usually the $\dot{V}/\dot{Q}$ ratio is considered for various areas of the lungs and not for the lungs as a whole. Alveolar ventilation and blood flow vary independently throughout the lung. Ventilation of lung units depends on their compliance and the patency of the airways; blood flow is unequally distributed and is dependent on the principles described by the zones of West or the patency of blood vessels. In an upright person blood flow is less than ventilation at the lung apex because some of the capillaries are compressed (zone I of West). The $\dot{V}/\dot{Q}$ ratio is high. At the base of the lung, ventilation is three times greater but blood flow is 10 times greater than that at the apex. The $\dot{V}/\dot{Q}$ at the bases is low. In chronic obstructive pulmonary disease large areas of the lung may have reduced ventilation because of blockage of the bronchioles by secretions. Large areas of low $\dot{V}/\dot{Q}$ ratios result.

In areas of the lung with low $\dot{V}/\dot{Q}$ ratios, the renewal of the alveolar oxygen supply is insufficient to oxygenate adequately the blood flowing through the pulmonary capillaries. The end-capillary blood is not fully oxygenated. This is termed a "physiological intrapulmonary shunt" (Fig. 10-31). The poorly oxygenated blood from these areas mixes with blood from other better ventilated areas. The total oxygen content of the mixed blood is reduced. In lung disease, the presence of large areas of the lung with low $\dot{V}/\dot{Q}$ ratios is the most common cause of low arterial oxygen (hypoxemia). Although the carbon dioxide concentrations in the poorly ventilated alveoli are increased when mixing occurs with blood from other areas, the carbon dioxide tension of the final mixture in the aorta is usually within normal limits. This normal carbon dioxide tension occurs for two reasons: the venous-arterial gradient for carbon dioxide is small, and so there is a small increase in Pa_{CO_2} from the areas with low $\dot{V}/\dot{Q}$ ratios, and the neural

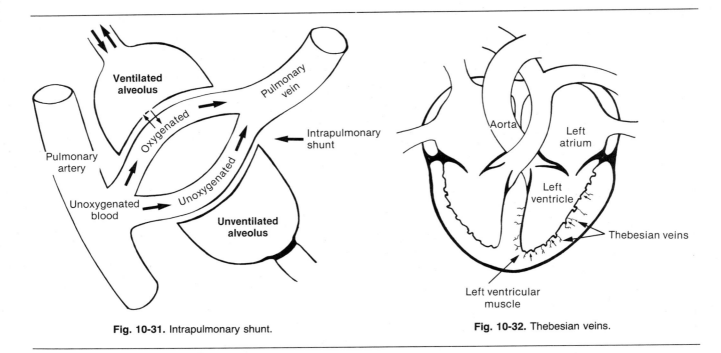

Fig. 10-31. Intrapulmonary shunt.   **Fig. 10-32.** Thebesian veins.

respiratory controls adjust the alveolar ventilation to maintain a normal Pa_{CO_2}.

When ventilation exceeds blood flow, the $\dot{V}/\dot{Q}$ ratio is high. There is excess alveolar ventilation and not all of the ventilated air takes part in gas exchange. This produces an "alveolar dead space" and is often termed "wasted" ventilation.

The end pulmonary capillary blood from all areas of the lung mixes as it flows into the left side of the heart. Blood from areas with low $\dot{V}/\dot{Q}$ ratios usually exerts more influence on the final oxygen tension than blood from areas with high $\dot{V}/\dot{Q}$ ratios (Fig. 10-31). A small amount of blood from bronchial and thebesian veins also flows directly into the pulmonary veins and the left side of the heart. This venous admixture also lowers the oxygen tension of the blood (Fig. 10-32). Because of these mixtures, the oxygen tension of the blood ejected into the aorta never equals the alveolar oxygen tension. This difference is known as the "alveolar-arterial difference," or the "A-a gradient."

In normal persons the A-a gradient is small, amounting to about 6 to 10 mm Hg when room air is breathed. In pulmonary disease, large areas with low $\dot{V}/\dot{Q}$ ratios may be present, and the A-a gradient may be as much as 30 to 40 mm Hg in room air. In congenital heart disease, abnormal openings in the atrial or ventricular septum may occur (Fig. 10-33). Large volumes of blood may be shunted directly from the right side of the heart into the left side, creating a large venous admixture, a large A-a gradient, and very low arterial oxygen tensions.

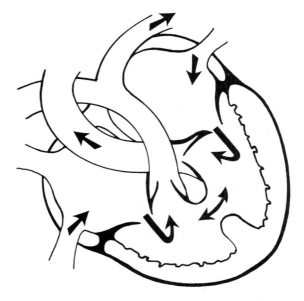

Fig. 10-33. Septal defect between the right ventricle and left ventricle.

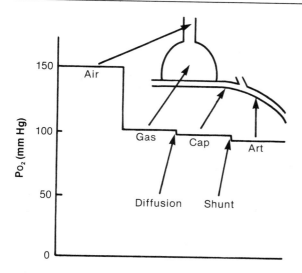

Fig. 10-34. Changes in the partial pressure of O_2 as oxygen moves from inspired air to the arterial blood. (From West, J.B.: Ventilation/blood flow and gas exchange, ed. 3, 1977, Blackwell Scientific Publications.)

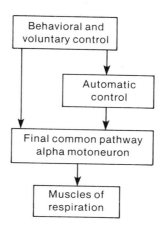

Fig. 10-35. Relationship between voluntary and automatic respiratory control pathways.

Testing and evaluation

Examination of the arterial blood gases is a means of determining the overall adequacy of the gas-exchange mechanisms. Blood is obtained by arterial (radial, brachial, femoral) puncture. The oxygen tension (PaO_2) and the carbon dioxide tension ($PaCO_2$) are measured. The normal PaO_2 ranges from 90 to 110 mm Hg. A reduction in PaO_2 could be caused by reduced oxygen tension in the inspired air (PIO_2), hypoventilation, inadequate diffusion across a thickened tissue barrier, or an abnormal $\dot{V}/\dot{Q}$ ratio (Fig. 10-34). If at the same time the arterial sample is taken the alveolar oxygen tension (PAO_2) is calculated, using the modified alveolar air equation, the A-a gradient can be determined. The modified alveolar air equation is as follows:

$$PAO_2 = PIO_2 - PaCO_2 \,(1.25)$$

The diffusion difficulty can be studied with a diffusing capacity (D_L) evaluation. If the increased A-a gradient is attributable to areas of low $\dot{V}/\dot{Q}$, giving the patient 100% oxygen to breathe will reduce the calculated apparent intrapulmonary shunt. If the large A-a gradient is attributable to right-to-left shunting through a cardiac septal defect, 100% oxygen will not change the calculated shunt.

The arterial PCO_2 is also very helpful. Since there is virtually no gradient for PCO_2 between the alveolar air and the arterial blood, the arterial PCO_2 represents the alveolar PCO_2. Normal PCO_2 ranges from 38 to 42 mm Hg. A high arterial PCO_2 (over 44 mm Hg) reflects a high alveolar PCO_2 and is caused by hypoventilation; a low arterial PCO_2 represents a low alveolar PCO_2 and indicates hyperventilation.

CONTROL OF BREATHING
Automatic and voluntary mechanisms

Control of respiratory muscle activity arises from within the central nervous system. The rate and depth of respiration are regulated by two control systems—the automatic and the voluntary mechanisms—which usually interact with each other (Fig. 10-35). Both systems terminate in a final common pathway, the spinal motor neurons, which innervate the respiratory muscles. Any disease process that involves either the motor nerves or the respiratory muscles will interfere with both sets of controls.

The most important control system is the automatic mechanism that originates in the brainstem. It produces spontaneous, cyclical respiration. Voluntary or behavioral control, important during verbal communication, arises from the cerebral cortex. This control typically exerts a modifying influence on the automatic activity. However, there is a direct pathway from the cortex to the spinal motor neurons, which can, on occasion, function independently of the automatic control system.

The spontaneous neuronal activity that produces cyclic breathing originates in the respiratory centers in the dorsal region of the medulla (Fig. 10-36). These neurons drive the ventral medullary centers. Together the centers drive contralateral respiratory muscles. Destruction of these medullary centers, associated with bulbar poliomyelitis, eliminates all automatic breathing though voluntary respiratory activity is still possible. Breathing produced by the medullary centers is weak and irregular. When the activity of the two pontine centers (the apneustic and the pneumotaxic) is superimposed on that of the medullary centers, breathing becomes strong, regular, and effective. This ac-

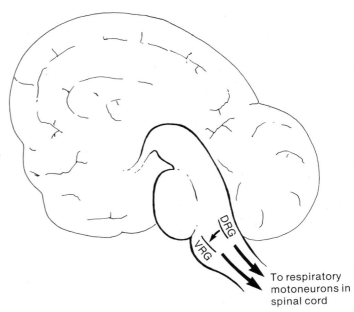

Fig. 10-36. Lateral view of the medulla. *DRG,* Dorsal respiratory group of neurons; *VRG,* ventral respiratory group of neurons.

tivity is further modified by the central and peripheral chemoreceptors, peripheral reflexes from the lungs and other parts of the body, and by the cortical centers.

Central and peripheral chemoreceptor mechanisms

The dominant regulation of the respiratory centers usually arises from the chemoreceptors. This mechanism modifies alveolar ventilation to ensure that the blood gases remain within normal limits. Of the two respiratory gases, carbon dioxide is most tightly controlled. The central chemoreceptors, which lie just below the surface of the ventrolateral aspects of the medulla, monitor the carbon dioxide levels of both the arterial blood and the cerebrospinal fluid. Carbon dioxide rapidly diffuses out of the cerebral capillaries into the interstitial tissue of the brain. It reacts with water to produce free hydrogen ions:

$$CO_2 + H_2O \rightarrow H_2CO_3 \rightarrow H^+ + HCO_3^-$$

It is the hydrogen ions that stimulate the central chemoreceptor cells, which in turn stimulate the medullary centers. Thus a rise in Pa_{CO_2} produces an increase in alveolar ventilation, which restores the Pa_{CO_2} levels to the normal (40 mm Hg) range.

A second group of chemoreceptors, the peripheral chemoreceptors, are found in the carotid and aortic bodies that lie outside the walls of the carotid sinus and the aortic arch (Fig. 10-37). They are stimulated by low arterial oxygen tensions, high arterial carbon dioxide tensions, and acidosis. The stimulation is carried through the afferent sensory nerves (cranial nerves IX and X) to the brainstem.

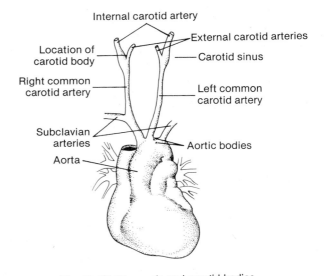

Fig. 10-37. The aortic and carotid bodies.

The medullary centers are stimulated, and ventilation is increased.

The peripheral chemoreceptors demonstrate low-grade tonic activity, which contributes to normal ventilation. However, stimulation by arterial oxygen tensions below 60 mm Hg produces a strong respiratory drive. High arterial carbon dioxide tensions and acidosis act synergistically with low oxygen tensions. The reflex drive, from the carotid body in particular, can stimulate brainstem centers, which are depressed by narcotics or anoxia, into activity and thus maintain breathing. At high altitudes, when inspired oxygen tensions are reduced, peripheral chemoreceptor stimulation overrides the central chemoreceptor regulation. A person hyperventilates in an attempt to maintain normal arterial oxygen levels at the expense of reduced arterial carbon dioxide levels.

Lung and peripheral reflex mechanisms

The lungs contain sensory receptors, which stimulate reflex respiratory activity. Although these reflexes are not usually active, they can override the normal chemical control of breathing.

The longest known lung reflex is the Hering-Breuer reflex (inflation reflex) which is stimulated by inflation of the lung during inspiration. The reflex response is inhibition of inspiration. This reflex is too weak to control the depth of the tidal volume during normal breathing. It is only during very deep inspiration, under anesthesia, in newborns, or in some patients with lung disease, that the signals become strong enough to inhibit inspiration and thus regulate the depth of breathing.

A more important reflex is that produced by stimulation of the irritant receptors. This is one of the lung's defense mechanisms against noxious materials. The receptors lie in the epithelial lining of the airways. They are stimulated by inhaled particles, by irritant gases, or by excessive amounts of sticky mucus produced by the respiratory tract itself. The reflex response is a sneeze if the stimulus occurs in the upper airways or a cough if the stimulus is in the lower airways.

A less well understood lung reflex is that produced by the "J receptors," which lie within the lung parenchyma. These are stimulated by interstitial edema and by some inhaled gases. The response is rapid, shallow breathing (tachypnea).

In asthma, pulmonary embolism, and heart failure, a frequent finding is a low Pa_{CO_2}. This is probably produced by the reflex hyperventilation caused by stimulation of either the irritant or the J receptors.

Stimulation of peripheral pain receptors will also produce reflex hyperventilation, accompanied by tachycardia, and a rise in blood pressure. Visceral pain may produce the opposite effect: inhibition of breathing, a slow pulse, and a fall in blood pressure.

Control mechanisms during exercise and sleep

The control of breathing during both sleep and exercise is worthy of further examination. During slow-wave sleep, sensory stimuli are reduced. Behavioral modifications are minimal. Chemical control of breathing is dominant. The situation is very different during REM (rapid eye movement) sleep. Breathing becomes irregular. Muscular activity is greatly reduced; indeed the skeletal muscles, including those of the larynx and pharynx, relax. This may

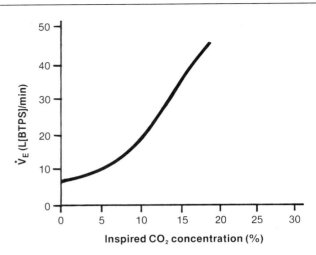

Fig. 10-38. Diagram of the ventilatory response to increasing CO_2 concentrations in the alveolar air and in the arterial blood. *BTPS,* Body temperature, ambient pressure, saturated with water vapor. (Modified from Slonim, N.B., and Hamilton, L.H.: Respiratory physiology, ed. 4, St. Louis, 1981, The C.V. Mosby Co.)

produce upper airway obstruction and apnea. Arousal usually occurs when the deranged blood gases stimulate the peripheral chemoreceptors. This type of "sleep apnea" is seen in all persons; however, it is especially frequent in older males. In patients with chronic obstructive pulmonary disease whose normal ventilation is severely reduced, further reduction attributable to apneic episodes may be extremely detrimental.

During exercise the utilization of oxygen and the production of carbon dioxide increase. Yet the control of respiration is such that alveolar ventilation is correspondingly increased and the blood gas levels remain within normal limits, except during the most severe exercise. The central chemoreceptors are certainly involved in this control, as are peripheral reflexes from muscles and joints, but the whole picture is not clear; perhaps other chemoreceptors, as yet undefined, in the lungs or the pulmonary vasculature are involved.

Testing and evaluation

Evaluation of the central chemoreceptors involves breathing increasing concentrations of CO_2 in 100% O_2. As the concentration of inspired CO_2 is increased, ventilation should increase (Fig. 10-38). One can test the function of the peripheral chemoreceptor by having the person breathe gas mixtures with reduced oxygen concentrations. The difficulty with these tests is that so many other stimuli (auditory, visual, etc.) can alter respiration and the pure effect of the altered respiratory gases may be obscured.

SUGGESTED READINGS

Bouhuys, A.: The physiology of breathing, New York, 1977, Grune & Stratton, Inc.

Cherniack, R.M., Cherniack, L., and Naimark, A.: Respiration in health and disease, ed. 2, Philadelphia, 1972, W.B. Saunders Co.

Clausen, J.L., editor: Pulmonary function testing: guidelines and controversies, New York, 1982, Academic Press, Inc.

Comroe, J.H.: Physiology of respiration, ed. 2, Chicago, 1974, Year Book Medical Publishers.

Comroe, J.H., Forester, R.E., Dubois, A.B., and others: The lung, clinical physiology and pulmonary function tests, Chicago, 1962, Year Book Medical Publishers.

Fishman, A.P.: Assessment of pulmonary function, New York, 1980, McGraw-Hill Book Co.

Green, J.F.: Fundamental cardiovascular and pulmonary physiology: an integrated approach for medicine, Philadelphia, 1982, Lea & Febiger.

Kryger, M.H., editor: Pathophysiology of respiration, New York, 1981, John Wiley & Sons, Inc.

Slonim, N.B., and Hamilton, L.G.: Respiratory physiology, ed. 3, St. Louis, 1976, The C.V. Mosby Co.

Spearman, C., and Sheldon, R.: Egan's fundamentals of respiratory therapy, ed. 4, St. Louis, 1982, The C.V. Mosby Co.

Tisi, G.M.: Pulmonary physiology in clinical medicine, Baltimore, 1980, The Williams & Wilkins Co.

Vander, A., Sherman, J.H., and Luciana, D.: Human physiology, ed. 3, New York, 1980, McGraw-Hill Book Co.

West, J.B.: Pulmonary pathophysiology: the essentials, ed. 2, Baltimore, 1982, The Williams & Wilkins Co.

West, J.B.: Respiratory physiology: the essentials, ed. 2, Baltimore, 1979, The Williams & Wilkins Co.

11

DAVID JAMES HENSON
WILLIAM L. MORRISSEY

Acute respiratory failure: mechanisms and medical management

DEFINITION

Respiratory failure can be defined as the inability of the respiratory system to perform its basic functions of eliminating carbon dioxide (CO_2) from the body and assimilating oxygen (O_2). Under normal conditions, the level of alveolar ventilation is so well adjusted that the arterial blood carbon dioxide tension ($Paco_2$) and pH are held nearly constant even when the rate of production of CO_2 varies widely. Failure of the delicate adjustment mechanisms may lead to failure of carbon dioxide excretion, with a consequent rise in the $Paco_2$.[51] When this failure occurs acutely, there is also a depression of the arterial pH and Pao_2, which results in the clinical signs and symptoms of acute respiratory failure as discussed below. Generally, acute respiratory failure is said to exist when the Pao_2 falls below 50 mm Hg (torr) at sea level. This value is considerably below the normal range of 85 to 100 torr which is slightly influenced by the patient's age and prevalent barometric pressure. The rise of the $Paco_2$ above 50 torr is also a commonly identified criterion for acute respiratory failure.[45] Arterial blood gas aberrations of lesser magnitude are difficult to clearly label as acute respiratory failure in an individual patient.[25]

Although the classification is somewhat artificial, one can subdivide respiratory failure into those situations associated with hypercapnia and concomitant hypoxemia and those with hypoxemia alone.

HYPERCAPNIC RESPIRATORY FAILURE

The partial pressure of CO_2 in arterial blood can be approximated by the formula:

$$Paco_2 = \frac{k \dot{V}co_2}{f(V_T - V_D)}$$

where $\dot{V}co_2$ is the amount of CO_2 produced per minute, or the expired amount of CO_2 under steady-state conditions; V_T is the tidal volume or ventilation per breath; V_D is the physiological dead space or wasted ventilation; f is the frequency or respiratory rate; and k is a constant. An increase in the $\dot{V}co_2$ is never a primary cause of an elevated $Paco_2$ though it may be a secondary or contributing factor. Thus the major determinants of hypercapnia are a decrease in tidal volume or respiratory rate and an increase in wasted ventilation.[31]

Depression of minute ventilation

The common causes for depressed minute ventilation leading to hypercapnic respiratory failure include disorders of the central nervous system (CNS) leading to reduction in the respiratory drive, neuromuscular diseases resulting in an inability of the ventilatory apparatus to respond to the respiratory drive from the central nervous system, and thoracic-cage deformities resulting in a diminished ability to move air into or out of the lungs.

Central nervous system respiratory drive. Respiratory failure from a decreased drive from the central nervous system is frequently attributable to a depression of the respiratory center from an overdose of sedatives as may be seen with suicide attempts. The need for ventilatory support is often apparent because the patient is frequently comatose and may be unresponsive to even painful stimuli. With increasing sedation, there may be gradual but relentlessly progressive depression of the respiratory center, leading to a reduction in the respiratory rate. The major exception to this situation occurs with glutethimide, which may cause sudden apnea despite a previously normal respiratory rate.[44] Ventilatory drive can also be depressed by diseases of the central nervous system, such as vascular insufficiency, tumors, and infections.

Neuromuscular diseases. Neuromuscular diseases can produce respiratory failure by causing a devastating reduction in the minute ventilation. Diseases in this category include poliomyelitis, amyotrophic lateral sclerosis, myopathies, spinal cord injuries, multiple sclerosis, and myasthenia gravis. Both lung and chest wall compliance are reduced in these disorders, requiring an increased work of breathing to maintain ventilation. Inability to meet this increased demand for muscular work may lead to CO_2 retention, right-sided congestive heart failure, and cor pulmonale. Little is known, however, concerning the latter circulatory derangements because these disorders either fail to cause abnormal blood gas values or deteriorate so rapidly that insufficient time elapses for the development of these hemodynamic complications. Patients with chronic poliomyelitis have been noted to develop cor pulmonale and congestive heart failure, but the precise interpretation of these clinical findings is complicated by the frequency of systemic hypertension in this disorder.[7]

Thoracic cage abnormalities. Diseases of the thoracic cage can lead to a reduction in minute ventilation with resultant respiratory failure. These disorders include scoliosis, the obesity-hypoventilation syndrome, fibrothorax, thoracoplasty, and ankylosing spondylitis. Increased pulmonary resistance and right-sided congestive heart failure occur in all these disorders except for ankylosing spondylitis whose victims are either spared these complications or develop them very late in the course of the disease. Lung and chest wall compliance are reduced in all thoracic-cage disorders, which may lead to increased work of breathing and CO_2 retention. Increased pulmonary vascular resistance, believed to be caused by proliferative changes in the pulmonary vessels, contributes to cor pulmonale. These patients also frequently have a decreased ventilatory response to inhaled CO_2. This poor response may result from a pharmacological "tolerance" to the high levels of CO_2 usually present.[7]

Increased physiological dead space

The alveolar gas equation is a method of determining whether an increased oxygen gradient exists between the alveolar air and the arterial blood. This equation is as follows:

$$\begin{aligned} P_{A}O_2 - P_aO_2 = &[\text{Barometric pressure (760 torr at sea level)} \\ &- \text{Water-vapor pressure (47 torr at body temperature)}] \\ &\times F_{I}O_2 \text{ (Concentration of inspired oxygen, 0.21 in room air)} \\ &- 1.25 \, (P_aCO_2) - P_aO_2 \end{aligned}$$

Inspection of the above equation indicates that a reduced P_AO_2 can result from the increased P_aCO_2 associated with hypoventilation. A common factor linking the hypercapnia in diseases of the central nervous system, neuromuscular systems, and thoracic cage is that they all produce CO_2 retention primarily by hypoventilation. Although these groups of patients will have an increased P_aCO_2 and de-

creased P_aO_2, there will be a normal alveolar-arterial oxygen gradient.

The physiological dead space can be thought of as consisting of areas of the lung that are well ventilated but poorly perfused or unperfused with blood (high ventilation/perfusion ratio, $\dot{V}/\dot{Q}$). Therefore much of the patient's ventilation to these areas is "wasted" by not participating in gas exchange. Nonetheless, energy is required to ventilate the dead space. If this dead space is large enough, the energy required to maintain its ventilation will be greater than what can be sustained. Both chronic bronchitis and pulmonary emphysema, considered under the term "chronic obstructive pulmonary disease," or COPD, can lead to respiratory failure through this mechanism. Pure emphysema and chronic bronchitis are very different entities but are often found to varying degrees in the same patient. Emphysema is not commonly associated with hypercapnia until late in its course, whereas hypercapnia occurs much earlier in the progression of chronic bronchitis. COPD causes hypercapnia through many poorly understood mechanisms including decreased respiratory drive, decreased mechanical efficiency, increased buffering in the central nervous system, and possibly a genetic predisposition for acquired hypersensitivity to increasing levels of CO_2.[22,38]

Compared to the hypercapnia seen with pure hypoventilation, that associated with COPD has an increased oxygen gradient between the alveolar air and the arterial blood. Just as there are regions of the lung in patients with COPD that have high $\dot{V}/\dot{Q}$ ratios resulting in increased physiological dead space, there are also regions that receive little ventilation but normal perfusion, thereby producing a low $\dot{V}/\dot{Q}$ ratio or a shunt-like effect. A shunt permits poorly oxygenated venous blood to bypass the lungs and causes arterial hypoxemia by contaminating arterial blood with blood that is poorly oxygenated. A large alveolar-arterial oxygen gradient can help distinguish between diseases with a large physiological dead space and those with hypoventilation in which the oxygen gradient is normal.

HYPOXEMIC RESPIRATORY FAILURE

Hypoxemic respiratory failure without hypercapnia defines a group of diseases with varied causes and prognoses. They may be divided into those with low oxygen gradients and those with high oxygen gradients.

Respiratory failure may present as hypoxemia without hypercapnia or metabolic acidosis. Two groups of patients commonly present with this form of hypoxemia and can be distinguished by the response of their hypoxemia to the administration of supplemental oxygen. The first group will show a significant response with an increase in P_aO_2 of 2 to 5 torr for each percentage increase in the $F_{I}O_2$. These patients will often have an oxygen gradient of less than 60 torr. The pathophysiology is believed to result from an excessive number of low $\dot{V}/\dot{Q}$ units with those areas that are well perfused but poorly ventilated producing shunts from the venous to arterial side of the system. Examples of these diseases include obstructive pneumonia, acute asthma, pneumothorax, and atelectasis.[31]

The second group of patients with almost pure hypoxemia and increased oxygen gradients without hypercapnia represents some of the sickest patients with respiratory failure—those with adult respiratory distress syndrome (ARDS). These patients will often have an oxygen gradient much greater than 60 torr and show very little response to increased FIO_2.[31] ARDS can be caused by a plethora of seemingly unrelated insults to the patient, including oxygen toxicity, septicemia, massive blood transfusions, aspiration pneumonitis, inhaled irritants, drug overdose, fat embolism, severe or prolonged hypotension, acute pancreatitis, certain medications such as aspirin, and chest trauma. The underlying pathophysiology is not completely understood and may vary with the underlying disease process though the result is the same. Even though the initiating factors may be heterogeneous, there appears to be two fundamental disturbances that characterize ARDS—pulmonary edema and atelectasis. While the patient is alive, the manifestations of pulmonary edema predominate and are responsible for many signs and symptoms of the disease. The pulmonary edema is not associated with cardiac disease, and the diagnosis of ARDS is particularly perplexing when there is coincident congestive heart failure.[22] The cause of the pulmonary edema in ARDS is believed to be attributable to an increase in the permeability of the capillary endothelial cells, which allows extravasation of plasma and some erythrocytes into the interstitial spaces and alveoli. The alveolar fluid contains granulocytes, macrophages, and erythrocytes and has a protein composition similar to plasma.[18]

In addition to the noncardiogenic pulmonary edema seen with ARDS, there is also widespread atelectasis, believed to be caused by damaged type II alveolar lining cells and subsequent reduction in surfactant production. Surfactant, secreted by the type II alveolar cells, reduces the alveolar surface tension, and without surfactant the alveoli tend to collapse, resulting in atelectasis.[19] Pulmonary edema results in alveolar fluid and cellular debris, and atelectasis produces alveolar collapse both of which cause a low $\dot{V}/\dot{Q}$ ratio and severe hypoxemia. Other mechanisms postulated to produce capillary endothelial and alveolar epithelial cell damage include release of inflammatory mediators within the lung, microvascular thrombosis, and activation of complement by its alternate pathway.[18]

DIAGNOSIS OF ACUTE RESPIRATORY FAILURE
Clinical setting

When it occurs in the usual clinical setting, respiratory failure is often a simple diagnosis. The cause of respiratory failure is most often chronic obstructive pulmonary disease (COPD), but other common causes include drug overdose, asthma, trauma, pulmonary embolism, and severe pneumonia. The fragile patient with COPD is particularly susceptible to an acute exacerbation of the disease from the slightest provocation such as a viral illness, sedative drug, or respiratory muscle fatigue with overt respiratory failure then ensuing.

Signs and symptoms

When first examined, the patient with respiratory failure has symptoms specific to the underlying disease, with superimposed symptoms of hypoxemia and hypercapnia. For example, the patient with COPD may have loud, audible wheezing, whereas the patient with a drug overdose may be somnolent and difficult to arouse.

Acute hypoxemia often produces multisystem disorders, affecting not only the respiratory system, but the circulatory, neuromuscular, and central nervous systems as well as causing generalized electrolyte imbalance. Specifically, there may be increased dyspnea, tachypnea, tachycardia, hypertension, weakness, asterixis (a flapping tremor), tremor, euphoria, seizures, and coma, along with retention of sodium and water. If respiratory failure is allowed to progress, severe bradycardia and myocardial depression will occur, leading eventually to shock and death.

Hypercapnia will produce many of the same symptoms, with confusion, drowsiness, and apprehension predominating. There is frequently increased activity of the sympathetic nervous system resulting in peripheral vasoconstriction. Local hypercapnia may result in peripheral vasodilatation. The resulting blood pressure will be determined by the balance of these competing factors.[16]

Respiratory abnormalities

The further clinical assessment of a patient who appears to be developing respiratory failure includes obtaining an analysis of arterial blood gases. As previously stated, hypoxemia is almost invariable, but hypercapnia and acidosis may or may not occur, depending on the cause. The thoughtful interpretation of hypoxemia should provide clues regarding the cause of the respiratory problem. Determination of which of the five causes of hypoxemia is present may lead to a better understanding of the underlying disease process responsible for the respiratory failure as shown in Table 11-1.[34,47] Hypercapnia is present with any disorder causing hypoventilation such as COPD, drug overdose, cerebral vascular accident, metabolic alkalosis, and the primary hypoventilation syndrome. The arterial pH can be determined by use of the Henderson-Hasselbalch equation as shown below:

$$pH = 6.1 + \left(\frac{\log HCO_3^-}{0.03 \times PaCO_2} \right)$$

During an episode of acute respiratory decompensation with hypercapnia, the pH of arterial blood will fall until

Table 11-1. The five causes of hypoxemia and example, method of determination, and results of oxygen therapy for each cause

Cause	Example	Determination	Results of oxygen therapy
Decreased oxygen intake	High altitude, rebreathing expired air	Low ambient inspired oxygen, no oxygen gradient	Rapid increase in PaO_2
Ventilation/perfusion ratio ($\dot{V}/\dot{Q}$) imbalance	Chronic obstructive pulmonary disease	Oxygen gradient, correction of PaO_2 with 100% oxygen	Moderately rapid increase in PaO_2
Shunt	Adult respiratory distress syndrome, ventricular septal defect, pulmonary arteriovenous fistula	Oxygen gradient, incomplete correction of PaO_2 with 100% oxygen	Moderately rapid, variable increase in PaO_2 depending on size of shunt
Diffusion impairment	Interstitial pneumonia, scleroderma	Normal oxygen gradient at rest; increased gradient with exercise	Moderately rapid increase in PaO_2
Hypoventilation	Chronic obstructive pulmonary disease, drug overdose, cerebral vascular accident	Hypercapnia	Early increase in PaO_2; variable later response

renal compensation elevates the bicarbonate level to buffer the CO_2. This buffering will raise the arterial pH toward normal (7.38 to 7.42). The renal compensation may take several days, and so during the acute episode the pH may reach dangerously low levels leading to hypotension, cardiac arrhythmias, and even death.

MANAGEMENT OF ACUTE RESPIRATORY FAILURE
Conservative management

Proper oxygen therapy is an integral part of the management of any patient with acute respiratory failure, and this therapy should be guided by arterial blood-gas determinations, with repeated analyses of the pH, PaO_2, and $PaCO_2$. High concentrations of oxygen should be avoided, especially in patients with CO_2 retention. These patient's primary ventilatory drive is chronic hypoxemia, which may be too quickly corrected by a high concentration of supplemental oxygen, leading to further ventilatory depression. Administration of oxygen is usually begun with either nasal cannulas or a loose-fitting face mask and delivery of a low flow of oxygen (about 2 to 3 liters per minute). Although this therapy is often successful at relieving some hypoxemia, the FIO_2 with low-flow oxygen therapy is difficult to predict accurately. With patients who breathe at higher minute ventilation levels, the FIO_2 is often reduced because of dilution of the oxygen concentration with room air. At an oxygen flow of 2 to 3 liters per minute, the patient with a minute ventilation of 12 liters could have an FIO_2 of about 28%, whereas a similar patient with a minute ventilation of only 5 liters could receive an FIO_2 of about 40%. In those with COPD and

chronic CO_2 retention, an FIO_2 of 28% could be acceptable, but 40% might be high enough to eliminate the hypoxic ventilatory drive, thereby worsening the hypercapnia.

Venturi masks are designed to deliver a fixed concentration of oxygen despite variations in the minute ventilation. This is accomplished by use of a special face mask that is flooded with a fixed concentration of oxygen at high flow so that no further dilution of the concentration occurs even with patients breathing at high minute ventilation.

High concentrations of oxygen can be delivered to patients without mechanical ventilation if they are not dependent on their hypoxic ventilatory drive. These high concentrations can be achieved with a tight-fitting face mask and an FIO_2 of up to 100%. Actual oxygen concentration to the patient depends on the volume of oxygen delivered, the amount of air that leaks into the mask, and the amount of exhaled gas rebreathed by the patient.

Management of an elevated $PaCO_2$ can also be difficult, since elevation of the $PaCO_2$ will tend to diminish the PaO_2 as shown in the alveolar gas equation. This diminution of PaO_2 can lead to overt respiratory failure, cardiac arrhythmias, and psychiatric changes. The patient should not receive respiratory depressants such as benzodiazepines or narcotics. Nutrition must be maintained, electrolytes adjusted properly, anemia corrected (with transfusions if necessary), magnesium and phosphate deficiencies minimized, thyroid function tested when indicated, infections treated, adequate bronchodilator therapy instituted if needed, psychiatric problems addressed, congestive heart failure controlled, adequate hydration maintained, and tracheobronchial secretions controlled as effectively as possible. If these conservative measures fail to improve respiratory function, endotracheal intubation may become necessary.

Endotracheal intubation

The endotracheal tube is a lifeline between the patient's lungs and a ventilator. One of the first decisions regarding intubation is whether the intubation will be performed orally or nasally. In general, a nasopharyngeal endotracheal tube is better tolerated and can be fully anchored to prevent tube migration. However, tracheal suctioning can be more difficult because of both the smaller sized tube that is commonly used and the greater angulation of the nasotracheal tube as compared with the orotracheal tube. The nasotracheal tube may also interfere with sinus drainage and is somewhat more difficult to insert, especially in emergency situations. The orotracheal tube is easier to insert, can be larger for easier suctioning and bronchoscopy if needed, but tends to migrate and be more uncomfortable to the patient.[44]

Tracheotomy and tracheostomy

The correct time at which to perform a tracheotomy after the initial endotracheal intubation is a matter of controversy. Whereas some physicians may routinely send their patients for tracheotomy after only a few days of intubation, recent studies have indicated that ''routine'' tracheotomies cannot be supported. Both endotracheal intubation and tracheotomy are associated with high incidences of complications. Indeed, complications occurring after tracheotomy may be more serious than those after intubation. In a recent study comparing these two procedures, the major complications of endotracheal intubation were excessive cuff-pressure requirements, self-extubations, and an inability to seal the airway. Tracheostomy complications included stomal infections, hemorrhages, excessive cuff-pressure requirements, and subcutaneous emphysema or pneumomediastinum. Importantly, the establishment of an inflexible time limit after intubation when tracheotomy should be performed could not be supported by the study, since some patients tolerated intubation for up to 22 days.[49] However, a tracheostomy is a valuable adjunct to patient care because it allows the patient to eat and drink, and it reduces the anatomical dead space, which may expedite and facilitate weaning from the mechanical ventilator.

Most complications arising from endotracheal intubation or tracheostomy are associated with improper care and lack of attention to detail. Proper humidity of the inspired air, prevention of trauma to the trachea, and proper suctioning techniques are critically important to minimize the complications associated with artificial airways. The air reaching the lungs of a normal person will be completely saturated with water vapor, primarily by the nasal mucosa, which adds approximately 650 ml of water per day to the inspired air. Both tracheostomy tubes and endotracheal tubes by-

pass the upper airway and do not permit the inspired gas to be adequately humidified unless that humidification is provided artificially. If this is not done, bronchial secretions will become viscous and thick, thereby increasing the airway resistance and work of breathing. Additionally, these secretions may dry out in the endotracheal or tracheostomy tube causing complete obstruction of the artificial airway and resulting in an emergency that endangers the patient's life. Prevention of trauma to the tracheal mucosa can be avoided only by scrupulous attention to detail in tube care. To avoid tracheal irritation, one should inflate the cuff on the tubes to a minimal pressure that will occlude or seal the airway outside the tube. If tracheal irritation occurs, it may be followed by tracheal stenosis because of scarring of the epithelium, or tracheal necrosis and subsequent tracheomalacia. The volume of air necessary to inflate the cuff should always be noted, and if an increased amount of air is needed at a later time, tracheal damage should be suspected. Suctioning of the tracheobronchial tree through the artificial airway is often necessary for secretion control, since most patients are unable to generate an effective cough while intubated. Aseptic technique is required for suctioning or the resultant contamination of the airway by the suction catheter will introduce pathogenic organisms into the airway. Additionally, suction catheters may produce epithelial damage and hypoxia if suctioning is performed too frequently. Excessive suctioning may also decrease ciliary activity in the trachea, and that decrease will reduce the patient's intrinsic ability to remove secretions and debris. Proper technique dictates that suction should be applied only when the catheter is being quickly withdrawn with a twisting motion. It is preferable to use a catheter with a single hole at the tip rather than one with many holes proximally. In the latter case, if the more distal holes become occluded with thick secretions, there may be a generation of very high pressures in the more proximal holes that can damage the tracheal mucosa. The material obtained through tracheal suctioning should be periodically examined for evidence of white blood cells and bacteria. These findings should be considered indications of infection, and, especially with fever, infiltrates on the chest radiograph and signs of lung consolidation should be treated with appropriate antibiotics.[16]

Mechanical ventilation

In some patients with respiratory failure, mechanical ventilation may become necessary despite efforts at conservative management using supplemental oxygen and secretion removal techniques. Judging the precise time for elective endotracheal intubation is often a difficult decision for the physician and is based upon numerous factors. Intubation is generally indicated when the respiratory failure is not improving and signs and symptoms of respiratory distress continue unabated. These signs and symptoms can be grouped under headings of mechanical failure, oxygenation failure, and ventilation failure.

Mechanical failure occurs when the patient appears to be working very hard to maintain ventilation and is often present when the respiratory rate exceeds 35 breaths per minute, when the vital capacity is less than 15 ml/kg (or 1 liter), and when the maximum inspiratory force is less than 20 cm H_2O.[20] If these above criteria exist, it is likely that the patient will soon tire from the excessive effort being expended to maintain ventilation. Elective mechanical support of ventilation at this point is usually preferable to the continued effort of the patient.

Oxygenation failure occurs when the PaO_2 cannot be maintained above 60 to 70 torr with oxygen delivered by mask, or when the alveolar-arterial oxygen gradient exceeds 350. When these criteria exist, dangerously low levels of arterial oxygen will result unless toxic levels of supplemental oxygen are administered.

Ventilatory failure is defined as an elevated $PaCO_2$, or an abnormally high physiological dead space (V_D/V_T) of greater than 0.60. Acutely and severely high $PaCO_2$ with respiratory acidosis and hypoxemia is encountered as the ventilatory failure worsens.

The situation becomes especially difficult in the patient with chronic obstructive pulmonary disease (COPD), since high levels of oxygen may lead to CO_2 retention. The explanation for this phenomenon, stated earlier, is that the administered oxygen eliminates the hypoxic drive to breathe. An alternative explanation, however, may be that a worsening $\dot{V}/\dot{Q}$ ratio develops with the additional oxygen. The physician attempts, if possible, to avoid intubating patients with COPD because of the higher incidence of complications such as tension pneumothorax, and the subsequent difficulty with extubation and weaning from the ventilatory support. Because these patients are often acclimated to hypoxemia and therefore tolerant of low levels of oxygen, which could be lethal to nonacclimated patients, indications for intubation in the COPD population are more stringent. Therefore mechanical ventilation is postponed, if possible, until all other attempts to reverse hypoxemia are exhausted. These attempts may include aggressive treatment of infection, bronchial hygiene techniques, adequate hydration, treatment of congestive heart failure, correction of anemia, and the assessment and treatment of any metabolic abnormality that may be present.[45]

Oxygen toxicity

Oxygen toxicity can present difficulties during the treatment of acute respiratory failure. Although sufficient oxygen must be delivered to assure adequate tissue oxygenation, inhaled concentrations of oxygen greater than about 50% can produce lung damage. Numerous theories have been proposed to explain this phenomenon, but the most widely held view is that the damage is associated with the intracellular production of toxic free radicals. These radicals include hydrogen peroxide, hydroxyl radicals, superoxide anions, and single oxygen radicals, all of which are believed to produce lung damage because of lipid peroxidation. The toxic lipids produced cause cellular damage through loss of membrane integrity, enzyme inactivation, and nucleic acid damage. Pulmonary oxygen toxicity may result in tracheobronchitis, bronchopulmonary dysplasia in the newborn, or acute respiratory distress syndrome (ARDS) in the adult. It is indeed ironic that the high concentration of oxygen required to treat the severe hypoxemia of ARDS may itself lead to ARDS.[41]

Positive end-expiratory pressure (PEEP)

PEEP is very useful in selected diseases to decrease the percentage of supplemental oxygen required in the treatment of severe hypoxemia and is especially useful in the treatment of ARDS. PEEP is indicated in only a limited number of patients with acute respiratory failure. The strict indications recognize the potential dangers of PEEP in the critically ill patient. The dangers include barotrauma, neumothorax, pneumomediastinum, hypotension and tissue hypoxia from decreased cardiac output, and the increased accumulation of lung water at higher levels of PEEP. PEEP may worsen the status of the spontaneously breathing patient by increasing the work of breathing as the lungs are hyperexpanded to an artificially high functional residual capacity. This places the inspiratory muscles at a mechanical disadvantage, which may cause them to tire rapidly. In the mechanically ventilated patient, however, PEEP is believed to relieve hypoxemia by as yet poorly defined mechanisms. PEEP appears to decrease atelectasis by opening previously collapsed alveoli thereby improving $\dot{V}/\dot{Q}$ ratios and decreasing hypoxemia.[8] Since there is little evidence that an FIO_2 of less than 50% produces pulmonary oxygen toxicity, PEEP is generally reserved for the patient whose FIO_2 must exceed 50%.[24] However, PEEP must be used cautiously in patients with nonhomogeneous lung disease. Regions of the lung with high compliance will be preferentially ventilated when PEEP is used, and this could result in an overall deterioration of the $\dot{V}/\dot{Q}$ relationship. Additionally, patients with COPD may experience pneumothorax or pneumomediastinum with PEEP, since their lungs are already hyperinflated, their disease is often nonhomogeneous, and they may have many surface blebs (blisters), which can easily rupture. There has been some recent indication that PEEP may reduce mortality in patients with ARDS or in those believed to be at high risk for ARDS.[39,46,48] PEEP is usually applied when the FIO_2 exceeds 50% and is begun at 3 to 5 cm H_2O pressure and, if necessary, increased gradually in 3 to 5 cm H_2O pressure increments if there are no complications. Careful monitoring of the blood pressure, PaO_2, and mixed venous oxygen tension are all recommended.[8]

Medications

In the patient with acute respiratory failure, improvement of residual pulmonary function assumes paramount importance. Commonly employed medications include bronchodilators, antibiotics, and corticosteroids.

Bronchodilators. The mechanism by which most bronchodilators work is not precisely known, but there are several postulated methods whereby they may improve pulmonary function. Aminophylline has long been known to increase intracellular concentration of cyclic AMP, an intracellular chemical modulator, thereby causing smooth muscle relaxation and decreased airway resistance. Aminophylline has recently been shown to reverse the diaphragmatic fatigue associated with respiratory failure and may relieve some of the dyspnea associated with respiratory failure. Additionally, the mucociliary removal of secretions may be enhanced with aminophylline thereby aiding in the prevention of infection.

Antibiotics. Pulmonary infection is believed to be the precipitating factor in many episodes of respiratory failure. Although as many as 47% of these infections appear to be of viral or mycoplasmal origin, there is frequent bacterial colonization or superinfection present.[27] A gram stain of expectorated sputum should be part of the initial assessment of the patient with respiratory failure, and antibiotics are prescribed in accordance with the results. The routine use of broad-spectrum antibiotics should be avoided, since this practice may lead to superinfection with organisms resistant to many antibiotics.

Steroids. The use of corticosteroids during episodes of acute respiratory failure has been a controversy for many years, especially for patients with chronic obstructive pulmonary disease. Most controlled studies have shown little or no benefit from corticosteroids used for patients with COPD suffering from acute respiratory failure.[27,33] However, there are patients who may occasionally benefit from their use, and a recent controlled study documented spirometric improvement with steroids when given in high doses.[1] Efforts to identify patients for whom corticosteroids will be beneficial have indicated that those patients wheezing at the onset of their disease, or those with high eosinophil counts in their sputum or blood, are most likely to respond.[27]

Management of systemic illnesses

Patients with acute respiratory failure often have multiple organ system diseases, which may adversely affect their pulmonary status. Fever from any cause will increase minute ventilation and may either lead to intubation or increase the difficulty in weaning from mechanical ventilation. Left-sided congestive heart failure, even without progression to pulmonary edema, can produce respiratory failure in patients with marginal respiratory status. With increased left ventricular end-diastolic pressure, there is a progressive leakage of fluid into the interstitial spaces of the lungs, decreasing lung compliance and increasing the work of breathing. If this situation progresses to pulmonary edema with leakage of fluid into the alveoli, a $\dot{V}/\dot{Q}$ abnormality will result and produce progressive hypoxemia. Gastrointestinal bleeding is often seen in patients with acute respiratory failure and may lead to severe anemia, with subsequent high-output congestive heart failure, tissue hypoxia, metabolic acidosis, and respiratory failure. Metabolic abnormalities often associated with respiratory failure include hypophosphatemia and metabolic acidosis or alkalosis, each of which could lead to further pulmonary compromise. Malnutrition is common in very ill patients and may produce muscular weakness and predispose to infection. Sedatives, if given to calm the patient during acute respiratory failure, can reduce ventilation. The above examples indicate the complexity of medical care for these patients and show why they easily develop respiratory failure even without additional insults to the lungs.[4]

Bronchial hygiene

An important aspect of the care of patients with acute respiratory failure is the mobilization of secretions. Intuitively, the removal of bronchial secretions seems as important as the relief of bronchoconstriction because both may impede pulmonary function through interference with gas exchange. The effectiveness of mobilization of bronchial secretions has been studied objectively only in recent years despite its being employed for many decades.

Gravity-assisted bronchial drainage. Bronchial drainage for removal of secretions is frequently an important adjunct in the comprehensive care of patients with acute respiratory failure. It is intuitively pleasing to conceptually visualize the lung as a group of alveoli connected to large airways, which can become clogged with mucus. Likewise, the drainage of these clogged airways after chest percussion and vibration, assisted by gravity drainage of the lung segments, should provide mucus clearance and improve pulmonary function.

The question regarding the effectiveness of bronchial drainage and associated manual techniques is discussed in subsequent chapters that describe treatment for several major patient populations who periodically receive bronchial drainage techniques as part of their treatment regimens.

Intermittent positive-pressure breathing. Intermittent positive-pressure breathing (IPPB) has been used for many years in the treatment of impending respiratory failure in an attempt to deliver bronchodilator medications, or enhance sputum mobilization and thus prevent deterioration. Although IPPB has been used extensively for the above two indications, until recently there have been few objective studies evaluating its efficacy. One of the early studies used pulmonary function tests to compare the outcome of patients who used IPPB to those who did not. Those receiving IPPB at home showed an approximate twofold reduction of their 1-second forced expiratory volume (FEV_1) over a 4-year period when compared to those who did not use IPPB. Additionally those who used IPPB had fewer improvements in their FEV_1 than those who did not.[15]

Possibly because of the reported subjective improvement with IPPB used at home during chronic treatment, or when used during hospitalization for an acute exacerbation, these treatments appear to have become more popular over time. However, in addition to the early clinical studies there is now recent physiological data to indicate that IPPB has little value either in the treatment of impending respiratory failure or in chronic home care of patients with chronic obstructive pulmonary disease. These investigations showed that with IPPB treatments tidal volume was increased and acute improvement was noted in PaO_2 and $PaCO_2$. Because these improvements were transient, however, IPPB should not be expected to effect any lasting improvement in these values.[30] Pulmonary function testing in patients with COPD who used IPPB machines showed increased residual volume (RV), total lung capacity (TLC), and functional residual capacity (FRC) when compared to results in patients using air compressors or receiving no therapy.[15] Although vital capacity in postoperative patients frequently increased by 10% or more with IPPB treatments when compared with voluntary deep breathing, IPPB was shown to be no more effective in preventing postoperative pulmonary complications.[10] Although tidal volume during IPPB treatments may increase, the additional ventilation is often directed to lung areas already well ventilated, and this may produce deterioration in $\dot{V}/\dot{Q}$ ratios, increase the dead space, and cause a rise in the $PaCO_2$.[12] Distribution of ventilation is partially determined by the flow rate at which inspiration is provided and the lung volume at which inspiration occurs. Both inspiratory criteria can be rendered grossly abnormal with IPPB. These patients are frequently hyperinflated not only from their underlying disease process, but also from chronic therapy with IPPB. Additionally, excessive flow rates which increase ventilation of only the more compliant lung segments are often used. Also the distribution of ventilation is different with a positive-pressure breathing pattern than with a physiological (negative-pressure) breathing pattern. This difference may be the result of variations in diaphragmatic mechanics in these two different methods of breathing.[36] The work of breathing is often increased in patients using IPPB, especially in those patients with COPD. When using IPPB, the normal person tends to let the machine perform the work of breathing and decrease the patient's cost to almost zero. Patients with obstructive lung disease, however, tend to increase their work of breathing by beginning expiratory efforts before the machine has completed the inspiratory cycle. This incoordinated effort causes increased air trapping, premature airway closure, and higher lung volume.[12]

Additionally, the cardiac output in patients who use IPPB will frequently drop slightly, a drop that is probably attributable to decreased venous return secondary to increased intrathoracic pressure resulting from pulmonary hyperinflation and the effect of the positive pressure.[30] The drop in cardiac output could be more severe for the patient who is dehydrated or otherwise decompensated from a circulatory standpoint.

No significant difference between simple hand-held nebulizers and IPPB machines can be demonstrated in the relief of bronchospasm. However, the IPPB machine may have an advantage over the hand-held nebulizers in the delivery of bronchodilators for the patient who is unable to voluntarily inspire deeply and cannot therefore effectively use the hand-held nebulizer.[12,17]

Not only is there a lack of acute improvement in patients with COPD when IPPB is compared to air-compressor delivery of bronchodilating medications, but there is also no difference in days hospitalized, morbidity, or mortality.[13,27] When IPPB, used in association with bronchial hygiene techniques for one group of patients with pneumonia, was compared to no treatment in a similar group of patients, there was no significant difference in duration of fever, clearance of the chest radiograph, length of hospital stay, or mortality.[18] If the IPPB machine is not properly maintained and sterilized, it can become a source of infection from contamination of the mouthpiece, nebulizer, or tubing. This may prove to be a significant problem for the already debilitated patient receiving IPPB treatments at home.[32]

Aerosols. Bland aerosol treatments have been recommended for mobilization of the tenacious secretions that periodically complicate respiratory failure. This approach is conceptually sound and rests on attempts to decrease the viscosity of sputum and improve its mobilization by either mixing it with fluid or coating it with water. Early studies indicated the possibility that aerosolized substances such as saline solution or propylene glycol were very effective at mobilizing secretions.[32] Subsequent studies have shown that the original enthusiasm regarding bland aerosols may have been premature.[21] The FEV_1 was shown to be significantly reduced and airway resistance significantly increased in those patients who inhaled droplets of water for up to 10 minutes.[26] Deposition of aerosolized water was shown to be greater in COPD patients when compared with normals, but no concomitant improvement in bronchial clearance or sputum viscosity was noted in the patients. On the other hand, airway obstruction and hypoxemia may increase with bland aerosol use, and contamination of the equipment with gram-negative bacteria was common.[17] Thus the use of bland aerosols is questionable to improve secretion mobilization in COPD patients with tenacious secretions. However, the effective use of aerosols for the delivery of bronchodilators cannot be disputed.

The sympathomimetic medications have been found particularly useful as bronchodilators when delivered by aerosol. Despite potential cardiotoxic side effects from the fluorocarbon propellants when metered-dose inhalers are used to excess and possible paradoxical bronchoconstriction occurs in some patients, sympathomimetic aerosol bronchodilators have been found generally safe and useful when incorporated into a respiratory therapy regimen. Parasympathetic drugs have also shown bronchodilator properties when delivered by aerosol inhalation, but they are still in the experimental stage of development.

Steroids can be administered in aerosol form but are usually reserved for the patient with stable COPD or asthma, not for those with acute respiratory failure.[17]

Acetylcysteine is a nonenzymatic mucolytic agent that is very effective in the in vitro reduction of sputum viscosity. This medication has a reactive sulfhydryl group, which is believed to dissolve the polysaccharide bond of mucin. Although acetylcysteine is considered innocuous, some question its use because of reports of mucosal irritation and bronchoconstriction. When used, it should always be accompanied by an adequate dosage of bronchodilator.[17,32]

Breathing exercises

Diaphragmatic breathing exercises have been used in an attempt to improve distribution of inspired gas. Maneuvers to increase diaphragmatic excursion have included the head-down position, elbows-on-knees position to relax accessory muscles of respiration, and voluntary use of the abdominal muscles rather than the accessory muscles. Although diaphragmatic breathing reduces minute ventilation, increases tidal volume, and reduces dead space, there occurs no demonstrable improvement in air mixing when this technique is used in patients with COPD.[21,35] Whereas the head-down position has been shown to increase diaphragmatic movement[5] and may be able to increase oxygen saturation,[50] gas distribution and lung volume do not change.[42] Leaning forward on the elbows has been proposed as a means to rest the accessory muscles while improving diaphragmatic excursion and tidal volume and reducing minute ventilation.[40]

The clinical effects of diaphragmatic breathing have been found disappointing. A comparison among breathing exercise, chloramphenicol, and placebo showed that the exercises did not influence duration of fever, sputum volume, PaO₂, or ventilatory function.[40] Some authors have been so pessimistic as to suggest that breathing exercises have no substantial effect on either ventilatory capacity or PaO₂ in patients with COPD.[29] This pessimism must be tempered with the realization that frequent subjective improvement is noted in patients with COPD after the use of breathing exercises. It is possible that the measures used to assess ventilatory capacity in these patients are not sufficiently sensitive to demonstrate an objective improvement.[27]

Physical training

After the patient has recovered from an episode of acute respiratory failure, emphasis should be upon physical rehabilitation in an attempt to prevent subsequent episodes of failure. The effects of physical training on cardiopulmonary performance in patients with COPD has become an intensively studied area. Aerobic training exercise such as bicycle or treadmill work have produced equivocal results. Although there appears to be improved exercise tolerance after a period of exercise training, there is no appreciable change in heart rate, cardiac index, peripheral vascular resistance, cardiac output, stroke volume, right- and left-sided cardiac pressures, lung volumes, or arterial blood gases. There is noted, however, a decrease in oxygen consumption. Apparently oxygen consumption diminishes primarily through either more efficient muscle use or greater skill and not through improved cardiopulmonary performance.[2,14,43] More recent investigations of ventilatory muscle training in patients with COPD have shown that with endurance training, there occurred a 31% increase in the maximal sustained ventilatory capacity. This improvement appears to persist after the exercise program is completed.[6]

Oxygen therapy

Oxygen therapy has also been proved useful in some patients after an episode of acute respiratory failure. Early studies examined the benefits of continuous oxygen therapy with the goal of maintaining a PaO₂ between 65 and 70 torr. No side effects were found, and there was clinical improvement characterized by improved clinical status, increased exercise tolerance, reversal of secondary erythrocytosis, and a significant fall in the pulmonary arteriolar resistance.[28] Subsequent investigations attempted to define more clearly the benefits of oxygen therapy and to determine the least amount of oxygen that would be beneficial. It was noted that hypoxemia could lead to right ventricular dysfunction primarily through two mechanisms. These mechanisms were by a direct toxic effect upon the heart and by pulmonary vasoconstriction, which increases the resistance against which the right ventricle must pump. Animals maintained at low PaO₂ developed both right and left ventricular hypertrophy, which was reversible with improved oxygenation. Additionally, early investigations recognized little benefit from oxygen delivered for 12 hours per day and recommended longer periods of oxygen therapy for added benefit.[3] Further refinements showed that while oxygen for 12 hours each day did not lower the pulmonary artery pressures or decrease pulmonary vascular resistance, 15 hours of oxygen per day could achieve those results.

During exercise with supplemental oxygen in patients with severe but stable COPD, a greater amelioration occurred in pulmonary artery pressure than when these same patients were studied in the resting state.[9] Too, it was noted that oxygen therapy increased platelet survival time, possibly decreasing the risk of thromboembolism.[23] It was not until recently, however, that parameters for oxygen use were refined. In a large nationwide cooperative study, a comparison was made between continual oxygen therapy (COT) and nocturnal oxygen therapy limited to 12 hours daily (NOT). These patients received oxygen by nasal cannulas at the rate of 1 to 4 liters per minute during sleep and during exercise. These results showed a significant decrease in mortality in both groups, but especially in the COT group. Also there was a significant decrease in the hematocrit and a significant change in the pulmonary vascular resistance in only the COT group. Probably, oxygen therapy is beneficial only in the group of patients with COPD who manifest rather severe arterial hypoxemia with a PaO_2 of less than 55 torr and only when the oxygen is given for all, or at least a major portion, of the day.[37]

REFERENCES

1. Albert, R., Martin, T., and Lewis, S.: Methylprednisolone improves chronic bronchitics with acute respiratory insufficiency, Chest **77** (suppl.):314-315, 1980.
2. Alpert, J.S., Bass, H., Szucs, M.M., and others: Effects of physical training on hemodynamics at rest and during exercise in patients with chronic obstructive pulmonary disease, Chest **66**:647-651, 1974.
3. Anderson, P.B., Cayton, R.M., Holt, P.J., and Howard, P.: Long-term oxygen therapy in cor pulmonale, Q. J. Med. **167**:563-573, 1973.
4. Andrews, J.L.: Treatment of hypoxemia and hypercapnia, Pract. Cardiol. **8**:148-184, 1982.
5. Barach, A.L., and Beck, G.J.: The ventilatory effects of the head-down position in pulmonary emphysema, Am. J. Med. **16**:55-60, 1954.
6. Belman, M.J., and Mittman, C.: Ventilatory muscle training improves exercise capacity in chronic obstructive pulmonary disease patients, Am. Rev. Respir. Dis. **121**:273-280, 1980.
7. Bergofsky, E.H.: Respiratory failure in disorders of the thoracic cage, Am. Rev. Respir. Dis. **199**:643-669, 1979.
8. Bone, R.C.: Treatment of severe hypoxemia due to the adult respiratory distress syndrome, Arch. Intern. Med. **140**:85-89, 1980.
9. Burrows, B.: Arterial oxygenation and pulmonary hemodynamics in patients with chronic airways obstruction, Am. Rev. Respir. Dis. **110**:64-70, 1974.
10. Cheny, R.W., Nelson, E.J., and Horton, W.G.: The function of IPPB related to breathing patterns, Am. Rev. Respir. Dis. **110**:183-192, 1974.
11. Cherniack, R.M.: The management of acute respiratory failure, Chest **58**:427-436, 1970.
12. Cherniack, R.M.: Intermittent positive pressure breathing in the management of chronic obstructive pulmonary disease, Am. Rev. Respir. Dis. **110**(suppl.):188-192, 1974.
13. Cherniack, R.M., and Svanhill, E.: Long-term use of intermittent positive pressure breathing (IPPB) in chronic obstructive pulmonary disease, Am. Rev. Respir. Dis. **113**:721-728, 1976.
14. Chester, E.H., Belman, M.J., Bahler, R.C. and others: Multidisciplinary treatment of chronic pulmonary insufficiency, Chest **72**:695-702, 1977.
15. Curtis, J.K., Liska, A.P., Rasmussen, H.K., and Cree, E.M.: IPPB therapy in chronic obstructive pulmonary disease, J.A.M.A. **206**:1037-1040, 1968.
16. Divertie, M.B.: The adult respiratory distress syndrome, Mayo Clin. Proc. **57**:371-378, 1982.
17. Fox, M.J., and Snyder, G.L.: Respiratory therapy, current practice in ambulatory patients with chronic airflow obstruction, J.A.M.A. **241**:937-940, 1979.
18. Hauser, M.J., and Sprung, C.L.: Noncardiogenic pulmonary edema and the adult respiratory distress syndrome, Res. Staff Phys. **28** (suppl.):67-72, 1982.
19. Henry, J.: The effect of shock on pulmonary alveolar surfactant; its role in refractory respiratory insufficiency of the critically ill or severely injured patient, J. Trauma **8**:756, 1968.
20. Hinshaw, C., and Murray, J.F., editors: Diseases of the chest, Philadelphia, 1980, W.B. Saunders Co., p. 987.
21. Hodgkin, J.E., Balchum, O.J., and Kass, I., and others: Chronic obstructive airway diseases: current concepts in diagnosis and comprehensive care, J.A.M.A. **232**:1243-1260, 1975.
22. Hurewitz, A., and Bergofsky, E.H.: Adult respiratory distress syndrome, physiologic basis of treatment, Med. Clin. North Am. **65**:33-51, 1981.
23. Johnson, T.S., Ellis, E.H., and Steele, P.P.: Improvement of platelet survival time with oxygen in patients with chronic obstructive airway disease, Am. Rev. Respir. Dis. **117**:255-257, 1977.
24. Kirby, R.R., Downs, J.B., Civetta, J.M., and others: High level positive end-expiratory pressure (PEEP) in acute respiratory insufficiency, Chest **67**:156-163, 1975.
25. Lanken, P.N.: Weaning from mechanical ventilation. In Fishman, A.P., editor: Update: pulmonary diseases and disorders, New York, 1982, McGraw-Hill Book Co.
26. Lefcoe, N.M., and Paterson, N.A.M.: Adjunct therapy in chronic obstructive pulmonary disease, Am. J. Med. **54**:343-348, 1973.
27. Lertzman, M.M., and Cherniack, R.M.: Rehabilitation of patients with chronic obstructive pulmonary disease, Am. Rev. Respir. Dis. **114**:1145-1165, 1976.
28. Levine, B.E., Bigelow, D.B., Hamstra, R.D., and others: The role of long-term continuous oxygen administration in patients with chronic airway obstruction with hypoxemia, Ann. Intern. Med. **66**:639-649, 1967.
29. Levy, D.: Therapy of obstructive bronchial diseases: the physiochemical approach, J. Asthma Res. **8**:161, 1971.
30. Loke, J., and Anthonisen, N.R.: Effect of IPPB on steady state chronic obstructive pulmonary disease, Am. Rev. Respir. Dis. **110**:178-182, 1974.
31. Mann, S.J.: Acute respiratory failure. In Bordow, R.A., Stool, E.W., and Moser, K.M., editors: Manual of clinical problems in pulmonary medicine, Boston, 1980, Little, Brown & Co.
32. Miller, W.F.: Aerosol therapy in acute and chronic respiratory disease, Arch. Intern. Med. **131**:148-155, 1973.
33. Mintz, S., Davies, G., Rostum, H., and others: A double-blind, cross-over study of beclomethasone diproprionate in asthmatic patients with and without chronic bronchitis, Postgrad. Med. J. **51** (suppl. 4):76-79, 1975.
34. Mithofer, J.C., Ramirez, C., and Cook, W.: The effect of mixed venous oxygenation on arterial blood in chronic obstructive pulmonary disease, Am. Rev. Respir. Dis. **117**:259-264, 1978.
35. Motley, H.L.: The effects of slow deep breathing on the blood gas exchange in emphysema, Am. Rev. Respir. Dis. **88**:485-492, 1963.
36. Murray, J.F.: Review of the state of the art in intermittent positive pressure breathing therapy, Am. Rev. Respir. Dis. **110**(suppl):193-199, 1974.
37. Nocturnal Oxygen Therapy Trial Group: Continuous or nocturnal oxygen therapy in hypoxemic chronic obstructive lung disease, a clinical trial, Ann. Intern. Med. **93**:391-398, 1980.
38. Park, S.S.: Respiratory control in chronic obstructive pulmonary diseases, Clin. Chest Med. **1**:73-84, 1980.
39. Perel, A., Olschvang, D., Eimerl, D., and others: The variable effect of PEEP in respiratory failure associated with multiple trauma, J. Trauma **18**:218-220, 1978.

40. Petersen, E.S., Esmann, V., Honcke, P., and Munker, C.: A controlled study of the effect of treatment on chronic bronchitis, Acta Med. Scand. **182:**293-305, 1967.
41. Petty, T.L., and Fowler, A.A.: Another look at ARDS, Chest **82:**98-104, 1982.
42. Petty, T.L., and Guthrie, A.: The effects of augmented breathing maneuvers on ventilation in severe chronic airway obstruction, Resp. Care **16:**104-111, 1971.
43. Petty, T.L., Nett, L.M., Finigan, M.M., and others: A comprehensive care program for chronic airway obstruction, Ann. Intern. Med. **70:**1109-1119, 1969.
44. Pierce, A.K.: Acute respiratory failure. In Guenter, C.A., and Welch, M.H., editors: Pulmonary medicine, Philadelphia, 1977, J.B. Lippincott Co.
45. Pontoppidan, H., Geffin, R., and Lowenstein, E.: Acute respiratory failure, N. Engl. J. Med. **287:**690-696, 1972.
46. Schmidt, G.B., O'Neill, W.W., Kotb, K., and others: Continuous positive airway pressure in the prophylaxis of the adult respiratory distress syndrome, Surg. Gynecol. Obstet. **143:**613-618, 1976.
47. Snider, R.L., and Rinaldo, J.E.: Oxygen therapy: oxygen therapy in medical patients hospitalized outside of the intensive care unit, Am. Rev. Respir. Dis. **122:**29-36, 1980.
48. Springer, R.R., and Stevens, P.M.: The influence of PEEP on survival of patients in respiratory failure, a retrospective analysis, Am. J. Med. **66:**196-200, 1979.
49. Stauffer, J.L., Olson, D.E., and Petty, T.L.: Consequences and complications of endotracheal intubation and tracheostomy, Am. J. Med. **70:**65-75, 1970.
50. Tucker, D.H., and Sieker, H.O.: The effect of change in body position on lung volumes and intrapulmonary gas mixing in patients with obesity, heart failure, and emphysema, Am. Rev. Respir. Dis. **82:**787-791, 1960.
51. Williams, H.M., and Shim, C.S.: Ventilatory failure, Am. J. Med. **48:**477-483, 1970.

12

NANCY HUMBERSTONE

Respiratory assessment

The physical therapy assessment of patients with pulmonary disease has two parts. Part one assesses the patient clinically through the chest examination. Part two completes the evaluation through objective assessment of the arterial blood gases, pulmonary function tests, chest radiography, graded exercise tests, and bacteriological studies.

CHEST EXAMINATION

The chest examination is administered by almost all health care professionals providing services to the patient with pulmonary disease. Although the examination may be conducted in a similar manner by all, the objectives for the examination may differ.

The physical therapist has four objectives for the chest examination. First, the therapist identifies the pulmonary problems acknowledged by the patient. Often the problems uppermost in the patient's mind are the cardinal symptoms of pulmonary disease: dyspnea, cough, sputum, and chest pain.[9] Second, the therapist assesses the coexisting signs of pulmonary disease. For example, the therapist identifies the patient's symptom of chest pain. Through further evaluation the therapist determines that the pain is localized to a small area of chest wall, exquisitely tender to palpation, associated with both a grating sound during breathing and a shallow, door-step breathing pattern, and aggravated by coughing and respiratory movements. At this point the co-existing signs suggest the presence of a rib fracture. Third, the therapist determines the need for further evaluative procedures when the results of the chest examination are unclear. In the preceeding example, further evaluation by chest radiography not only may confirm the assessment by the therapist but may also localize the problem anatomically. Fourth, the therapist identifies treatment goals and formulates a plan to track progress toward realization of the goals identified. Using the previous example, the therapist identifies pain reduction and improved ventilation as treatment goals. Pain reduction could be monitored by palpation, and improvement in ventilation could be monitored through auscultation.

Despite any difference in objectives, the chest examination administered by any health-care professional should be reliable and valid. For the examination to be reliable and valid the examiner must have intact sensory apparatus and well-developed observational skills, the patient must follow directions exactly, and the examination room must be warm, well lit, and quiet.

COMPONENTS OF THE CHEST EXAMINATION

The chest examination has four components: inspection, auscultation, palpation, and percussion.

Inspection

This phase of the chest examination documents the clinical characteristics associated with the presenting symptoms. During inspection the therapist detects problems previously unidentified. The results of the inspection determine what other components of the examination are necessary.

Part (1) of the inspection consists of evaluation of the patient's general appearance. In part (2) the therapist closely inspects the head and neck. The therapist inspects the chest in parts (3) and (4) and evaluates the breath, speech, cough, and sputum in part (5).

1. Evaluation of general appearance

In evaluating the general appearance of the patient the therapist assesses the state of consciousness in reference to seven somewhat ill-defined and often overlapping stages.[23] Following are the seven stages of consciousness from highest to lowest level:

1. Alert
2. Automatic
3. Confused
4. Delirious
5. Stuporous
6. Semicomatose
7. Comatose

The alert patient is oriented, attends to the therapist's

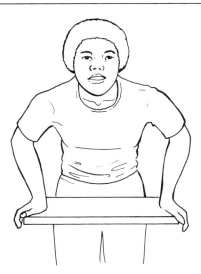

Fig. 12-1. The forward bent or professorial posture.

Table 12-1. Guidelines for the recognition and interpretation of the clinical signs associated with evaluation of the head and neck

Characteristic evaluated	Clinical sign	Interpretation
Facial expression	Alae nasi flaring Dilatation of pupils Sweating Pallor	Severe distress
Color of mucus membranes	Blue	Severe arterial oxygen desaturation
Facial color	Plethoric Cherry red	Possible hypertension Possible carbon monoxide poisoning
Size of neck veins	Distended above clavicle when sitting	Central venous pressure may exceed 15 cm H_2O

instructions, and cooperates in carrying them out. The automatic patient is irritable, shows impaired judgment, and retains instructions poorly. The confused patient is disoriented, illogical and able to respond to simple commands only. The delirious patient is totally irrational, often agitated, sometimes hostile, and generally uncooperative. The stuporous patient is unresponsive to the environment and often incontinent. The semicomatose patient is unconscious but rouses to painful stimuli. The comatose patient is both unconscious and unarousable.

The therapist evaluates body type as normal, obese, or cachectic. In assessing posture the therapist takes particular note of any spinal malalignment or unusual postures. In this part of the exam the therapist documents kyphosis, scoliosis, and forward bent or professorial postures. Fig. 12-1 illustrates the professorial posture.

During the extremity evaluation the therapist notes nicotine stains on the fingers, digital clubbing, painful swollen joints, tremor, and edema. Nicotine stains suggest a history of heavy smoking and are important in the evaluation of the unconscious patient. Clubbing of the fingers or toes is associated with cardiopulmonary and small bowel disease.[20] Painful swollen joints may indicate pseudohypertrophic pulmonary osteoarthropathy rather than the osteoarthritis or rheumatoid arthritis more familiar to physical therapists. The presence of asterixis (flapping tremor of the wrists when the arms are extended) may suggest hypercapnia.[5] Bilateral pedal edema suggests right-sided heart failure.

To complete the evaluation of the patient's appearance, the therapist notes all equipment used in managing the patient. For example, the use of a cardiac monitor, a Swan-Ganz catheter, or an intra-aortic balloon pump suggest potential or actual cardiac rhythm disturbances, or hemodynamic or cardiac output problems respectively.

2. Specific evaluation of head and neck

In evaluating the head and neck the therapist assesses the face to detect signs of distress, signs of oxygen desaturation, carbon monoxide poisoning, or hypertension. The therapist completes this part of the evaluation by observing the neck veins to detect signs of elevated central venous pressure. Table 12-1 presents guidelines for the recognition and interpretation of clinical signs associated with the evaluation of the head and neck.

3. Evaluation of the unmoving chest

During this part of the chest the physical therapist evaluates the condition of the skin and the shape and symmetry of the chest. Inspection of the skin assures documentation of incisions, scars, and trauma. Evaluation of the shape of the chest permits documentation of congenital defects like pectus carinatum, pectus excavatum, or Harrison's sulcus.[8] Evaluation of the chest in both the anteroposterior and transverse planes facilitates identification of the barrel-chest abnormality, a feature of obstructive lung disease. A barrel chest exists when the anteroposterior diameter is greater than or equal to twice the transverse diameter.[17]

Therapists next evaluate rib angles and intercostal spaces. Normally rib angles measure less than 90 degrees and attach to the vertebrae at an angle of about 45 degrees. The spaces between them are broader posteriorly than anteriorly. Widening of the rib angles and broadening of the

Table 12-2. Breathing patterns commonly encountered in the assessment of patients with respiratory problems

Pattern of breathing	Description
Apnea	Absence of ventilation
Fish-mouth	Apnea with concomitant mouth opening and closing; associated with neck extension and bradypnea
Eupnea	Normal rate, normal depth, regular rhythm
Bradypnea	Slow rate, shallow or normal depth, regular rhythm; associated with drug overdose
Tachypnea	Fast rate, shallow depth, regular rhythm; associated with restrictive lung disease
Hyperpnea	Normal rate, increased depth, regular rhythm
Cheyne-Stokes (periodic)	Increasing then decreasing depth, periods of apnea interspersed; somewhat regular rhythm; associated with critically ill patients
Biot's	Slow rate, shallow depth, apneic periods, irregular rhythm; associated with central nervous system disorders like meningitis
Apneustic	Slow rate, deep inspiration followed by apnea, irregular rhythm; associated with brainstem disorders
Prolonged expiration	Fast inspiration, slow and prolonged expiration yet normal rate, depth, and regular rhythm; associated with obstructive lung disease
Orthopnea	Difficulty breathing in postures other than erect
Hyperventilation	Fast rate, increased depth, regular rhythm; results in decreased arterial carbon dioxide, tension; called "Kussmaul breathing" in metabolic acidosis; also associated with central nervous system disorders like encephalitis
Psychogenic dyspnea	Normal rate, regular intervals of sighing; associated with anxiety
Dyspnea	Rapid rate, shallow depth, regular rhythm; associated with accessory muscle activity
Doorstop	Normal rate and rhythm; characterized by abrupt cessation of inspiration when restriction is encountered; associated with pleurisy

anterior intercostal spaces suggests hyperinflation of the lungs.

Evaluation of the musculature around the chest may reveal bilateral trapezius muscle hypertrophy, which may be associated with chronic dyspnea. Finally comparison of the symmetry of the hemithoraces permits detection of abnormalities like apical retraction.

4. Evaluation of the moving chest

Evaluation of the moving chest begins with assessment of the ventilatory rate, which normally ranges from 12 to 20 breaths per minute. This normal, or eupneic, pattern of breathing supplies one breath for every four heart beats. Tachypnea refers to a ventilatory rate faster than 20 breaths per minute. Bradypnea refers to a ventilatory rate slower than 10 breaths per minute. Fever affects ventilatory rate by adding four breaths per minute for every one Fahrenheit degree of fever.[22]

Next, the therapist evaluates the ratio of inspiratory and expiratory time, the I:E ratio. Normally, expiration is twice as long as inspiration, a ratio of 1:2. In obstructive lung disease reports of I:E ratios of 1:4 are common.

When evaluating the moving chest, one also evaluates the noise of breathing. Detection of *stridor,* a crowing sound during inspiration, suggests upper airway obstruction. Stridor may indicate laryngospasm. Another noise detected during inspiration is stertor. *Stertor* is a snoring noise created when the tongue falls back into the lower palate. Stertor may be heard in patients with depressed consciousness. During expiration one may also hear grunt-

ing sounds, particularly in children with pulmonary disease. Expiratory *grunting* may be a physiological attempt to prevent premature airway collapse. *Gurgling* sounds heard during both ventilatory phases are often called "death rattles."

The therapist then evaluates the pattern of breathing. This pattern reflects not only the rate but also the depth and regularity of the ventilatory cycle. Some commonly encountered ventilatory patterns appear in Table 12-2.

After evaluating the pattern and noise of breathing the therapist evaluates the symmetry and synchrony of ventilation. The timing and relative motion of one hemithorax to the other and to the abdomen is compared during both tidal and deep breathing. One may find asymmetrical, asynchronous chest motion during deep breathing in hemiplegia. In patients with flail-chest deformity expansion of one part of the chest may occur simultaneously with retraction of the other, a condition creating the basis for a paradoxical breathing pattern also known as *Pendelluft* ('pendulum air'). In chronic obstructive lung disease the chest and abdomen may move as a unit, hence the term "en bloc" motion. At least one exploratory study suggests that asynchronous, or seesaw, motion between the rib cage and the abdomen has prognostic significance.[16]

Next to be evaluated are the muscles of breathing. Gross observation permits detection of deviations from the normal, diaphragmatic breathing pattern used by men and children and the costal breathing pattern used by women. Close inspection facilitates detection of accessory inspiratory or expiratory muscle activity. Moreover, careful ob-

Table 12-3. Guidelines for evaluating cough

Cough characteristics	Associated features	Interpretation
Nonspecific	Sore throat, runny nose, runny eyes	Acute lung infection; tracheobronchitis
Productive	Preceded by an earlier, painful, nonproductive cough associated with an upper respiratory infection	Lobar pneumonia
Dry or productive	Acute bronchitis	Bronchopneumonia
Paroxysmal; mucoid or blood-stained sputum	Flu-like syndrome	*Mycoplasma* or viral pneumonia
Purulent sputum	Sputum formerly mucoid	Acute exacerbation of chronic bronchitis
Productive for more than 3 months consecutively and for at least 2 years		Chronic bronchitis
Foul-smelling, copious, layered purulent sputum	Long-standing problem	Bronchiectasis
Blood-tinged sputum	Month long	Tuberculosis or fungal infection
Persistent, nonproductive		Pneumonitis, interstitial fibrosis, pulmonary infiltrates
Persistent, minimally productive	Smoking history, injected pharynx	"Smoker's cough"
Nonspecific; minimal hemoptysis	Long standing	Neoplastic disease
Nonproductive	Long standing; dyspnea	Mediastinal neoplasm
Brassy		Aortic aneurysm
Violent cough	Sudden; onset at the same time as signs of asphyxia; localized wheezing	Aspiration of foreign body
Frothy sputum	Worsens in supine position; dyspnea	Heart failure, pulmonary edema
Hemoptysis	Sudden; simultaneous dyspnea; pleural effusion	Pulmonary infarct

Adapted from Fishman, A.P.: Pulmonary diseases and disorders, New York, 1980, McGraw-Hill Book Co., vol. 1.

servation of the intercostal spaces may reveal inspiratory retraction associated with decreased pulmonary compliance[7] or expiratory bulging associated with expiratory obstruction.[17]

5. Evaluation of speech, breath, cough, and sputum

Inspection of the chest proceeds with evaluation of speech, breath, cough, and sputum. Conversation with the patient facilitates recognition of various speech patterns or breath problems. Limited word patterns, frequently interrupted for breath, are known collectively as "dyspnea of phonation." Poor voice-volume control is associated with muscular incoordination and can be found in central nervous system disorders like cerebral palsy. Bad breath detected during the conversation may indicate anaerobic infection of the mouth or respiratory tract.[16]

After evaluating speech and breath, one identifies the characteristics of the cough. The therapist determines if cough is persistent, paroxysmal, or occasional; dry or productive; and finally notes the circumstances associated with the onset or cessation of the cough. Identification of

the characteristics of the cough as well as the conditions associated with it enables the therapist to interpret its significance (Table 12-3). Assessment of the voluntary cough permits evaluation of its constituent parts and its sequencing as well. For example, the cough of a surgical patient is often associated with a poor inspiratory effort followed by negligible abdominal muscle compression. These findings contribute to a "poor" nonproductive cough. They provide important clues for the treatment plan.

Sputum evaluation often follows cough assessment. The source of the sputum sample and the quantity of expectorate raised per day should be noted. Normally, persons are unaware of the 100 ml of mucus raised daily. Conscious awareness of any sputum production is significant. In addition to quantity, the color and consistency of any sputum raised should be evaluated. Table 12-4 presents some guidelines for evaluating sputum samples.

The inspection phase of the chest examination closes with a brief evaluation of the abdomen to detect any impedance to diaphragmatic descent such as ascites, pregnancy, or a paralytic ileus.

Table 12-4. Guidelines for evaluation of sputum samples	
Source	Upper airway
	Lower airway
Quantity	Milliliters or cupsful per day
Color	Red: Blood
	Rust: Pneumonia
	Purple: Neoplasm
	Yellow: Infected
	Green: Pus
	Pink: Pulmonary edema
	Flecked: Carbon particles
Consistency	Thin, watery
	Gritty
	Thick, mucous
	Layered

Further evaluation of the signs and symptoms discussed during inspection are presented during the second phase of the chest examination, auscultation.

Auscultation

Auscultation either confirms the findings of inspection or identifies areas of impaired ventilation or impaired secretion clearance. In addition, auscultation provides important feedback about the effectiveness of a treatment program in resolving pulmonary problems.

The stethoscope

Readiness for auscultation requires preparation of the equipment, the patient, and the therapist. A stethoscope is the only piece of equipment necessary for auscultation. The stethoscope should have binaural earpieces connected to a removable diaphragm by tubing of sufficient length to permit examination of the patient in either the supine or seated posture. Excess tubing creates extraneous noise. Improper tubing, for example, Foley catheter tubing, may not conduct sound adequately to permit valid and reliable evaluation of all sounds produced.

Two styles and several sizes of earpieces are available to assure comfortable fit. Earpieces may be made of hard, molded plastic or soft, flexible plastic. Directing the earpieces forward into the external auditory canals assures proper position. Occasional wiping with conventional alcohol maintains earpierce cleanliness.

Most authors agree that the diaphragm rather than the bell of the stethoscope most accurately evaluates lung sounds. Prolonged use or frequent cleaning may break the diaphragm. Although exposed x-ray film can temporarily substitute for a broken diaphragm, manufacturers suggest that sounds are less accurately assessed with this substitute and strongly urge their customers to order appropriate replacements.

Stethoscopes equipped with both diaphragm and bell have a valve that may be turned toward either the bell or diaphragm to listen.

Preparing the patient for auscultation involves teaching the patient the importance of deep breathing through the mouth and of reporting dizziness or undue fatigue.

Nomenclature

Before auscultating, the therapist must be aware that there is disagreement concerning the nomenclature pertaining to breath sounds. In 1974 the Joint Committee on Pulmonary Nomenclature (JCPN) of the American College of Cardiologists and the American Thoracic Society recommended the adoption of a standardized nomenclature for describing variations in the quantity and quality of breath sounds.[1]

The JCPN suggests interpreting the quantity of breath sounds as absent, decreased, normal, or bronchial. Normal, or vesicular, breath sounds rustle. The intensity of this rustling sound increases rapidly reaching a maximum shortly after inspiration is begun. This sound persists during the transition to expiration and disappears shortly thereafter.[3,18] Bronchial or tubular breath sounds are loud and harsh. Their initial intensity is maintained through both phases of ventilation but is conspicuously absent during the transition from inspiration to expiration. Decreased breath sounds are merely less intense than normal breath sounds.

The recommendations of the JCPN further suggest adopting a uniform nomenclature for interpreting the quality of abnormal breath sounds. The committee recognizes two categories of abnormal breath sounds: crackles or rales (French *râles*), and wheezes or rhonchi. Crackles are defined as nonmusical sounds whose further subclassification serves no useful purpose. Inspiratory crackles or rales may be heard throughout inspiration or only at its termination. Inspiratory crackles are common at the bases of the lungs in an erect subject. Crackles may represent the sudden opening of airways previously closed by gravity and therefore may be a sign of abnormal lung deflation.[14,21] Expiratory crackles or rales are rhythmical and nonrhythmical. Rhythmical crackles may indicate the reopening of previously closed airways. Nonrhythmical sounds are generally low pitched and occur throughout the ventilatory cycle. They may represent fluid in the large airways.

Rhonchi, or wheezes, are both continuous and musical. Rhonchi are probably produced by air flowing at high velocities through apposed airways. Their pitch varies directly with the velocity of airflow. Rhonchi may be monophonic or polyphonic. They may be heard in either inspiration or expiration. Inspiratory rhonchi unaccompanied by expiratory rhonchi are usually monophonic. These rarely occuring rhonchi suggest that the airway is rigid. Inspiratory rhonchi may be caused by stenosis produced, for example, by bronchospasm or foreign-body impaction. End-inspiratory rhonchi occur when the inspiratory traction

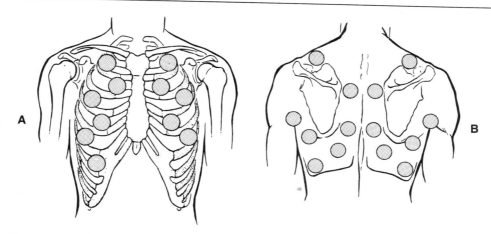

Fig. 12-2. One method of auscultating the chest. **A,** The chest. **B,** The back. (From Buckingham, E.B.: A primer of clinical diagnosis, ed. 2, New York, 1979, Harper & Row, Publishers, Inc.)

forces, initially insufficient to allow some airways to open, are suddenly overcome. This results in high-velocity air-flow across the still-apposed lumens producing a musical sound of short duration. Expiratory rhonchi are encountered more frequently. They tend to be low pitched and polyphonic and may reflect unstable airways that have collapsed. Expiratory rhonchi are associated with diffuse airway obstruction. Monophonic expiratory rhonchus occurs when only one airway reaches the point of collapse. The bagpipe sign describes a persistent monophonic wheeze occurring at end expiration.[7]

During auscultation the sounds produced by vocalization are also evaluated. The JCPN further recommends that all voice-generated sounds, whether whispered or spoken, be evaluated as decreased, normal, or increased. Bronchophony, egophony, and pectoriloquy are voice-generated sounds. They each reflect the clarity and intensity of sound transmission in the lung.

Other adventitious sounds detected during auscultation include rubs and crunches. Rubs are coarse, grating, leathery sounds occurring with either the ventilatory or the cardiac cycle. Pleural rubs are heard concurrently with the ventilatory cycle, whereas pericardial rubs are heard during the cardiac cycle. Rubs generally indicate inflammation.

Crunches are crackling sounds heard over the pericardium during systole. Detection of such crunches suggests the presence of air in the mediastinum, called mediastinal emphysema.

The examination

With the aforementioned concepts in mind, the therapist compares the quality, intensity, pitch, and distribution of the breath and voice sounds of homologous bronchopulmonary segments of the anterior, lateral, and posterior as-

pect of the chest. Fig. 12-2 presents one method of sequential auscultation of the chest. Following are the steps for this method of auscultation:

1. Instruct the patient to sit forward (where sitting is not possible, place patient in side-lying position).
2. Expose the anterior chest sufficiently to permit evaluation of the upper and middle lung zones.
3. Remind patient to breathe in and out through the mouth.
4. Evaluate at least one breath in each pulmonary segment comparing the intensity, pitch, and quality of the breath sounds heard between the right and left lungs.
5. Proceed craniocaudally in a systematic manner.
6. At the completion of the examination of the anterior chest, readjust draping to cover the anterior chest and expose the back (Fig. 12-2, B).
7. Proceed as in step A. Close gown. Indicate you are finished, and instruct the patient to relax.

Interpretation of the examination

Upon completion of auscultation the therapist must record and interpret the findings in a nomenclature acceptable to the institution. Table 12-5 presents some guidelines for the documentation and interpretation of breath sounds.

Normal breath and voice sounds in all bronchopulmonary segments suggests a normal examination. If inspection was also negative and the patient denied all pulmonary symptoms, one considers the chest examination normal, and further evaluation is deferred. If breath sounds are abnormal or if adventitious sounds are present, the examination is positive but at this point inconclusive. Generally, decreased or absent breath sounds or inspiratory crackles suggest reduced ventilation. Rales during both ventilatory

Table 12-5. Guidelines for the documentation and interpretation of auscultated sounds

Type of sound	Nomenclature	Interpretation
Breath sound	Normal	Normal, air-filled lung
	Decreased	Hyperinflation in chronic obstructive pulmonary disease Hypoinflation in acute lung disease, e.g., atelectasis, pneumothorax, pleural effusion
	Absent	Pleural effusion Pneumothorax Severe hyperinflation Obesity
	Bronchial	Consolidation Atelectasis with adjacent patent airway
	Crackles	Secretions, if biphasic Deflation, if monophasic
	Wheezes	Diffuse airway obstruction, if polyphonic Localized stenosis, if monophonic
Voice sound	Normal	Normal, air-filled lung
	Decreased	Atelectasis Pleural effusion Pneumothorax
	Increased	Consolidation Pulmonary fibrosis
Extrapulmonary adventitious sounds	Crunch	Mediastinal emphysema
	Pleural rub	Pleural inflammation or reaction
	Pericardial rub	Pericardial inflammation

Table 12-6. Conditions associated with shifts of the mediastinum

	Direction of shift	
Condition	Ipsilateral	Contralateral
Atelectasis	+	
Lobectomy	+	
Pneumonectomy	+	
Pleural effusion		+
Pneumothorax		+
Herniation of abdominal viscera		+

evaluation of the mediastinum and evaluation of chest motion. It detects signs of increased work of breathing by palpation of the scalene muscles and evaluation of the diaphragm. It provides information concerning the amount of air in the chest through evaluation of fremitus, and finally it further describes chest pain through palpation of the painful area.

Evaluation of the mediastinum

Fig. 12-3 presents one method of evaluating the mediastinal position by tracheal location. Following are the steps for this method of evaluating the mediastinum:

1. Place the patient in the sitting or recumbent position.
2. Flex the neck slightly to relax the sternocleidomastoid muscles.
3. Position the chin in the midline.
4. Place the top of the index finger in the suprasternal notch medial to the left sternoclavicular joint.
5. Push inward toward the cervical spine.
6. Repeat from step 4 to evaluate along the right sternoclavicular joint.

Another equally acceptable method consists in either palpating or auscultating the point of maximal impulse of the heart. This point is normally located in the fifth intercostal space in the midclavicular line (5 ICS MCL).

Shifts in the mediastinum occur when intrathoracic pressure or lung volume is disproportionate between the hemithoraces. The mediastinum shifts toward the affected side when lung volume is unilaterally decreased. The mediastinum shifts toward the unaffected side or contralaterally when pressure or volume is unilaterally high. Mediastinal shifts to the right because of pressure exerted by the ascending aorta may be seen in the elderly. Table 12-6 provides some examples of problems that result in mediastinal shifts. This evaluation informs the examiner of the consequences of any disproportionate expansion detected during inspection.

cycles suggest impaired secretion clearance. Monophonic, biphasic wheezing suggests stenosis or bronchial smooth-muscle spasm. Polyphonic wheezing suggests diffuse airway obstruction. The absence of crackles and wheezes does not, however, assure the absence of acute disease for some patients with chronic obstructive lung disease have lungs hyperinflated so much that adventitious sounds cannot be heard.

Palpation

In general, palpation refines the information gained previously. It further evaluates any thoracoabdominal asymmetry or asynchrony detected during inspection through

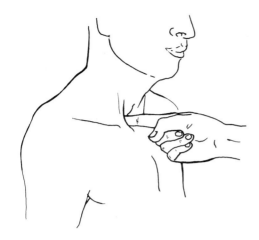

Fig. 12-3. Palpation of the mediastinum. (From Cherniack, R.M., and others: Respiration in health and disease, ed. 2, Philadelphia, 1972, W.B. Saunders Co.)

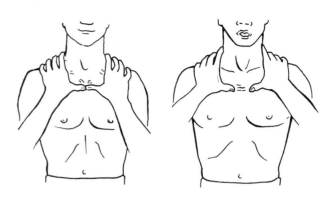

Fig. 12-4. Palpation of upper lobe motion. (From Cherniack, R.M., and others: Respiration in health and disease, ed. 2, Philadelphia, 1972, W.B. Saunders Co.)

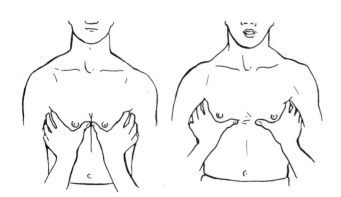

Fig. 12-5. Palpation of right middle and left lingula lobe motion. (From Cherniack, R.M., and others: Respiration in health and disease, ed. 2, Philadelphia, 1972, W.B. Saunders Co.)

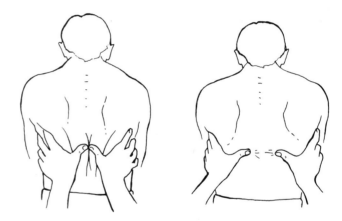

Fig. 12-6. Palpation of lower lobe motion. (From Cherniack, R.M., and others: Respiration in health and disease, ed. 2, Philadelphia, 1972, W.B. Saunders Co.)

Evaluation of chest motion

Palpation also permits comparative evaluation of upper, middle, and lower lobe expansion during quiet and deep breathing. In each case the therapist compares the timing and extent of movement of each hand. Lobar motion is considered normal when each hand moves the same amount at the same time. One method of evaluating chest motion appears in Figs. 12-4 to 12-6.[9]

Following are the steps for palpating the lobes:

Upper lobe motion

1. Face the patient.
2. Instruct the patient to turn his or her face away from yours.
3. Drape to expose the upper lobes of both lungs.
4. Place the palms of the hand firmly over the anterior aspect of the chest from the fourth rib cranially.
5. Hook the fingers over the upper trapezii.
6. Stretch the skin downward until the palms are in the infraclavicular areas.
7. Draw skin medially until the tips of the extended thumbs meet in the midline.
8. Relax the elbows and shoulders.

9. Instruct the patient to inspire.
10. Allow your hands to reflect the movement of the lobe of the lung underneath.

Right middle and left lingula lobe motion
1. Face the patient.
2. Instruct the patient to turn his or her face away from yours.
3. Drape to expose the right middle lobe or left lingula with males (may permit light clothing on females).
4. Hook fingers over posterior axillary folds.
5. Place palms firmly against chest wall.
6. Draw skin medially until extended thumbs meet in the midline.
7. Draw skin medially until the tips of the extended thumbs meet in the midline.
8. Relax the elbows and shoulders.
9. Instruct the patient to inspire.
10. Allow your hands to reflect the movement of the lobe of the lung underneath.

Lower lobe motion
1. Position client with his or her back toward you.
2. Drape to expose back.
3. Hook fingers around the anterior axillary fold.
4. Draw skin medially until extended thumbs meet at the midline.
5. Relax the elbows and shoulders.
6. Instruct the patient to inspire.
7. Allow your hands to reflect the movement of the lobe of the lung underneath.

This phase of palpation allows the therapist to localize any disproportionate expansion observed during inspection. For example, if inspection reveals asymmetrical chest expansion, palpation may not only localize the problem to the right upper lobe but also uncover a resultant ipsilateral shift of the mediastinum. Together these signs suggest that the problem is either a loss of right upper lobe lung volume or a volumetric gain in the left upper lobe.

Evaluation of fremitus

Fremitus is the vibration produced by either the voice or secretions and transmitted to the chest wall where it is detected by the hand, that is, tactile fremitus. Fig. 12-7 presents one method of evaluating fremitus.

Following are the steps for performing this method of palpating the fremitus:
1. Place palms lightly in symmetrical areas of the chest, or alternatively place the hypothenar eminence of each hand over symmetrical areas of the chest.
2. Instruct the patient to say "99."
3. Compare the intensity of the vibrations detected by each hand in the apical, anterior, lateral, and posterior areas of the chest.

Other methods for evaluation of fremitus are by substitution of the hypothenar eminences or fingertips for the palms.[6]

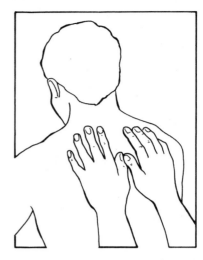

Fig. 12-7. Palpation of tactile fremitus.

The therapist evaluates fremitus by comparing the intensity of the vibrations detected by each hand during quiet breathing and speech. A normal evaluation occurs when equal and moderate vibrations are perceived during speech. Fremitus is abnormal when it is increased, decreased, or present during quiet breathing. Increased fremitus suggests a loss or decrease in ventilation. Decreased fremitus suggests a gain in the amount of air within the chest. "Rhonchal fremitus" is the term describing vibrations detected during quiet breathing.

Evaluation of fremitus permits the therapist to locate secretion problems or to define further the decreased breath sounds found during auscultation (Fig. 12-8).

Evaluation of scalene muscles

Palpation also permits specific evaluation of muscle activity identified grossly during inspection. One method of detecting activity of the scalene muscles is presented in Fig. 12-9.

Following are the steps for performing this method of palpating scalene muscle activity:
1. Position the patient with his or her back toward you.
2. Place thumbs over spinous process so that fingers reach around to the anterolateral aspects of the neck.
3. Evaluate the area during at least two resting respiratory cycles to detect activity of the scalenes.

Normally, the scalene muscles are inactive during quiet breathing. Palpation of scalene muscle activity indicates that the tertiary muscles of inspiration are functioning and therefore the work of breathing is increased.

Evaluation of chest pain

Palpation also permits assessment of chest pain. The results of this assessment determine the safety of continuing

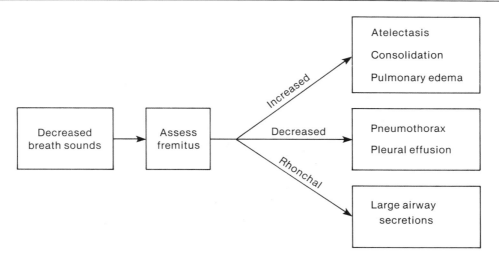

Fig. 12-8. Role of fremitus assessment in further defining the sign of decreased breath sounds. In the example, if breath sounds are decreased and fremitus is increased, alveolar airlessness is most likely caused by atelectasis, consolidation, or pulmonary edema. If both breath sounds and fremitus are decreased, pneumothorax or pleural effusion may be most likely. Rhonchal fremitus suggests large airway secretions.

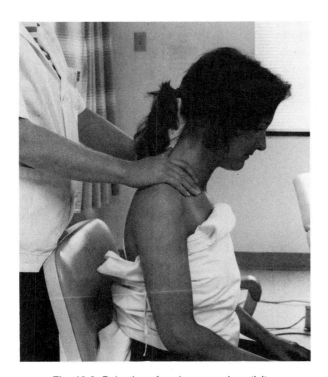

Fig. 12-9. Palpation of scalene muscle activity.

further evaluation or treatment. In addition, palpation facilitates identification of those characteristics associated with the pain for more complete and effective communication with the attending physician. One method of evaluating chest pain is illustrated in Fig. 12-10.

Following are the steps for performing this method of palpating the chest wall:

1. Request the patient to describe the type, extent, distribution, characteristics of onset, and characteristics of diminution of the pain.
2. Request the patient to point to the painful area. Expose the area and drape accordingly.
3. Starting distant from the painful area identified, palpate the ribs and intercostal spaces by pressing downward firmly.
4. Determine the effect of deep breathing and coughing on the pain.
5. Determine the effect of breath holding and ipsilateral arm motion on the pain.

Palpation provides information regarding the source of chest pain, which may be caused by musculoskeletal problems, coronary artery disease, malignancy, cervical disk or nerve root disease, thoracic outlet syndrome, shoulder-hand syndrome, herpes zoster, and pulmonary embolism.[19] Identifying the probable anatomical source of chest pain requires associating the type of pain and its stimulus (Table 12-7).

Matching the sensory distribution of the pain to the appropriate anatomical structure may also help the therapist identify the anatomical source of the pain. Table 12-8 pre-

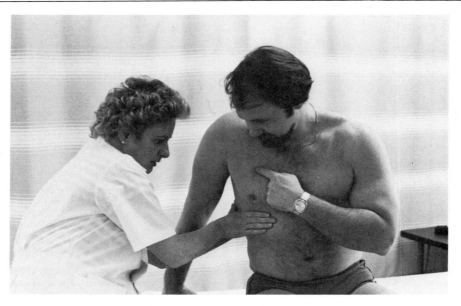

Fig. 12-10. Palpation of painful areas of the chest wall.

Table 12-7. Guidelines for identifying the probable source of chest pain*

Symptom characteristics	Effective stimulus	Anatomic source
Sharp Superficial Burning Precisely localized	Fine touch Pinprick Heat Cold	Skin
Dull or sharp Intermediate depth Aching Generally localized	Movement Deep pressure	Chest wall
Dull Deep Aching Diffuse, vaguely localized	Ischemia Distention Muscle spasm	Thoracic viscera

*Adapted from Edmeads, J., and Billings, R.F.: In Levine, D.L., editor: Chest pain: an integrated diagnostic approach, Philadelphia, 1977, Lea & Febiger.

Table 12-8. The segmental innervation of the chest and abdomen*

Cord segments	Structure
T1-T4	Mediastinal contents: heart, aorta, pulmonary vessels
T3-T8	Descending aorta
T4-T8	Esophagus
T3-T5	Trachea and bronchi
T7-T9	Upper abdominal viscera
C5-T1	Chest wall; apical parietal pleura
T2-T8	Remainder parietal; upper pericardial pleura
T6-T8	Peripheral diaphragm
C3-C5	Central diaphragm; lower pericardial pleura
T2-T10	Intercostal muscles; ribs
C5-T1	Pectoral muscles
C3-C4	Skin overlying shoulders
T1-T2	Upper arms, inner surface
T3-T8	Skin on chest wall

*Adapted from Edmeads, J., and Billings, R.F.: In Levine, D.L., editor: Chest pain: an integrated diagnostic approach, Philadelphia, 1977, Lea & Febiger.

sents the segmental innervation of the structures of the chest and abdomen. Fig. 12-11 illustrates the distribution of the cervical and thoracic dermatomes.

Exquisite localized tenderness accompanied by grating during the ventilatory cycle characterizes the pain associated with rib fracture. Subluxation of the costal cartilage generates local tenderness over the intercostal space and

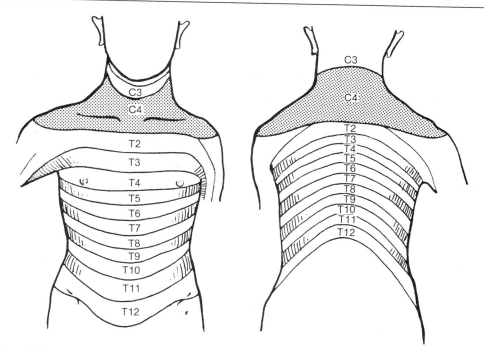

Fig. 12-11. Cervical and thoracic dermatomes. (From Cherniack, R.M., and others: Respiration in health and disease, ed. 2, Philadelphia, 1972, W.B. Saunders Co.)

suggests intercostal fibrositis. Pleuritic pain is sharp, usually localized and aggravated by breathing and coughing. Pleuritic pain is often associated with bacterial pneumonia, but when accompanied by hemoptysis and restricted activity, it may indicate pulmonary embolism.

Chest wall pain resulting from musculoskeletal problems is common. This pain is usually nonsegmental, localized to the anterior chest and aggravated by deep breathing. Chest wall pain is usually unrelated to exercise and differs from angina pectoris. Angina is a viselike, crushing, midline pain that radiates to the jaw and arm and is aggravated by any exercise. Chest pain from undiagnosed tumor is commonly associated with other pulmonary symptoms such as cough and hemoptysis. Disk and nerve root pain follow dermatomal distribution.

Evaluation of diaphragmatic movement

During this last phase of palpation, movement of the diaphragm is evaluated as normal or abnormal. Fig. 12-12 presents one method of evaluating diaphragmatic motion.

Following are the steps for performing this method of palpating diaphragmatic motion:

1. Direct the patient to assume the supine, flat position.
2. Drape to expose the costal margins of the anterior chest.
3. Stand beside the patient.
4. Place both hands lightly over the anterior chest wall

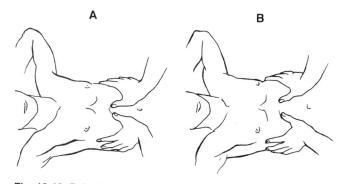

Fig. 12-12. Palpation of diaphragmatic motion. **A,** At rest. **B,** At the end of a normal inspiration. (From Cherniack, R.M., and others: Respiration in health and disease, ed. 2, Philadelphia, 1972, W.B. Saunders Co.)

with thumbs over costal margins so that the tips almost meet at the xyphoid.
5. Instruct the patient to take a deep breath.
6. Allow thumbs to move with the breath.

Motion of the normal diaphragm results in equal, upward motion of each costal margin. Inward motion of the costal margins during inspiration has been associated with a poor prognosis for the survival of patients with chronic obstructive lung disease.[15]

Percussion

Percussion is the fourth and final part of the chest examination. It enables the therapist to associate any symptoms and signs previously uncovered with changes in lung density. In addition, it enables the therapist to establish the borders of abnormally dense lung areas and normally occurring organs. Finally, percussion allows the therapist to evaluate the extent of diaphragmatic motion.

Evaluation of lung density

In assessment of lung density any of three sounds or notes may be produced.[1] A normal note is produced when resonant lung of normal density is percussed. A dull note is soft, brief, high pitched, and thudlike. It can be simulated by percussion of the liver or the thigh. A tympanic note, on the other hand, is loud, lengthy, low pitched, and hollow. It can be simulated by percussion of the empty stomach.

Normally dense, resonant lung can be found from the clavicle to the sixth rib anteriorly, the eighth rib laterally, and the tenth rib posteriorly (Fig. 12-13).

Fig. 12-14 presents the correct hand position for percussion. One technique for examining lung density is presented in Fig. 12-15.

Following are the steps for performing this technique for evaluating lung density:

1. Position the patient supine for evaluation of the density of the upper and middle lobes and sitting for evaluation of the lower lobes.
2. Expose the suspicious area and drape accordingly.
3. Lightly place the terminal phalanx of the middle finger of the nondominant hand between the ribs of the area to be evaluated.
4. Lift the rest of the middle finger as well as the others from the surface of the chest.
5. Using the wrist as the fulcrum, strike the middle finger of the nondominant hand in rapid succession, recoiling instantly after each blow.
6. Percuss the unaffected lungs before percussing the affected lung wherever possible, proceeding from apex to base, and right to left in 2-inch intervals.
7. Compare the pitch of the sound produced during percussion, as well as its intensity and duration.
8. Notice the limits of the abnormality both vertically and horizontally.

In a normal evaluation the resonance is similar across homologous lung segments. Moreover, to be normal, the resonance must extend throughout the anatomical limits of the lungs.

Abscesses, tumors, cysts, and areas of atelectasis and pneumonia produce changes in lung resonance. To be detected in this manner, however, the lesion must be at least 2 or 3 cm in diameter and no more than 5 cm in depth.[22]

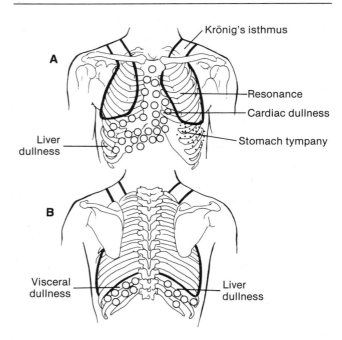

Fig. 12-13. Normal resonance pattern of the chest. **A,** Anteriorly. **B,** Posteriorly. *Circles,* Areas of dullness; *small dots,* tympanic areas.

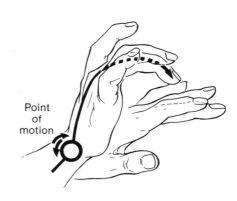

Fig. 12-14. The correct hand position for percussion. (From Buckingham, E.B.: A primer of clinical diagnosis, ed. 2, New York, 1979, Harper & Row, Publishers, Inc.)

Lung borders are affected by volume changes in either the abdomen or lungs. Abnormally high lung bases are associated with increased abdominal volume as is seen in pregnancy and ascites. Abnormally low lung bases are associated with increased lung volumes as is typical chronic obstructive lung disease.

Evaluation of diaphragmatic excursion

Percussion also quantifies diaphragmatic motion. Evaluation of diaphragmatic excursion requires that the patient

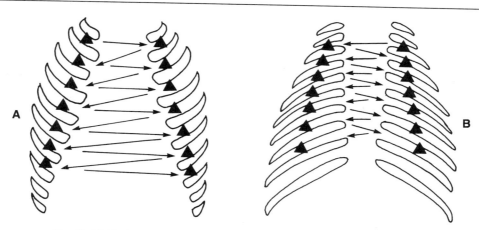

Fig. 12-15. Technique for evaluating lung density. **A,** Anteriorly. **B,** Posteriorly.

be seated. After exposing the posterior thorax, the therapist percusses the rib interspaces from apex to base. When dullness is encountered, the therapist stops percussing and asks the patient to exhale fully. The examiner uses percussion to track the motion of the diaphragms, marking the limit of their ascent. The patient then inspires fully. Once again diaphragmatic motion is tracked by percussion and the limit of descent is identified. Diaphragmatic excursion is the distance traveled between maximum inspiration and maximum expiration.

Diaphragmatic excursion is normally from 3 to 5 cm and is commonly decreased bilaterally in chronic obstructive lung disease.

LABORATORY EVALUATION

In addition to the chest examination, the complete clinical evaluation of a pulmonary patient requires interpretation of arterial blood gases, pulmonary function tests, chest radiographs, exercise tests, and bacteriological tests. Interpretation of arterial blood gases permits assessment of oxygenation, ventilation, and acid-base balance.

Arterial blood gases
Assessment of oxygenation

Oxygenation is adequate when the partial pressure of oxygen in the arterial blood, PaO_2, is sufficiently intense to bind most of the hemoglobin with a net quantity of oxygen fast enough to meet tissue needs.[12] Aberrations in PaO_2 reflect abnormal oxygenation also known as "hypoxemia." The therapist may suspect hypoxemia when inspection reveals any of the following clinical signs: pallor, cyanosis, skin coolness, or unexplained behavioral changes. A blood gas report of a low PaO_2, that is, less that 80 mm Hg, the lower limit of normal, may confirm clinical suspicions. In persons over 60 years of age lower oxygen tensions are acceptable, however if they do not exceed an additional 1 mm decrement in oxygen tension

Table 12-9. Examples of estimated arterial oxygen tensions in persons over 60 years of age*

Age (years)	PaO_2 (mm Hg)
60	80
65	75
70	70
75	65
80	60
85	55

*Adapted from Shapiro, B.A., and others: Clinical interpretation of blood gases, Chicago, 1977, Year Book Medical Publishers.

Table 12-10. Criteria for interpreting the severity of acute hypoxemia*

PaO_2 (mm Hg)	Interpretation
60-80	Mild hypoxemia
40-60	Moderate hypoxemia
<40	Severe hypoxemia

*Adapted from Shapiro, B.A., and others: Clinical interpretation of blood gases, Chicago, 1977, Year Book Medical Publishers.

for each year of age over 60.[24] Examples of some estimated arterial oxygen tensions in persons over 60 years of age in Table 12-9. Criteria for interpreting the magnitude of acute hypoxemia are presented in Table 12-10.

Regardless of its severity, arterial hypoxemia suggests abnormal cardiopulmonary function. Hypoxemia is often the earliest sign of atelectasis, embolism, or infiltrate. In response to hypoxemia, the body increases total ventilation. However, this increase in total ventilation is minimally effective at improving oxygenation because it may cause a simultaneous increase in oxygen consumption because of increased energy cost of breathing at higher rates. Persistent arterial hypoxemia may also increase cardiac output though this response may be more common in stagnant and anemic hypoxemia than in hypoxic hypoxemia.[12]

The most effective method of correcting arterial hypoxemia is oxygen therapy. Oxygen therapy is adequate when normal arterial oxygen tensions are approximated. Arterial hypoxemia is overcorrected when the arterial oxygen tension exceeds the upper limit of the normal range, 100 mm Hg.

Assessment of ventilation

Assessment of ventilation requires evaluation of alveolar ventilation, which is reflected by the arterial carbon dioxide tension, $PaCO_2$. Under normal or steady-state conditions, the relationship between carbon dioxide production and elimination results in $PaCO_2$ of 35 to 45 mm Hg. When the lungs eliminate carbon dioxide faster than the body produces it, the arterial carbon dioxide tension decreases. Conversely, when carbon dioxide production exceeds elimination, $PaCO_2$ increases.

Arterial pH is inversely related to the $PaCO_2$, and acute changes in $PaCO_2$ have a predictable impact on pH. Generally, in acute situations, every 10 mm Hg decrease in $PaCO_2$ increases pH by approximately 0.10 units. Conversely, a 20 mm Hg increase in $PaCO_2$ decreases arterial pH by approximately 0.10 units.[24]

The relationship between minute ventilation and alveolar ventilation additionally allows the therapist to predict how changes in the rate and depth of breathing, that is, the minute ventilation, will affect the $PaCO_2$ and therefore the pH. Table 12-11 illustrates these relationships.

Ventilation is abnormal when the $PaCO_2$ falls out of the normal range. Hyperventilation exists when the $PaCO_2$ is not only less than normal, but also less than the clinically tolerable lower limit of 30 mm Hg.[24] This condition is commonly called "respiratory alkalosis." If accompanied by a simultaneous increase in pH, it is called "respiratory alkalemia." Pain and pulmonary emboli often induce respiratory alkalemia. Hypoventilation exists when the $PaCO_2$ exceeds not only the upper range of normal but also the clinically tolerable limit of 50 mm Hg.[24] This condition is called "respiratory acidosis" and implies acute ventilatory failure. When pH is simultaneously decreased, it is called "respiratory acidemia." Acute airway obstruction may induce acute alveolar hypoventilation.

When hypoventilation or hyperventilation is not associated with acute changes in pH, that nonassociation may indicate that the condition is chronic. In chronic alveolar hyperventilation, for example, the pH falls within the range of normal. The reason is that the kidneys have had time to compensate for the increased elimination of carbon dioxide by increasing their elimination of bicarbonate,

Table 12-11. Approximate relationship among minute ventilation, alveolar ventilation ($PaCO_2$), and acid base status (pH)*

Minute ventilation	PaCO₂ (mm Hg)	pH
Normal	40	7.40
Twice normal	30	7.50
Four times normal	20	7.60

*Adapted from Shapiro, B.A., and others: Clinical interpretation of blood gases, Chicago, 1977, Year Book Medical Publishers.

HCO_3. Similarly, in chronic alveolar hypoventilation the normality of the pH is obtained by counteraction of the acid gain from ventilatory failure with reduced bicarbonate excretion by the kidneys. Chronic alveolar hypoventilation is most usually associated with chronic obstructive pulmonary disease.

Assessment of acid-base balance

A complete interpretation of arterial blood gases requires evaluation of the acid-base status in addition to evaluation of the respiratory status. The preceding section described the relationship between minute ventilation, $PaCO_2$, and pH. This section describes the additional impact of metabolic factors on pH.

Metabolic factors directly influence the pH because of the action of the kidneys on the serum bicarbonate. As the serum bicarbonate increases or decreases from its normal range of 22 to 28 milliequivalents per liter, mEq/L, the pH becomes more alkalotic or acidotic respectively. When the bicarbonate concentrate is less than 22 mEq/L, the pH is less than 7.30, and the alveolar ventilation ($PaCO_2$) is normal, the problem is uncompensated or primary metabolic acidemia.

When the serum bicarbonate concentration is more than 28 mEq/L, the pH is greater than 7.50, and the alveolar ventilation is normal, the acid-base problem is uncompensated or primary metabolic alkalemia. Table 12-12 presents some conditions known to be associated with primary acid-base disturbances.

Because the lungs compensate for metabolic disturbances, changes in alveolar ventilation often occur simultaneously with acid-base problems. For example, the lungs will hyperventilate to assist in correcting metabolic acidemia or hypoventilate to assist in correcting metabolic alkalemia.

Further analysis of blood gas aberrations is beyond the scope of this chapter. However, a description of the role of blood gases in cardiopulmonary physical therapy is essential. Clinicians use arterial blood gases to determine the need for physical therapy intervention, to generate appropriate therapeutic regimens, and to monitor treatment ef-

Table 12-12. Conditions associated with primary acid-base disturbances of metabolic origin

Acid-base disturbances	Clinical problem
Metabolic acidosis	Renal failure
	Ketoacidosis
	Lactic acidosis
	Shock
	Severe diarrhea
	Dehydration
	Poisoning: alcohol, paraldehyde
	Acetazolamide therapy (Diamox)
	Ammonium chloride
	Pancreatic drainage
	Ureterosigmoidostomy
Metabolic alkalosis	Hypokalemia
	Hypochloremia
	Vomiting
	Nasogastric suction
	Steroid therapy with Cushing's disease
	Aldosteronism

Table 12-13. Condition associated with abnormal ventilatory regulation*

Chronic hypoxemia
Encephalitis
Bulbar palsy
Cerebrovascular disease
Parkinson's disease
Anemia
Tabes dorsalis
Hypothyroidism
Carotid body endarterectomy
Familial dysautonomia
Idiopathic hypoventilation
Obesity
After adult respiratory distress syndrome
Athleticism
Narcotic addiction
Chronic obstructive pulmonary disease

*Adapted from Wanner, A.: In Sackner, M.A., editor: Diagnostic techniques in pulmonary disease, Part 1, New York, 1980, Marcel Dekker, Inc.

Table 12-14. The relationship between predicted ventilatory function and respiratory impairment*

Percent impairment	Percent predicted ventilatory function
0	>85
20-30	70-85
40-50	55-70
60-90	55

*Adapted from American Medical Association Committee on Rating of Mental and Physical Impairment: Guidelines to evaluation of permanent impairment: the respiratory system, J.A.M.A. **194:**919, 1965.

fectiveness. For example, postoperative atelectasis and mild hypoxemia, despite routine nursing care, warrants cardiopulmonary physical therapy. The effectiveness of this and any other therapy may be reflected by changes in arterial oxygen tension.

Pulmonary function tests

Pulmonary function tests (PFT's) evaluate ventilation by allowing assessment of factors that affect the movement of gas into and out of the lungs. PFT's serve as a guide to physicians for diagnosis of problems, formulating of treatment plans, and prognostication of outcomes. This same information helps the therapist identify realistic therapeutic goals and generate measureable therapeutic interventions appropriate to the pulmonary problems identified and the permanent respiratory impairment present.

Guidelines for interpretation of pulmonary function tests

Pulmonary function tests evaluate airway responsivity, ventilatory regulation, and ventilatory mechanics. Bronchial provocation tests document the response of the airway to the introduction of an allergen. In asthmatic patients a normal or nonallergic response is one where inhalation of potential allergen fails to induce a decrease in expiratory flow rate.

In assessment of ventilatory regulation PFT's allow examination of the effect of hypoxic or hypercapneic stimulation on the rate and depth of breathing. Normally, either type of stimulation will produce hyperventilation. Conditions that have been associated with regulatory dysfunction are listed in Table 12-13.

The assessment of ventilatory mechanics include the measurement of lung volumes and flow rates. It facilitates the categorization of all pulmonary problems into restrictive or obstructive patterns where decreases in lung volume are consistent with restrictive patterns and decreases in forced flow rates are consistent with obstructive patterns. Assessment of ventilatory mechanics also permits evaluation of the effectiveness of therapy, the general progression of the disease process, and the determination of pulmonary impairment. By administering tests of ventilatory mechanics before and immediately after the administration of a drug, one can objectively assess the effect of that drug. Serial tests, administered over several years, demonstrate the stability or instability of the disease process. Finally, by relating a patient's actual to predicted performance, the extent of permanent respiratory impairment can be estimated. Table 12-14 presents some guidelines recommended for this estimation.

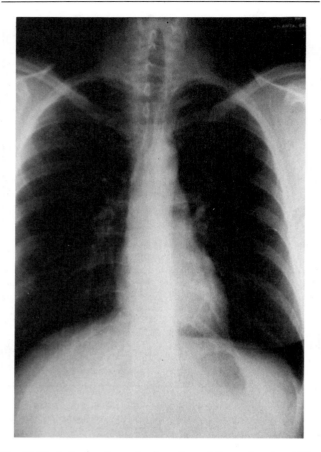

Fig. 12-16. A chest radiograph where the soft tissue, heart and hilar structures, diaphragms and lungs are all normal.

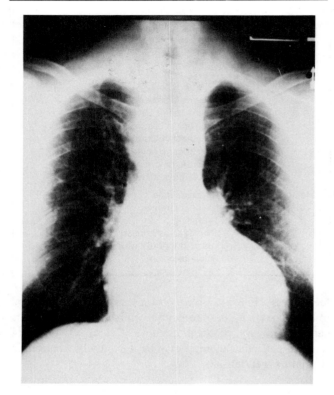

Fig. 12-17. A chest radiograph illustrating normal hilar configuration.

Chest radiography

Clinicians involved in pulmonary care frequently encounter chest radiographs taken to update the condition of their patients. The therapist uses this information to modify the physical therapy program to reflect any changes documented. Because resources for the interpretation of radiographs are not always readily available, physical therapists should develop a familiarity with the basic principles of radiology. An understanding of those principles can be acquired quickly through programmed learning.[11]

Evaluation of the chest radiograph

Interpretation of the chest radiograph involves evaluation of the bones, soft tissue, heart and hilar structures, the diaphragm, and the lungs.

First, one evaluates the dense radiopaque bony structures. Normally the ribs are uniformly dense, their margins are smooth and free of deformity, and they articulate with thoracic vertebrae only.

Next, the soft tissue of the neck and chest wall is evaluated. Here one examines the position of the trachea, car-

ina, and mainstem bronchi. Normally, the tracheal shadow falls in the midline, the carina overlies the fourth thoracic vertebra, and the right mainstem bronchus branches slightly higher and more vertically than the left mainstem bronchus. Fig. 12-16 presents a chest radiograph where the bones and soft-tissue structures are all normal.

Evaluation of the heart and hilar structures follows the soft-tissue evaluation. Normally the borders of the right atrium, superior vena cava, aortic knob, aortic appendage, and left ventricle are visible, and the left hilum is higher than the right. Fig. 12-17 illustrates the normal relationship between the left and the right hilum.

Next, one evaluates the diaphragms. Normally, both diaphragms are visible and well rounded. They lie at the level of the tenth rib posteriorly, and the right diaphragm is about one interspace higher than the left. Both costophrenic angles (CPA) should be clear and sharp. In Fig. 12-16 the diaphragms are also normal.

To summarize, interpretation of the chest radiograph requires a systematic evaluation of the structures contained within. Fig. 12-18 summarizes this evaluation by relating

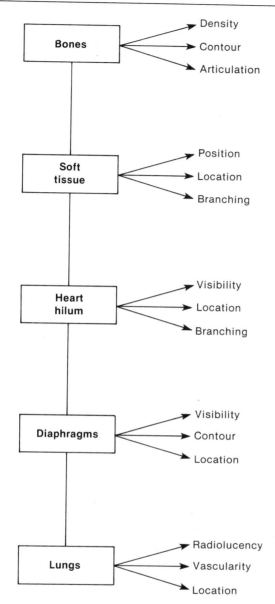

Fig. 12-18. Guideline for systematic evaluation of chest radiograph. Parallelograms identify structures, and arrows indicate criteria for each assessment.

Table 12-15. The radiographic signs of collapse associated with specific lobes of the lung*

Lobe	Radiographic sign
Left upper lobe	Elevated left hilum Ipsilateral tracheal shift Bowing of major fissures
Left lingula	Slight left hilar displacement downward obliteration of left heart border
Left lower lobe	Left hilar displacement downward Elevated left hemidiaphragm Major fissure displacement caudally Triangular opacity adjacent to spine
Right upper lobe	Elevated right hilum Ipsilateral tracheal shift Minor fissure displacement upward
Right middle lobe	Slight right hilar displacement down-ward Obliteration of right heart border Minor fissure displacement downward
Right lower lobe	Right hilar displacement downward Elevated right hemidiaphragm Major fissure displacement caudally Triangular radiopacity adjacent to spine

*Adapted from Felson, B., and others: Principles of chest roentgenology: a programmed text, Philadelphia, 1965, W.B. Saunders Co.

the structure evaluated to the criteria for its assessment. Abnormal chest radiographs require further examination to determine their impact on the physical therapy program.

Guidelines for interpretation of abnormal chest radiographs

Radiographic abnormalities commonly encountered in respiratory treatment include changes in the size, shape, or density of the lungs, heart, or diaphragms. Changes in the size of the lungs usually indicate a loss of lung volume

and may indicate atelectasis. Additional signs of atelectasis include any of the following: displacement of the transverse or oblique fissures, nonuniform radiolucency, vascular crowding, displacement of the hilum toward the collapsed side, tracheal or hemidiaphragmatic shift toward the collapsed side, or inequality of intercostal spaces. The radiological characteristics associated with atelectasis of specific lobes are summarized in Table 12-15. Fig. 12-19 illustrates right upper lobe collapse where the minor fissure is displaced upward and the right middle and lower lobes are more radiolucent than the left. Fig. 12-20 illustrates right lower lobe collapse where the major fissure is displaced caudally and the right hilum is displaced downwardly.

Changes in the normal shape of the heart or diaphragms usually indicate that a border, formed by the abutment of structures of unlike density, has been obliterated. The change in shape induced by the loss of a border is called the "silhouette sign." In the absence of signs of atelectasis, the silhouette sign is closely associated with lobar pneumonia. Table 12-16 associates some silhouette signs with the probable site of the responsible lobar pneumonia. Figs. 12-21 to 12-23 present chest radiographs with silhouette signs suggesting pneumonia of the right middle lobe, right lower lobe, and left lower lobe respectively.

Changes in lung density occur in pneumothorax. Addi-

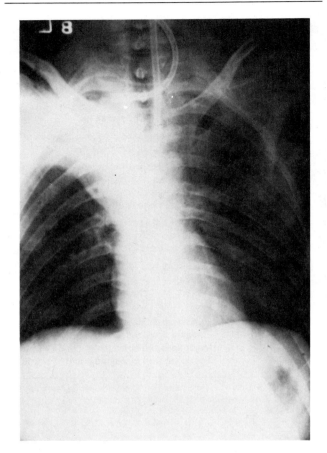

Fig. 12-19. A chest radiograph illustrating a right upper lobe collapse.

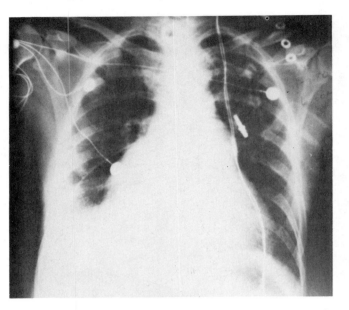

Fig. 12-20. A chest radiograph illustrating a right lower lobe collapse.

Table 12-16. The silhouette signs associated with various lobar pneumonias*

Silhouette sign	Site of pneumonia
Loss of aortic knob or appendage	Left upper lobe
Loss of left ventricular border	Left lingula
Loss of left hemidiaphragm	Left lower lobe
Loss of upper right heart border; loss of ascending aorta	Right upper lobe
Loss of most of right heart border	Right middle lobe
Loss of right hemidiaphragm	Right lower lobe

*Adapted from Felson, B., and others: Principles of chest roentgenology: a programmed text, Philadelphia, 1965, W.B. Saunders Co.

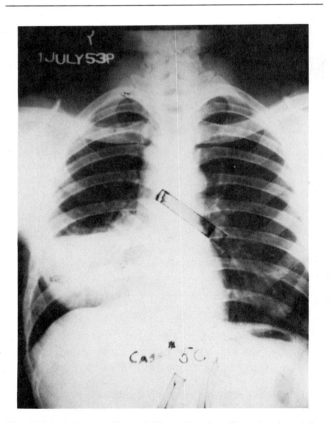

Fig. 12-21. A chest radiograph illustrating the silhouette sign at the right middle lobe.

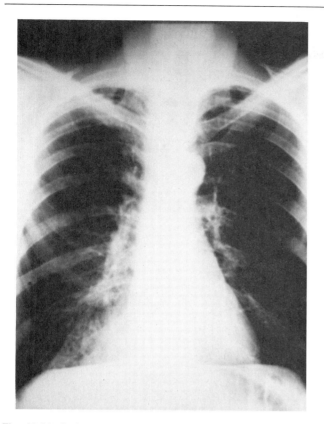

Fig. 12-22. A chest radiograph illustrating a silhouette sign at the right lower lobe.

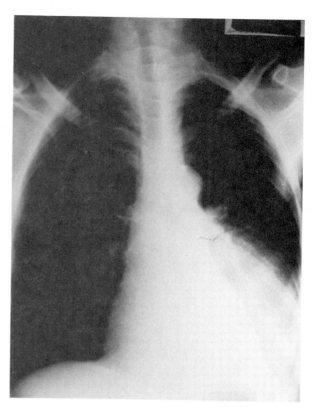

Fig. 12-23. A chest radiograph illustrating a silhouette sign at the left lower lobe.

tional radiographic signs of pneumothorax include failure of the vascular markings to extend to the chest wall and the existence of an extreme radiolucency between the termination of the vascular markings and the chest wall. Fig. 12-24 presents a radiograph of a left pneumothorax.

The radiological characteristics associated with pleural effusion also include failure of vascular markings to extend fully to the chest wall. However, pleural effusion also blunts the costophrenic angles and may be associated with the presence of an air-fluid level. Fig. 12-24 is also an example of a left pleural effusion.

In summary, interpretation of a chest radiograph helps the therapist differentiate atelectasis and pneumonia. In addition, the skill assists in locating problems and directing treatment anatomically.

Graded exercise tests

As in cardiac disease, exercise testing facilitates the diagnosis of disease, assists in quantifying disability, provides an appropriate basis for exercise prescription, and permits objective evaluation of general progress. In pa-

tients with lung disease, however, limited exercise tolerance may be the result of impaired oxygen transport, impaired pulmonary circulation, metabolic disturbances or disturbances of respiratory regulation, and the sensation and result of impaired cardiac function.[4]

The role of the physical therapist in exercise testing and prescription is described elsewhere in this book. Because the principles and practice of exercise testing and prescription do not differ greatly in pulmonary disease, the subject will not be discussed further here except to note that patients with known pulmonary hypertension or whose arterial oxygen tension is less than or equal to 50 mm Hg at rest generally require oxygen supplementation for both initial testing and subsequent training.[26]

Bacteriological and cytological tests

Therapists may be requested to obtain from their patients sputum samples for cytological or bacteriological evaluation. The validity and reliability of the results of these tests depends largely on the collection technique used when the specimen is obtained.

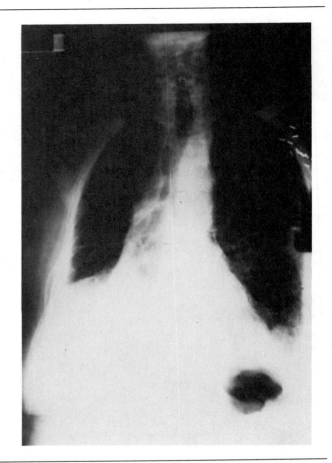

Fig. 12-24. A chest radiograph illustrating a left pneumothorax and a left pleural effusion.

Table 12-17. Characteristics of the infective process associated with the staining properties of sputa*

	Characteristics of infective process			
Staining property	**Type of infection**	**Probable infecting organism**	**Most probable type of pneumonia**	**Potential complications**
Gram positive	Primary	*Pneumococcus*	Lobar	Empyema, bacteremia, meningitis
	Secondary	*Staphylococcus*	Lobar	Empyema, bronchopleural fistula, pyopneumothorax, bacteremia
Gram negative	Secondary	*Klebsiella*	Upper lobes	Suppuration, destruction of lung tissue, bacteremia

*Adapted from Cherniack, R.M., and others: Respiration in health and disease, ed. 2, Philadelphia, 1972, W.B. Saunders Co.

Technique for specimen collection

Appropriate collection technique requires no preparation beyond assurance that the patient's nasopharynx and oropharynx are free of contaminents. The therapist therefore directs the patient to clear the nose and throat and rinse the mouth thoroughly before expectorating the sputum sample. The therapist then directs the patient to inhale maximally and cough forcefully, expectorating secretions into a sterile receptable. This process may be repeated as many as five times on five successive days for cytological evaluations. Bacteriological evaluations, however, require fewer samples.

Clinical significance of test results

Bacteriological evaluation of the sputum sample assures the institution of appropriate antibiotic therapy by allowing identification of the infecting organism and the antimicrobial drug to which the organism is sensitive. This knowledge along with the symptoms and signs of the disease provides valuable clues concerning the pneumonic process and its potential complications. Table 12-17 demonstrates how, if the staining property and type of infection are known, one can predict the probable infecting organism, type of pneumonia, and its potential complications.

Cytological evaluation contributes to the differential diagnosis. For example, the discovery of lymphocytes in the sputum supports the differential diagnosis of tuberculosis. The discovery of erythrocytes supports the diagnosis of pneumonia. The discovery of malignant cells supports the diagnosis of carcinoma.

REFERENCES

1. American College of Chest Physicians–American Thoracic Society, Joint Committee on Pulmonary Nomenclature: Pulmonary terms and symbols, Chest **67**:583, 1975.
2. American Medical Association, Committee on rating of mental and physical impairment: Guidelines to evaluation of permanent impairment: the respiratory system, J.A.M.A. **194**:919, 1965.
3. Banaszak, E.F., and others: Phonopneumography, Am. Rev. Resp. Dis. **107**:449, 1973.
4. Berglund, E.: Limiting factors during exercise in patients with lung disease, Bull. Europ. Physiopath. Resp. **15**:15, 1979.
5. Bouchier, I.A.D., and Morris, J.S.: Clinical skills, London, 1976, W.B. Saunders, Ltd.
6. Buckingham, E.B.: A primer of clinical diagnosis, ed. 2, New York, 1979, Harper & Row, Publishers.
7. Burnside, J.W.: Adams's physical diagnosis, ed. 15, Baltimore, 1974, The Williams & Wilkins Co.
8. Chamberlain, W.N., and Ogilvie, C.: Symptoms in clinical medicine: an introduction to medical diagnosis, ed. 9, Chicago, 1974, Year Book Medical Publishers.
9. Cherniack, R.M., and others: Respiration in health and disease, ed. 2, Philadelphia, 1972, W.B. Saunders Co.
10. Edmeads, J., and Billings, R.F.: Neurological and psychological aspects of chest pain. In Levine, D.L., editor: Chest pain: an integrated diagnostic approach, Philadelphia, 1977, Lea & Febiger.
11. Felson, B., and others: Principles of chest roentgenology: a programmed text, Philadelphia, 1965, W.B. Saunders Co.
12. Filley, G.F.: Acid base and blood gas regulation, Philadelphia, 1971, Lea & Febiger.
13. Fishman, A.P.: Pulmonary diseases and disorders, vol. 1, New York, 1980, McGraw-Hill Book Co.
14. Forgacs, P.: Lung sounds, Br. J. Dis. Chest **63**:1, 1969.
15. Gilbert, R., and others: Clinical value of observations of chest and abdominal motion in patients with pulmonary emphysema, Am. Rev. Resp. Dis. **119**:155, 1979.
16. Lorber, P.: ''Bad breath'': presenting manifestation of anaerobic infection, Am. Rev. Resp. Dis. **112**:875, 1975.
17. Malasanos, L., and others: Health assessment, St. Louis, 1977, The C.V. Mosby Co.
18. McKusick, V.A., and others: Acoustic basis of chest examination: studies made by means of sound spectography, Am. Rev. Resp. Dis. **72**:12, 1955.
19. Miller, R.D.: The medical history. In Sackner, M.A., editor: Diagnostic eachniques in pulmonary disease, Part 1, New York, 1980, Marcel Dekker, Inc.
20. Mills, P.: The significance of physical signs in medicine, London, 1971, H.K. Lewis & Co., Ltd.
21. Nath, A.R., and Capel, L.H.: Inspiratory crackles and mechanical events of breathing, Thorax **29**:695, 1974.
22. Prior, J.A., and Silberstein, J.S.: Physical diagnosis: the history and examination of the patient, ed. 5, St. Louis, 1977, The C.V. Mosby Co.
23. Roddie, I.C., and Wallace, W.F.M.: Physiology of disease, Chicago, 1975, Year Book Medical Publishers.
24. Shapiro, B.A., and others: Clinical interpretation of blood gases, Chicago, 1977, Year Book Medical Publishers.
25. Wanner, A.: Interpretation of pulmonary function tests. In Sackner, M.A., editor: Diagnostic techniques in pulmonary disease, Part 1, New York, 1980, Marcel Dekker, Inc.
26. Woolf, C.R.: A rehabilitation program for improving exercise tolerance of patients with chronic lung disease, Can. Med. Assoc. J. **106**:1289, 1972.

13

NANCY HUMBERSTONE

Respiratory treatment

Proper management of the patient with a pulmonary problem requires an understanding of both the physiological derangement present and the effectiveness of a given treatment within the context of that problem. Historically, the effects of various therapeutic measures were not validated by rigorous scientific evaluation.[98] As a result, therapists must be prepared to amend their thinking in response to the continual influx of new information.

This chapter reviews those therapeutic measures commonly administered by physical therapists to patients with pulmonary problems. The review both describes the therapeutic measure and discusses its effectiveness; that is, the treatment is described in relation to the therapeutic goal, and documentation is presented to support the desired therapeutic effects.

To facilitate the resolution of pulmonary problems, physical therapists administer treatments to improve ventilation and increase oxygenation, decrease oxygen consumption, improve secretion clearance, maximize exercise tolerance, and reduce pain.

Because changes in the amount of effective ventilation are best reflected in the arterial carbon dioxide tension, $PaCO_2$, the most accurate measure of the effectiveness of treatments given to improve ventilation is the $PaCO_2$. The most accurate measure of the effectiveness of treatments administered to improve oxygenation is the arterial oxygen tension, PaO_2. Oxygen consumption is difficult to measure directly at bedside. Consequently, the effectiveness of treatments administered to reduce oxygen consumption is assessed indirectly also as a reduction in the symptoms exhibited during the performance of a given activity.

In clinical medicine changes in secretion clearance are assessed directly by changes in the volume or the chemical composition of sputum expectorated, and indirectly by changes in the chest examination, the arterial blood gases, or the chest radiograph. The effectiveness of treatments administered to improve secretion clearance should therefore be assessed similarly.

Exercise tolerance is most accurately assessed by graded exercise tests. These tests therefore are the most accurate method of assessing the effectiveness of treatments administered to improve exercise tolerance.

Perceived pain depends not only on the quality, quantity, and duration of noxious stimulation, but also on one's emotional reaction. Therefore treatments administered to relieve pain, if effective, should modify at least one of these characteristics.

If the intent of physical therapy is to attain any of the therapeutic goals identified above, the effectiveness of the treatment must be measured by the suggested criteria. These criteria should serve as guidelines for interpreting the reviews of treatment effectiveness that follow.

TREATMENTS ADMINISTERED TO INCREASE VENTILATION AND OXYGENATION

Alveolar ventilation depends on the magnitude of tidal volume and dead space.[18] Decreases in alveolar ventilation are the result of decreased tidal ventilation or increased dead-space ventilation. Therefore physical therapy strategies administered to increase alveolar ventilation should increase tidal ventilation, decrease dead space ventilation, or both. If successful, these strategies should decrease the arterial carbon dioxide tension, $PaCO_2$.

Physical therapy strategies that increase alveolar ventilation should also increase alveolar oxygen tension, PaO_2. Therefore strategies that increase tidal ventilation or decrease dead space ventilation should also improve oxygenation. If successful, these strategies should increase PaO_2. Measures administered to increase ventilation and oxygenation include positioning techniques and breathing exercises.

Positioning techniques

Research using small numbers of patients indicates that postural changes may improve ventilation and oxygenation. In one study of five patients with adult respiratory

Table 13-1. Objectives and potential outcomes of position changes	
Therapeutic objective	Alleviate dyspnea
Physiological objective	Increase oxygenation
	Improve ventilation
Potential outcome	
Prone	Increased arterial oxygen tension in bilateral lung disease
Supine	Decreased arterial oxygen tension in bilateral lung disease
Lateral	Decreased arterial oxygen tension lying on the affected lung in unilateral lung disease
	Decreased arterial oxygen tension lying on the left side in bilateral lung disease
	Improved arterial oxygen tension lying on the unoperated side after thoracotomy (relative to supine)

distress syndrome the prone position improved arterial oxygen tension.[68] Another study of six patients with adult respiratory distress syndrome had similar results.[22] Improvement in PaO₂ occurred whenever patients were turned from supine to prone. Turning from prone to supine, however, decreased arterial oxygen tension in 12 of 14 trials.

Lateral decubitus positioning also affects ventilation and oxygenation. In 1974 Zack and colleagues studied the effect of decubitus postures on oxygenation.[104] Their results suggest that patients with unilateral lung disease lying with the affected lung dependent had significant decreases in oxygenation. When the disease process affected both lungs equally, turning onto the left side impaired oxygenation more than turning onto the right. Later research explored the effects of decubitus postures on oxygenation after thoracotomy.[78] The results of this later research suggest that lying on the unaffected side provides better oxygenation than supine-lying. A comparison of oxygenation when the surgical side was either dependent or uppermost was inconclusive. These results then indicate that changes in patient position may significantly alter a patient's arterial oxygenation. The objective and possible outcomes of changes in patient position are summarized in Table 13-1.

Breathing exercises

To achieve the goal of increased ventilation, therapists teach breathing exercises that presumably influence the rate, depth or distribution of ventilation or muscular activity associated with breathing. Although these exercises may affect the variables in the desired way, they may not necessarily result in improved alveolar ventilation or oxygenation.[98] Moreover, they may have unexpected negative effects. For example, maximal inspiratory efforts in asthmatics may result in bronchoconstriction.[26]

The breathing exercises administered to improve ventilation and oxygenation are diaphragmatic breathing, pursed lip breathing, segmental breathing, low-frequency breathing, and sustained maximal inspiration breathing exercises. The effectiveness of these breathing exercises in treating ventilatory problems of the acutely ill has been reviewed extensively elsewhere.[47,105] This review examines the effectiveness of each of these treatments.

Diaphragmatic breathing exercises

The diaphragm is the principle muscle of inspiration. Historically, when muscles other than the diaphragm assumed a role in inspiration, therapeutic efforts were directed toward restoring a more normal, diaphragmatic pattern of breathing. The return to diaphragmatic breathing was seen as relieving dyspnea.

Diaphragmatic breathing exercises allegedly enhance diaphragmatic descent during inspiration and diaphragmatic ascent during expiration. Diaphragmatic descent is assisted by directing the patient to protract the abdomen gradually during inhalation. One assists diaphragmatic ascent by directing the patient to allow the abdomen to retract gradually during exhalation or by directing the patient to contract the abdominal muscles actively during exhalation. Although the exact techniques used to teach diaphragmatic breathing vary, in principle they are similar. That is, they all indicate the patient should assume a comfortable position, usually sitting, before beginning. In addition, they recommend that the patient's hips and knees be flexed to relax the abdominal and hamstring muscles respectively. Diaphragmatic breathing exercises are then taught. One method of teaching diaphragmatic breathing exercises is described in Fig. 13-1.

Following are the steps for teaching diaphragmatic breathing exercises.

1. Place the patient's dominant hand over the mid–rectus abdominis area.
2. Place the patient's nondominant hand on the mid-sternal area.
3. Direct the patient to inhale slowly through the nose.
4. Instruct the patient to watch the dominant hand as inspiration continues.
5. Encourage the patient to direct the air so that the dominant hand gradually rises as inspiration continues.
6. Caution the patient to avoid excessive movement under the nondominant hand.

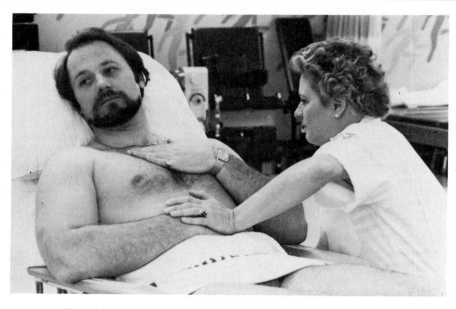

Fig. 13-1. One method of teaching diaphragmatic breathing exercises.

7. Apply firm counterpressure over the patient's dominant hand just before directing the patient to inhale.
8. Instruct the patient to inhale as you lessen your counterpressure as inspiration continues.
9. Practice the exercise until the patient no longer requires the manual assistance of the therapist to perform the exercise correctly.
10. Progress the level of difficulty by sequentially removing auditory, visual, and tactile cues. Thereafter, progress the exercise by practicing seated, standing, and walking.

Diaphragmatic breathing exercises have also been administered to eliminate accessory muscle activity and strengthen the diaphragm. In the past, increased diaphragmatic strength was assumed when increased resistance to abdominal protraction was tolerated. However, recent evidence[59] may indicate that in normals this assumption may be invalid. Moreover, the inference that strong diaphragms provide increased ventilation has not been validated.

The validation of diaphragmatic breathing exercises is the objective of much research. One study explored the effect of diaphragmatic breathing on the ventilation of erect normal subjects, two of whom were physical therapists and were presumably well-trained in the technique.[81] The results suggested that diaphragmatic breathing increased lower lung zone ventilation when certain subjects inhaled diaphragmatically after a maximal exhalation. This effect, however, was limited to the physical therapists, an indication that proper execution of diaphragmatic breathing may require substantial training. Later research repeated the above study using different instrumentation and an experimental group of subjects with chronic obstructive pulmonary disease.[75] The results of this subsequent study supported the previous findings of improved lower lung zone ventilation only in well-trained normals inhaling after a maximal expiration.

This failure of diaphragmatic breathing to alter the distribution of ventilation in chronically obstructed patients has been corroborated in subsequent studies.[10,30] However, its effect in normals continues to be unclear.[10,74]

The effect of diaphragmatic breathing on oxygenation is also unclear. An early study reported significant improvement in arterial oxygen saturation during diaphragmatic breathing in selected subjects.[60] Sinclair later failed to substantiate such improvement.[82] Recent evidence, however, suggests that diaphragmatic breathing may affect oxygenation indirectly by altering regional pulmonary perfusion.[37]

The effect of diaphragmatic breathing on the mobility of the diaphragm is also controversial. Early research reported no increase in diaphragmatic motion whether normals[96] or patients with chronic obstructive lung disease[82] breathed diaphragmatically. However, the recent report of improved diaphragmatic excursion in selected patients has fueled the controversy.[27]

Finally, and perhaps most notably, although the literature has frequently associated a reduced rate of postoperative pulmonary complications with breathing exercises,[89,93,100] the

Table 13-2. Objectives and potential outcomes of diaphragmatic breathing exercises	
Therapeutic objectives	Alleviate dyspnea
	Reduce the work of breathing
	Reduce the incidence of postoperative pulmonary complication
Physiological objectives	Improve ventilation
	Improve oxygenation
Potential outcomes	Eliminate accessory muscle activity
	Decrease respiratory rate
	Increase tidal ventilation
	Improve distribution of ventilation
	Decreased need for postoperative therapy

exact contribution of diaphragmatic breathing to this association has yet to be described.

Diaphragmatic breathing exercises will continue to be used as research progresses. The objectives and potential outcomes of diaphragmatic breathing are summarized in Table 13-2.

Pursed-lips breathing exercises

Pursed-lips breathing is another method suggested for improving ventilation and oxygenation. This breathing pattern, used spontaneously by patients with chronic obstructive lung disease, was first recommended for therapeutic use in this country around 1935.[77] Since that time the technique has enjoyed wide popularity for the relief of dyspnea.

Two methods of pursed-lips breathing have been reported. One method advocates passive expiration,[60] whereas the other recommends abdominal muscle contraction to prolong expiration.[99] Because abdominal muscle contraction and excessively prolonged expiration may promote airway collapse,[9,40] contemporary application of this technique usually encourage passive expiration only.

Following are the steps for one method of teaching pursed-lips breathing:

1. Position the patient comfortably.
2. Review the objectives of the exercise: relief of dyspnea of improved ventilation.
3. Explain that the benefit of the technique varies among subjects.
4. Explain why abdominal muscle contraction is undesirable.
5. Place your hand over the mid–rectus abdominis area to detect activity during expiration.
6. Direct the patient to inhale slowly.
7. Instruct the patient to purse the lips before exhalation.
8. Instruct the patient to relax the air out through the pursed lips and refrain from abdominal muscle contraction.
9. Direct the patient to stop exhaling when abdominal muscle activity is detected.
10. Progress the intensity of the exercise by substituting the patient's hand for yours, removing tactile cues, and having the patient perform the exercise while standing and exercising.

How this pattern of breathing affects ventilation and oxygenation has been the object of research since the mid-1960s. Thoman and colleagues studied the effect of pursed-lips breathing on ventilation in subjects with chronic obstructive lung disease.[88] They found that this breathing pattern significantly decreased the respiratory rate and increased the tidal volume. In addition, pursed-lips breathing improved alveolar ventilation, as measured by $PaCO_2$, and enhanced the ventilation of previously underventilated areas. The authors postulated that these beneficial effects might be attributed solely to slowing the respiratory rate.

Further research[39] was prompted by the clinical observation that, with pursed-lips breathing, the symptomatic relief of dysnea occurs before changes in ventilation. Ingram[39] explored the short-term effects of pursed-lips breathing, which was found to reduce both the peak and mean expiratory flow rates. Moreover, those who claim to benefit from this technique obtained a greater reduction in "nonelastic" resistance across the lung than those who denied such benefit.

A later study reported significant decreases in respiratory rate during simulated pursed-lips breathing.[1] However, these reductions in respiratory rate were associated with reduction of tidal volume. Moreover, these investigators could not substantiate improvements in alveolar ventilation or oxygenation despite a decrease in physiological dead space.

Mueller and colleagues reevaluated the effect of pursed lips breathing on ventilation and oxygenation.[62] Their results supported the previous findings of decreased respiratory rate and increased tidal volume. Moreover, they found that these effects persisted during exercise. At rest, pursed-lips breathing consistently improved alveolar ventilation and oxygenation, whereas during exercise the effect could not be sustained. Finally, like Ingram,[39] the authors reported a positive association between symptomatic relief and magnitude of objective improvement.

Later research evaluated the effect of pursed-lips breathing on exercise tolerance in patients with severe chronic obstructive pulmonary disease.[14] The study reported that pursed-lips breathing improved exercise tolerance without incurring increased metabolic cost; that is, it improved performance without increasing the respiratory rate or decreasing the PaO_2.

This discussion indicates that research has failed to explain fully the symptomatic benefits some patients ascribe

Table 13-3. The objectives and potential outcomes of pursed-lips breathing exercises

Therapeutic objectives	Alleviate dyspnea Increase tolerance
Physiological objectives	Increase alveolar ventilation Increase oxygenation Reduce the work of breathing
Potential outcomes	Elimination of accessory muscle activity Reduced respiratory rate Increased arterial oxygen tension Decreased carbon dioxide tension Increased exercise tolerance

to pursed-lips breathing. At the very least, pursed-lips breathing appears to reduce the respiratory rate without compromising minute ventilation. It may also improve ventilation and oxygenation not only during rest, but also during exercise.

Physical therapists should continue to teach pursed-lips breathing exercises to patients complaining of dyspnea. The objectives and potential outcomes of this therapy are presented in Table 13-3.

Segmental breathing exercises

Segmental breathing is the third exercise used to improve ventilation and oxygenation. This exercise, also known as localized breathing, presumes that inspired air can be directed to a predetermined area.[71]

This treatment has been recommended to prevent the accumulation of pleural fluid, to reduce the probability of atelectasis, to prevent the accumulation of tracheobronchial secretions, to decrease paradoxical breathing, to prevent the panic associated with uncontrolled breathing, and to improve chest mobility.

Although contemporary methods of administering segmental breathing exercises differ from those described earlier,[33] the rationale is essentially the same. Each technique uses manual counterpressure to encourage the expansion of a specific part of the lung.

Following are the steps for one method of administering segmental breathing exercises:

1. Identify the surface landmarks demarcating the affected area.
2. Place the therapist's hand or hands on the chest wall overlying the bronchopulmonary segment or segments requiring treatment.
3. Apply firm pressure to that area at the end of the patient's expiratory maneuver. (Pressure should be equal and bilateral across a median sternotomy incision.)
4. Instruct the patient to inspire deeply through his

mouth attempting to direct the inspired air toward your hand, saying "Breathe into my hand."
5. Reduce hand pressure as patient inspires. (At end inspiration, the instructor's hand should be applying no pressure on the chest.)
6. Instruct the patient to hold his breath for 2 to 3 seconds at the completion of inspiration.
7. Instruct the patient to exhale.
8. Repeat sequence until patient can execute breathing maneuver correctly.
9. Progress the exercises by instructing the patient to use his own hands or a belt to execute the program independently.

Evaluation of the effectiveness of segmental breathing begins with validation of its underlying premise that ventilation can be directed to a predetermined area.

In 1955, Campbell and Friend studied the effect of lateral basal expansion exercises on ventilation.[13] They concluded that this type of segmental breathing exercise failed to improve ventilation in patients with emphysema. A more recent study also failed to find any change in the distribution of ventilation when subjects with lung restriction breathed segmentally.[56]

Still another study reported that, in a population of patients at high risk for the development of pulmonary complications, those treated with segmental breathing exercises suffered fewer postoperative pulmonary complications than those not similarly treated.[93] Because more than one type of breathing exercise was administered, the exact contribution of segmental breathing to this beneficial effect is uncertain. This meager evidence may indicate that the effect of segmental breathing exercises on ventilation is still unclear.

The lack of objective evidence linking segmental breathing and the other therapeutic effects identified in the introduction signifies that these associations are still uncertain. The objectives and potential outcomes of segmental breathing are listed in Table 13-4.

Low-frequency breathing exercises

Several researchers[61,66,69] report that slow, deep breathing improves alveolar ventilation and oxygenation. However, the improvement reported seem to be sustained only as long as the low-rate breathing pattern is maintained. The objectives and potential outcomes of low-frequency breathing are presented in Table 13-5.

Sustained maximal breathing exercises

Breathing exercises where a maximal inspiration is sustained for about 3 seconds have also been associated with improved oxygenation.[97] The objectives and potential outcomes of sustained maximal inspiration breathing are also presented in Table 13-5.

Table 13-4. Objectives and potential outcomes of segmental breathing exercises

Therapeutic objective	Alleviate dyspnea
Physiological objectives	Increase alveolar ventilation Increase oxygenation
Potential outcomes	Prevent accumulation of pleural fluid Prevent accumulation of secretions Decrease paradoxical breathing Decrease "panic" Improve chest mobility

Table 13-5. Objectives and potential outcomes of both low-frequency and sustained maximal inspiration breathing

Therapeutic objective	Alleviate dyspnea
Physiological objectives	Increase ventilation Increase oxygenation
Potential outcome	Slow respiratory rate

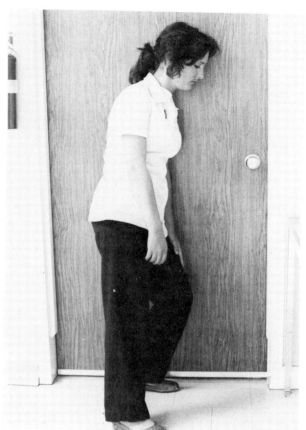

Fig. 13-2. The forward-leaning posture.

TREATMENTS ADMINISTERED TO REDUCE OXYGEN CONSUMPTION

The amount of oxygen consumed in a given activity depends, in part, on the type of work performed. To sustain work, the oxygen supply must meet the oxygen demand. When the supply of oxygen cannot be expanded to meet work requirements, continued work depends solely on the reduction of oxygen demand. Theoretically the physical therapist can reduce oxygen demand by eliminating all work extraneous to the desired activity.

Following are several strategies for reducing oxygen consumption[83]:
1. Reduce basal metabolic rate
2. Minimize unsupported body position
3. Minimize extrabasal body function
4. Minimize antigravity work
5. Minimize work to accelerate or decelerate body parts

Physical therapy treatments administered for this purpose reflect those strategies by adjustment of either the work of breathing or general body work.

Treatments administered to reduce the work of breathing
Breathing exercises

The work of breathing may be reduced by either reduction of the rate or depth of ventilation or by elimination of accessory muscle activity. Because the breathing exercises previously discussed have been associated with both the elimination of accessory muscle activity and the slowing of the respiratory rate, they are often incorporated in programs designed to reduce the work of breathing. Because they have been discussed previously, they are not discussed here.

Forward-leaning postures

The forward-leaning posture shown in Fig. 13-2 is also recommended to reduce the work of breathing.[5] In patients who are unable to tolerate functional walking in the forward-leaning posture, the use of a high walker, adapted to permit forward leaning, can eliminate sufficient work to permit the desired activity (Fig. 13-3).

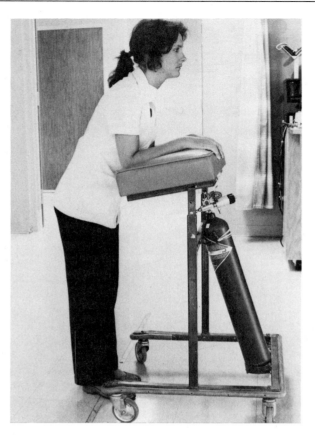

Fig. 13-3. A high-wheeled walker that permits assumption of the forward-leaning posture.

Table 13-6. Objectives and potential outcomes of treatment programs designed to reduce oxygen consumption	
Therapeutic objectives	Improve the quality of life by increasing functional activity tolerance
Physiological objectives	Reduce the oxygen consumption associated with a given activity
Potential outcomes	Elevate the dyspnea threshold for a given activity. Broaden the functional activity tolerance Improve the quality of life Elevate the functional activity tolerance

5. Proceed as above relaxing the major muscle groups of the extremities.
6. Monitor relaxation periodically by moving the limbs or palpating muscle tension.
7. Provide appropriate feedback or cues.
8. Contract then relax each accessory muscle of inspiration and expiration.
9. Direct the patient to inhale slowly and deeply and then ''relax'' the air out.
10. Monitor relaxation of specific respiratory muscles by palpation.
11. Progress the exercise by proceeding with self-monitoring. Advance the exercise as tolerated by requiring relaxation, while seated and standing and while ambulating.

This method incorporates the principles of relaxation as described by Benson[7] and Jacobsen.[42]

Work adjustment

Another method of reducing general body work uses the strategies presented previously to modify the conditions of work. For example, if a patient wants to perform all oral hygiene activities independently but becomes dyspneic standing at the sink, the therapist may eliminate the unnecessary work done to stand erect and direct the patient to assume the seated position.

Treatments administered to reduce oxygen consumption by a decrease in the work of breathing or general work, though apparently sound and widely practiced, require further objective evaluation. The objectives for and potential outcomes of treatments are summarized in Table 13-6.

TREATMENTS ADMINISTERED TO IMPROVE SECRETION CLEARANCE

Normal secretion clearance requires effective mucociliary transport and an effective cough. When either of these

The effectiveness of these treatments in reducing the work of breathing has not been substantiated objectively. It has been based largely on the observation that they eliminate accessory muscle activity. More objective evaluation is needed to update this observation.

Treatments administered to reduce general body work
Relaxation exercises

The treatment most frequently administered to reduce general body work is relaxation.

Following are the steps for one method of facilitating total body relaxation:
1. Minimize auditory and visual distractions.
2. Position the patient in a posture that provides maximum support and minimal discomfort.
3. Direct the patient to refrain from generating mental images.
4. Instruct the patient to contract and then relax the major muscle groups of the lower extremities proceeding distally to proximally.

mechanisms functions improperly, secretions accumulate. Early clinical signs of accumulated secretions include changes in body temperature, respiratory rate, pulse, blood pressure, and breath sounds.[2]

The consequences of accumulated secretions include inflammation, infection, airway obstruction, atelectasis, and pneumonia. Identification and treatment of the underlying cause of the excessive secretions may help reduce the likelihood of these consequences.

Secretion accumulation may be caused by either impaired mucociliary transport or impaired cough. Impairment of mucociliary transport results from altered ciliary function or altered mucus composition.

Following are some causes of impaired mucociliary transport:

1. Hypoxia or hyperoxia
2. Cuffed endotracheal tube
3. Dehydration
4. Electrolyte imbalance
5. Infection
6. Loss of ciliated respiratory epithelium
7. Inhalation of dry gases
8. Cigarette smoke
9. Anesthetics and analgesics
10. Pollutants

Impaired cough may result from pain, weakness, incoordination, or structural abnormality.

Following are some conditions that may be associated with impaired cough:

1. Coma
2. Neuromuscular disease
3. Debilitation
4. Morphological abnormality
   a. Bronchiectasis
   b. Bronchomegaly
   c. Tracheomalacia
   d. Endotracheal tube
   e. Obstruction by tumor
5. Pain
   a. Associated with trauma
   b. Associated with incisions

Impaired secretion clearance is best treated by administration of the therapy most appropriate to the problem identified. Postural drainage enhances mucociliary transport. Hydration, humidity, aerosol, and drug therapy alter mucus composition, ciliary motility, or bronchial caliber. Where indicated, these treatments should precede postural drainage because thickened secretions moving slowly through constricted bronchi may not respond readily, if at all, to gravity. Physical therapy treatments that are administered to improve an inadequate cough include positioning, forced expiration, pressure, manual ventilation, mechanical stimulation, and neuromuscular facilitation.

Improved secretion clearance may be inferred clinically from either increased volume or viscosity of secretions expectorated or from changes in the clinical signs associated with retained secretions.

Treatments administered to enhance mucociliary transport
Classical postural drainage

The technique of postural or bronchial drainage classically aligns the segmental bronchi with gravity.[87] In this way, theoretically, secretions accumulated in a bronchopulmonary segment move toward a central, segmental bronchus from which they can be removed by coughing and then easily expectorated. Figs. 13-4 to 13-6 illustrate the postural drainage positions for each bronchopulmonary segment of both lungs. Therapists commonly direct patients to maintain each posture for about 20 minutes and to cough before assuming a new position. If, however, the adjunctive techniques of percussion and vibration are administered simultaneously, the postures can be changed after approximately 2 minutes.

Modified postural drainage

Following are adverse physiological consequences that may be associated with postural drainage:

1. Increased intracranial pressure
2. Decreased arterial oxygen tension
3. Decreased cardiac output
4. Decreased forced expired volume in 1 second
5. Decreased specific airway conductance
6. Pulmonary hemorrhage

The following is an example of modified postural drainage. The positions described for the postural drainage of the lingula, right middle lobe, or lower lobes (except the superior segments) require elevation of the foot of the bed. This can increase venous return to the heart. In situations where this effect may be undesirable, the positions can be modified. One method of modifying these positions declines only the chest (Figs. 13-7 to 13-11.) A different modification is required immediately after open heart surgery, when the chest itself must remain horizontal. Modified postural drainage, in this example, uses classical patient positioning in the horizontal position only.[35]

Finally, the modification of classical postural drainage positions to avoid adverse effects may require the avoidance of certain positions altogether. For example, in severe unilateral lung disease prolonged lying on the affected lung may be unadvisable.[104]

In the past 20 years postural drainage has been widely discussed. Researchers have studied the effects of postural drainage alone[4,23,43,52,54,102] and when augmented by percussion,[25,43] vibration, or both.[12,36,67,86]

Postural drainage has been evaluated by determination of its effect on the transport of secretions in animals[15] and in humans.[6] Investigators have evaluated postural drainage

Text continued on p. 242.

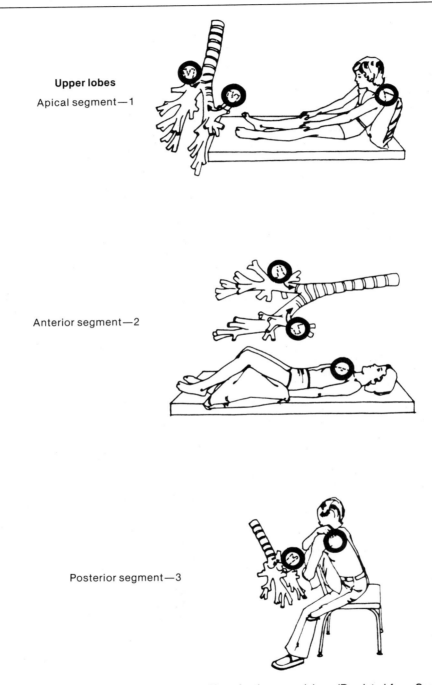

Upper lobes

Apical segment—1

Anterior segment—2

Posterior segment—3

Fig. 13-4. The classical postural drainage positions for the upper lobes. (Reprinted from Segmental bronchial drainage slide chart, New York, 1976, Breon Laboratories, Inc., with permission from the publisher.)

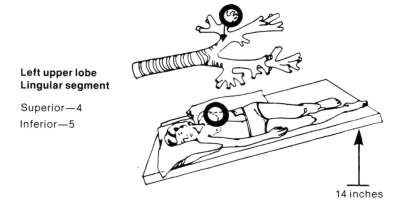

Left upper lobe
Lingular segment

Superior—4
Inferior—5

14 inches

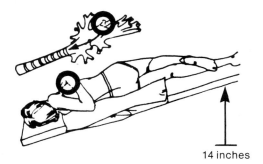

Right middle lobe

Lateral segment—4
Medial segment—5

14 inches

Fig. 13-5. The classical postural drainage positions for the right middle lobe and the left lingula. (Reprinted from Segmental bronchial drainage slide chart, New York, 1976, Breon Laboratories, Inc., with permission from the publisher.)

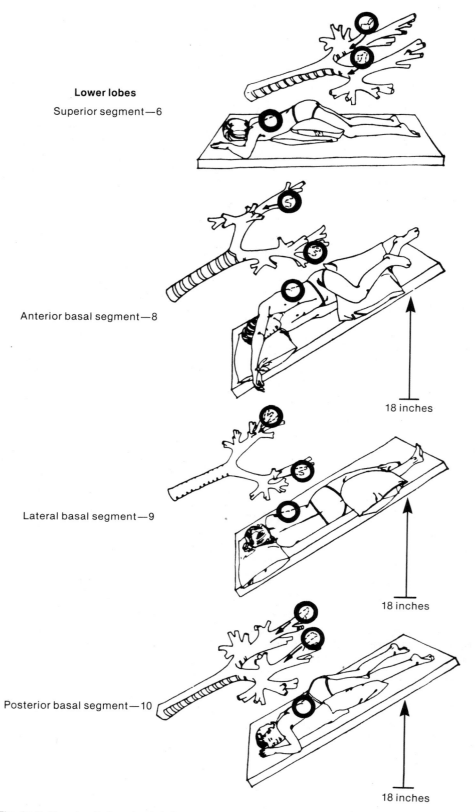

Lower lobes

Superior segment—6

Anterior basal segment—8

18 inches

Lateral basal segment—9

18 inches

Posterior basal segment—10

18 inches

Fig. 13-6. The classical postural drainage positions for the lower lobes. (Reprinted from Segmental bronchial drainage slide chart, New York, 1976, Breon Laboratories, Inc., with permission from the publisher.)

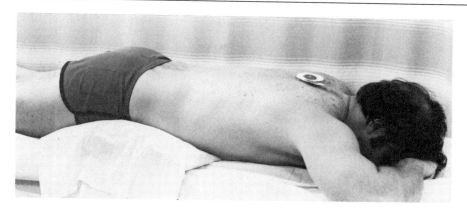

Fig. 13-7. Modification of the position classically recommended for postural drainage of the superior segment, both lower lobes.

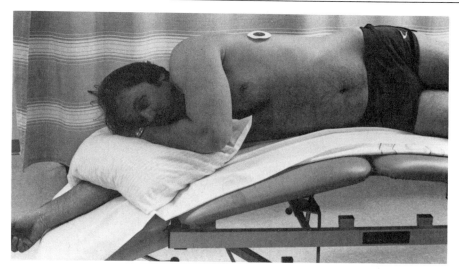

Fig. 13-8. Modification of the position classically recommended for postural drainage of the left lateral basal segment.

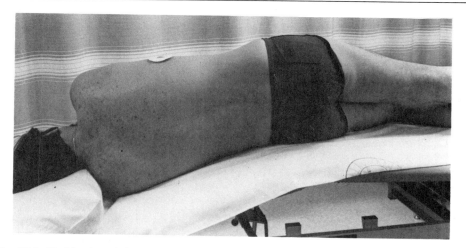

Fig. 13-9. Modification of the position classically recommended for postural drainage of the right lateral basal segment.

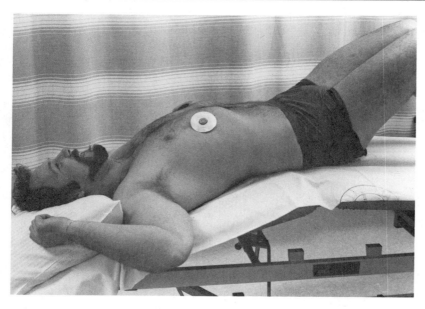

Fig. 13-10. Modification of the position classically recommended for postural drainage of the anterior basal segments, both lower lobes.

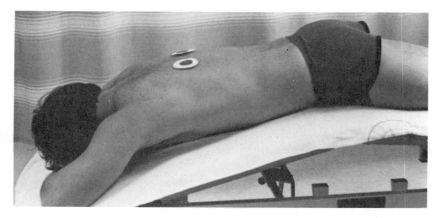

Fig. 13-11. Modification of the position classically recommended for drainage of both posterior basal segments.

in neonates,[25] children,[52] and adults. In addition, investigations have explored both the long-[23] and short-term[19] effects of drainage. The effects of drainage have been evaluated in a variety of conditions including chronic bronchitis,[12] cystic fibrosis,[54,73,86] respiratory failure,[55] and pneumonia.[29,52] Researchers have evaluated the effects of postural drainage in patients with acute exacerbations of chronic disease[4,12,65] and in patients with stable chronic disease.[6,23,67]

Postural drainage has been evaluated according to its effects on sputum volume[4,54] and composition.[67] Its effects on the resolution of fever[4,23,29,52] and abnormal chest radiographs,[29,52,53,55] has been examined. Its effect on forced expired volume in 1 second,[12,35,43,65] maximum midexpiratory flow rate,[86] and peak expiratory flow rates[86] has also been assessed. Other investigators have evaluated postural drainage according to its effect on lung compliance,[101] specific airway conductance,[65] vital capacity,[65] functional residual capacity,[65] and oxygenation.[4,55,65,102] Finally, researchers have assessed postural drainage by evaluating its effect on the rate of postoperative pulmonary complications[53] and the length of hospital stay.[29]

Because these studies contain few similarities in experimental design, it is difficult to draw firm conclusions. At the very least, it appears that postural drainage augmented by percussion and vibration enhances mucociliary transport better than postural drainage alone. However, percussion may be associated with an immediate bronchospasm that lasts for 20 to 30 minutes. The onset of this transient bronchospasm may be avoided by the administration of bronchodilators before treatment.[12] Postural drainage may be more effective when secretions are abundant, rather than when they are scanty.[63]

Although fatal hemoptysis has been associated with postural drainage administered to patients with end-stage disease,[32,84] the nature and frequency of this association is unclear. Physical therapists should exercise caution when administering postural drainage to any patient with end-stage disease until this association is clarified. Caution is also recommended when administering therapeutic percussion.

Following are some cardiovascular conditions in which caution in the application of therapeutic percussion has been recommended:

1. Chest-wall pain
2. Unstable angina
3. Hemodynamic lability
4. Low platelet count
5. Anticoagulation therapy
6. Unstable or potentially lethal dysrhythmias

Following are some orthopaedic conditions in which caution in the application of therapeutic percussion has been recommended:

1. Osteoporosis
2. Prolonged steroid therapy
3. Costal chondritis
4. Osteomyelitis
5. Osteogenesis imperfecta
6. Spinal fusion
7. Rib fracture or flail chest

Following are some pulmonary conditions in which caution in the application of therapeutic percussion has been recommended:

1. Bronchospasm
2. Hemoptysis
3. Severe dyspnea
4. Untreated lung abscess
5. Pneumothorax
6. Immediately after chest-tube removal
7. Pneumonia or other infectious process
8. Pulmonary embolus

Following are some oncological conditions in which caution in the application of therapeutic percussion has been recommended:

1. Cancer metastatic to ribs or spine
2. Carcinoma in the bronchus
3. Resectable tumor

Following are miscellaneous conditions in which caution in the application of therapeutic percussion has been recommended:

1. Recent skin grafts
2. Burns

3. Open thoracic wounds
4. Skin infection thorax
5. Subcutaneous emphysema head and back
6. Immediately after cataract surgery

The basis for the above recommendations is not always clear.

In summary, the conventional role of postural drainage and its adjunctive techniques of percussion and vibration is to facilitate clearance of excess secretions. This role is summarized in Table 13-7.

Treatments administered to enhance cough

A reflex cough has four phases: irritation, inspiration, compression, and expulsion. A voluntary cough does not require the first phase. To be effective either cough must generate enough force to clear secretions from the first through the seventh generation bronchi.[51] Decreased secretion clearance results when any phase of coughing fails to meet this objective.

The physical therapist improves an impaired cough by counseling the patient in proper cough technique and by administering treatments that either increase the volume inspired, augment the compression force generated, or elicit a cough reflex. Proper cough technique requires that the patient inspire maximally, close the glottis, "bear down" by tightening the abdominal, perineal, gluteal, and shoulder depressor muscles, and cough no more than two times during each expulsive, expiratory phase. Proper cough technique after surgery additionally requires the application of incisional splinting.

Table 13-7. Objectives and potential outcomes of postural drainage and adjunctive techniques like percussion and vibration

Therapeutic objective	Eliminate retained secretions
Physiological objective	Improve mucociliary transport
Potential outcomes	Increase volume expectorated
	Improve clearance of thick secretions
	Reduce airway resistance
	Improve compliance
	Reduce the work of breathing
	Improve oxygenation and ventilation
	Reduce the rate of postoperative pulmonary complications
	Shorten hospitalization

Following are techniques used to improve cough:

1. Positioning

   Sitting in the forward leaning posture with the neck flexed, the arms supported, and the feet firmly planted on the floor promotes effective coughing.[48] (Fig. 13-12).

2. Forced expiration or huffing

   Forceful rapid expiration, or huffing, may induce a reflex cough by stimulation of the pulmonary mechanoreceptors.

3. Pressure

   Pressure applied to the extrathoracic trachea may elicit a reflex cough. Pressure applied to the mid–rectus abdominis area after inspiration may improve cough effectiveness if the pressure is suddenly released. Pressure applied along the lower costal borders during exhalation may also improve the effectiveness of an impaired cough.

4. Manual ventilation

   The high inspiratory flow rates produced by the forceful compression of a manual ventilator may stimulate the pulmonary mechanoreceptors and produce a reflex cough.[16]

5. Mechanical stimulation and suctioning

   The direct application of mechanical stimulation to the airway may also induce a reflex cough.[91] However, if this direct stimulation fails to clear the airway, endotracheal suctioning is advisable.

6. Neuromuscular facilitation

   The intermittent application of ice for 3 to 5 seconds along the paraspinal areas of the thoracic spine may also improve cough.[34] Because the application of ice has been associated with hypertension, candidates for this technique should be chosen carefully and monitored closely.

Although the literature describes several techniques to improve cough few have scientifically evaluated cough effectiveness. Langlands compared the effectiveness of voluntary and reflex coughs to forced expiration in a small population of normals and patients with chronic bronchitis.[50] The results of this study suggest that nonvoluntary or reflex coughs are stronger than those voluntarily produced. Therefore patients who suffer from the following complications of cough should be taught controlled voluntary coughing or forced expiration to minimize the risk of complications:

1. Serum creatinine phosphokinase elevation
2. Rectus abdominis muscle rupture
3. Rib fracture
4. Pneumothorax
5. Fainting
6. Bradycardia
7. Vascular rupture
8. Heart block
9. Headache
10. Exhaustion

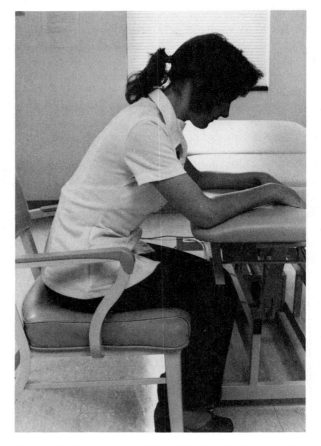

Fig. 13-12. The recommended position for effective coughing.

11. Vomiting
12. Urinary incontinence
13. Wound dehiscence
14. Sore throat

The physical therapy techniques administered to improve cough play a central role in the current practice of chest physical therapy. The objectives and potential outcomes of these techniques are summarized in Table 13-8.

TREATMENTS ADMINISTERED TO IMPROVE EXERCISE TOLERANCE

Patients with pulmonary disease often experience dyspnea on exertion. To avoid dyspnea, they may refrain from participating in any activity that precipitates this unpleasant sensation. The continued avoidance of activity may further decrease their exercise tolerance and, in turn, lower their dyspnea threshold. The physical therapy strategy most commonly used to break this vicious cycle is exercise. Because during exercise the work of breathing in patients with pulmonary disease may constitute a major portion of their oxygen consumption, the work load administered must be applied judiciously.[45]

Table 13-8. Objectives and potential outcomes of treatments administered to improve cough

Therapeutic objective	Eliminate excessive retained secretions
Physiological objective	Increase the positive pressure developed during cough
Potential outcomes	Expectoration Production of a reflex cough Avoidance of cough complication Elimination of the clinical signs of retained secretions Appearance of a cough complication

Exercise programs

Physical therapy programs administered to increase exercise tolerance vary widely. They may be formal, based on a strictly derived exercise prescription, or informal, started from an arbitrary point and progressed according to a patient's tolerance.[25] They may require special equipment like treadmills[69] or bicycle ergometers or merely require enough space to permit obstacle-free walking.[44] Participants may have either subacute pulmonary disease or chronic pulmonary disease of varying severity. Exercise may be administered while the patient breaths room air or supplemental oxygen.[8,11,95,108] Finally, completion of the programs may require several days, several months,[58] or as long as a year.[31]

Before administering any exercise program, the therapist must evaluate the medical history and the most recent clinical and laboratory data to identify any contraindications or precautions for exercise as well as any indications for oxygen supplementation during exercise. The absolute and relative contraindications for any exercise testing are published elsewhere[3] and are not discussed here.

Following are some indications for oxygen-supplemented exercise[103]:

1. Right heart failure, cor pulmonale
2. Resting PaO_2 at 50 mm Hg
3. Inability to tolerate exercise while breathing room air

When patients tolerate 30 consecutive minutes of oxygen-supplemented exercise, one may progress the program by decreasing the level of supplemental oxygen.

Preparation for any exercise program also requires determining the degree of monitoring sophistication indicated to preserve the patient's safety. No formal guidelines that establish the monitoring requirements for informal exercise programs have been published; this determination must be made according to individual circumstances.

Final preparation for any exercise program requires that the therapist and patient identify a mutually acceptable goal for the program, develop a plan for periodically evaluating progress toward that goal, and, in asthmatics, discuss how the risk of exercise-induced bronchospasm[46] will be managed.

Bicycle ergometry to improve exercise tolerance is one technique that has been used successfully in formal programs. In addition to the preparation described above, a formal bicycle ergometry program requires a previously administered graded exercise test to determine the load at which the patient achieves his or her maximum oxygen consumption.

Following are steps for one method of implementing a conditioning program using bicycle ergometry:

1. Review the conditioning program with the patient. The review should include the purpose, expectations (risk to benefit), cost, and duration of the program (three 25-minute sessions per week for 4 weeks)
2. Differentiate between the roles and responsibilities of the patient and therapist.
3. Attach the ECG electrodes and obtain a base-line strip.
4. Measure the blood pressure with the patient lying supine and sitting.
5. Identify the symptoms that the patient should report immediately.
6. Direct the patient to mount the bicycle.
7. Cycle at 25 to 40 watts for 5 minutes to warm up.
8. Cycle at 75% of the previously determined maximum load.
9. Monitor the ECG every 5 minutes during the first exercise session and any time the patient reports chest pain, severe dyspnea, nausea, or palpitations.
10. Terminate the exercise in the presence of the following:
    Premature ventricular contractions in pairs, runs, or increasing frequency
    Atrial dysrhythmias: tachycardia, fibrillation, flutter
    Heart block, second or third degree
    Angina
    ST-segment changes of greater than or equal to 2 mm in either direction
    Persistent heart rate or blood pressure decline
    Elevation of diastolic pressure of more than 20 mm Hg greater than resting or more than 100 mm Hg.
    Dyspnea, nausea, fatigue, dizziness, headache, blurred vision
    Intolerable musculoskeletal pain
    Heart rate greater than target
    Patient pallor, diaphoresis

Physical therapy can improve exercise tolerance. Six weeks of submaximal bicycle ergometry increased symptom-limited maximal oxygen uptake in 11 patients with moderate to severe chronic obstructive lung disease.[20] Vyas and colleagues[94] supported this finding, and Pierce[69] from his research suggests that objective improvement is

Table 13-9. Objectives and potential outcomes of conditioning exercise administered to improve exercise tolerance

Therapeutic objectives	Heighten dyspnea threshold
	Increase exercise tolerance
Physiological objective	Improved maximum oxygen uptake
Potential outcomes	Increase walking, stepping, and cycling distance
	Precipitation of dyspnea
	Inability to progress breathing room air

not specific to the bicycle but can also be associated with the treadmill.

The objectives and potential outcomes of physical therapy administered to improve tolerance are summarized in Table 13-9.

TREATMENTS ADMINISTERED TO REDUCE PAIN

Pain is perceived when tissue is being damaged. The intensity of that perception depends on both the extent of tissue damage and the emotional reaction to the injury. To be effective, treatments administered to reduce pain must influence either the pathophysiological or the psychological aspects of pain, or both.

Physical therapists use many strategies in the management of pain. This section describes the use of one particular strategy, transcutaneous electrical nerve stimulation, TENS, in the management of the pain most frequently encountered in patients treated by chest physical therapists, postoperative pain.

Transcutaneous electrical nerve stimulation (TENS)

TENS is a nonaddictive, noninvasive, non–habit forming, relatively low-cost alternative to pharmaceutically induced analgesia for the management of acute postoperative pain. TENS may be most effective when a stimulator with dual-channel, variable voltage capability[76] applies a controlled, constant-current pulse[57] by way of crossed-channel electrodes.[76]

Ideally the electrodes would be placed close to the painful area[38,80] with the anode placed distally.[70] Because there may be some delay before the onset of the analgesia,[70] the stimulation would begin in the operating room and, ideally, be maintained constantly for at least 24[80] to 48[76] hours.

Because the only adverse effect associated with TENS is skin irritation,[49] any patient experiencing incisional pain may be a candidate for TENS. However, those who require electrocardiographic monitoring or artificial cardiac pacing should be offered other alternatives because TENS may affect monitoring feedback or pacemaker function.

Following is one method of administering TENS postoperatively:

1. Connect the leads to each channel according to the color code indicated on both the leads and the receptacles.
2. Abrade the electrode site with an alcohol scrub and then dry with gauze or clean toweling to lower skin resistance.
3. Coat electrodes with electrode gel.
4. Attach electrodes in crosswise fashion paraincisionally so that one electrode of channel 1 is, for example, on the upper right margin of the incision and the second electrode of channel 1 is on the lower left margin of the incision.
5. Secure electrodes in place with hypoallergenic tape.
6. Inform the patient and the nurse that you are initiating the treatment.
7. Instruct the patient to report any sensation perceived.
8. Ensure that the pulse rate is high.
9. Turn on the unit very slowly by increasing the intensity in both channels.
10. Continue to increase the intensity of both channels until a sensation is reported.
11. Increase the intensity slowly in both channels until the paraincisional area is numb; ideally this intensity should be below contractile threshold and be comfortable.
12. Maintain stimulation at this level until the treatment is ended.
13. Slowly decrease the intensity of stimulation in both channels until the unit is off.

Several investigators have evaluated the effectiveness of TENS in relieving postoperative pain. In their study of acute pain after thoracic and abdominal surgery, Hymes and others[38] reported a lower incidence of atelectasis in patients treated with TENS than in similar control groups. In addition, they discovered that TENS therapy was associated with reduced intensive care unit days and for the most part decreased length of hospital stay. In another study of acute pain, Vander Ark and McGrath[92] reported a high incidence of pain relief, 77%, associated with TENS. They additionally noted that in one third of the thoracic surgery patients studied TENS lessened incisional pain by 50% and, as a result, obviated the need for analgesics. The finding that TENS decreased the narcotic requirement of postoperative patients was later supported by Rosenberg, Curtis, and Bourke,[72] whose research additionally uncovered a patient preference for TENS-induced analgesia over that which was pharmaceutically induced. This study could not, however, associate a lower incidence of atelectasis with TENS.

The impact of TENS on variables other than pain has

Table 13-10. Objectives for and potential outcomes of the postoperative application of transcutaneous electrical nerve stimulation (TENS)

Therapeutic objective	Pain relief
Physiological objective	Physiological pain relief
Potential outcome	Decreased narcotic requirement No change of lower incidence of atelectasis Increased forced vital capacity Skin irritation ECG or pacemaker interference

also been explored. Noting that patients often associated a feeling of warmth with TENS, Dooley and Kasprak[21] examined the relationship between TENS and blood flow. Their results indicate that application of TENS along the peripheral nerve does not increase peripheral blood flow but TENS applied more centrally does. The effect of TENS on pulmonary function has also been explored. Stratton and Smith[85] reported higher forced vital capacities in patients treated with TENS after open thoracotomy than in a comparable control group.

This discussion suggests that TENS is an appropriate therapeutic strategy for postoperative pain management. The objectives and potential outcomes of this treatment are summarized in Table 13-10.

REFERENCES

1. Abboud, R.T., and others: The effect of added expiratory obstruction on gas exchange in chronic airways obstruction, Br. J. Dis. Chest 62:36, 1968.
2. Amborn, S.A.: Clinical signs associated with the amount of tracheobronchial secretions, Nurs. Res. 25:121, 1976.
3. American College of Sports Medicine: Guidelines for graded exercise testing and exercise prescription, ed. 2, Philadelphia, 1980, Lea & Febiger.
4. Anthonisen, P., and others: The value of lung physiotherapy in the treatment of acute exacerbations in chronic bronchitis, Acta Med. Scand. 175:715, 1964.
5. Barach, A.L.: Chronic obstructive lung disease: postural relief of dyspnea, Arch. Phys. Med. Rehabil. 55:404, 1974.
6. Bateman, J.R.M., and others: Regional lung clearance of excessive secretions during chest physiotherapy in patients with stable chronic airways obstruction, Lancet 1(811):294, 1979.
7. Benson, H.: The relaxation response, New York, 1975, William Morrow & Co., Inc.
8. Block, A.J., and others: Chronic oxygen therapy treatment of chronic obstructive pulmonary disease at sea level, Chest 65:279, 1974.
9. Bolton, J.H., and others: The rationale and results of breathing exercises in asthma, Med. J. Aust. 2:675, 1956.
10. Brach, B.B., and others: Xenon washout patterns during diaphragmatic breathing: studies in normal subjects and patients with chronic obstructive pulmonary disease, Chest 71:735, 1977.
11. Bradley, B.L., and others: Oxygen assisted exercise in chronic obstructive lung disease, Am. Rev. Respir. Dis. 118:239, 1978.
12. Campbell, A.H., and others: The effect of chest physiotherapy upon the FEV1 in chronic bronchitis, Med. J. Aust. 1:33, 1975.
13. Campbell, E.J.M., and Friend, J.: Action of breathing exercise in pulmonary emphysema, Lancet 19:325, 1955.
14. Casiari, R.J., and others: Effects of breathing retraining in patients with chronic obstructive pulmonary disease, Chest 79:393, 1981.
15. Chopra, S.K., and others: Effects of hydration and physical therapy on tracheal transport velocity, Am. Rev. Respir. Dis. 115:1009, 1977.
16. Clement, A.J., and Hubsch, S.C.: Chest physiotherapy by the "bag squeezing" method: a guide to technique, Physiotherapy 54:355, 1968.
17. Cochrane, G.M., and others: Effects of sputum on pulmonary function, Br. Med. J. 2:1181, 1977.
18. Comroe, J.H.: Physiology of respiration, ed. 2, Chicago, 1974, Year Book Medical Publishers.
19. Connors, A.F., and others: Chest physical therapy: the immediate effect on oxygenation in acutely ill patients, Chest 78:559, 1980.
20. Degre, S., and others: Hemodynamic responses to physical training in patients with chronic lung disease, Am. Rev. Respir. Dis. 110:395, 1974.
21. Dooley, D.M., and Kasprak, M.: Modification of blood flow to the extremities by electrical stimulation of the nervous system, South. Med. J. 69:1309, 1976.
22. Douglas, W.W.: Improved oxygenation in patients with acute respiratory failure: the prone position, Am. Rev. Respir. Dis. 115:559, 1977.
23. Emirgil, C., and others: A study of the long term effect of therapy in chronic obstructive pulmonary disease, Am. J. Med. 47:367, 1969.
24. Fergus, LC., and Cordasco, E.M.: Pulmonary rehabilitation of the patient with COPD, Postgrad. Med. 62:282, 1978.
25. Finer, N.N., and Boyd, J.: Chest physiotherapy in the neonate: a controlled study, Pediatrics 61:141, 1977.
26. Gayrard, P., and others: Bronchoconstrictor effects of a deep inspiration in patients with asthma, Am. Rev. Respir. Dis. 111:433, 1975.
27. Gimenez, M., and others: Exercise training with oxygen supply and directed breathing in patients with chronic airway obstruction, Respiration 37:157, 1979.
28. Gormenzano, J., and Branthwaite, M.A.: Effects of physiotherapy during intermittent positive pressure ventilation, Anaesthesia 27:258, 1972.
29. Graham, W.C.B., and Bradley, D.A.: Efficacy of chest physiotherapy and intermittent positive pressure breathing in the resolution of pneumonia, N. Engl. J. Med. 299:624, 1978.
30. Grimby, G., and others: Effects of abdominal breathing on the distribution of ventilation in lung disease, Clin. Sci. Molec. Med. 148:193, 1975.
31. Guthrie, A.G., and Petty, T.L.: Improved exercise tolerance in patients with chronic airway obstruction, Phys. Ther. 50:335, 1970.
32. Hammon, W.E., and Martin, R.J.: Fatal pulmonary hemorrhage associated with chest physical therapy, Phys. Ther. 59:1247, 1979.
33. Harmony, W.: Segmental breathing, Phys. Ther. Rev. 36:106, 1956.
34. Hedges, J., and Bridges, C.J.: Stimulation of the cough reflex, Am. J. Nurs. 68:347, 1968.
35. Howell, S., and Hill, J.D.: Chest physical therapy procedures in open heart surgery, Phys. Ther. 58:1205, 1978.
36. Huber, A.W., and others: Effect of chest physiotherapy on asthmatic children, J. Allergy Clin. Immunol. 53:109, 1974.
37. Hughes, R.C.: Does abdominal breathing effect regional gas exchange? Chest 76:258, 1979.

38. Hymes, A.C., and others: Acute pain control by electrostimulation: a preliminary report, Adv. Neurol. **4:**761, 1974.

39. Ingram, R.H., Jr., and Schilder, D.P.: Effect of pursed lips expiration on the pulmonary pressure-flow relationship in obstructive lung disease, Am. Rev. Respir. Dis. **96:**381, 1967.

40. Innocenti, D.M.: Breathing exercises in the treatment of emphysema, Physiotherapy **52:**437, 1966.

41. Irwin, R.S., and others: Cough: a comprehensive review, Arch. Intern. Med. **137:**1189, 1977.

42. Jacobsen, E.: Progressive relaxation, Chicago, 1938, University of Chicago Press.

43. Kang, B., and others: Evaluation of postural drainage with percussion in chronic obstructive lung disease, J. Allergy Clin. Immunol. **53:**109, 1974.

44. Kass, I., and Rubin, H.: Chest physiotherapy for chronic obstructive pulmonary disease, Postgrad. Med. **48:**145, 1970.

45. Keens, T.G.: Exercise training programs for pediatric patients with chronic lung disease, Pediatr. Clin. North Am. **26:**517, 1979.

46. Khan, A.U., and Olson, D.L.: Physical therapy and exercise induced bronchospasm, Phys. Ther. **55:**878, 1975.

47. Kigin, C.M.: Chest physical therapy for the postoperative or traumatic injury patient, Phys. Ther. **61:**1724, 1981.

48. Lagerson, J.: The cough: its effectiveness depends on you, Respir. Care **18:**434, 1973.

49. Lampe, G.N.: Introduction to the use of transcutaneous electrical nerve stimulation devices, Phys. Ther. **58:**1450, 1978.

50. Langlands, J.: The dynamics of cough in health and in chronic bronchitis, Thorax **22:**88, 1967.

51. Leith, E.E.: Cough. In Hislop, H., and Sanger, J.O., editors: Chest disorders in children, New York, 1968, American Physical Therapy Association.

52. Levine, A.: Chest physical therapy for children with pneumonia, J. Am. Osteopath. Assoc. **78:**101, 1978.

53. Lord, G.M., and others: A clinical, radiologic and physiologic evaluation of chest therapy, J. Maine Med. Assoc. **60:**143, 1972.

54. Lorin, M.I., and Denning, C.R.: Evaluation of postural drainage by measurement of sputum volume and consistency, Am. J. Phys. Med. **50:**215, 1971.

55. Mackenzie, C.F., and others: Chest physiotherapy: the effect on arterial oxygenation, Anesth. Analg. **57:**28, 1978.

56. Martin, D.J., and others: Chest physiotherapy and the distribution of ventilation, Chest **69:**174, 1976.

57. Mason, C.P.: Testing of electrical transcutaneous stimulators for suppressing pain, Bull. Prosthet. Res. **25:**38, 1976.

58. McGavin, C.R., and others: Physical rehabilitation for the chronic bronchitic: results of a controlled trial of exercises in the home, Thorax **32:**307, 1977.

59. Merrick, J., and Axen, K.: Inspiratory muscle function following abdominal weight exercises in healthy subjects, Phys. Ther. **61:**651, 1981.

60. Miller, W.P.: A physiological evaluation of the effects of diaphragmatic breathing training in patients with chronic pulmonary emphysema, Am. J. Med. **17:**471, 1954.

61. Motley, J.C.: The effects of slow deep breathing on the blood gas exchange in emphysema, Am. Rev. Respir. Dis. **88:**484, 1963.

62. Mueller, R.E., and others: Ventilation and arterial blood gas changes induced by pursed lips breathing, J. Appl. Physiol. **28:**784, 1970.

63. Murray, J.F.: The ketchup-bottle method, N. Engl. J. Med. **300:**1155, 1979.

64. Newhouse, M.T.: Factors affecting sputum clearance, Proceedings of the Thoracic Society, Thorax **28:**262, 1973.

65. Newton, D.A., and Stephenson, A.L.: Effect of physiotherapy on pulmonary function, Lancet 2(8083):228, July 1978.

66. Paul, G., and others: Some effects of slowing respiration rate in chronic emphysema and bronchitis, J. Appl. Physiol. **21:**877, 1966.

67. Pham, Q.T., and others: Respiratory function and the rheological status of bronchial secretions collected by spontaneous expectoration and after physiotherapy, Bull. Pathophysiol. Resp. **9:**295, 1973.

68. Piehl, M.A., and Brown, R.S.: Use of extreme position changes in acute respiratory failure, Crit. Care Med. **4:**13, 1976.

69. Pierce, A.K., and others: Responses to exercise training in patients with emphysema, Arch. Intern. Med. **173:**28, 1964.

70. Pike, P.M.G.: Transcutaneous electrical stimulation: its use in the management of post-operative pain, Anaesthesia **33:**165, 1978.

71. Reed, J.M.W.: Localized breathing exercises in surgical chest conditions, Br. J. Phys. Med. **16:**111, 1953.

75. Rosenberg, M., and others: Transcutaneous electrical nerve stimulation for the relief of post-operative pain, Pain **5:**129, 1978.

73. Rossman, C.M., and others: Effect of chest physiotherapy on the removal of mucus in patients with cystic fibrosis, Am. Rev. Respir. Dis. **126:**131, 1982.

74. Roussos, C.S., and others: Voluntary factors influencing the distribution of inspired gas, Am. Rev. Respir. Dis. **116:**457, 1977.

75. Sackner, M.A., and others: Distribution of ventilation during diaphragmatic breathing in obstructive lung disease, Am. Rev. Respir. Dis. **109:**331, 1974.

76. Santiesteban, A.M., and Sanders, B.R.: Establishing a postsurgical TENS program, Phys. Ther. **60:**789, 1980.

77. Schutz, K.: Muscular exercise in the treatment of bronchial asthma, N.Y. J. Med. **55:**635, 1935.

78. Seaton, D., and others: Effect of body position on gas exchange after thoracotomy, Thorax **34:**518, 1979.

79. Sergysels, R., and others: Low frequency breathing at rest and during exercise in severe chronic obstructive bronchitis, Thorax **34:**536, 1979.

80. Shealy, C.M., and Maurer, D.: Transcutaneous electrical stimulation for control of pain, Surg. Neurol. **2:**45, 1974.

81. Shearer, M.C., and others: Lung ventilation during diaphragmatic breathing, Phys. Ther. **52:**139, 1972.

82. Sinclair, J.D.: The effect of breathing exercises in pulmonary emphysema, Thorax **10:**246, 1955.

83. Slonim, N.B., and Hamilton, L.H.: Respiratory physiology, ed. 2, St. Louis, 1971, The C.V. Mosby Co.

84. Stern, R.C., and others: Treatment and prognosis of massive hemoptysis in cystic fibrosis, Am. Rev. Respir. Dis. **117:**825, 1978.

85. Stratton, S.A., and Smith, M.M.: Postoperative thoracotomy: effect of transcutaneous electrical nerve stimulation on forced vital capacity, Phys. Ther. **60:**45, 1980.

86. Tecklin, J.S., and Holsclaw, D.S.: Evaluation of bronchial drainage in patients with cystic fibrosis, Phys. Ther. **55:**1081, 1975.

87. Thacker, W.E.: Postural drainage and respiratory control, London, 1947, Lloyd-Luke.

88. Thoman, R.L., and others: The efficacy of pursed-lips breathing in patients with chronic obstructive pulmonary disease, Am. Rev. Respir. Dis. **93:**100, 1966.

89. Thoren, L.: Post-operative pulmonary complication: observations on their prevention by means of physiotherapy, Acta Chir. Scand. **107:**193, 1954.

90. Tyler, M.L.: Complications of positioning and chest physiotherapy, Respir. Care **27:**458, 1982.

91. Ungvarski, P.: Mechanical stimulation of coughing, Am. J. Nurs. **71:**2358, 1971.

92. Vander Ark, G.D., and McGrath, K.A.: Transcutaneous electrical stimulation in the treatment of postoperative pain, Am. J. Surg. **130:**338, 1975.

93. Vraciu, J.K., and Vraciu, R.A.: Effectiveness of breathing exercises in preventing pulmonary complications following open heart surgery, Phys. Ther. **57:**1367, 1977.

94. Vyas, M.N., and others: Response to exercise in patients with chronic airway obstruction: effects of exercise training, Am. Rev. Respir. Dis. **103:**390, 1977.

95. Vyas, M.N., and others: Response to exercise in patients with chronic airway obstruction. II. Effects of breathing 40 per cent oxygen, Am. Rev. Respir. Dis. **103:**401, 1971.

96. Wade, O.L.: Movements of the thoracic cage and diaphragm in respiration, J. Physiol. **124:**193, 1954.

97. Ward, R.J., and others: An evaluation of postoperative respiratory maneuvers, Surg. Gynecol. Obstet. **123:**51, 1976.

98. Watts, N.: Improvement of breathing patterns. In Hislop, H.E., and Sanger, J.O., editors: Chest disorders in children, New York, 1968, American Physical Therapy Association.

99. Westreich, N., and others: Breathing retraining, Minn. Med. **53:**621, June 1970.

100. Wiklander, O., and Norlin, U.: Effect of physiotherapy on post-operative pulmonary complications: a clinical and roentgenographic study of 200 cases, Acta Chir. Scand. **112:**246, 1957.

101. Winning, T.J., and others: A simple clinical method of quantifying the effects of chest physiotherapy in mechanically-ventilated patient, Anaesth. Intensive Care **3:**237, 1975.

102. Winning, T.J. and others: Bronchodilators and physiotherapy during long term mechanical ventilation of the lungs, Anaesth. Intensive Care **5:**48, 1977.

103. Woolf, C.R.: A rehabilitation program for improving exercise tolerance of patients with chronic lung disease, Can. Med. Assoc. J. **106:**119, 1972.

104. Zack, M.B., and others: The effect of lateral positions on gas exchange in pulmonary disease, Am. Rev. Respir. Dis. **110:**49, 1974.

105. Zadai, C.C.: Physical therapy for the acutely ill medical patient, Phys. Ther. **61:**1746, 1981.

14

MARGARET E. KLEINFELD
PATRICE CASTLE

Physical therapy for patients with abdominal or thoracic surgery

Postoperative pulmonary complications (PPC) have plagued patients and their surgeons for years. Statistically they are the leading cause of morbidity and mortality in surgical patients.[25] So goes the old addage, "The surgery was a success but the patient died."

Initially chest physical therapy was exclusively utilized for medical chest patients and polio victims.[24] Prompted by the research of Palmer, Sellick, and others, physicians began to consider pulmonary hygiene a postoperative adjunct to surgical management.[29] In 1970 Stein and Cassara broadened the scope of chest physical therapy to include presurgical involvement.[39]

This chapter presents the aspects of chest physical therapy involving the patient who has had thoracic and high abdominal surgery.

The practice and scope of chest physical therapy varies from institution to institution. Respiratory therapists, nurses, or physical therapists provide the service. It is our opinion that physical therapists are best suited to administer chest physical therapy.

Care of the surgical patient is multifaceted and must be delivered by professionals who have expertise in a number of treatment areas. A rehabilitation component in most patient's postoperative course must be addressed. This component includes the preventive aspects of care and a strong emphasis on patient education.

Physical therapists can address these needs because of their experience with pain modulation, pulmonary hygiene, patient education, mobilization, and their background in basic medical sciences. Physical therapists alone cannot be the sole providers of respiratory care. They work with physicians, nurses, and respiratory therapists. The common goal of the team is to return patients to their prior level of function.

The specific goals of chest physical therapy treatment for the surgical patient include the following:

1. Promote pulmonary hygiene
2. Restore range of motion and strength
3. Prevent phlebitis
4. Modify pain
5. Provide patient education
6. Decrease patient anxiety

FACTORS CONTRIBUTING TO POSTOPERATIVE PULMONARY COMPLICATIONS

Patients undergoing surgery requiring general anesthesia are at risk for postoperative pulmonary complications. Anesthesia, surgery, and trauma have a detrimental effect on pulmonary function by altering a patient's breathing pattern. This alteration is attributable to a decrease in respiratory drive, depressed cough reflex, and pain associated with the surgery or trauma. Increased mucus pooling results from decreased ciliary activity. This factor alone supports preoperative emphasis of deep breathing.

A preexisting pulmonary, cardiac, or other condition that affects pulmonary reserve clearly increases the risk of pulmonary complications after surgery.[4] Anesthesia and surgery are the most common causes of respiratory failure in patients with chronic obstructive pulmonary disease.[13]

The surgery or trauma may involve the thorax, lung, or cardiac tissue making the patient susceptible to localized complications such as empyema, air leak, or lesions of the pleura.[4]

A patient's mentation postoperatively may be altered from the effects of anesthesia, pain, metabolic changes, and emotional stress, thus limiting their comprehension and cooperation.

Muscle spasm associated with pain limits the patient's ability to breathe deeply and move. For some surgical procedures muscles may have been incised; others are in spasm in response to pain. Even if the patient wants to cooperate, the muscular effort is diminished.

Recently, transcutaneous electrical nerve stimulation (TENS) has been found helpful in the management of postoperative incisional pain. In 1974 Hymes and associates used TENS for postoperative pain and found a significant decrease in the incidence of atelectasis and considerable increase in shoulder range of motion after a 15-minute treatment.[18]

In 1975 a study was performed by Vander Ark and McGrath, who examined 100 patients with thoracic or abdominal surgery. Seventy-seven percent of the patients treated with TENS reported maximum pain relief after the first treatment; however there was no difference of incidence of atelectasis noted between the test group and the control group.[46]

Stratton and Smith measured forced vital capacity in thoracotomy patients and found that those patients receiving TENS had significantly greater values than those who did not.[40]

All patients are deconditioned as a result of prolonged bed rest. Physiologically, inactivity causes decreased efficiency of the use of oxygen, muscle weakness, and increased energy expenditure for normal activities, and clinically patients will show decreased exercise tolerance.

CARDIAC SURGERY
Preoperative testing

Reviewing the findings from preoperative laboratory studies and testing procedures will provide additional information on the cardiopulmonary status of the patient and aid in predicting the postoperative course.

Cardiac catheterization. Before surgery every patient undergoes cardiac catheterization to determine the presence and severity of atherosclerotic lesions in the coronary arteries and of most other intracardiac abnormalities.

During this procedure, the patient usually remains awake. Using fluoroscopy, the physician inserts a catheter into the femoral, brachial, or axillary artery, and advances the catheter through the aorta to the heart. Before passing through the aortic valve, the catheter releases dye, which will go into the coronary arteries. Dye in the coronary arteries can define specific lesions and areas of low perfusion. When dye is released in the left ventricle, changes in heart size during systole and diastole can be observed and ventricular aneurysms will be outlined.

Pulmonary function tests. The results of pulmonary function tests provide information regarding the efficiency of the lung and the integrity of viable lung tissue. These studies differentiate restrictive from obstructive lung disease. Patients with preexisting pulmonary disease are at high risk for postoperative complications. The respiratory department may use these studies as a base line to determine mechanical ventilation settings for postoperative care.

Arterial blood gases. Arterial blood gases are arterial blood samples that allow one to measure the acid-base balance and partial pressures of oxygen, carbon dioxide, and bicarbonate in the blood. These values describe the metabolic relationship between the lungs and the kidneys, as well as oxygen uptake and oxygen saturation. This is shown by the values for PO_2, PCO_2, HCO_3^-, pH, and O_2 saturation.

Electrocardiogram. An electrocardiogram (ECG) shows the electrical conduction through the cardiac muscle. Voltage variations are produced by depolarization and repolarization of individual muscle cells and are represented in graph form. An preoperative ECG will provide a base line for postoperative comparison. This will help identify any changes that may have resulted from or occurred during the surgery. Surgery is stressful to the heart, and ischemia may occur during or after the procedure. Often there will be an improvement in the ECG after coronary bypass graft surgery. This results from increased blood flow to various areas of the heart.

Surgical considerations

Incision placement. The most common incision used in cardiac surgery is the median sternotomy. This is also referred to as a "split sternotomy," or "sternal split." The incision extends from the sternoclavicular notch to the xyphoid. The sternum is then split and retracted to expose the thoracic cavity[9] (Fig. 14-1, *A*).

The alternative incision for cardiac surgery is the thoracotomy. This incision follows the path of the fourth intercostal space and is primarily used if valve surgery is indicated. This approach affords greater accessibility to the mitral valve[9] (Fig. 14-1, *A*).

Extracorporeal circulation. The extracorporeal circulation is the means, during cardiac surgery, by which blood is oxygenated, filtered, and warmed or cooled by an external system. The heart-lung bypass pump needed for cardiac surgery allows the surgeons to work on a bloodless heart for an extended period of time.

Venous blood is siphoned through a catheter from the superior and inferior venae cavae, passes through the pump, and is returned to the aorta or femoral artery. Coronary circulation must be maintained if the bypass time exceeds 40 minutes. This is accomplished by use of catheters inserted in the main coronary arteries through which the myocardium is nourished.

Cardiac surgeries

Coronary artery bypass graft (CABG). This procedure is used to promote increased circulation to the myocardium when there is a major coronary artery occlusion. Surgery is indicated in patients with (1) stable angina pectoris that is severe enough to significantly alter their life-style, (2) initial angina pectoris with episodes at rest, despite treatment, (3) myocardial ischemia with or without ST-segment changes of the ECG, (4) stable angina pectoris associated

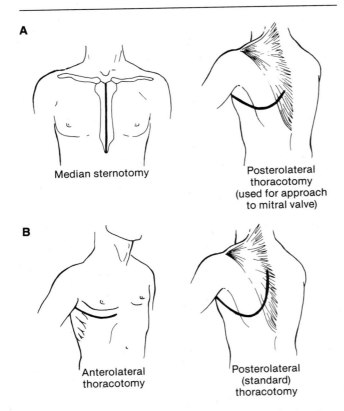

Fig. 14-1. Surgical incisions. **A,** Common incisions for heart surgery. *Left,* Median sternotomy; *right,* posterolateral thoracotomy used for approach to mitral valve. **B,** Common incisions for lung surgery. *Left,* Anterolateral thoracotomy; *right,* posterolateral (standard) thoracotomy.

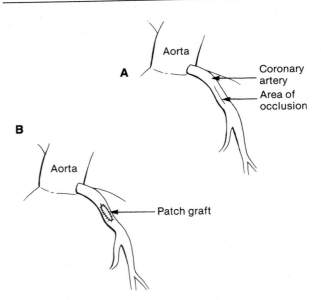

Fig. 14-2. Patch vein grafting. **A,** An incision is made in the area of the occlusion. **B,** The patch graft enlarges the lumen of the artery to allow patency.

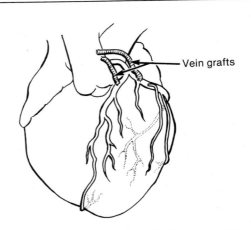

Fig. 14-3. Coronary artery bypass graft. The vein graft is attached to the aorta and distal to the occlusion of the coronary artery.

with ST changes of 2 mm during a stage I or stage II treadmill stress test.[15]

Two techniques are commonly used to improve myocardial circulation—patch grafting and vein grafting.

Patch grafting is performed by utilization of a patch of pericardium or a patch of vein to widen the lumen of an obstructed artery. A linear incision that extends above and below the obstructed site is made in the coronary artery. The patch is then sutured in place (Fig. 14-2).

Vein grafting is the most commonly used technique and involves using segments of a large vein, usually the saphenous vein, to bypass diseased segments of the coronary artery. End-to-end or end-to-side anastomoses are used to reestablish blood flow from the aorta to the coronary artery below the occlusion (Fig. 14-3). There can be any number of bypasses done. Usually one to four are performed, but up to six have been performed.

Extracorporeal circulation is required for both procedures, and a split sternotomy is the most commonly used incision.

Valvular surgery. The first successful open-heart surgery was not performed on man until 1953 though extra-

corporeal circulation was being investigated up to 20 years before. This operation was first done by Gibbon on a patient with a diseased mitral valve.[22,34]

Mentioned below are a commissurotomy, annuloplasty, and replacement, the most common valvular surgeries. Until recently, the commissurotomy was performed under fluoroscopy, a closed procedure. Now they are all done by open-heart surgery.

A commissurotomy involves cutting or splitting the commissures of the valve that have become hardened and

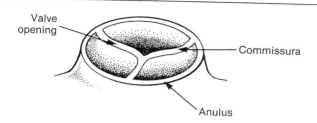

Fig. 14-4. Heart valve. Tricuspid valve showing commissura and surrounding fibrous anulus.

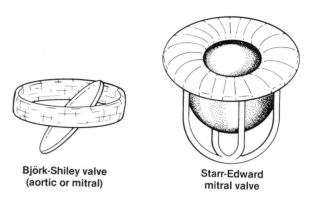

Björk-Shiley valve
(aortic or mitral)

Starr-Edward
mitral valve

Fig. 14-5. Valve replacements. *Left,* Björk-Shiley valve (aortic or mitral); *right,* Starr-Edward valve (mitral).

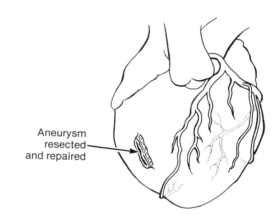

Aneurysm
resected
and repaired

Fig. 14-6. Ventricular aneurysmectomy. Resected aneurysm with suture reinforcement.

less mobile because of the accumulation of plaque. The commissure is the junction between the adjacent cusps of the valves of the heart (Fig. 14-4). The plaque formation will cause a stenosis, that is, narrowing in the size of the orifice, and therefore inadequate blood flow. The commissure is simply split surgically.

An annuloplasty is another procedure that will improve the function of the valve. The anulus (formerly annulus), in reference to the heart, is one of a number of dense fibrous rings that are found around the four major valves of the heart (Fig. 14-4). With hypertrophy of the heart chambers, these anuli will also increase in size, making valve closure difficult. The surgery involves implantation of a C ring around the diseased valve and pulling the anulus in, therefore allowing the cusps to close properly. These two preceding surgeries require little time on the heart-lung pump and seldom have major postoperative complications.[27] Good recovery is expected.

Valve replacements are performed more frequently than the above two surgeries. The most common valve replacements are mitral, aortic, and tricuspid.

The first valve replacement model was developed in 1961. The two designs of valve replacements are the ball valve and the disk valve (Fig. 14-5).

The surgical procedure involves either a split sternal incision or, occasionally, a lateral thoracotomy when only the mitral valve is being replaced. The heart is incised, the diseased valve is removed, and the replacement valve is inserted. Because the artificial valve is a foreign body, there is a risk of blood clotting in the area. These patients are started on anticoagulation therapy before surgery and must continue taking anticoagulants permanently.[15]

Valve replacements are indicated when there is a valve insufficiency or stenosis. Calcifications and plaque accumulation not only cause clinical symptoms secondary to insufficiency, but also present a risk of embolus formation. The destination of these emboli is usually cerebral.[34]

Aneurysmectomy. Aneurysmectomy of the ventricles of the heart is occasionally performed with a coronary artery bypass graft. The surgical procedure involves incision of the aneurysm and then approximation and suturing together of the two sides of the resultant opening thereby creating one straight suture line[41] (Fig. 14-6).

An aneurysm occurs when there is a localized loss of cardiac muscle tone and contractility because of an infarction. The muscle tissue will dilate and form a bulging sac with increased pressure in the full chamber during systole. This bulging decreases the cardiac output and increases the residual volume and the turbulence within the chamber. Repair of this disturbance will improve ventricular function and decrease the chance of emboli forming in the heart.

Pericardiectomy. Pericardiectomy and pericardotomy are excision and incision of the percardium respectively. These procedures, done with a median sternotomy, are performed to relieve constricting pressure on the heart. The increased pressure can be attributable to an accumulation of fluid, usually blood, in the pericardial sac around the heart or by fibrosis or calcification of the pericardial sac resulting from chronic pericarditis.[10,41]

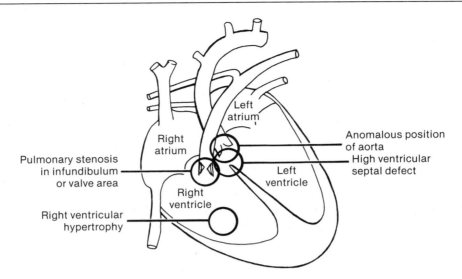

Fig. 14-7. Tetralogy of Fallot. *Left top,* Pulmonary stenosis in the infundibulum or valve area; *left bottom,* right ventricular hypertrophy; *right top,* anomalous position of the aorta; *right bottom,* high ventricular septal defect.

Repair of atrial septal defect. An atrial septal defect is a common congenital lesion and accounts for 15% of the cardiac lesions.[2] An atrial septal defect is characterized by an abnormal opening in the interatrial septum resulting in decreased systemic blood flow and increased pulmonary blood flow. Children with this defect present with dyspnea on exertion and pulmonary hypertension.

Recommended management is surgical closure, usually during childhood, if pulmonary flow is more than one and a half to two times systemic flow.[2,41]

An anterior right thoracotomy through the fourth intercostal space or a median sternotomy is used. These incisions facilitate entrance to the right atrium. If the defect is greater than 1.5 to 2 cm, a pericardial patch of fabric is surgically applied.[15]

Repair of ventricular septal defect. A ventricular septal defect is characterized by communication between the two ventricles and may involve the muscle or membrane of the septum. This is the most frequent congenital circulatory lesion and accounts for 20% to 25% of all children with cardiac disease.[2,41]

The left-to-right shunt, which usually forms, results in pulmonary blood flow greater than systemic flow. Secondary pulmonary vascular changes may lead to an increase in right ventricular pressure. If great enough, the right ventricular pressure will reverse the shunting, thereby mixing unoxygenated blood with oxygenated aortic blood. Depending on the size of the defect, patients may exhibit cyanosis, digital clubbing, dyspnea on exertion, and right ventricular failure.

Surgical repair is indicated after 3 years of age. A me-

dian sternotomy is used to enter the heart through the right ventricle. Small defects are corrected with sutures. Larger defects may require a Dacron polyester patch.[15]

Tetralogy of Fallot. The lesion tetralogy of Fallot accounts for most of the patients with congenital heart disease with accompanying cyanosis. It is characterized by (1) a high ventricular septal defect, (2) pulmonary stenosis because of valve or infundibular involvement or both, (3) deviation of the aorta, and (4) right ventricular hypertrophy (Fig. 14-7).

A right-to-left interventricular shunt results from pulmonary outflow tract obstruction in the right ventricle. Inadequate blood flow to the lungs and the shunting of blood from the right ventricle to the aorta allows unoxygenated blood to enter the systemic circulation.

Clinically, cyanosis and syncope are seen. Children are usually small framed and present with digital clubbing and dyspnea on exertion.

Surgical correction can be accomplished through left thoracotomy, median sternotomy, or submammary incision. A pulmonary valvotomy or resection of the infundibular defect is done. A suture or patch repair of the ventricular septal defect is necessary.[15]

Patent ductus arteriosus. The defect patent ductus arteriosus accounts for 15% of all congenital cardiovascular defects.[15,41] It is characterized by a conduit from the pulmonary artery to the aorta that persists from fetal life.

Blood flow from the aorta to the pulmonary system results, increasing the work of both ventricles. If the volume of blood flow through the shunt exceeds normal cardiac

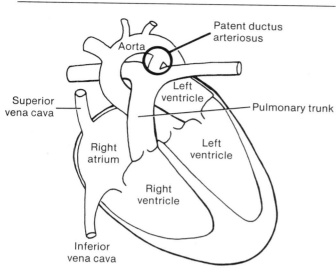

Fig. 14-8. Patent ductus arteriosus. Conduit between the pulmonary trunk and the aorta.

output, an abnormal blood load results in the left ventricle with increased pulmonary vascular resistance. Patients may be asymptomatic, or exhibit dyspnea on exertion. Subacute bacterial endocarditis or pulmonary hypertension may occur.

Surgery after 2 years of age is recommended. A left posterolateral thoracotomy incision through the fourth intercostal space, or median sternotomy, is used. The ductus is surgically divided and closed off from the aorta[15] (Fig. 14-8).

Atresias. Atresias are defined as the congenital absence or closure of a normal body orifice, and they account for less than 1% of congenital cardiac defects.[15]

Pulmonary atresias involving a severe narrowing of the opening of the pulmonary artery and right ventricle can be lethal. Cardiomegaly, decreased pulmonary vascularity, and right ventricular atrophy result.

A pulmonary valvotomy is the recommended surgical procedure.[15]

PULMONARY SURGERY
Preoperative testing

In addition to the standard preoperative studies, the prospective pulmonary surgery patient undergoes additional tests. Special attention should be given to pulmonary function studies, radiographs, and bronchoscopy reports if available.

A bronchoscopy may be a diagnostic or therapeutic procedure. A flexible fiber-optic tube is inserted nasotracheally into the major bronchi and large airways. This method allows observation and inspection of the airways.

Brushings and tissue biopsies may be performed through the scope. If necessary, aspiration of secretions is done. These studies provide the practitioner with information regarding the area of involvement, the type and extent of the pathological condition, and the apparent viability of the remaining lung.

Lung resections

Surgical intervention by resection may be the treatment of choice for a multitude of pulmonary disorders. The most common include tuberculosis, neoplasm, benign tumors and cysts, fungal infections, emphysematous blebs, spontaneous pneumothoraces, or pleuritis. Lung resections can vary in extent and are usually approached by a standard thoracotomy incision (see Fig. 14-1, *B*), with the level of the incision depending on the lobe, segment, or area involved.[9] The extent of surgery may range from clamping a small bleb in a segment to removal of an entire lung. Before surgery, one must determine that the patient will be able to ventilate adequately with the remaining lung tissue, be it healthy or diseased.[41]

Blebectomy

In most cases a blebectomy is the least extensive of the lung resections. A bleb, or bulla, is a bubble or sac formed by destruction and expansion of the alveoli distal to the terminal bronchioles. These can be minute or large enough to be seen on a radiograph by even an untrained person. Blebs frequently occur in the base of the lungs in patients with emphysema. A standard thoracotomy is made, and the bleb is either resected or plicated. Plication is folding or taking a tuck in the tissue (Fig. 14-9). This procedure will decrease the dead space and residual volume and relieve the pressure of the bleb on adjacent tissue or structures. This technique is sometimes performed to prevent the bursting of a bleb, which can cause a spontaneous pneumothorax.

Although pneumothorax is also discussed under postoperative complications, spontaneous pneumothorax is mentioned here to clarify the differences and causes. A pneumothorax is gas or air in the chest cavity, outside the lung, that causes displacement of lung tissue. A spontaneous pneumothorax can be life threatening because the entire lung may collapse. Chest tubes (p. 262 and 282) must be inserted immediately to remove air and assist with reinflation of the lung. These will remain until no or little air leak is detected. If spontaneous pneumothorax is a recurring problem, surgical intervention is indicated.

Segmental resection

Segmental resection involves removal of lung tissue distal to the segmental bronchus. This procedure is performed to remove either severely diseased lung tissue or an invading process such as a tumor or fungal cyst. The approach is by standard thoracotomy (Fig. 14-1).

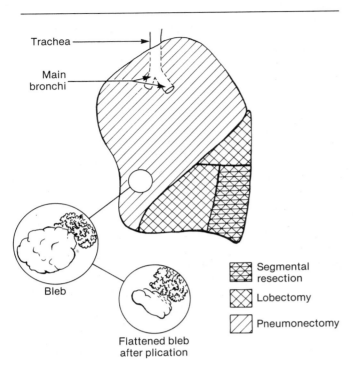

Bleb

Flattened bleb
after plication

	Segmental resection
	Lobectomy
	Pneumonectomy

Trachea

Main bronchi

Fig. 14-9. Lung resections. Various selections and segments are plicated or removed for blebectomy, segmental resection, lobectomy, or pneumonectomy.

Lobectomy

A lobectomy is removal of a lobe of lung, which is usually performed by standard thoracotomy. The indications may be similar to those for a segmental resection but with more extensive involvement. The bronchus leading into the involved lobe is cut and stapled, and the entire lobe is removed.

With these three procedures, the pleural sac remains intact. After resection, the remaining lung will expand to fill much of the space left by the resection.

Pneumonectomy

In some cases a pneumonectomy, removal of an entire lung, is required. This is usually indicated in cases of extensive carcinoma. The lung and visceral pleura are removed, and the main bronchus leading into that lung is stapled shut.[41] This procedure leaves the patient with a large cavity of mostly air and some body fluids. Postoperatively, the diaphragm rises, and the remaining thoracic structures shift toward the operative side, resulting in decreased rib excursion on that side. The cavity eventually fills with normal body fluids, and the air is removed by chest tubes. This procedure is done by thoracotomy.

Immediately after pneumonectomy patients should not be placed on the operative side. This position places undue stress on the mediastinal structures, since they are no longer supported by the lung. Also, since ventilation and perfusion are greatest in the dependent area of the remaining lung, PaO_2 will decrease with the greater alveolar density superior.[21,45]

In all the above procedures, except for pneumonectomy, chest tubes are inserted at the time of surgery through two small incisions caudal to the thoracotomy incision. The chest tubes are connected to a closed system of continuous suction. They aspirate excess air or fluid from the chest cavity. These tubes remain in the chest postoperatively until there is little or no fluid drainage, air leaks have closed, and all residual air in the cavity has been suctioned out or reabsorbed. Any void left after surgery becomes filled with normal body fluids that eventually coagulate. The chest cavity is smaller because of mediastinal shift, elevation of the hemidiaphragm, and decreased rib excursion.

Pleurectomy

A pleurectomy is the removal of the pleural sac of a segment or of an entire lung. This procedure results in adherence of the lung tissue to the internal chest wall. In normal respiration, the pleural sac allows for easy movement of the lung within the thoracic cavity. After a pleurectomy, the lung will move with the chest wall.

This surgery is indicated for recurrent spontaneous pneumothorax. The adherence of the lung to the chest wall will have a sealing affect on the lungs and prevent further pneumothoraces.[41]

Pleurodesis

Pleurodesis can be either artificial, abrasive, or chemical. It involves stimulation of a reaction of the pleural lining that creates adhesions of the visceral and parietal pleural layers. The artificial procedure is usually done with other thoracic surgery, such as lung resection. Chemical pleurodesis involves instillation of an abrasive drug such as tetracycline into the pleural space. This is done through the chest tube. This procedure prevents further collapse of the lung and eliminates the space for potential fluid accumulation.[14,41]

Decortication

Decortication is the removal from the surface of the lung of any restrictive membrane that significantly limits pulmonary function. A thickened pleura caused by empyema is one indication. This surgery is performed only if a significant improvement in respiratory function is expected.

OTHER SURGERIES AFFECTING THE THORAX
Thoracic aortic aneurysm

Thoracic aortic aneurysms are second in incidence to infrarenal abdominal aneurysms. They usually occur in the sixth, seventh, and eighth decades of life because of atherosclerosis. Trauma, hypertension, or inflammation can also account for the formation of the aneurysm.

Unlike abdominal aortic aneurysms, thoracic aneurysms expand slowly and do not usually rupture. However, thoracic aneurysms can be lethal by enlarging and surrounding vital structures such as the trachea or great vessels.

Symptoms may vary according to the pressure imposed in the surrounding structure. Dyspnea, cough from pressure on the trachea or bronchi, and venous engorgement caused by pressure on the superior vena cava or right atrium are common symptoms.

Surgical management is by a median sternotomy or left thoracotomy. Correction is accomplished by resection of the aneurysm by anastomosis or Dacron polyester grafting. The patient undergoes cardiopulmonary bypass if there is involvement of the ascending aorta or aortic arch.

Mediastinotomy

Mediastinotomy is usually an exploratory procedure used to provide tissue for a definitive diagnosis in mediastinal lesions.

A right or left thoracotomy at the appropriate interspace is used. One approaches thyroid and thymus lesions by splitting the upper half or the entire sternum.

Trauma

Trauma, either open or closed, to the chest cavity, is a serious situation. A forceful blow to the chest may damage various organs and structures including the esophagus, trachea, diaphragm, chest wall, lungs, heart, and great vessels.[15] Chest and lung injuries are discussed.

After a lung contusion, there occurs localized edema, hemorrhage into the parenchyma, and increased secretion production. Ventilation-perfusion mismatching occurs because of parenchymal congestion and increased fluid in the alveoli. Contusion to the lungs does not usually require surgical intervention. However, mechanical ventilation may be necessary until the lungs are cleared of fluid and can be ventilated effectively by the patient.[38]

Another type of closed chest injury is flail chest. This occurs when several ribs are fractured in at least two places and no longer provide a rigid chest wall. The severity of the injury depends on the number of ribs fractured and whether the lung has been punctured causing hemothorax, pneumothorax, or both (see pp. 268 and 269). Because of the negative intrathoracic pressure during inspiration, the ribs are pulled inward and the chest cannot expand. As a result, ventilation is severely compromised, and the patient will require oxygen therapy, usually delivered by mechanical ventilation.

Laminectomy

Although thoracic spine laminectomy surgery does not involve entering the thorax, patients may develop pulmonary problems secondary to immobility. Deep breathing

may be painful, and rolling from side to side is seldom carried out without encouragement. Early mobilization can prevent most pulmonary problems, but positioning and segmental breathing may be necessary. By instructing patients in bed mobility, one may prevent complications secondary to immobility.

Burns and skin grafts

The range-of-motion limitations from burns and skin grafts are well known to the therapist. Thoracic burns or grafts have similar effects on decreasing rib excursion and ventilation. The patients must be instructed to breathe deeply hourly from the beginning of the burn injury. The movement of the chest wall is not great enough to cause damage to any grafts, but can make a significant difference in improving pulmonary hygiene.

UPPER ABDOMINAL SURGERY
Surgical considerations

The proximity of the abdominal cavity to the diaphragm and lungs increases the risk for pulmonary problems in patients who have high abdominal surgery. Up to 70% of all patients undergoing high abdominal surgery will experience postoperative pulmonary complications.[45]

Incision placement, the organs involved, postoperative inflammation, and pain at the operative site will all compromise normal pulmonary function. Even without preexisting pulmonary disease, the location of the surgery will directly affect the pulmonary function.

The major problem is hypoventilation from splinting secondary to pain. The abdomen lacks bony support to stabilize the incision, resulting in increased movement and increased pain. Patient immobility and pressure on the diaphragm from edema in the involved area may also contribute to increased pain.

Preoperative testing

A review of the patient's pulmonary function studies for any signs of impaired function is helpful. X-ray reports of the lungs and abdomen will provide additional information.

Patients with concomitant diseases, such as chronic obstructive pulmonary disease and renal or cardiac disease should be considered potential high risks for postoperative pulmonary problems.

Gastrectomy

Gastrectomies can be either partial, subtotal, or total. Most are performed for gastric neoplasm or gastric ulcer.

A radical subtotal gastrectomy is the most widely used procedure and involves removal of a major portion of the stomach, proximal duodenum, greater omentum, and subpyloric lymph node tissues.[15,41]

Total gastrectomy requires removal of the spleen and the entire stomach. Sometimes surgical construction of a res-

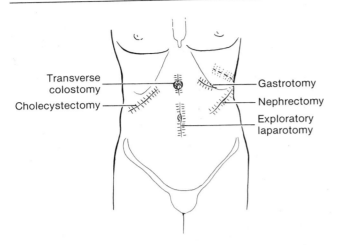

Fig. 14-10. Incision placements for various high abdominal surgeries.

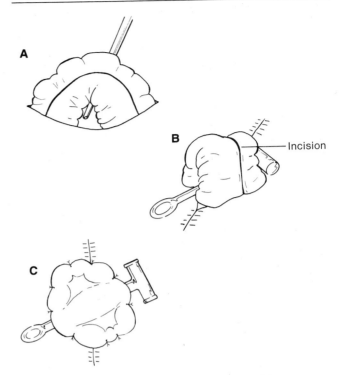

Fig. 14-11. Transverse loop colostomy. **A,** Section of the transverse colon is looped over a glass rod. **B,** The colon is incised and the abdominal incision is closed to the colon. **C,** The wall of the colon is sutured to the skin.

ervoir pouch for nutritional advantage is performed.

Reconstruction by anastomosis of the jejunum to the esophagus provides a diversion for irritating alkaline juices away from the esophagus, thus inhibiting esophagitis.

A thoracic or thoracoabdominal incision is used.[41]

Cholecystectomy

Removal of the gallbladder is the most common mode of treatment in patients with calculus disease. Many cholecystectomies are performed as preventive procedures that enhance a favorable prognosis.

A right subcostal incision extending from the xyphoid process to the right flank is commonly used (Fig. 14-10). Because of the proximity of the gallbladder to the diaphragm and the incisional placement, these patients are at particularly high risk for pulmonary congestion. They also demonstrate poor inspiratory effort and greatly decreased coughing ability. However, with increased mobility, improvement in their pulmonary status is observed.[37,41]

Laparotomy

This procedure, usually exploratory, is used to identify and determine the extent of an abdominal injury. These usually large incisions are in the midline and periumbilical area to provide extended exposure to the abdominal structures. A transverse incision may be considered when a specific diagnosis is available, such as a spleenectomy (Fig. 14-10).

Transverse colostomy

A transverse colostomy is indicated for patients with diverticulitis, penetrating trauma, or obstructions in the colon, rectum, or bowel. The purpose of a colostomy is two-fold: (1) decompressive, to release obstruction, and (2) divertive, to allow complete diversion of intestinal flow.

The procedure may be done as a temporary divertive or decompressive function, or the colostomy may be needed permanently.

A high stoma is created by use of a superior midline incision (Fig. 14-10). A loop of colon is brought through the abdominal wall and suspended over a glass rod. The colon is incised and opened to allow a wide separation of the functional and nonfunctional ends. The longitudinal abdominal incision is closed to the protruding colon, and then the wall of the colon is sutured to the skin to form the stoma[41] (Fig. 14-11). This will allow drainage of fluid through the proximal stump.

Nephrectomy

Nephrectomy is a surgical procedure indicated for patients with tuberculosis of the kidney, pyelonephritis, kidney calculi, or tumor.

A simple nephrectomy involves removal of the kidney from the capsule, with transection of and clamping the ureter and excision of the kidney. A radical nephrectomy involves excision of the entire kidney and its capsule.[41]

There are several incisions used, depending on the patient's diagnosis.

1. *Translumbar flank incisions* are the most commonly used incisions. They follow the costovertebral angle of the twelfth rib, downward and toward the abdomen (see Fig. 14-10). This incision is used in patients with flexible spines and normally placed kidneys.

2. *Transabdominal incisions* are indicated in elderly patients with impaired pulmonary function.

3. *Transthoracic incisions* are indicated for patients with pathological lesions of the superior aspect of the kidney, or with kidneys positioned high.[41]

PATIENT TREATMENT
Preoperative preparation

The opportunity to work with a patient preoperatively has proved beneficial for the patient and therapist. Thoren's study in 1954 demonstrated a 12% incidence of postoperative atelectasis in patients instructed in deep breathing preoperatively, as compared to a 27% incidence in patients with postoperative follow-up only.[44]

Gracey and others studied the number of postoperative complications in 157 COPD patients who had a standard preoperative program of postural drainage, percussion, and vibration. Patients were seen at a minimum of 48 hours before surgery. There was a 17% incidence of pulmonary complications postoperatively. The rate of complications was highest in patients with upper or long abdominal incisions.[13]

Tarhan and others looked at the incidence of pulmonary complications in 357 men with COPD and found a 43% incidence without preoperative involvement and 24% with preoperative preparation.[42]

Stein and Cassara found that preoperative chest physical therapy was valuable not only in reducing the number of postoperative complications but also in decreasing the severity of those complications.[39]

Preoperative patient contact aids the therapist in determining postoperative expectations and treatment. Gracey and others found that patients who produced greater than 2 ounces of sputum daily preoperatively demonstrated increased postoperative respiratory difficulty.[13]

Preoperative assessment

1. *Chart review.* The chart should be reviewed with special attention to tests and studies related to the type of pending surgery.

2. *Patient interview.* The patient interview can contribute useful information regarding a patient's family history, occupation, and habits such as smoking and use of alcohol. The patient should be questioned specifically regarding pulmonary symptoms and their frequency and pattern. Functional activities must be assessed for determination of appropriate postoperative goals for the patient.

3. *Physical assessment.* Physical assessment includes five areas: observation, palpation, auscultation, percussion, and range of motion.

    a. *Observation.* Observation of the patient provides much information before a "hands-on" examination, including the following:
    (1) Color
    (2) Breathing pattern: rate, amplitude, rhythm
    (3) Mentation
    (4) Posture
    (5) Body build
    (6) Supportive equipment
    (7) Secretions
    (8) Patients ability to move
    (9) Skin: scars, turgor

    b. *Palpation.* Bilateral palpation of the thorax allows comparison of the symmetry of the following physical signs:
    (1) Equality of thoracic movement
        (a) Lateral costal expansion
        (b) Apical expansion
        (c) Posterior thorax: basal expansion
        (d) diaphragmatic excursion
    (2) Vocal fremitus

    c. *Auscultation and percussion.* Auscultation and percussion are necessary to establish a base-line assessment of chest sounds. If adventitious breath sounds are noticed, treatment preoperatively is indicated to improve pulmonary status before surgery.

    d. *Range of motion.* With thoracic surgery it is important to observe preoperative ROM to determine goals of postoperative mobility. Special emphasis should be placed on joints that will be affected by incised musculature.

Preoperative patient education

Preoperative patient education can strongly influence the postoperative course. Semanoff, Kleinfeld, and Castle found that two or more preoperative sessions decreased (1) the patient's length of stay from surgery to discharge, (2) the number of postoperative complications, and (3) the number of physical therapy treatments required postoperatively. They also noted that patients with valve surgeries treated with preoperative chest physical therapy were discharged 8 days sooner than their counterparts who were not treated preoperatively.[36]

Postoperatively a patient's mentation can be altered from the effects of anesthesia, emotional stress, and pain, thereby limiting comprehension and cooperation. Preoperative sessions afford the therapist the opportunity to prepare the patient for the surgery. Major points to be covered during preoperative sessions are the following:

1. *Rationale for treatment.* One should explain the rationale in detail covering the effects of bed rest and immobility on pulmonary status, respiratory depression from anesthesia, and, when appropriate, the lung's response to thoracic surgery. All of these may result in decreased aeration and increased mucus production.
2. *Surgical procedure.* A brief description of the surgical procedure is offered, including incision placement and length of surgery. The detail depends on the patient's level of understanding.
4. *Monitoring and support devices.* Explanation of the monitoring and support devices the patient can expect to encounter postoperatively is very important and may include the following:
   a. *Foley catheter* to collect urine output and monitor kidney function
   b. *Chest tubes* to drain the thoracic cavity of any accumulation of air or fluid
   c. *Intravenous tubes* to maintain nutrition and hydration
   d. *Cardiac monitor and electrodes* to follow cardiac status
   e. *Arterial line* to provide an access for arterial blood samples for blood gas analysis and for injection of medications
   f. *Left atrial pressure line* to measure cardiac function
   g. *Endotracheal tube* to provide an artificial airway for respiratory assistance by a ventilator
   h. *Nasogastric tube* to drain gastric secretions

Preoperative treatment

A standard postoperative treatment is demonstrated with the patient. Rolling, positioning for bronchial drainage, percussion, vibration and splinted coughing are practiced. This practice provides the patient with an example of what will be expected after surgery. The therapist may find little time to instruct the patient before surgery. These are five areas that must be covered:

1. *Deep breathing.* Changes in the mechanics of breathing, lung volume, and gas exchange have been noted to occur postoperatively. These changes are attributable to a decrease in the respiratory drive from general anesthesia and narcotics and a decrease in thoracic expansion from pain and accompanying muscle spasm. Persistence of these abnormal changes facilitates alveolar collapse and after several hours results in gross atelectasis.[5] Decreased lung capacity and compliance result, thereby increasing the work of breathing.

   For reversal of these processes, deep breathing to improve alveolar ventilation is very important. Deep breathing is taught with the patient in a semi-Fowler position, in which the abdominal muscles are on slack. This position allows greater diaphragmatic excursion. Deep diaphragmatic breathing is taught and is emphasized as the most important modality for postoperative pulmonary hygiene.

   Some patients breathe effectively with their diaphragm and need only encouragement to aerate their lungs fully, whereas others find the technique difficult and need additional cues.

   Hand placement on the substernal area over the diaphragm may be helpful for patients to feel where motion should occur. Three strong ''sniffs'' will cause the diaphragm to ''pop up'' to demonstrate diaphragmatic movement. By extending the sniff, the patient will have taken a good diaphragmatic breath. Deep breathing also promotes relaxation, which may be useful to reduce anxiety.

2. *Rolling.* Rolling is a technique that allows patient mobility while minimizing trunk movement. The patient is encouraged to flex at the hip and knees and roll with the shoulders and hips simultaneously. Even though CABG patients have incisions on their lower extremities, hip and knee flexion is usually allowed.

3. *Coughing.* Decreased cough effectiveness is related to anesthesia and surgery. Compared to preoperative pressures generated with coughing, postoperative values may be diminished for as long as 1 month.[23]

   Byrd and Burns found that narcotics did not significantly alter a patient's ability to produce an increased cough pressure and were not effective in decreasing pain associated with coughing. They also noted that patients with median sternotomies had severely reduced cough pressures.[8]

   Bateman and colleagues noted that coughing with bronchial drainage, vibration, shaking, and percussion accelerated central and peripheral lung clearance.[6]

   Proper coughing involves a two-stage cough preceded by a full, deep diaphragmatic breath. (The bigger the breath, the stronger the cough.) The first cough raises the secretions, the second facilitates expectoration.

   Because a cough will jar the thorax and cause pain, splinting of the incision is taught. Patients are instructed to apply pressure over the incision by using pillows or their hands.

   Yamazaki and others found that higher cough pressures were achieved when thoracotomy patients in a sitting position had additional manual compression of the thorax by a nurse or therapist. Compression of the abdominal wall with the patient supine was also effective.[48]

   Starr studied cough effectiveness and positioning in cholecystectomy patients. She found that patients in an upright position attained greater flow rates than those in side-lying or semi-Fowler's positions.[37]

Patients who have difficulty coughing even with splinting techniques can be taught huffing. This maneuver is reportedly a less painful method of airway clearance.

Studies involving patients with asthma, cystic fibrosis, and chronic obstructive lung disease have shown that huffing provides increased stabilization of the airways. Huffing is an effective mode of secretion mobilization and may be used as an alternative in patients who demonstrate an ineffective cough.[16,32,43]

Huffing is accomplished by forceful expiration through an open glottis. The patient is asked to say the word "huff" and attempt to elongate the *h*. Eventually, repetition of this maneuver may stimulate a spontaneous cough.

4. *Incentive spirometry.* Incentive spirometry is an adjunct to breathing exercises that provides the patient with visual feedback of the volume of air inspired during a deep breath. Patients are encouraged to practice deep inspiration every hour in addition to their chest physical therapy sessions. Cardiac patients are instructed not to hold their breath at the end of expiration. Bartlett showed that maximal inhalation with incentive spirometry successfully inflated the alveoli and, as a result, decreased postoperative pulmonary complications.[5]

Other adjuncts to deep breathing include "blow bottles," intermittent positive-pressure breathing (IPPB), and positive end-expiratory pressure (PEEP).

Bartlett and co-workers in 1973 noted that blow bottles were ineffective in preventing alveolar collapse in surgical patients. They cited the lack of efficacy of IPPB as a prophylactic mode of treatment. Incentive spirometry, as stated above, was found to decrease postoperative pulmonary complications.[5]

In 1980, Jung and colleagues compared the effectiveness of IPPB, incentive spirometry, and resisted breathing in 126 patients with upper abdominal surgery. They concluded that there was no significant difference between the three treatments in reducing postoperative pulmonary complications.[20]

Craven and associates compared incentive spirometry and chest physical therapy in 70 upper abdominal surgery patients. The patients who received chest physical therapy had a 63% incidence of postoperative pulmonary complications as compared to 37% incidence in those receiving incentive spirometry. Note that deep breathing was not emphasized in the chest physical therapy protocol.[22]

Paul and Downs recently compared IPPB, incentive spirometry, and positive end-expiratory pressure (PEEP) in patients who had a coronary artery bypass graft. No additional chest physical therapy was ad-

ministered. Transpulmonary pressure was measured in each mode of treatment. Although PEEP significantly increased expiratory transpulmonary pressure more than either incentive spirometry or IPPB, there was little residual effect on the transpulmonary pressure.[30]

Overall, there is little evidence that any of these modes of treatment significantly decrease postoperative pulmonary complications.

5. *Ankle circles.* Use of ankle pumps are taught to the patient to minimize the incidence of phlebitis and facilitate venous return.

These preoperative sessions strengthen the patient-therapist relationship. Patients feel confident meeting the therapist who will treat them through their hospital course. In the recovery room, some patients open their eyes for the first time and are thrilled to see their therapist. They know they're not in heaven!

Postoperative treatment
Considerations of postoperative treatment

A full assessment should be performed with each session, since a patient's status may change from one treatment to the next. Routine chart review should provide current vital signs, lab results, procedures performed, and the postoperative course. Often some of these values may be recorded on flow sheets at the bedside. Close attention should be paid to postoperative changes in heart rate and rhythm, blood pressure, respiratory rate, and temperature. These measures will indicate the hemodynamic stability and general condition of the patient. Hemodynamic stability is most important when treating the cardiac surgery patients. Patients undergoing upper abdominal and pulmonary surgery tend to be more stable hemodynamically than the cardiac surgery patients.[5,23] During extracorporeal circulation trauma to the red blood cells induces anemia and hemolysis. There is a decrease in pulmonary perfusion and a decrease in the oxygen level of the blood going to bronchial arteries. All these changes can contribute to hypoxia, which can lead to dysrhythmias.[17,31] The ability of the heart to maintain adequate cardiac output and therefore manage body fluid levels is compromised. This results in a decreased blood pressure. Close monitoring of blood pressure and heart rhythm is required during treatment.

It is helpful to discuss the patient's status with the nurse and physicians. Know the medications the patients are receiving. Cardiac patients may receive antiarrythmics, antihypotensives, and pain medications, and valvular surgical patients commonly receive anticoagulation therapy. Other surgical patients may be treated with only pain medications and broad spectrum antibiotics. Postoperative pain is a major factor in commonly seen postoperative pulmonary complications and severely limits the ability of the patient to produce an effective cough. This is especially true for thoracotomy patients.[24,35] The most commonly seen postoperative pulmonary complications include atelectasis because of surgical technique, fluid imbalances, and immobility and pneumonia. The physical therapy treatment for these problems is more effective and less uncomfortable for the patient if timed with the administration of pain medications. Twenty to 30 minutes after the drug is given is the optimal time for treatment.

At the bedside the therapist must take time to examine the placement and patency of various lines and tubes. The therapist should check them all again before leaving the patient's room to assure that they were not disrupted or displaced. All patients will be receiving intravenous fluids, and most will have drainage tubes of some type. The high abdominal wounds will be draining either by gravity (straight drainage) or with a low level of suction. Thoracotomy and cardiac patients will have chest tubes (p. 255 and 282). To avoid dislodging the chest tubes in patients with lateral thoracotomies, one should not flex the shoulder on the side of the surgery more than 80 degrees.

All patients in the intensive care unit will be connected to an ECG monitor, and many will have an arterial line, an indwelling catheter, and intravenous tubes. In addition, the cardiac surgery patient will have several central pressure lines. Many surgeons routinely place pacemaker wires perioperatively. These wires can be attached to a temporary external pacemaker or a permanent internal pacemaker or can be removed a few days after surgery if they are not needed.

Recently the intra-aortic balloon pump (IABP) has been utilized preoperatively and postoperatively to improve coronary artery circulation and prevent or reduce myocardial ischemia.[28] Using a deflated balloon whose size depends on the patient's size, the IABP is threaded through the femoral artery to the descending thoracic aorta. Its instantaneous inflation is synchronized with the period just after systole to create a backflow or counterpulsation of blood into the coronary arteries, therefore improving perfusion to the myocardium.[7,28] With the IABP in place, hip flexion at the insertion sight is prohibited, and the head of the bed cannot be elevated above 15 to 30 degrees so that the balloon does not migrate upward and occlude the subclavian artery. The patient should be rolled at least every 2 hours, with hip extension being maintained on the side of the insertion. Chest percussion and vibration are not contraindicated unless the patient is otherwise medically unstable.[7]

Last, if the patient is being mechanically ventilated, the ventilator settings must be checked before initiation of the treatment. Values recorded on the bedside flow sheet should correspond to those set on the ventilator. Next, check that the patient is receiving the proper number of breaths and the full volume. Notify those in charge of maintaining the ventilator if changes are needed rather than making changes yourself.

Physical assessment

Physical assessment should include observation, palpation, auscultation and percussion, and range of motion as discussed previously in the section on preoperative assessment (p. 259). You should immediately determine the patient's level of alertness and ability to cooperate. Questioning a patient about any pain he or she may be experiencing and if he or she is receiving enough oxygen will give a clue about the alertness and ability to cooperate.

Chest physical therapy

Promoting pulmonary hygiene is the primary goal in treatment of postsurgical patients. Assessment criteria will determine the aggressiveness used to reach this goal.

The point at which treatment is initiated will vary from institution to institution. Some therapists start in the recovery room reassuring the patient and encouraging them to breathe deeply and do ankle circles. This early intervention will often depend on the anesthesiologist's protocol and how soon after surgery the anesthesiologist chooses to reverse the anesthesia. Many programs do not allow initiation of chest physical therapy until one day postoperatively.[22] Physical assessment can be done when it has been determined that the patient is stable enough to tolerate a treatment.

Before the patient is moved in any way there are a few precautions to consider:

1. Tubes and lines must be free to move with the patient and must be checked for patency when the patient is repositioned.
2. Condensation collected in the ventilator tubing should be drained so that it does not flow into the endotracheal tube and cause the patient to cough unexpectedly.
3. To decrease patient discomfort, splinting pillows for incisional pain or pillow support for maintaining positions may be required.
4. Be aware of changes in vital signs when a patient's position is altered.

Note again that patients undergoing pneumonectomies should not be positioned on the operative side for any length of time during the first few days after surgery (p. 259).

It is not unusual for patients to have clear breath sounds during their early postoperative course: therefore percussion and vibration are not commonly needed. The patient is encouraged to assist the ventilator and to aerate their lungs fully by using the diaphragmatic and segmental breathing techniques taught preoperatively. It is helpful to provide added tactile stimulation to the areas you want the patient to expand.[22] Although the ventilator is supplying the volume, the patient may be able to determine actively the segments to which the volume will go by selectively expanding the chest wall adjacent to those segments.

There is no formula for treating postoperative pulmonary patients. Many things that must be considered have been mentioned above. The treatments may be very short or may last up to an hour or more. They might be very aggressive involving many modalities or include only breathing exercises. These factors will be determined by thorough assessment, patient tolerance, and hospital protocol. Various modalities and their place in treating postoperative patients are described below.

Breathing exercises. Breathing exercises are the most used and versatile modalities for chest physical therapy treatments. Other treatment modalities such as bronchial drainage, percussion, or vibration may be a priority during a specific treatment session, but breathing exercises will be used with every treatment. More importantly, if properly instructed and responsible enough, the patient can be taught to carry out these maneuvers between treatments. This process can speed the patient's recovery.

The therapist should not assume that a patient will attain complete lung excursion when asked to take a deep breath. Proper instruction, preferable preoperatively, is required. Vraciu and Vraciu pointed out the importance of thorough teaching of breathing exercises. The only difference between the control and experimental group in their study was that the latter group received instruction in breathing exercises from physical therapists as well as standard treatment regimen. The patients instructed by the physical therapists had significantly fewer postoperative pulmonary complications.[47]

The patient should be instructed while sitting upright or in a semi-Fowler position with the abdominal muscles relaxed. The therapist places a hand just below the xiphoid process and asks the patient to take a breath in through the nose. The descent of the diaphragm is noticed, and the patient is taught to palpate for this action. Lateral and posterior basilar excursion is then pointed out to the patient to increase the awareness of different types of chest expansion. The tactile stimulus of the therapist's hand is very important. Once the patient understands the requests, review deep breathing by encouraging the patient to inspire fully and then exhale through the mouth. The patient will attempt to use this breathing technique while in the bronchial drainage positions to ventilate more fully the various lung segments. The patient is instructed to practice this breathing technique between treatments and while using the incentive spirometer.

There are some contraindications to breathing exercises. Patients with cardiac or hemodynamic instability may not be candidates for physical therapy. Patients with a pneumothorax resulting in a moderate or large air leak should not participate in deep breathing until that leak has been closed. All other patients who are able should perform deep-breathing exercises as part of each treatment, including the alert patient being mechanically ventilated. This

latter group can use segmental and diaphragmatic breathing to deliver the inspiratory volume to bases of the lungs.

Bronchial drainage. Bronchial drainage, or postural drainage as it has been called, is employed to enhance mucus transport to the trachea for easier expectoration. Classical bronchial drainage positions can be stressful to the cardiovascular system and are seldom used for surgical or traumatic patients. The Trendelenburg position, with the head down at 30 degrees, will cause blood pressure changes and is contraindicated for hemodynamically unstable patients. Increased intracranial pressure is a relative contraindication, especially for patients who have had craniotomies.[3,14] Incision placement will also prevent many patients from assuming classical positions; therefore modified drainage positions are used to assist the removal of excess secretions.[17] These modified positions include side-lying and Trendelenburg positions of approximately 15 degrees. If the patient does not tolerate the head-down position, as shown by blood pressure changes, increased respiratory rate, or complaints of headache, positioning with the bed flat or even slightly elevated can be used.

For proper bronchial drainage the patient should be placed in the optimal position to allow drainage of the involved segment without causing any ill effects to the patient.

With the patient positioned, other treatment modalities such as percussion and vibration can be employed to expedite transport of secretions. The length of time positioned for bronchial drainage will depend on the quantity, tenacity, and location of the secretions as well as patient tolerance. This time is usually approximately 20 minutes. While the patient is in drainage positions, breathing exercises should be done. Tactile stimulation to the chest wall or a quick stretch to the intercostal muscles before the initiation of the breath may increase the patient's awareness of what area to expand. The quick stretch to the intercostals may enhance inspiration by a stretch reflex.

During bronchial drainage the air and blood flow are greatest to the dependent, and often healthier, lung. Remaining on the same side for longer periods of time will inhibit this somewhat desirable effect because excursion of the dependent lung decreases.[22] These patients must be assisted with rolling at least every 1 to 2 hours so that the dependent lung does not become atelectatic and to assure that both lungs are adequately ventilated.

Percussion. Percussion involves striking the thorax with a cupped hand over a specific segment of the lung. This technique is believed to break up and loosen mucus within the lungs.[11] Percussion is often considered the distinctive feature of chest physical therapists because it is the most visible and audible aspect of the treatment. It is also the modality most often practiced by other medical professionals when they believe the patient's pulmonary status needs improvement. This belief is unfortunate because there is much more involved in assessment of the patient and provision of a worthwhile treatment. Percussion should be used in patients unable to mobilize and expectorate excess secretions or to assist in reexpanding an area atelectasis.[9,11,17,26] Only the lung area involved needs to be percussed. The patient should be positioned to allow optimal drainage and excursion of the involved lobe. For postsurgical patients this is usually a modified position. Of course no percussion will be done in the area of the incision. If the patient has had abdominal surgery, it is helpful to place one hand between the incision and the area percussed to make the treatment more tolerable. A pillow held over the incision will also accomplish this splinting effect.

Percussion may not be tolerated by some postoperative patients because of pain or hemodynamic instability. Arrhythmias have been noticed during percussion.[14,22] If arrhythmias occur a less vigorous treatment of drainage with deep breathing and possibly vibration should be attempted with close monitoring of the heart rate and rhythm.

The length of time for percussion will depend on patient tolerance and response. It has been our experience that early postoperative patients respond better to shorter and more frequent treatments with the nurse turning the patient and working on deep breathing between sessions.

Vibration. Vibration is a rapid shaking back and forth, not downward, of the thorax over a segment of a lung causing mucus to flow toward the trachea. Vibration is less traumatic to the patient than percussion. Often the patient can tolerate vibration and not percussion while in a full or modified drainage position. Patients are instructed to exhale as they are vibrated.[19] There are few patients who cannot tolerate vibration when done properly. Optimally, vibration should follow percussion while the patient is in a bronchial drainage position.[22] These techniques with gravity will promote loosening and flow of secretions toward the trachea. The secretions can then be coughed up or suctioned out if the patient is intubated.

Cough and suctioning. Postsurgically many patients will be intubated. They often complain more about the discomfort of the endotracheal tube than about the incision. Explaining that improved ventilation, with their efforts, will result in removal of the endotracheal tube provides additional incentive to the patient. While the patient is intubated, excess secretions are aspirated through the endotracheal tube using a suction catheter. This is called "endotracheal suctioning." Patients who are not intubated may also require suctioning if they have a weak or ineffective cough. In this case the catheter will be inserted nasally or sometimes orally. This is very uncomfortable for the patient. Every effort should be made to help the patient produce an effective cough. The best cough is produced while the patient is sitting upright, a position in which the highest cough pressures are attained. If the cough is still not strong with the patient sitting, manual pressure to the

rib cage and abdomen can produce greater pressure.[48] Pain greatly limits the ability to achieve a strong cough.[8] Many hospitals use splinting pillows to support the wound. Patients can also be encouraged to flex their hips to allow the abdominal muscles to relax, thereby decreasing the stress to the abdominal incision during the cough.

As mentioned above, the patient with an endotracheal tube will not be able to cough and will need endotracheal suctioning. Significant drops in PaO_2 and resultant cardiac arrhythmias have been noticed during endotracheal suctioning.[1,31] In 1978, Adlkofer and Powaser found that preoxygenation of the patient prevented the sudden drop of PaO_2 and strongly suggested postoxygenation to hasten the return of oxygen values to an adequate level.[1] In 1979, Peterson, Pierson, and Hunter strongly supported this practice as well as oxygenation between catheter passes.[31] If suctioning is done properly, hypoxemia can be avoided so that the chances of cardiac arrhythmias are reduced.[12] Below are the suggested considerations for safe suctioning procedure:

Sterile technique

Correct catheter size, usually No. 14 French for adults. Too large a catheter will traumatize the airways; a small one may not remove thick secretions.

Vacuum level, 120 mm Hg for adults.[31] Too high will remove more oxygen and may traumatize airways; too low will not remove thick secretions.

Prepare the patient: explain the procedure and prepare to splint during cough.

Preoxygenate the patient to prevent hypoxemia.[1,31]

Enter airway slowly with suction off.[24]

Apply suction-release-suction technique as catheter is removed[24,26]

Suction for no longer than 10 to 15 seconds.[47]

Postoxygenate the patient.[24]

Auscultation of the lungs and palpation of the upper chest should be performed before, during, and after suctioning. The patient may require lengthy suctioning because of a large quantity of secretions. Allow for periods of rest, and oxygenate between catheter passes. Very thick secretions may require the instillation of small amounts of sterile wetting agents such as saline solution or water. These liquids will frequently loosen the secretions in the upper airways. Remember to monitor closely the patient's heart rate and rhythm during these techniques.

Patients are extubated when their arterial blood gas levels and respiratory parameters are adequate to maintain spontaneous ventilation. Respiratory parameters, measured usually by the respiratory therapist, include minute volume, respiratory rate, forced inspiratory pressure, and forced inspiratory volume. It is helpful for the therapist to be present during extubation. Removal of the tube causes strong coughing and gagging while the patient expectorates secretions that had accumulated around the distal end of the tube. Encouraging the patient and assisting with splinting during this coughing may prevent added discomfort.

Mobilization. Strong emphasis is placed on mobilizing the patient to promote pulmonary hygiene and decrease the incidence of pulmonary embolism secondary to phlebitis.[33,35] Initially, mobilization may involve only rolling side to side at least every 2 hours and the use of ankle circles and shoulder shrugs. As the patient becomes hemodynamically stable and gains strength, trunk mobility, sitting, and eventually ambulation will be added. Physicians usually allow foot dangling at the bedside or sitting out of bed early in the postoperative course if the patient is stable. Upper extremity and trunk exercises are incorporated into the treatment to prevent loss of motion and muscle atrophy. In addition, these exercises demonstrate to patients that they can move despite their incision, thereby fostering normal unsplinted posture. The patient must be reassured that coughing and movement will not harm the incision site. Special attention should be paid to shoulder range of motion on the involved side of patients who have had thoracotomy. This is also true for standing posture in patients who have had abdominal surgery. Neither group should be quickly forced into full range of motion or erect posture, rather one should encourage them to stretch slowly. Full range of motion and erect posture should be attained before discharge.

By the third or fourth postoperative day the patients who have had cardiac surgery begin slow ambulation.[17] Some of the other surgical patients begin sooner. Ambulation is increased daily until discharge.

Physical therapy should continue until the patient's lungs are clear, full preoperative range of motion and posture is attained, and ambulation is functional or at the preadmission level. Patients should be encouraged to continue breathing and trunk mobility exercises when they return home. In some hospitals cardiac surgery patients are also seen by a cardiac rehabilitation team that teaches them about medication, diet, and physical activity and offers them psychological support. These patients will return home with a better understanding of their abilities and limitations. Patients not involved with such a program should be instructed by their physician and physical therapist regarding stair climbing, driving, diet, and other activities of daily living.

POSTOPERATIVE COMPLICATIONS

Postoperative complications that can occur in patients who have experienced abdominal or thoracic surgery are summarized in Table 14-1. A detailed discussion of these complications follows.

Atelectasis

Atelectasis is incomplete expansion of the lung because of collapse of the alveoli. Hypoventilation is the most common postoperative cause. This decrease in lung volume occurs for a number of reasons:

1. Anesthesia and narcotic drugs decrease ciliary function and limit the patient's inspiratory effort, thus facilitating secretion pooling in the alveoli.
2. Pain and fear associated with the surgery impair the strength of the patient's cough and the patient's mobility and thus impede secretion removal.
3. Fluid or air that collects in the pleural cavity exerts pressure on the lungs, decreases thoracic expansion, and promotes alveolar collapse.
4. Irritation of the lung tissue from the mechanics of surgery or infection can cause increased sputum production.

Patients with atelectasis will develop a low-grade fever, and rales will be heard on auscultation. The radiograph will show a plate-like atelectasis usually adjacent to the diaphragm.

Good preoperative teaching and postoperative care can prevent atelectasis. The patient should be made aware of the responsibility to roll from side to side and should be able to move the diaphragm slowly and fully. The patient should be motivated to participate in his own postoperative care.

Cardiac arrhythmias

Cardiac arrhythmias are variations from the normal rhythm of the heart. They include rapid or slow rhythms, tachycardia or bradycardia, irregular rhythms, atrial or ventricular beats. Arrhythmias are caused by diminished blood supply or anoxia to the heart muscle, electrolyte imbalance, or surgical intervention. It is not uncommon to see various arrhythmias after open-heart surgery. Other surgical patients may also exhibit arrhythmias depending on their presurgical status and the seriousness of the surgery. Patients who have had open-heart surgery and some who have had high-risk thoracic or abdominal surgery will be monitored for a few days after surgery.

Obviously, treatment is held or modified if the patient's status is unstable. If the arrhythmias include sinus tachycardia of less than 140 beats per minute or occasional premature ventricular contractions (PVC), treatment is modified with postural drainage performed in the bed-flat position. If the arrhythmias are more serious such as a rapid sinus tachycardia, sinus bradycardia, frequent PVC's, first-degree or second-degree heart blocks, or rare PVC's, the treatment may be modified more. Emphasis on segmental breathing with the patient in a side-lying, bed-flat position without percussion or vibration may be an option. With more serious arrhythmias, such as frequent PVC's or third-degree heart blocks, further assessment for treatment modification is needed. Treatment is discontinued if six or more PVC's per treatment minute are noted. If the patient is receiving antiarrhythmic drugs, the treat-

Table 14-1. Possible postoperative complications that can occur in patients who have experienced abdominal or thoracic surgery

Complications	Definition	Clinical signs	Treatment modification or emphasis
Atelectasis	Incomplete expansion of lung and collapse of alveoli	Low-grade temperature rales on inspiration	Deep diaphragmatic breathing
Cardiac arrest	Cessation of function of heart	Breathless, pulseless, pale, unresponsive	Cardiopulmonary resuscitation, immediate medical attention recovery: No Trendelenburg position Segmental breathing, bed-flat or deep breathing in cardiac position (45 to 60 degrees, head elevated)
Cardiac arrythmias	Irregularity in normal rhythm of heart	Irregular pulse, vary with arrhythmia	Modified with deep breathing, bed-flat drainage, side-to-side rolling with PVC's, SVT, 1- to 2-degree block, or 6 PVC's per minute, or any more serious arrhythmias, or modify with deep breathing in cardiac position
Cardiac tamponade	Fluid in pericardial sac limiting ventricular filling	$\downarrow$ Cardiac output $\downarrow$ Blood pressure $\uparrow$ Heart rate $\pm$ Shortness of breath	No treatment if in severe distress Modified postural drainage, No percussion, vibration, or suctioning if arrhythmias present
Congestive heart failure	Effusion of serous fluid in the interstitial tissues of the lungs	Shortness of breath $\pm$ Diaphoresis $\pm$ Peripheral edema	Modified postural drainage Relaxation exercises Decrease respiratory rate
Empyema	Accumulation of pus in the pleural cavity	Those seen with infection; fever, weight loss, malaise, $\downarrow$ breath sounds, and dull percussion over area	Segmental breathing Deep diaphragmatic breathing $\uparrow$ Mobility
Hemothorax	Blood in the pleural space, usually seen with pneumothorax (called "hemopneumothorax")	$\pm$ Shortness of breath $\pm$ Pain $\pm$ Dyspnea $\pm$ Hypertension $\pm$ Diaphoresis $\pm$ "Shocky"	When stabilized: segmental breathing on involved side
Hypercapnia	Increase of CO_2 concentration in arterial blood	Change in mental status	Proper O_2 therapy
Hypoxia	Low O_2 content in the body from hypoventilation, ventilation/perfusion imbalance or underlying pulmonary disease	$\pm$ Mental fatigue $\pm$ Headache Poor judgment $\pm$ $\downarrow$ Breath sounds	Medical treatment Teach effective breathing
Pleural effusion	Fluid in pleural space	$\pm$ Shortness of breath $\pm$ Pain $\pm$ Dyspnea $\downarrow$ Breath sounds over pleural effusion with tubular breath sounds from 1 or 2 intercostal spaces above effusion	No postural drainage if shortness of breath $\uparrow$ Mobility Deep diaphragmatic and segmental breathing

$\uparrow$, Increasing; $\pm$, positive; $-$, negative; $\downarrow$, decreasing; *PVC*, premature ventricular contractions; *SVT*, supraventricular tachycardia.

Table 14-1. Possible postoperative complications that can occur in patients who have experienced abdominal or thoracic surgery—cont'd

Complications	Definition	Clinical signs	Treatment modification or emphasis
Pneumonia	Inflammation of alveoli, usually from a blood-borne organism	+ Fever and rales + Chills and tubular breath sounds + Dyspnea, dull percussion ± Painful inhalation	Deep breathing and cough Postural drainage Percussion and vibration when productive
Pneumothorax	Gas, usually air, in the pleural space	± Shortness of breath ± Dyspnea ± Diaphoresis No breath sounds over upper lobe area	Segmental breathing Postural drainage
Postcardiotomy syndrome	Combination of pericarditis, pleurisy, pneumonitis, and pleural effusion	Thoracic pain ± Dyspnea ± Shortness of breath	Treat dyspnea ↓ Respiratory rate with controlled expiration No percussion because of pleuritic pain Segmental breathing for pleural effusion Reorient patient to person, place, and time

Pulmonary embolism	Obstruction of pulmonary artery or one of its branches by a clot	Acute:
		  Pain
		  Shortness of breath
		  Dyspnea
		  Tachycardia
		Subacute:
		  ± Hemoptysis
		  ± Pleural effusion
		  ± Friction rub
		  ↓ Breath sounds over involved area
			When stabilized:
			  Deep breathing, segmental breathing
			  Extended expiration
			  Postural drainage if hemodynamically stable
			  Percussion and vibration after 6 days of anticoagulation therapy

Respiratory arrest	Cessation of respiratory function	↑ To no respiratory rate ± Hypoxic symptoms ± Diaphoresis	CPR Immediate medical treatment
Respiratory distress	Noticeable difficulty in breathing	↑ Respiratory rate ± Diaphoresis ± Hypoxic symptoms Anxiety ± ↑ Secretions throughout lungs	Medical: O_2 therapy, drug therapy Intubated: preoxygenate and suction, full treatment as indicated Extubated: relax and reassure patient; teach effective cough to clear secretion; treat fully as indicated; ± suction, ± intubate by doctor
Subcutaneous emphysema	Collection of air in subcutaneous tissue	Swelling in area involved, "crackle" upon palpation	Avoid deep breathing with large air leak, no percussion over swollen areas

ment should include at least diaphragmatic breathing in cardiac position.

The decision whether to treat patient's with arrhythmias and how vigorously to treat should depend on information from the physician or nurse caring for the patient and your assessment of the medical data. The physical therapist must have a good basic understanding of arterial blood gases (ABG), electrolyte levels, cardiac drugs, and hemodynamics. The goal of treatment is to maintain good aeration to prevent pulmonary complications.

Cardiac tamponade

Cardiac tamponade is a limitation of ventricular filling during diastole because of fluid collection within the pericardial sac. If the percardium is intact and the fluid continues to collect, the pressure inside continues to increase and further restricts cardiac function. Cardiac output and blood pressure will fall. Cardiac arrest is imminent unless the percardium can be incised to relieve the pressure.

Because of the overall instability of the vital signs in these patients, modifications will have to be made in all areas of treatment. Chest physical therapy may be contraindicated with this complication.

Cardiogenic shock

Cardiogenic shock results from sudden diminution of cardiac output. The cardiac output may fall very low immediately after cardiac damage. Therefore this phenomenom is usually seen after myocardial infarction, but may occur after open-heart surgery, usually in the intensive care unit. These patients will be seriously hypotensive, and immediate medical and drug therapy is required. Treatment should be discontinued until the patient becomes stabilized.

Deep vein thrombosis

Deep vein thrombosis, venous thrombosis, is a coagulation or clot of blood that remains at the site of origin. If it detaches, the clot can travel to the right side of the heart and enter the lung—a pulmonary embolism.

The causes for venous thrombosis include venous stasis, increased platelets secondary to surgery, trauma, or dehydration. The therapist can assist with prevention of the thrombosis by teaching and encouraging patients to perform ankle pumps preoperatively and postoperatively. Patients at bed rest should perform a series of 10 to 15 ankle pumps every hour.

If the patient has developed a thrombus, care is taken when positioning him or her. Avoid flexing the knee and hip. If the leg shows signs of inflammation (thrombophlebitis), excessive movement, even rolling, should be avoided until sufficient anticoagulation therapy is given (4 or 5 days).

Hemothorax

Hemothorax is a collection of blood in the pleural cavity usually after trauma and often associated with a pneumothorax. When they are both present, it is called a "hemopneumothorax." It will also occur with the rupture of an aneurysm in the pleural cavity.

The patient will experience varying degrees of symptoms depending on the severity of the hemorrhage. If it is extensive, the patient will become hypotensive, tachycardiac, tachypneic, and diaphoretic. In light of the blood loss the patient must be given fluid replacements. Because the blood in the pleural cavity can clot rapidly and compromise lung function, it must be aspirated. With a significant fluid accumulation, a chest tube may be placed in the lower pleural space in the area of the sixth intercostal space.

When the patient becomes stabilized, treatment emphasis will be on increasing respiratory effort to improve lung expansion on the involved side. When these patients are positioned, care should be taken not to flex the shoulder on the side when the chest tube above 80 degrees since the tube may be dislodged.

Hypercapnia

Hypercapnia is increased partial pressure of carbon dioxide in the arterial blood. Generally the partial pressure should be about 50 mm Hg. Of the many causes for hypercapnia, it is most often caused by hypoventilation or a circulatory deficiency. The physical therapist's role is to assist the patient with "blowing off" CO_2 by teaching extended expiration. These patients will exhibit an altered mental status, irritability, and lethargy. In addition, the patient may be cyanotic, dyspneic, and tachycardiac.

Hypoxia

Hypoxia is low oxygen content within the tissues of the body. It can result from ventilation-perfusion imbalance or underlying pulmonary disease, but it is seen most often postoperatively as a result of inadequate transport and delivery of oxygen to the tissues.[14] Usually a PaO_2 below 60 mm Hg with a person at rest constitutes hypoxia. In the case of patients who have had open-heart surgery the heart lung machine destroys blood cells thereby leaving the patient anemic and with decreased blood hemoglobin levels. This anemia will decrease O_2 transport to the body tissues and, more significantly, to the brain. These patients may demonstrate mental fatigue, headaches, poor judgment and in some cases hallucinations have been reported in intensive care settings. Oxygen therapy is indicated to increase oxygen tension in the tissues. Efforts should be made to keep the patient oriented and cooperative so that necessary treatments can be carried out. If the hypoxia is caused by hypoventilation, one deals with it simply by encouraging deep breathing.

Pleural effusion

A pleural effusion is an accumulation of fluid in the pleural space. The fluid may be called a "transudate" if it is not infected, or an "exudate" if it is infected. Transudates occur with changes in capillary pressure, membrane permeability, and plasma colloid osmotic pressure. These changes occur with congestive heart failure or diseases of the liver or kidney, or after heart or lung surgery. The fluid is clear and will usually be reabsorbed with treatment of the primary physiological disorder. Exudates tend to be straw colored and cloudy and are a response to inflammation or neoplasm. They must be treated medically and sometimes require thoracentesis. Thoracentesis is aspiration of fluid from the pleural space. This is done also if the amount of fluid is so large it is compromising respiration or if the effusion is slow in dissipating. If the fluid remains in the pleural space long enough, it will become fibrotic and will not be reabsorbed into the system.

Some pleural effusions are painful, but the patient may notice discomfort only when taking a full deep breath and during shortness of breath, or dyspnea. If the patient is immobile, atelectasis may develop in the lung tissue adjacent to the pleural effusion. On auscultation, the breath sounds will be greatly decreased or absent over the effusion and tubular or bronchial breath sounds can be heard one to two intercostal spaces above the fluid level.

The therapist can aid in reabsorption of the effusion by having the patient concentrate on deep breathing in postural drainage positions and encouraging increased mobility. The pressure exerted on the fluid by a forceful deep breath will disperse the fluid over as much of the pleural membrane as possible, a process that will aid in its reabsorption. The patient should be placed in postural drainage positions for the lower lobes with emphasis on segmental breathing. In most cases, the breath sounds improve as the fluid flows to the dependent side of the pleural space. Rales may be heard if an atelectasis has developed. Atelectasis should be treated accordingly, and the patient encouraged to roll side to side every 2 hours and ambulate if allowed.

Pneumonia

Pneumonia is an infection of the alveolar spaces of the lungs. With early postoperative mobilization, the incidence of postoperative pneumonia has declined. Of all types of pneumonia, those most commonly seen postoperatively are lobar and bronchopneumonia. The former is confined to one or more lobes and usually brought on by blood-borne organisms. Bronchopneumonia is often patchy in distribution throughout the lungs and caused by airborne organisms. The patient develops fever, chills, dyspnea, and often pain in the involved hemithorax. Sputum production may occur in the early stages and is classically rust in color. The involved alveoli become plugged with fibrin and red blood cells, and the alveolar capillaries are congested. There is poor air exchange, and the bronchi to the affected area may be plugged. This filling of alveoli is called ''consolidation.'' Tubular or bronchial breath sounds will be heard on auscultation because the normal sounds of the large airways are more fully transmitted through these fluids. Percussion will be dull. Sputum cultures indicate the type of infection present, and antibiotic therapy is started. Physical therapy will concentrate initially on removal of secretions and expansion of the involved lung area. Initial treatment should also include teaching diaphragmatic breathing, lateral costal breathing, and basilar expansion. Instruction in efficient cough techniques, controlled breathing to decrease shortness of breath, and positioning to drain the lung is included. If the patient is productive of sputum and in the less acute stages of the disease, percussion and vibration in the postural drainage positions is indicated.

Pneumothorax

A pneumothorax is an accumulation of gas or air in the thoracic cavity. It can be therapeutic, spontaneous, or traumatic.

A therapeutic pneumothorax may be performed to equalize pressure in the thorax or to immobilize the lung for treatment of tuberculosis. Spontaneous pneumothorax is discussed on p. 255 with blebectomy. Traumatic pneumothorax may be caused by trauma, surgical damage to the chest wall, rupture of a peripheral bleb with coughing or artificial ventilation, or perforation and fistulas in the trachea and esophagus.

In almost all cases, patients will experience shortness of breath, pain, diaphoresis, and dyspnea. They may appear cyanotic, have decreased excursion of the involved hemithorax, and have decreased or no breath sounds ipsilaterally. These signs depend on the size of the pneumothorax, which is commonly estimated by the percentage of the lung displaced. If there is air in the thoracic cavity, it tends to show on the radiograph as a loss of tissue in the area of the upper lobes. These patients usually need immediate medical care. A needle or chest tube will be inserted in the area of the second intercostal space to measure pressure and withdraw the accumulated gas or air. If any degree of lung collapse has occurred, the chest tube with continuous suction should assist reexpansion in a day or two.

Physical therapy begins when the chest tubes are inserted and the patient is stabilized. If the pneumothorax was not large enough to necessitate chest tubes, early physical therapy will assist with reexpansion. Emphasis should be on segmental breathing exercises with careful positioning.

Postcardiotomy syndrome

Postcardiotomy syndrome is a relatively uncommon complication and occurs in only 3% to 4% of the cardiac patient mix. The cause is not fully established, but viral infection has been proposed. The theory of autoimmunity is most widely accepted. Antiheart antibodies have been found in the blood sera of these patients. This is a result of cardiac necrosis from myocardial infarction or surgery.

Characteristic signs and symptoms include pericarditis, pleurisy, pneumonitis, and pleural effusion. A pattern of recurrent fever can precede or coincide with chest pain. The chest pain mimics that of myocardial infarction; however, the pain usually intensifies with movement of the thorax with deep inspiration. Dyspnea accompanies the pleuritis, pneumonitis, and the pleural effusion. These symptoms may last from 2 days to 12 weeks.

Treatment should address the dyspnea primarily and concentrate on decreasing respiratory rate by utilizing controlled expirations and improving aeration in the area of the pleural effusion with segmental breathing. Percussion is usually contraindicated in light of the existing pleuritic pain. If there is an infiltrate, every effort to drain secretions should be made using postural drainage, deep breathing, and good hydration until pleuritic pain subsides.

Pulmonary embolism

Pulmonary embolism is obstruction of a pulmonary artery or one of its branches by a clot. The embolus most frequently arises from a deep vein in the leg or pelvis though other origins include deep veins in the arms, mural thrombi from the right atrium or ventricle, or fat emboli from the marrow of a fractured long bone. The occlusion of the blood supply to the lung parenchyma will cause hemorrhagic consolidation with possible necrosis, pulmonary edema, and pulmonary hypertension. These along with the decrease in the oxygen exchange will cause varying hemodynamic changes depending on the size of the embolus and the patient's preexisting cardiopulmonary status.

Clinically, the patient may exhibit dyspnea, pleuritic pain, tachycardia, cyanosis, diaphoresis, hemoptysis, and a pleural effusion may develop. Immediate treatment includes anticoagulation drugs and oxygen therapy. As the patient becomes stabilized, physical therapy is employed to improve oxygen exchange and mobilization of secretions. If the patient still has dyspnea, instructions in segmental breathing, slow extended expiration, and deep diaphragmatic breathing with a few seconds of breath holding at the end of inspiration will be helpful.

If the patient is productive of sputum and hemodynamically stable, postural drainage is indicated. There has been some controversy regarding the use of percussion with these patients. Some practitioners believe the clot may be dislodged during percussion. We believe that a safe guideline is to wait until the sixth day of anticoagulant therapy. Of course, percussion would not be used if the patient is still experiencing pleuritic pain. Otherwise, it may be used to mobilize secretions.

Respiratory arrest

Respiratory arrest is cessation of respiratory function because of airway obstruction, respiratory depression, or cardiac arrest.

Some causes include partial or complete airway obstruction by the tongue, a foreign body, secretions, or edema. Respiratory depression can be attributable to trauma to the central nervous system, drug overdose, asphyxiation, severe shock, and others. In the case of respiratory depression, hypoxia and hypercapnia occur, and they will in turn worsen the depression. Cardiac arrest will always lead to respiratory arrest if the circulation is not restored in a short period of time.

Physical therapy involvement is aimed at prevention. When dealing with patients in respiratory distress, we want to prevent respiratory arrest. Cardiac arrest will soon follow respiratory arrest if emergency medical care does not intervene.

The most common cause of postoperative respiratory arrest with which we are concerned is airway obstruction secondary to secretions. Secretions may develop from the lungs' normal response to surgery, from pneumonia, or from severe preexisting pulmonary disease. If the patient is having difficulty clearing secretions, there will be compromise of oxygenation and resulting cardiac arrhythmias, altered mental status, and other symptoms of hypoxia (p. 268). If cardiac arrhythmias occur, the therapist must determine the cause and proceed with appropriate treatment.

If the patient is intubated, suctioning and oxygenating can make a noticeable and immediate difference in the patient's alertness and cardiac rhythm if the cause of hypoxia was secretions. The patient's status should be reassessed and treatment should be continued to clear secretions from the involved segments of the lung by positioning, oxygenating, deep-breathing exercises, percussion, and vibration.

Time should be spent relaxing and reassuring the nonintubated patients who are having difficulty clearing secretions. Full patient cooperation is needed for effective expectoration. First, the patient should breathe in through the nose and blow out through the mouth with the lips slightly pursed and minimal back pressure. This will decrease the respiratory rate and stop nonproductive spasmodic coughing. If the patient responds well to this relaxed breathing, encourage deep but slow diaphragmatic breathing to prepare for coughing. An effective coughing technique is three to four slow large breaths through the nose expired through slightly pursed lips to allow the secretions to move up the trachea closer to the glottis. A subsequent breath should be as large as possible, followed by two strong staged coughs. The first cough moves the secretions; the second expectorates them. Slow controlled nasal breathing follows until the patient can no longer raise secretions. Should the patient's mental status limit cooperation, oropharyngeal suctioning or use of the Trendelenburg position will both assist secretion movement. Again, the status of the patient must be reassessed and further treatment given. Some patients have large amounts of secretions, and frequent treatments or suctioning may be required. The patient's understanding of the technique for effective coughing should be emphasized.

Subcutaneous emphysema

Subcutaneous emphysema is a collection of air in the interstices of the subcutaneous tissues.[34] This can be caused by the rupture of marginal alveoli or an airway. This rupture can permit air to escape into the subpleural spaces and move to the mediastinum and upwards to the neck and chest.

Clinically the face, neck, and chest may appear swollen. On palpation, the tissues "crackle" and air will move under the tissues. Patients may experience dyspnea and appear cyanotic depending on the extent of the air leak. If severe enough, the tissue may have to be incised to allow air to escape and relieve the pressure, which could cause vascular compression and pain.

REFERENCES

1. Adlkofer, R.M., and Powaser, M.M.: The effect of endotracheal suctioning on arterial blood gases in patients after cardiac surgery, Heart Lung 7(6):1011-1014, 1978.
2. Anson, B.J., and McVay, C.B.: Surgical anatomy, ed. 5, vol. 1, Philadelphia, 1971, W.B. Saunders Co.
3. Barrell, S.E., and Abbas, H.M.: Monitoring during physiotherapy after open heart surgery, Physiotherapy 64(9):272-273, 1978.
4. Bartlett, R.H.: Pulmonary pathophysiology in surgical patients, Surg. Clin. North Am. 60(6):1323-1337, 1980.
5. Bartlett, R.H., Gazzaniga, A.B., and Geraghty, T.R.: Respiratory maneuvers to prevent post-operative pulmonary complications, J.A.M.A. 224(7):1017-1021, 1973.
6. Bateman, J.R.M., Newman, S.P., Daunt, K.M., and others: Is cough as effective as chest physiotherapy in the removal of excessive tracheobronchial secretions? Thorax 36:683-687, 1981.
7. Bricker, P.L.: The intense nursing demands of the intra-aortic balloon pump, RN 43(7):23-29, July 1980.
8. Byrd, R.B., and Burns, J.R.: Cough dynamics in the post-thoracotomy state, Chest 67(6):654-657, 1975.
9. Cash, P., editor: Cash's textbook of chest, heart and vascular disorders for physiotherapists, ed. 3, London, 1979, Faber & Faber, Ltd.
10. Cooper, P.: The craft of surgery, ed. 2., vol. 1, Boston, 1971, Little, Brown & Co.
11. Frownfelter, D.: Chest physical therapy and pulmonary rehabilitation: an interdisciplinary approach, Chicago, 1978, Year Book Medical Publishers, Inc.
12. Gaskell, D.V., and Webber, B.A.: The Rompton Hospital guide to chest physiotherapy, ed. 4, Oxford, London, 1980, Blackwell-Scientific Publications.
13. Gracey, D., Divertie, M., and Didier, E.: Preoperative pulmonary preparation of patients with chronic obstructive pulmonary disease: a prospective study, Chest 76:2, 123-129, Aug. 1970.
14. Hammon, W.E., and Martin, R.J.: Chest physical therapy for acute atelectasis: a report on its effectiveness, Phys. Ther. 61:217-220, 1981.
15. Hardy, J.D.: Rhoads' textbook of surgery, ed. 5, Philadelphia, 1977, J.B. Lippincott Co.
16. Hieptas, B.G., Roth, R.D., and Jensen, W.M.: Huff coughing and airway patency, Respir. Care 24(3):710-713, 1979.
17. Howell, S., and Hill, J.D.: Chest physical therapy procedures in open heart surgery, Phys. Ther. 58:1205-1214, 1978.
18. Hymes, A.C., Raale, D.E., Yonehino, E.G., and others: Electrical surface stimulation for control of acute post-operative pain and prevention of ileus, Surg. Forum 24:447-449, 1973.
19. Ingwersen, V.: Respiratory physical therapy and pulmonary care, New York, 1976, John Wiley & Sons, Inc.
20. Jung, R., Wight, J., Nusser, R., and others: Comparison of three methods of respiratory care following upper abdominal surgery, Chest 78(1):31-35, 1980.
21. Kaneko, K., Milie-Emili, J., Dolovich, M.B., and others: Regional distributions of ventilation and perfusion as a function of body position, J. Appl. Physiol. 21:767-777, 1966.
22. Kigin, C.M.: Chest physical therapy for the post-operative or traumatic injury patients, Phys. Ther. 61(12):1724-1736, 1981.
23. Latimer, R.G., Dickman, M., Day, W.C., and others: Ventilatory patterns and pulmonary complications after upper abdominal surgery determined by pre-operative and post-operative computerized spirometry and blood gas analysis, Am. J. Surg. 122:622-632, 1971.
24. Lewis, S.: Intensive care—7: physiotherapy in the intensive therapy unit, Nurs. Times 74(13):534-537, 1978.
25. Lord, G., Clement, A., and Francis, C.: A clinical, radiologic, and physiologic evaluation of chest physiotherapy, J. Maine Med. Assoc. 63:142-150, July 1972.
26. MacKenzie, C., editor, and others: Chest physiotherapy in the intensive care unit, Baltimore, 1981, The Williams & Wilkins Co.
27. Nakhjavahn, F.K.: Cardiologist at Albert Einstein Medical Center, personal communication, 1982.
28. Olson, H.G., Aronow, W.S., and Stemmer, E.A.: Clinical use of intra-aortic balloon counterpulsation in the treatment of coronary artery disease, Cardiologist Dig., pp. 12-18, Feb. 1977.
29. Palmer, K.N.V., and Sellick, B.A.: The prevention of post-operative pulmonary atelectasis, Lancet 1:164-168, 1953.
30. Paul, W.L., and Downs, J.B.: Post-operative atelectasis: intermittent positive pressure breathing, incentive spirometry, and face-mask positive end-expiratory pressure, Arch. Surg. 116:861-863, 1981.
31. Peterson, G.M., Pearson, D.J., and Hunter, P.M.: Arterial oxygen saturation during nasotracheal suctioning, Chest 76(3):283-287, Sept. 1979.
32. Pryor, J.A., and Webber, B.A.: An evaluation of the forced expiration technique as an adjunct to postural drainage, Physiotherapy 65(10):304-307, 1979.
33. Rose, S.D.: Prophylaxis of thromboembolic disease, Med. Clin. North Am. 63(6):1205-1223, 1979.
34. Sabiston, D.C., and Spencer, F.C.: Gibbon's surgery of the chest, ed. 3, Philadelphia, 1976, W.B. Saunders Co.
35. Schmidt, G.B.: Prophylaxis of pulmonary complications following abdominal surgery, including atelectasis, ARDS, and pulmonary embolism, Surg. Annu. 9:29-73, 1977.
36. Semanoff, T., Kleinfeld, M., and Castle, P.: Chest physical therapy as a preventive modality in cardiac surgery patients, Arch. Phys. Med. 62:506, Oct. 1981.
37. Starr, J.A.: The influence of posture and cumulative trails on the effectiveness of coughing in post-operative cholecystectomy patients, doctoral thesis, Boston, 1980, Boston University.
38. Stein, A.M., Mandell, D., and Ferguson, J.: Multiple fractures: look out for those pulmonary complications, Nursing'74, pp. 26-32, Nov. 1974.
39. Stein, M., and Cassara, F.L.: Pre-operative pulmonary evaluation and therapy for surgery patients, J.A.M.A. 211(5):787-790, 1962.
40. Stratton, S.A., and Smith, M.M.: Post-operative thoracotomy: effect of transcutaneous electric nerve stimulation on forced vital capacity, Phys. Ther. 60:45-47, 1980.
41. Swartz, S.I., and others: Principles of surgery, ed. 3, vols. 1 & 2, New York, 1969, McGraw-Hill Book Co.
42. Tarhan, S., Moffit, E.A., Sessler, A.D., and others: Risk of anesthesia and surgery in patients with chronic bronchitis, and chronic obstructive pulmonary disease, Surgery 74:720-726, 1973.
43. Thompson, B., and Thompson, H.T.: Forced expiratory exercises in asthma and their effect on FEV, N.Z. J. Physiother. 3(15):19-21, 1968.
44. Thoren, L.: Post-operative pulmonary complications: observations on their prevention by means of physiotherapy, Acta Chir. Scand. 107:193-205, 1954.
45. Tisi, G.M.: State of the art: pre-operative evaluation of pulmonary function, Am. Rev. Respir. Dis. 119:293-310, 1979.
46. Vander Ark, G.D., and McGrath, K.A.: Transcutaneous electrical stimulation in treatment of post-operative pain, Am. J. Surg. 130:338-340, 1975.
47. Vraciu, J.K., and Vraciu, R.A.: Effectiveness of breathing exercises in preventing pulmonary complications following open heart surgery, Phys. Ther. 57:1367-1371, 1977.
48. Yamazaki, S., Ogawa, J., Shohzu, A., and others: Intra-pleural cough pressures in patients after thoracotomy, J. Thorac. Cardiovasc. Surg. 80:600-604, 1980.

WILLY E. HAMMON

Physical therapy for the acutely ill patient in the respiratory intensive care unit

In many hospitals across the country, the physical therapist may be a relative newcomer to the critical care team.[72] Unfortunately, student physical therapists receive minimal if any exposure to the intensive care unit (ICU). As a result, the request to provide care in the ICU may cause anxiety in many therapists. The area is viewed as foreboding and crisis oriented. The majority of patients are perceived to be medically unstable and perhaps close to death. The unit is full of unfamiliar equipment. The patients are frequently semiconscious, with multiple central and peripheral monitoring and therapeutic lines. The many monitors and their sensitive alarms can contribute to the therapist's uneasiness.

However, a more realistic viewpoint is important. The severity of illness in these patients spans the spectrum from medically stable in good condition to the unstable whose survival is in question; however, the majority fall somewhere in between.

The numerous monitors should be viewed as "friends," not "foes," because they can provide rapid objective data on the patient's condition and tolerance to treatment. Like any area the physical therapist is unfamiliar with, the most important aspect for gaining confidence in the ICU is spending time there learning about the various monitors and gaining experience treating those who are critically ill.

The purpose of this chapter is to describe the various physical therapy techniques that can be effectively used in treating the medical patient in the respiratory intensive care unit (RICU). Conditions requiring caution and special consideration are identified. Alterations of the normal respiratory defense mechanisms that predispose the critically ill

to respiratory complications and frequently encountered pulmonary conditions are discussed. Also included is information regarding psychological disorders the critically ill occasionally suffer.

The physical therapist can make a valuable contribution in caring for the medical patient in the RICU. Our training in chest physical therapy and rehabilitative medicine adds an important element to the comprehensive treatment of the critically ill. To be excluded from this area is neither in our professions nor in the patient's best interests, and such exclusion would certainly omit an important aspect of their care.

RESPIRATORY DEFENSE MECHANISMS

The respiratory system can be divided into the upper and lower airways. The upper airway consists of the nose, mouth, pharynx, and larynx. The lower airway consists of the tracheobronchial tree and lung parenchyma. The major upper and lower airway defense mechanisms and their alterations in critically ill patients are described below.

The upper airway

The first respiratory defense mechanisms are encountered in the upper airway, particularly in the nose.[82] Inspiration draws air into the nostrils past the anterior nasal hairs and nasal turbinates with an airflow pattern that provides maximal exposure with the mucosa.[46] The nasal hairs and mucus covering the mucosa filter foreign particles from the inspired air. Ciliary action propels the particles posteriorly and eventually into the oropharynx where they are swallowed. Large particles are expelled from the anterior nasal passages by sneezing or nose blowing.

Two other important functions of the upper airway are warming the air to body temperature and saturating it with water vapor.

The author acknowledges the invaluable assistance of Janis Baird and Barbara Tucker in the preparation of this chapter. I am also grateful to Paula Freeman, R.P.T., Leslie Simcox, R.P.T. and Lyn Hobson, R.P.T., R.R.T., for reviewing the manuscript and providing suggestions.

The larynx

The larynx connects the upper and lower airways. The glottis is located at the opening of the larynx and has an important function during the cough reflex (p. 273). The mucosa of the larynx has receptors that are sensitive to mechanical or chemical irritation. Stimulation of these receptors will elicit the cough reflex to expel the irritant.[56] The cough reflex and the epiglottis (during swallowing) are the two major defense mechanisms that prevent aspiration and contamination of the lower respiratory tract.[56,82]

Alterations by artificial airways

Critically ill patients frequently have artificial airways placed for adequate ventilation or effective removal of secretions. However, placement of an artificial airway bypasses the normal upper airway function and defense mechanisms, resulting in bacterial contamination of the tracheobronchial tree.[82] Air being delivered to the patient must be warmed and humidified to maintain adequate mucociliary function.[93] The presence of a foreign object (the artificial airway) in the trachea causes an increased production of secretions. Cuffed endotracheal tubes are known to reduce the clearance rate of tracheal mucus.[77] The effectiveness of the cough reflex is diminished because the glottis cannot close during the compressive phase of the cough. Also the potential for pulmonary aspiration is increased and has been reported in 15% to 20% of intubated critically ill patients.[10] For these reasons critically ill patients with artificial airways generally benefit from postural drainage, percussion, and vibration, which enhance the drainage of secretions.

The mucociliary escalator

The mucociliary escalator is a important defense mechanism for clearing the airways of unwanted material.[38,68,86] The term "mucociliary escalator" describes the interrelationship between the mucus secretions and the cilia that propel the mucus. The airways are coated with a double (sol-gel) layer of mucus secreted by mucus glands and goblet cells. The outer layer is the viscous (gel) layer and the inner is the liquid (sol) layer in which the cilia beat. The cilia beat in unison, sweeping mucus and any material in the airways toward the larynx at a rate of 1 to 2 cm per minute. Approximately 10 ml of mucus are cleared from the respiratory tract daily.[46]

The mucus blanket is composed of numerous substances that in combination probably have a role in the defense of the respiratory tract against infection.[30] These include secretory immunoglobulins (especially IgA), polymorphonuclear leukocytes, lysozymes, interferon, and others. For example, it is known IgA antibodies have a viral neutralizing activity, and a deficiency of IgA is commonly associated with recurrent sinopulmonary infections. However, the precise activity of these substances in the defense of the respiratory system remains ill defined.

Altered mucociliary transportation

The mucociliary transport rate can be affected by multiple factors.[93] Dehydration and the inhalation of dry gases cause the secretions to become more viscous and difficult to move.[19] Impaired ciliary activity has been demonstrated in cystic fibrosis,[92] chronic bronchitis,[46] and asthma and in cigarette smokers.[91] Numerous drugs, including narcotics and acetylcysteine (Mucomyst),[92,93] breathing elevated concentrations of oxygen,[51,76] intubation with cuffed endotracheal tubes,[77] and intermittent suctioning[50] slow mucociliary transportation. By contrast, hydration,[19] bronchial drainage,[19] and some drugs (i.e., aminophylline, acetylcholine, etc.)[93] can increase the rate at which secretions are cleared. An increased production of secretions can be caused by tracheobronchial inflammation from a variety of causes. The most frequent acute causes are infection and inhalation of noxious gases or materials. Many persons with chronic lung disease, especially chronic bronchitis or bronchiectasis, have long-standing hypersecretions of mucus.

These secretions can usually be removed adequately by the mucociliary escalator or by coughing, a second important clearance mechanism of the respiratory system. When performed properly, a cough propels secretions and foreign material through the airways toward the mouth. However, if respiratory clearance mechanisms become ineffective, the inability to remove secretions becomes clinically significant.

Cough

An effective cough is an important mechanism for clearing the airways of secretions or foreign material.[54,56] A cough has three distinct phases.[44] First is a deep inspiration. The second, or compressive, phase begins with closure of the glottis. Both intrathoracic and intra-abdominal pressure build with contraction of the expiratory respiratory muscles. The final, or expulsive, phase begins with opening of the glottis and expulsion of the trapped air. The diaphragm relaxes to provide for the transmission of the increased intra-abdominal pressure into the lung. Usually airways above the fourth-generation bronchi are compressed by the high intrathoracic pressure.[61] The narrowed lumen of the airways is important for maintaining the high linear velocity of airflow required for an effective cough. The high lung volume, along with the increased static lung elastic recoil and the reduced airway frictional resistance, contribute to maximal expiratory flow rate during the final cough phase. The lung volume attained during inspiration also determines which airways are compressed during the expulsive phase. Coughing at large lung volumes compresses large airways, but coughing at lower lung volumes compresses smaller airways. This observation has caused some to postulate that a series of coughs is more effective than a single cough.[60] After a deep breath, the initial cough would clear the secretions from the larger airways, and the following coughs at successively lower lung volumes would advance the secretions from smaller airways to larger ones. Another deep inspiration and series of coughs would begin clearing the most proximal secretions and continue advancing the secretions from smaller to larger airways.

The cough of the critically ill patient can be inadequate for a number of reasons.[44] Some chronic respiratory diseases such as advanced chronic ostructive pulmonary disease (COPD)[57] and bronchiectasis[60] reduce cough effectiveness by limiting the maximal expiratory airflow rate. Pain,[16,26] depression of the central nervous system,[17] small tracheostomy tubes,[53] paralysis,[84] and weakness[89] have each been shown to alter one or more cough phases. This alteration can have especially serious implications in patients with an increased production of secretions. Therapists should analyze the quality of patient's coughs and try to improve their effectiveness. Some techniques we have found helpful for improving coughs are discussed on p. 278.

The alveolar macrophage

The most important defense mechanism in the alveoli is the macrophage.[30,33] The alveolar macrophage is a large mononuclear ameboid cell that scavenges the surface of the alveolar epithelium.[82] Any foreign particles or organisms encountered by the macrophage are engulfed and digested. These cells are then removed from the alveoli either through the lymphatics or by migration to the terminal bronchioles where they become attached to the mucus. The mucus transports the macrophages up the respiratory tract, and they are eventually expectorated or swallowed.

The rate of phagocytosis by the alveolar macrophage is reduced by multiple factors[30] including acute hypoxia, alcohol ingestion,[12] cigarette smoking, starvation, corticosteroids, air pollutants, and oxygen.

COMPLICATIONS OF RETAINED SECRETIONS

Chest physical therapy is indicated in the removal of retained secretions and treatment of their complications. One of the most common complications is hypoxemia caused by secretions that partially occlude airways and cause ventilation-perfusion mismatching. We have found bronchial drainage and percussion effective in rapidly correcting this type of hypoxemia (Fig. 15-1).[21,34] In patients with copious secretions, improved oxygenation can result from treatment as frequent as every 2 hours (Fig. 15-2).

Atelectasis attributable to secretions completely occluding airways causes hypoxemia by shunting blood past nonventilated alveoli. This complication can also be reversed by bronchial drainage and percussion (Fig 15-3).[21,34,36,62]

On occasion, the inability to remove secretions effectively can present life-threatening problems. We have previously described in a 21-year-old quadriplegic a cardio-

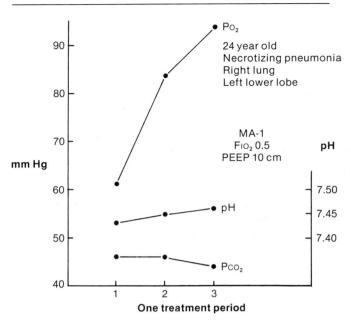

Fig. 15-1. This graph shows a dramatically improved P_{O_2} during and after a single 15-minute bronchial drainage, percussion, and vibration treatment in this critically ill patient. It was productive of copious amounts of sputum. *Point 1,* Reclining head up immediately before treatment; *point 2,* at the end of 15 minutes of treatment in the Trendelenburg position; *point 3,* reclining head up 30 minutes after treatment.

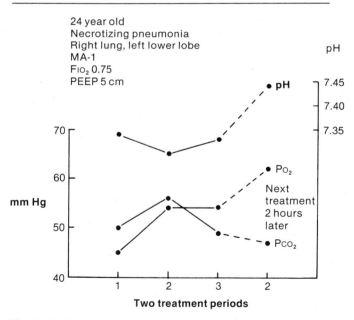

Fig. 15-2. The same patient in Fig. 15-1. *Point 1,* Reclining head up immediately before treatment; *point 2,* at the end of 15 minutes of treatment, in Trendelenburg position; *point 3,* reclining head up 30 minutes after treatment. The second point 2 was drawn at the end of a second 15-minute treatment, in Trendelenburg position, 2 hours after the first treatment. The further improvement in his P_{O_2} over the previous level *(point 3)* indicates some patients with copious secretions can benefit from treatments every 2 hours.

A

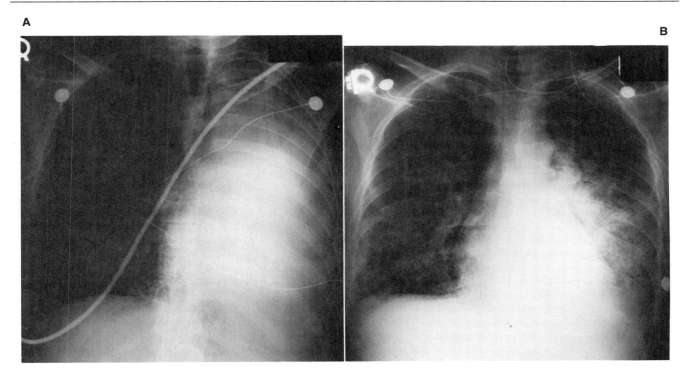

B

Fig. 15-3. A, A radiograph taken immediately before treatment shows complete left lung atelectasis in this 42-year-old man with dermatomyositis and left lower lobe pneumonia. **B,** A radiograph taken immediately after bronchial drainage, percussion, and vibration shows reexpansion of the left lung.

pulmonary arrest attributable to complete occlusion of the trachea by a large volume of mucus.[34] One confirmed death has occurred at this medical center because of inspissated secretions. At the postmortem examination a large mucus plug was found obstructing the trachea of a young asthmatic patient. Therapists should be aware of the importance of draining secretions from seriously ill patients, especially those with impaired respiratory clearance mechanisms.

PATIENT ASSESSMENT

A complete review of the medical chart should precede the initial treatment. The therapist should briefly check the chart before each treatment to be certain the patient's status has not changed significantly. Ascertain the patient's state of health before he was admitted to the RICU. Note his chronic diseases as well as acute episodes that caused him to be admitted to the critical care area. A history of acute and chronic cardiovascular disease should alert the therapist to the increased possibility of poor tolerance to treatment. The likelihood of any increased production of or difficulty in clearing secretions should be considered, as was discussed in the previous sections of this chapter.

Laboratory results should be reviewed to rule out coagulopathies that would contraindicate treatment. Any reference to thorax or rib-cage abnormalities should be noted. Therapists should be aware that long-term steroid use may contribute to osteopenia and may predispose to easily fractured ribs. The chest radiographs should be read. Is there any central nervous system or spinal cord disorder? If there is also an acute pulmonary problem, this patient will need aggressive chest physical therapy. In short, carefully review the chart to glean as much information as possible about the patient.

Examine the most recent chest radiograph to visualize any infiltrates and determine if atelectasis is present.[34] Make a mental note of anatomic landmarks and their relation to the involved lobe to locate the precise area on which to concentrate percussion and vibration. The film should be examined for signs of congestive heart failure (an enlarged heart, bilateral pleural effusions), rib lesions, or pneumothorax. The location of all lines and tubes should be noted.

Before treatment, take a couple of minutes to study the patient's base-line heart rate and rhythm on the cardiac monitor. This is important, since cardiac dysrhythmias during treatment may occur in 20% of patients receiving bronchial drainage and percussion.[32]

Identify the most recent arterial blood gas values. Is the patient hypoxemic? What is the acid-base status?

The nurse caring for the patient should be asked about the current condition of the patient. Explain that you have come to do a bronchial drainage treatment. If this is the first time to see the patient, the nurse can provide important additional information. Is he alert and cooperative? How many people are needed to turn him? Most importantly, has he become unstable since the last note was written on the medical chart? For example, if the patient has developed significant arrhythmias and is now receiving lidocaine, it probably would be best to allow him to become stabilized before the requested treatment is performed.

PHYSICAL ASSESSMENT

The chest should be inspected before treatment. Are any chest deformities present? Note the lateral and anteroposterior dimensions of the chest. An increase in the anteroposterior diameter suggests underlying chronic obstructive pulmonary disease (COPD).[15] Observe the patient's breathing. Normally during quiet breathing, inspiration is active and expiration passive, each lasting approximately the same length of time. However, use of the sternocleidomastoids and other accessory muscles of inspiration indicate an increased work of breathing. This increased inspiratory work and a prolonged forced expiration with contraction of the abdominal muscles is commonly seen during an exacerbation of COPD.[14] Next, inspect the skin for abnormalities. Are there any scars from previous trauma or surgery? Are there needle marks or areas of ecchymosis present? These, or a Band-Aid on the back, may indicate that a thoracentesis has been performed recently. If this procedure has been done within the past few hours, examine the postthoracocentesis chest radiograph to rule out a residual pneumothorax before proceeding. (See the discussions on precautions and special considerations, p. 281, and on thoracentesis, subclavian lines, and chest tubes, p. 282.)

With your hands, palpate for symmetrical bilateral expansion of the chest. There is diminished chest movement over the area of lung disease.[20] Auscultate the chest, not only to locate the most congested segments,[67] but also to establish a base line for determining the effectiveness of your treatment.[33] When breath sounds are diminished or absent, percussion is important to differentiate the conditions that may cause these findings, as these true examples illustrate.

EXAMPLE 1. A 19-year-old man with quadriplegia is noted to suddenly become diaphoretic and short of breath. Auscultation reveals absent breath sounds in the left lung, and there is dullness to percussion. A chest radiograph shows complete left-lung atel-

ectasis.[34] Bronchial drainage and percussion to the left lung is productive of several mucus plugs. Auscultation then indicates breath sounds in the previously silent lung and a normal resonance to percussion. The posttreatment chest radiograph shows resolution of the atelectasis. Dullness to percussion is most often found in pleural effusions, pneumonia, and atelectasis.[20]

EXAMPLE 2. A 23-year old man is evaluated for bronchial drainage 1 day after laparotomy for an abdominal gunshot wound. Auscultation reveals normal breath sounds in the left lung, but absent breath sounds in the right. Percussion to the right lung was hyperresonate. A chest radiograph taken a few minutes earlier was read by the therapist and showed a large right pneumothorax. The physician was notified, and he inserted a chest tube to treat the pneumothorax.

All acutely ill patients whether in the ICU or not should be examined for signs and symptoms of hypoxia and carbon dioxide retention (Table 15-1). These signs and symptoms should correspond with the previously reviewed arterial blood gases. If they do not, his condition may have deteriorated since the last sample was drawn. Before proceeding with treatment, ask the nurse if the patient's physical condition has changed in the past few minutes.

The majority of health professionals are familiar with cyanosis as a sign of hypoxia and can recognize central cyanosis by looking at the color of the patient's lips and tongue. However, the signs and symptoms of carbon dioxide (CO_2) retention are frequently poorly recognized. The patient may be dozing and difficult to arouse. The redness of the skin (especially the face), sclera, and conjunctiva, secondary to vasodilatation is striking. Persons with these signs of CO_2 retention have reduced respiratory effort and usually have a greater need for ventilatory assistance than for drainage of secretions.

Table 15-1. Signs and symptoms of hypoxia and carbon dioxide (CO_2) narcosis

Hypoxia
Symptoms
   Ethanol-like symptoms: confusion, loss of judgment, paranoia, restlessness, dizziness

Signs
   Sympathetic response: tachycardia, mild hypertension, peripheral vasoconstriction
   Nonsympathetic response: bradycardia, hypotension

CO_2 narcosis
Symptoms
   Headache
   Mild sedation→Drowsiness→Coma

Signs
   Vasodilatation: redness of skin, sclera, and conjunctiva secondary to increased cutaneous blood flow; sweating
   Sympathetic response: hypertension (systolic and diastolic); tachycardia

From Rogers, R.M.: Acute respiratory failure, Resident and Staff Physician 25(5):39, 1979.

TREATMENT PROCEDURES: BRONCHIAL DRAINAGE, PERCUSSION, VIBRATION

Introduce yourself to the patient. Tell him that you are a physical therapist. His physician has asked you to do a treatment to help his breathing by clearing his lungs of secretions. You will help him turn on his side and then percuss or clap his chest gently to help drain the secretions from his lungs. The head of his bed will be lowered to help the secretions drain toward his mouth so that he can cough them out more easily.

If the patient, in particular the intubated patient, tries to communicate with you, make a determined effort to understand.[2] This is an important aspect of developing rapport. Reading lips is the most ideal way to communicate because many seriously ill patients find writing quite tedious.

Be certain there is sufficient slack in all tubing and lines (heart monitor, central venous pressure [CVP], Swan-Ganz, arterial lines, etc.) before the patient is turned onto the side. Check the ventilator tubing for accumulation of water. Sometimes when the patient is turned, several milliliters of water in the tubing can be "spilled" down the patient's airway, triggering paroxyms of coughing. Although probably not harmful, to the anxious, alert patient it is very uncomfortable and frightening. Confidence in the therapist may be lost, and the patient may become uncooperative after such an episode.

One person can effectively turn most comatose patients on to the side. Stand on the side toward which the patient is to be turned. The patient's arm that will be uppermost when he is on his side should be adducted (with the elbow flexed) across his chest. With the patient supine, flex the patient's farthest hip and knee. Your hand is placed just above the knee, over the anterior lateral surface of the leg. Then pull the patient toward you until the side-lying position is achieved. Pillows may be placed behind the patient's back to maintain the position better. The uppermost hip and knee should remain flexed to most effectively maintain this side-lying position. Pillows can also be used to support the uppermost arm and leg.

Patients can be turned to the prone position in a similar manner. Stand on the side of the bed opposite from the direction he will be turned. Slide the patient toward you. Take the patient's arm farthest from you and adduct it against his side, with the elbow extended and the hand pronated. The arm closest to you is adducted across the patient's chest with the elbow flexed. The hip and knee closest to you is flexed. Roll the patient away from you, toward the prone position. Pull the dependent arm posteriorly, out from beneath the torso. One pillow can be placed under the uppermost shoulder, another under the flexed hip and knee.

Be certain none of the attached lines are pulled taut in this position. Check to be sure the intravenous (IV) lines are running. Observe the patient's heart rhythm and rate on the heart monitor. Allow him a minute to stabilize before placing the bed in the head-down position (Trendelenburg) for treatment of the middle, lingula, or lower lobes.

Begin percussion lightly over the involved lobe and gradually increase to the patient's tolerance. Generally, heavier persons tolerate more vigorous percussion than thinner persons do.

If the cardiac electrodes are in proximity to the area being treated, the percussion may register on the cardiac monitor as tachycardia or artifacts. These artifacts can simulate serious arrhythmias, such as ventricular tachycardia or flutter.[91] The brief conversation with the nursing staff before bronchial drainage can prevent an inappropriate emergency resuscitation being called. Observation of the heart rhythm as percussion is initiated is particularly helpful in distinguishing artifact from arrhythmias. Briefly halting percussion is also useful in distinguishing artifact from arrhythmias.

Continue percussion for 4 minutes. Then, after the patient has taken a deep breath, compress and vibrate the thorax during expiration. We repeat this for 6 consecutive breaths. Patients receiving mechanical ventilation can be given a deeper breath when the "sigh" button on the ventilator is pushed. Vibration can be performed during expiration and before triggering of another breath.

Remember the proper direction to compress and vibrate. During inspiration the lateral chest wall rises as the ribs move upward and outward (bucket-handle effect). Hence, during expiration the ribs are moving downward and inward. To vibrate in the proper direction, many therapists stand near the head of the bed to compress and vibrate in the approximate direction of the patient's opposite hip. However, if vibration is done improperly (toward the patient's head), injuries can result, especially in persons with less mobile or osteoporotic ribs.

Vibration is an important part of the treatment. It is noteworthy that many persons expectorate secretions during this maneuver. Secretions have been observed (by bronchoscopy) moving into larger airways during vibration.[96] The precise manner by which this technique advances the sputum is unclear. In addition to the effect that a vibratory force might have on advancing secretions, we believe that there are other important reasons for vibration. The airways dilate and expand on inspiration. Conversely, during expiration the airways constrict. If there is a bolus of mucus in an airway, the deep inspiration moves an increased volume of air distal to the mucus. Expiration narrows the airway around this mucus. Compression and vibration of the lung tissue and the "confined" air may have an effect similar to a Heimlich Maneuver by dislodgment of the bolus centrally. This would also explain, at least in part, the findings noticed during bronchoscopy.

Percussion is resumed for another 4 minutes before one repeats vibration. Length of treatment should be based, in part, on how productive bronchial drainage, percussion,

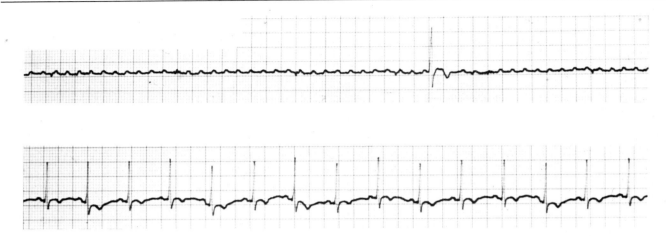

Fig. 15-4. The upper tracing shows an arrhythmia (ventricular standstill) induced by suctioning of an intubated 42-year-old man receiving 40% oxygen. Preoxygenation with 100% oxygen results in no arrhythmias during suctioning *(lower tracing)* of the same patient.

and vibration have been on removing secretions. A patient should be treated as long as sputum is produced provided that there are no signs of poor tolerance to treatment. Occasionally, patients with copious secretions may receive very lengthy treatments of 30 to 60 minutes. They may also benefit from frequent treatments done every 1 or 2 hours (Fig. 15-2). The majority of patients receive treatments that range from 10 to 20 minutes. Patients should be suctioned as needed during and after treatment before the head of the bed is elevated.

IMPROVING COUGH

The therapist should listen to and analyze the quality of a cough. When a cough is abnormal, try to determine which phase or phases are reducing its effectiveness.[20,44] When inspiration is too shallow, a deeper breath may be attained if the person is taught diaphragmatic or lateral costal breathing. Another method to improve inspiration for spontaneously breathing patients is to deliver a deep inspiration using intermittent positive-pressure breathing. The patient then closes the glottis, removes the mouthpiece, and contracts the abdominal muscles to deliver a productive cough.

Glottic closure is not essential for an adequate cough.[44] However, if indicated in persons with artificial airways, an Ambu bag (breathing bag) can be compressed to resist expiration for a few seconds after the end of inspiration. This technique increases intrathoracic pressure for a more force-

ful expulsive phase. Assisted coughing is a technique that is useful for increasing the force of the expulsive phase particularly in spontaneously breathing spinal cord–injured patients. Assisted coughing is often helpful when used with postural drainage and percussion.[84] The therapist places one hand in the epigastric region of the patient's abdomen and the other hand on the lateral chest wall. At the end of inspiration, the therapist compresses the chest downward and the abdomen toward the diaphragm increasing the expiratory velocity of air. It is very effective for mobilizing secretions and reduces the need for frequent suctioning. The patients are also convinced of its benefit, since they frequently request abdominal compression when congested.

SUCTIONING

Suctioning is an important procedure for removing secretions from patients with artificial airways and from those who cannot cough well. However, suctioning must be done carefully to avoid the complications of hypotension, hypoxemia, and cardiac arrest.[1,45,82] Use of catheters with "ringed tips" is advocated to reduce tracheal mucosal trauma associated with suctioning.[47,75]

Hyperoxygenation is very important to prevent arterial hypoxemia that can lead to myocardial hypoxia and arrhythmias. The effect of 100% oxygen on reducing arrhythmias has been reported.[83] Fig. 15-4 also demonstrates this reduction.

The suction catheter in the trachea may cause arrhythmias by vagal stimulation. To reduce this hazard, the catheter should not remain in the patient's trachea longer than 10 to 15 seconds.

The following procedure is recommended to suction patients:

1. Explain to the patient what you are going to do.
2. Set the wall-suction regulator at 100 to 120 mm Hg.
3. Using sterile technique, open the package containing the suction catheter and put the glove on. Then using the gloved hand, attach the catheter to the wall-suction tubing.
4. Hyperoxygenate the patient.
5. Pass the suction catheter through the airway, without vacuum, until resistance is met (usually the level of the carina).
6. Withdraw the tip of the catheter approximately 1 cm before applying intermittent suction.
7. The catheter should rotate between the thumb and forefinger as it is withdrawn, with intermittent suction being applied.
8. The catheter should not be in the airway longer than 10 to 15 seconds.
9. Hyperoxygenate the patient before reintroducing the suction catheter into the airway.
10. The tubing may be flushed with sterile water to clear it of secretions before reintroduction of the catheter into the airway.
11. The instillation into the airway of 5 to 10 ml of sterile water may be helpful in loosening especially tenacious secretions.
12. Reset the oxygen to the presuction value.
13. Wrap the suction catheter around the gloved fingers. Then, holding the catheter with the thumb, remove the glove over the suction catheter. The glove should be inside out with the suction catheter in the center, ready to be discarded.
14. The suction may be shut off.
15. Wash your hands.

TOLERANCE TO TREATMENT

The majority of patients receiving bronchial drainage, percussion, and vibration demonstrate no ill effects from treatment. Of concern are those patients who have side effects from treatment. The therapist must recognize signs of poor tolerance to treatment. Side effects and intolerance to treatment are often associated with positioning the patient with the head down to treat the lingula, right middle lobe, or lower lobe.[34]

CARDIAC ARRHYTHMIAS

Cardiac arrhythmias may be one of the earliest manifestations of poor tolerance to treatment. At times arrythmias occur transiently when the patient is placed in the Trendelenburg position, and the rhythm returns to normal

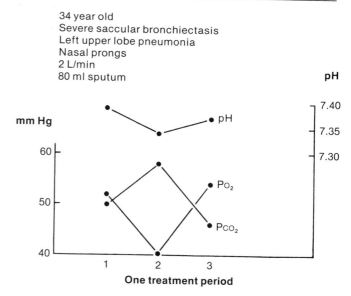

34 year old
Severe saccular bronchiectasis
Left upper lobe pneumonia
Nasal prongs
2 L/min
80 ml sputum

Fig. 15-5. Hypoxemia during a single bronchial drainage, percussion, and vibration treatment of a patient with severe bronchiectasis, which was productive of 80 ml of sputum. *Point 1*, Reclining head up immediately before treatment; *point 2*, at the end of 15 minutes of treatment, on his left side in Trendelenburg position; *point 3*, reclining head up 30 minutes after treatment. Note that the hypoxemia occurred at point 2 when the lobe involved with pneumonia was positioned dependent.

within 30 to 45 seconds. On other occasions arrhythmias occur after percussion is begun. In a series of consecutive treatments we found clinically significant arrhythmias in 9% of treatments.[32] Huseby and co-workers[42] observed arrhythmias, including ventricular tachycardia, in the seriously ill during treatment. Laws and McIntyre[52] were prompted to study the cardiac output in a group of patients after two episodes of sudden death during bronchial drainage. The investigators apparently suspected that a cardiovascular mechanism was responsible. Hypoxemia during treatment may play a role in precipitating some arrhythmias. However, we have documented arrhythmias in some critically ill persons with arterial blood gas values that showed Po_2 well above 80 mm Hg. Apparently there are other physiological mechanisms, besides hypoxemia, that cause arrhythmias during bronchial drainage. Hence, an important part of any treatment is close observation of the cardiac monitor to recognize arrhythmias that may occur.

HYPOXEMIA

Hypoxemia is another indication of poor tolerance to treatment. We have noticed that hypoxemia is more likely to occur in persons who do not expectorate sputum during treatment.[21] However, as Fig. 15-5 shows, hypoxemia can be seen in patients who expectorate large volumes of sputum. We have found hypoxemia during treatment to be caused most often by ventilation-perfusion mismatching or shunting. A fall in cardiac output has been shown in some instances[5,52] and may also contribute to a fall in Po_2.

Huseby and co-workers[42] noticed that some of their patients who received bronchial drainage to multiple lung segments had a fall in mean Po_2 of 19 mm Hg. This fall was noticed most often when the involved lung was dependent (Fig. 15-4). Remolina[71] and others[43] have also demonstrated a dramatically lower Po_2 when patients with unilateral acute lung disease were positioned with the involved lung dependent. Hence it is important to recognize that hypoxemia can occur or worsen during bronchial drainage. This is most likely when the involved lung segments are dependent. We try to emphasize the involved lung by placing it uppermost during treatments and by draining it thoroughly so that the incidence of this complication is reduced.

If on physical examination the patient with unilateral radiographic involvement has developed bilateral congestion, both lungs must be treated. Certain modifications of treatment may be necessary to ensure adequate oxygenation.

SYMPTOMS ASSOCIATED WITH POOR TOLERANCE TO TREATMENT

A striking fact is that most patients who complain of difficulties during treatment have a demonstrable reason for their complaint. They may become agitated, orthopneic, dyspneic, weak, or diaphoretic with arrhythmias. A change in blood pressure may also be noted. Agitation, shortness of breath, dyspnea, increased use of accessory muscles, and central cyanosis are often associated with hypoxemia. There are a few patients in whom arrhythmias or hypoxemia can be demonstrated who do not become symptomatic. Therefore, whether or not the patient has monitors attached, the therapist should carefully consider all complaints of difficulty and watch for signs of poor tolerance to treatment. Often modifications can be made to allow the patients to receive effective bronchial drainage.

MODIFICATIONS

If hypoxemia or arrhythmias are a problem during bronchial drainage, certain adjustments can be made to permit a less physically demanding treatment. Secretions can be effectively drained with the patient in the horizontal rather than the head-down position, or some physicians may permit a temporary increase in the percentage of oxygen delivered during bronchial drainage to reduce the chances of hypoxemia and thereby ensure a safer treatment. If signs of poor tolerance are noted several minutes after initiation of bronchial drainage, it may be beneficial to shorten the length of treatment. Although treatments are shorter, the time interval between treatment sessions can be reduced and effective bronchial hygiene can still be provided.

Some patients with chronic obstructive pulmonary dis-

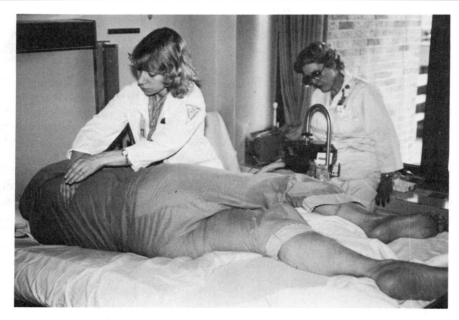

Fig. 15-6. A physical therapist *(left)* doing bronchial drainage with percussion to a patient who requires the assisted ventilation of an IPPB (intermittent positive-pressure breathing) machine operated by the respiratory therapist *(right)* to tolerate the head-down position.

ease or neuromuscular or spinal cord dysfunction have great difficulty maintaining adequate ventilation in the head-down posture. In addition, the presence of an increased amount of secretions and the patient's compromised cough can lead to atelectasis and life-threatening problems.[9,34] We have found it useful to coordinate treatment with a respiratory therapist who provides intermittent positive-pressure breathing (IPPB) as a means of assisted ventilation with the patient in the appropriate bronchial drainage position (Fig. 15-6). The patient is effectively ventilated with supplemental oxygen, and the necessary treatment can be performed with minimal distress.

PRECAUTIONS AND SPECIAL CONSIDERATIONS
Cardiac disease

It is particularly important to assess the intensive care unit patient for evidence of acute and chronic cardiac disease before bronchial drainage. Any signs of congestive heart failure such as jugular vein distention, pulmonary edema, and pitting edema of the lower extremities should be noted. The cardiac monitor should be observed for arrhythmias. Review the patient's electrocardiographic rhythm strips that have been recorded in the past 3 to 4 hours.

As expected, we noticed a significantly higher incidence of arrhythmias in patients with underlying cardiac disease.[32] For example, patients with irregular rhythms before treatment had a tendency to deteriorate with bronchial drainage (i.e., an increased number of premature atrial contractions). Others who had received antiarrhythmia drugs within the past 48 hours developed a significant number of premature ventricular contractions that necessitated the early termination of treatment. Patients with cardiac disease have an increased tendency to tolerate treatment poorly and should be closely monitored.

Congestive heart failure

Patients with significant congestive heart failure should not receive bronchial drainage in the Trendelenburg position. Experience has shown that these persons have increased respiratory distress and cardiac arrhythmias while reclining head down. Also this position increases venous return to the failing heart and can produce an increased amount of pulmonary edema. Posttreatment auscultation reflects this effect by a significant increase in rales throughout both lung fields. We prefer to treat patients with congestive heart failure in the horizontal (bed-flat) position rather than in the Trendelenburg position. After their cardiac status improves, they can often tolerate the standard bronchial drainage positions.

CO$_2$ retention

Occasionally therapists are asked to treat nonventilated patients who are acidotic (pH<7.30) with elevated carbon dioxide levels. These patients should also be treated

cautiously. If the patient ventilates inadequately in a sitting position, being placed in the Trendelenburg position, with the diaphragm working against both gravity and the abdominal contents during inspiration, can further increase respiratory distress. It may be possible to tolerate the bed-flat position for short periods of time (5 to 10 minutes). Diaphragmatic and pursed-lips breathing may be helpful[66,89] but these persons often require intubation and mechanical ventilation before effective bronchial drainage can be delivered.

Adult respiratory distress syndrome (ARDS)

Some patients with the adult respiratory distress syndrome (ARDS) have an improved Po$_2$ after bronchial drainage, whereas others show a fall in both their Po$_2$ and their lung compliance. It appears that the fall in Po$_2$ may be related to an increased amount of fluid "leaking" into the extravascular spaces in the lung from the pulmonary vessels, perhaps secondary to an increased venous return from being in the head-down position. Interestingly, similar findings have been noted in neonates with the respiratory distress syndrome.[81] The ARDS patient's response to treatment is individualized, and each should be assessed accordingly. If the cause of the ARDS is related to a pulmonary infection, these persons generally tolerate treatment better than those who develop the condition from pancreatitis, shock, or other extrathoracic insults.

Pleural effusions

Questions often arise regarding the efficacy of treatment of persons with pleural effusions. Pleural effusions are not an indication for bronchial drainage but accompany many cardiac and pulmonary conditions seen in critically ill patients. Some may believe that the increased pleural fluid between the lung and chest wall would significantly reduce the effectiveness of percussion during bronchial drainage. However, if the fluid is not loculated, when the patient is positioned on his side (with the involved lobe uppermost) the fluid will track away from the lateral chest wall and accumulate medially. This will usually allow effective percussion of the lingula, middle lobe, and lower lobe. Auscultation can confirm this change in the location of the fluid. Breath sounds are distant with the patient sitting up (with dullness to percussion), but when the patient is positioned for bronchial drainage, breath sounds can almost always be heard (with resonant percussion). If these persons have an underlying pulmonary condition that necessitates chest physical therapy, pleural effusions usually do not present a problem.

Pulmonary embolism

Pulmonary embolism is a frequent complication in critical illnesses.[13,14,69] On occasion therapists are asked to administer bronchial drainage to persons with increased secretions who also have a pulmonary embolism. Questions have arisen regarding the likelihood of bronchial drainage and percussion moving the embolus and causing further problems. It is important to remember that emboli lodge in the pulmonary artery system. These blood vessels become progressively smaller in diameter until they form the pulmonary capillary bed. Therefore the probability of advancing dislodged emboli along the narrowing pulmonary artery system is quite remote.

Most pulmonary thromboemboli originate from the deep veins of the legs or pelvis. One should weigh the possibility of causing additional emboli with the benefits of turning and positioning the patient for bronchial drainage. Three questions should be addressed before one proceeds. Is the patient anticoagulated? Has the nursing staff been turning the patient from side to side for nursing care? Does the patient have sufficient secretions to benefit significantly from bronchial drainage? If these questions can be answered affirmatively, the benefits generally outweigh the risks, and we proceed with the treatment.

Hemoptysis

Hemoptysis in all patients should be carefully evaluated. The cause must be known before initiation of bronchial drainage. Hemoptysis is a common finding after thoracic trauma with pulmonary contusion and bronchial hygiene does not present any risk to the patient.[58] Persons with bronchiectasis intermittently develop hemoptysis, but rarely is the bleeding of life-threatening proportions. We have seen patients with dysphagia develop hemoptysis from aspirating blood during nose bleeds resulting from trauma caused by nasotracheal suctioning. Other than not percussing the aforementioned bronchiectatics, treatments for this group do not ordinarily present an added risk to the patient. However, of major concern is hemoptysis in patients with coagulopathies caused by either anticoagulants or a very low platelet count (less than 20,000). Major bleeding from a lung abscess or a cavitating pulmonary carcinoma, especially after radiation therapy, has especially serious implications. At least two deaths have been reported during chest physical therapy in patients with pulmonary malignancies.[18,35] The therapist must be convinced that the benefits of treatment outweigh the risks before proceeding with the bronchial drainage.

Osteopenia and osteoporosis

Osteopenia, in particular when the ribs are involved, is another condition that necessitates precautions. On occasion patients with malignancies are admitted to the intensive care unit. It is important before chest percussion, to the extent possible, to rule out metastasis to the ribs.

Osteoporosis, a condition that affects an estimated 15 million persons in this country is most common in postmenopausal women. It is best to assume that elderly women, in particular those of slight body build, have some

bone demineralization and adjust treatment accordingly. Corticosteroids are used to treat asthma and many other nonthoracic conditions. Long-term steroid use may result in osteopenia and predispose the patient to rib fractures from mild stresses. One woman with lung disease treated for several years with steroids reported that she had fractured her ribs by pulling up a plant and trying to grab a gnat. Special caution must be used in treating these persons to determine an effective force that will not injure the ribs.

Intracranial pressure

Questions have been raised on the effect of Trendelenburg positioning on intracranial pressure in patients with intracranial lesions. Although some have alluded to an increased intracranial pressure during an unspecified chest physiotherapy treatment,[65] rarely have we seen this. In an on-going study, we have found that the greatest change in pressure occurs when the patient is repositioned from head up to supine.[32] The change from supine to Trendelenburg has been insignificant. Interestingly, as the intracranial pressure increases in the Trendelenburg position, so does the blood pressure. Hence cerebral perfusion pressure is not altered significantly. However, if the patient has suffered a spontaneous cerebral hemorrhage, one must weigh the risk of additional bleeding against the benefit of treatment. It is often best to position the patient bed flat with the head supported for more conservative treatment.

THORACENTESIS, SUBCLAVIAN LINES, AND CHEST TUBES

If the patient has had a thoracentesis, placement of subclavian lines, or placement of or removal of chest tubes, treatment should be withheld until the postprocedure chest radiograph rules out a pneumothorax. At times there will be a small residual pneumothorax, which the physicians elect to observe rather than reduce by inserting a chest tube. The therapist should view the untreated pneumothorax as a strict contraindication. Techniques that encourage the patient to cough will likely increase the size of a pneumothorax. One therapist treated a patient with an initially small pneumothorax. Thoracentesis had not been documented in the physician's or nurse's notes. The patient suffered a cardiopulmonary arrest. After successful resuscitation, the chest radiograph showed a much larger pneumothorax attributed to the increased intrathoracic pressure during coughing.

TUBE FEEDING

To reduce the potential for regurgitation, patients who receive tube feeding at regular intervals are best treated immediately before a feeding. Some therapists find it helpful to aspirate the stomach contents of these patients before placing the patient in the Trendelenburg position.

CONDITIONS FREQUENTLY TREATED IN THE RICU
Adult respiratory distress syndrome (ARDS)

The adult respiratory distress syndrome (ARDS) is a form of respiratory failure commonly encountered in the respiratory intensive care unit (RICU). It is characterized by respiratory distress (evidenced by severe dyspnea), hypoxemia that is unresponsive to high concentrations of oxygen (caused by intrapulmonary right-to-left shunting), decreased lung compliance, and a chest radiograph with diffuse bilateral pulmonary infiltrates (often sparing the costophrenic and cardiophrenic angles).[22] ARDS has been associated with a variety of conditions including the following:

1. Aspiration of gastric contents
2. Drug overdose
    a. Barbiturates
    b. Heroin
3. Infection
    a. Diffuse bacterial, fungal, or viral pneumonias
4. Inhalation of toxic gases
    a. Oxygen ($FIO_2 > 0.5$)
    b. Smoke
5. Near drowning
6. Shock
    a. Cardiogenic
    b. Hemorrhagic
    c. Septic (especially gram-negative)
7. Trauma
    a. Pulmonary contusion
    b. Head trauma

Regardless of the specific insult that precipitates ARDS, the resulting pulmonary pathological condition is similar— an alveolar-capillary membrane injury that increases the permeability of the pulmonary capillary bed.[22,41] An increased amount of fluid is allowed to flow into the interstitial and alveolar spaces, resulting in pulmonary edema and abnormalities of surfactant function. This abnormality causes a fall in lung compliance, and areas of atelectasis develop. The flow of blood past nonventilated alveoli (right-to-left shunt) results in hypoxemia. Severe hypoxemia is a leading cause of death in persons who do not respond to treatment.

Medical treatment. Treatment is directed primarily at maintaining adequate oxygenation and preventing additional complications.[22,41] All these persons require supplemental oxygen. Many must be mechanically ventilated to maintain acceptable arterial oxygen levels. Large tidal volumes (15 ml/kg of body weight) and frequent hyperinflations may help prevent atelectasis. Positive end-expiratory pressure (PEEP) may be used to lower the inspired oxygen fraction below 50% to reduce the toxic effects of oxygen on the respiratory system. PEEP is used carefully to avoid compromising the patient's cardiac output. Frequent turn-

ing, suctioning, and bronchial drainage are often effective in draining secretions and preventing atelectasis. However, one must carefully monitor each patient's tolerance to bronchial drainage (see the discussion on precautions for ARDS, p. 281). Infections and sepsis are treated with appropriate antibiotics. Corticosteriods may be administered, but their value remains controversial. The amount of fluid the patient receives is carefully regulated to prevent overhydration and worsening of the pulmonary problems. However, despite these aggressive measures the mortality remains high, between 20% and 75%.

Chronic obstructive pulmonary disease (COPD)

Chronic obstructive pulmonary disease (COPD) is the most frequently encountered respiratory diagnosis in the RICU. It is characterized by increased airway resistance and prolonged forced expiration.[36] COPD is a general description that usually includes chronic bronchitis, emphysema, and asthma. Although these diseases are described separately, the majority of patients admitted to the RICU have some combination of all three. These persons typically have a long history of cigarette smoking and a chronic productive cough. They usually report intermittent episodes of wheezing. On physical examination one notes an increased anteroposterior diameter of the chest. There is moderate to pronounced contraction of the accessory muscles of inspiration, depending on the degree of respiratory distress. On auscultation one often notices bibasilar crackles, with scattered to diffuse wheezes and rhonchi over both lung fields. With significant right-sided heart failure, neck-vein distention and pedal edema may be present. The chest radiograph shows hyperinflated lungs with flattened diaphragms. The other findings will vary according to each COPD patient's predominant disease process.

Chronic bronchitis. Chronic bronchitis is a disease characterized by a cough productive of sputum for at least 3 months and for 2 consecutive years.[37] The cause is prolonged exposure to nonspecific bronchial irritants, the most common of which is cigarette smoke.[82] The inhaled irritants cause hypersecretion of mucus and result in changes within the airways including tracheal mucus gland hypertrophy and goblet cell hyperplasia.[46,88] The abnormal ciliary function and a disrupted mucus blanket that accompanies this condition reduce the effective clearance of mucus. Hypersecretion of mucus combined with an impaired mucociliary transport system results in a chronic productive cough.

Because bronchitics often have a stocky body build and present with cyanosis (because of hypoxemia), they have been referred to as "blue bloaters."[82]

Emphysema. Emphysema is characterized by an irreversible destruction of interalveolar septal walls and of the connective tissue that provides much of the elastic recoil of the lung. This disease can be classified as centrilobular or panlobular. Centrilobular emphysema is characterized by destruction of the respiratory bronchiole and panlobular emphysema refers to a destructive enlargement of the alveoli.[88]

The cause of this disease remains obscure. Emphysema occurs more frequently in cigarette smokers than in nonsmokers, and its incidence increases with age. There are hereditary predispositions also, as evidenced by the severe panlobular emphysema that is found at a relatively early age in nonsmokers with an alpha₁-antitrypsin deficiency.

Emphysema patients tend to be thin with an increased anteroposterior chest diameter. Because of the increased work of breathing they must do to maintain relatively normal arterial blood gases, they have been referred to as "pink puffers."[82]

Asthma. Asthma is a disease characterized by reversible intermittent attacks of airway obstruction because of an increased responsiveness of the smooth muscle of the trachea and bronchi to various stimuli. Asthma can generally be divided into two types: allergic or immunological (formerly called "extrinsic") and nonallergic or non-immunological (sometimes called "intrinsic"), which is often associated with a history of recurrent respiratory tract infections.[37] Allergic asthma usually dates from early childhood, whereas the nonallergic type begins primarily in adulthood.[36]

During an acute attack, the lumen of the airways is narrowed by bronchial smooth muscle spasm, mucosal inflammation, and hypersecretions of mucus. This obstruction causes audible wheezing and rhonchi that persist despite frequent coughing.

Medical treatment. Most patients with COPD have elements of reversible airway obstruction. Therefore bronchodilators and corticosteroids are administered.[70] Antibiotics are given for respiratory infection.[13] Congestive heart failure is treated with diuretics. Arterial blood gases are closely monitored. Low-flow oxygen is given by nasal prongs or by Venturi mask to raise the Po_2 to approximately 60 mm Hg.[14,70,72] Carbon dioxide retention is initially treated with intermittent positive-pressure breathing (IPPB) for 15 minutes each hour.[11,37] Bronchial drainage, percussion, and vibration are given to aid in the expectoration of sputum, with the frequency varying according to the needs of the individual patient.[13,72] Diaphragmatic and pursed-lips breathing may also be useful to relieve dyspnea and improve arterial blood gases.[66,89] These measures are successful in 60% to 95% of patients with COPD in respiratory failure. If, however, the Po_2 falls below 40 mm Hg or the Pco_2 continues to climb with a corresponding deterioration in blood pH (< 7.20), the patient is intubated and mechanically ventilated.[13,72]

Disorders of the thoracic cage

Respiratory failure in patients with disorders of the thoracic cage is frequently seen in the RICU. The disorders can be divided into two major categories: a mechanical syndrome (scoliosis, obesity-hypoventilation, thoracoplasty, etc.) and a neuromuscular or paralytic syndrome (after poliomyelitis, spinal cord injury, etc.).[9] The common finding is alveolar hypoventilation at some time during the course of the disease.

The mechanical syndrome. The development of alveolar hypoventilation in patients with mechanical derangements differs from the neuromuscular category, in that it is preceded by significant dyspnea on exertion.[9] Symptoms increase with advancing age. In particular, those with a scoliosis that approaches a 70-degree angle (at the intersection of upper and lower limbs of the thoracic curvature) during youth are much more likely to become symptomatic with age. Although respiratory failure is common, the incidence of secretions, atelectasis, and pneumonia is increased only in those with obesity-hypoventilation or thoracoplasty (Table 15-2). However, cor pulmonale, congestive heart failure, and pulmonary hypertension occur almost exclusively in this group rather than the neuromuscular group. Infection and congestive heart failure are the most frequent reasons they require admission to the RICU.

The neuromuscular syndrome. The onset of respiratory failure in the neuromuscular group can be abrupt (Guillain-Barré), episodic (myasthenia gravis), or chronic (muscular dystrophy, spinal cord injury). Acute respiratory failure develops in a relatively predictable manner.[9] All the diseases in this category affect both the inspiratory and expiratory muscles of respiration. Therefore the patient's ability to perform maximal inspiratory and expiratory maneuvers is impaired. The cough becomes progressively less effective. The inspiratory capacity becomes progressively smaller, resulting in an inadequate sigh. As the inspiratory capacity falls to approximately one third the predicted value, alveolar hypoventilation becomes significant, causing hypoxemia and hypercapnia. The incidence of secretions, atelectasis, and pneumonia is increased within this entire group (Table 15-2) and, along with deteriorating arterial blood gases, frequently requires that the patient be admitted to the RICU.

Medical treatment. Treatment of disorders of the thoracic cage is similar to the treatment of chronic obstructive pulmonary disease.[9] It includes low-flow oxygen, intermittent positive-pressure breathing, antibiotics, bronchodilators, and diuretics. Bronchial drainage is indicated and effective for most patients in the neuromuscular category.[9,34,63,84] It should also be performed on patients with scoliosis,[53] obesity-hypoventilation, and thoracoplasty.

In addition, efforts to strengthen and increase the endurance of the respiratory muscles are often begun in the RICU. This topic is more fully discussed elsewhere in this text.

Pharmacological ventilatory stimulants such as proges-

Table 15-2. Clinical description of respiratory failure in derangements of the thorax

| Category | Respiratory failure | | Clinical course | Secretions, atelectasis, pneumonia |
	Incidence	Severity		
Mechanical				
Scoliosis	Common	+ + +*	Slow	NL†
Obesity-hypoventilation	Common	+ + +	Periodic	NL or ↑
Fibrothorax	Common	+ + +	Slow	NL
Thoracoplasty	Common	+ + +	Slow	NL or ↑
Ankylosing spondylitis	Rare	+	Slow	NL
Neuromuscular				
Postpoliomyelitis	Common	+ + +	Slow	↑
Amyotrophic lateral sclerosis	Common	+ + +	Fast	↑
Muscular dystrophies	Common	+	Slow	↑
Spinal cord injury	Common	+ +	Slow	↑
Multiple sclerosis	Uncommon	+	Slow	↑
Myasthenia gravis	Common	+ + +	Periodic	↑

* + = dyspnea on exertion; + + = dyspnea, mild hypoxemia, and hypercapnia only; + + + = severe hypoventilation.
†NL = normal lungs; ↑ = increased incidence.
From Bergofsky, E.H.: Am. Rev. Respir. Dis. **119**:694, 1979.

terone, caffeine, and theophylline may be administered though their use remains controversial. Long-term ventilatory assistance at home may be necessary in the management of chronic or sleep-induced hypoventilation (see the discussion of discharge planning, p. 287).[3,9,40] Also physical rehabilitation ' of the ventilator-dependent patient should be a major on-going effort, as described in a separate chapter.

RESPIRATORY MUSCLE DYSFUNCTION

There has been increased interest in the role of the respiratory muscles in the precipitation and management of respiratory failure.[7,73,74,80] Persons predisposed to respiratory muscle weakness or fatigue include those with neuromuscular conditions, spinal cord injuries, and thoracic and pulmonary conditions associated with respiratory failure.[29,59,73,74]

In addition, the respiratory muscles can atrophy in patients who require long-term mechanical ventilation. Inspiratory muscle fatigue in persons being weaned from mechanical ventilation is manifested by rapid shallow breathing, paradoxical abdominal motion, and inspirations that alternate between predominant abdominal and rib-cage movement.[59]

Studies in normal subjects have shown that both inspiratory muscle strength and endurance can be increased by appropriate training.[7,48,54] Respiratory muscle training has also been demonstrated in persons with cystic fibrosis,[48] COPD,[4] and quadriplegia.[28] Such training has special significance in the latter two groups because the prevention of respiratory failure depends to a large extent on the strength and endurance of the inspiratory muscles.[24,25]

Physical therapists will have the opportunity to be more

actively involved in designing and implementing exercise programs that strengthen weak respiratory muscles. Breathing against increased inspiratory resistance or progressively adding external resistance are the two methods most frequently used.[3,4,7,28] Another technique they may use is biofeedback, which has been used successfully to wean paralyzed patients from ventilators.[23] This topic is discussed comprehensively in a separate chapter.

PROGRESSIVE PHYSICAL ACTIVITY

The adverse effects of immobilization have been well documented. They include a decrease in circulating blood volume, which causes tachycardia and orthostatic hypotension when the patient is mobilized.[27] Immobilization also increases blood viscosity, which, along with venous stasis from the reduced use of the leg muscles, predisposes to thromboembolism.[94] The first week of bed rest reduces skeletal muscle mass, contractive strength, and efficiency by 10% to 15%. By the end of 3 weeks of bed rest, physical work capacity may be reduced by 20% to 25%.[78,94] Hence exercise can be very important to minimize the adverse inactivity.

Another important aspect of exercise and ambulation of alert patients in the intensive care unit is the psychological benefit derived from these activities. Reaching the point of recovery from a catastrophic illness where physical rehabilitation is indicated gives the patient immense reassurance. Progressive exercise and ambulation of these persons is rewarding, even though they require mechanical ventilation.

While the ventilated patient is confined to bed, we begin active exercises as soon as possible and progress to resistive exercises. When the patient is initially transferred to

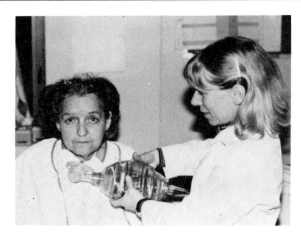

Fig. 15-7. This 62-year-old woman required mechanical ventilation for respiratory failure secondary to an exacerbation of her chronic obstructive pulmonary disease (COPD). The physical therapist is bagging her in preparation for walking around the intensive care unit.

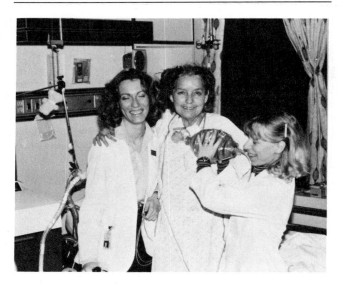

Fig. 15-8. Two physical therapists in the intensive care unit walking the patient shown in Fig. 15-7. The therapist on the left is supporting the patient and pulling the oxygen cylinder as the one on the right bags the patient.

the bedside chair, we prefer to be present to observe the strength and coordination of the lower extremities. As soon as the patient is medically stable and can sit and be away from the life-support system for a few minutes, we suggest short trips out of the ICU. If assisted ventilation is still necessary an Ambu bag (breathing bag) with supplemental oxygen from a small oxygen cylinder can be used. After the patient gains confidence in a bed-to-chair transfer, we prepare for ambulation by having him walk in place while still attached to the ventilator. If he does well for 20 to 30 seconds, arrangements are made to ambulate around the ICU during the next treatment, maintaining ventilation with the Ambu bag and supplemental oxygen. We try to increase the distance ambulated with each treatment session (Figs. 15-7 and 15-8).

If lack of motivation to walk is a problem,[90] we ask the patient to walk to the wheelchair placed 20 to 30 feet away, before he takes the wheelchair ride out of the ICU. After returning to the ICU, the wheelchair is stopped approximately the same distance away from the bed and the patient walks back to bed. In this way the patient benefits physically from exercise as well as emotionally from brief trips out of the critical care area. This topic is more fully discussed in Chapter 16.

PSYCHOLOGICAL ASPECTS OF CRITICAL ILLNESS

Patients with critical illnesses are anxious[2] and often terrified of their life-threatening conditions. The busy and crowded environment in the ICU has been implicated as contributing to their anxiety. The frequent procedures and vital-sign measurements permit only minutes of uninter-

rupted sleep at one time. The rooms are usually plain and filled with unfamiliar machinery. The patient's personal items and clothing have been removed. Many lines, tubes, and needles are attached to or inserted into the patient's body. Continuously irritating sounds are heard from the ventilator, cardiac monitor, or some other type of life-support equipment. Impersonal communication and treatment of the patient as an inanimate object take their psychological toll as well. Psychologically, the patient may cope with these threats by temporarily retreating from reality (neurosis or psychosis) or humanity (psychoplegia).[79]

Professionals working in the ICU should be aware that temporary psychological disturbances have been reported in approximately 12.5% of critically ill patients.[39] Among those in whom psychic disorders are frequently seen are those with respiratory failure or pulmonary insufficiency.[87] Alterations of memory, orientation, judgment, perception, concentration, or level of consciousness are common signs of psychological disturbance.

Those with a prolonged ICU stay may manifest a simple reactive apathetic depression when a significant improvement is made over their admission status.[90] They become apathetic and do not actively cooperate or participate in their own care. Although some have attributed this to sleep deprivation, there must be additional facts because it occurs even when sleep is minimally disturbed.[79] Explaining to the patient that the depression is normal, and consistent reassurance of recovery is helpful. Health professionals should be sympathetic but firm in dealing with persons with this type of disturbance.[90] Much less frequently, pa-

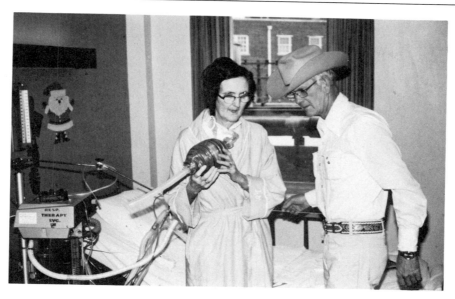

Fig. 15-9. This 55-year-old woman became ventilator dependent after an infarct to her brainstem, but she did not require oxygen. She was transferred to a general nursing floor and taught to bag herself for independence. The patient has just taken herself off the ventilator, has attached the Ambu bag (breathing bag) to her tracheostomy tube, and is going for a walk with her husband.

tients that have been weaned from ventilators may manifest great apprehension about going to sleep without ventilatory support. This is also transitory in most cases.

DISCHARGE PLANNING

Occasionally patients cannot be weaned from the ventilator. This poses a serious dilemma and considerable controversy in patients with progressive systemic diseases. However, regardless of the cause, if the physician and patient are committed to long-term ventilator support, it is important that the patient be weaned from supplemental oxygen. Then the patient can eventually be transferred to a nursing home or even home, despite being ventilator dependent. The persons we have seen make the choice to go home have been most appreciative of the assistance and support received in this effort.

A measure of independence can be achieved by teaching the ambulatory patient self-ventilation with an Ambu bag while walking (Figs. 15-9 and 15-10). This is also a good safe measure, in case mechanical problems occur with the ventilator after the patient has been discharged.

Volume ventilators are often used for home ventilation. Or a chest cuirass may be used, which appears like a turtle shell that covers the patient's abdomen and chest.[40] A suction tube protrudes from the center of the shell and creates a negative pressure at the desired inspiratory intervals. The diaphragm is pulled downward and the chest expands, drawing air into the lungs.

A pneumobelt can be used for assisted ventilation. It consists of an abdominal corset with an inflatable bladder

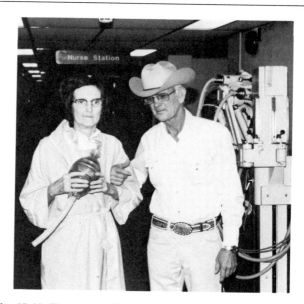

Fig. 15-10. The same patient as in Fig. 15-9, going down the hallway, past a nurse station, for a walk around the hospital.

anteriorly. When the bladder is inflated, it compresses the abdominal contents and moves the diaphragm upward, causing expiration. The bladder then deflates and allows the diaphragm to work more effectively during inspiration from this elevated position. It is especially useful in spinal cord–injured patients.[3]

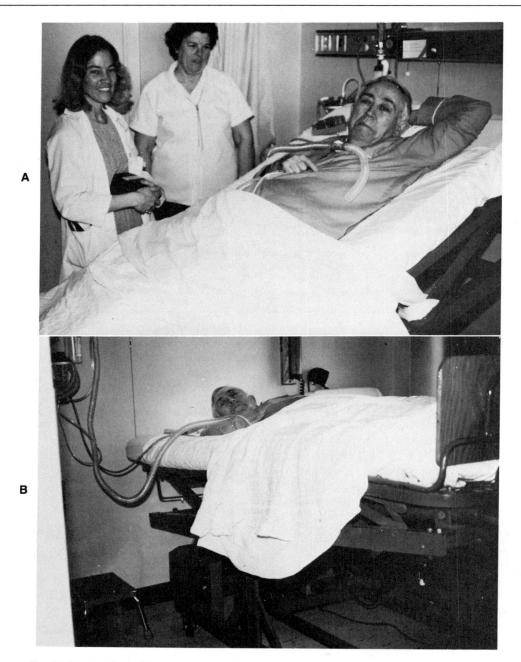

Fig. 15-11. A patient with respiratory muscle weakness secondary to polio in 1950, on the rocking bed. The bed oscillates between, **A,** 30 degrees head up and, **B,** 10 degrees head down. He has been followed for over 1 year using this bed primarily to sleep on at home, without recurrent respiratory failure.

The rocking bed is another means of assisted ventilation that was first used during the polio era. As it moves into the head-down position (about 10 degrees), the abdominal contents are pushed upward against the diaphragm, which moves upward and assists expiration. Then, as the bed moves into the head-up position, the abdominal contents and diaphragm descend, assisting inspiration (Figs. 15-11 and 15-12). The number of respirations per minute is adjusted to the patient's needs. Interestingly, the patients usually adjust quickly to the motion.

There are also portable ventilators available that can be mounted on wheelchairs to allow mobility of nonambulatory patients.[8]

The patient's family is instructed in the operation of the machines and how to trouble-shoot minor problems. They are also instructed in proper bagging and suctioning techniques. These duties are done by the family members many times in the hospital under the supervision of the health professionals. Training in exercises and ambulation is given to the family when appropriate. When the patient is discharged, the family members are competent in caring for him.

REFERENCES

1. Albanese, A.J., and Toplitz, A.D.: A hassle-free guide to suctioning a tracheostomy, RN, p. 24-29, April 1982.
2. Allen, C.B.: Just breathing, Nursing'74, p. 22-23, Nov. 1974.
3. Alvarez, S.E., and others: Respiratory treatment of the adult patient with spinal cord injury, Phys. Ther. **61**:1737, 1981.
4. Anderson, J.B., and others: Resistive breathing training in severe chronic obstructive pulmonary disease: a pilot study, Scand. J. Respir. Dis. **60**:151-156, 1979.
5. Barrell, S.E., and Abbas, H.M.: Monitoring during physiotherapy after open heart surgery, Physiotherapy **64**:272-273, 1978.
6. Bateman, J.R., and others: Is cough as effective as chest physiotherapy in the removal of excessive tracheobronchial secretions? Thorax **36**:683-687, 1981.
7. Belman, M.S., and Sieck, G.C.: The ventilatory muscles—fatigue, endurance and training, Chest **82**:751-766, 1982.
8. Benvenuti, C.S.: Independence for the quadriplegia: the Bantam respirator, Am. J. Nurs. **79**:918, 1979.
9. Bergofsky, E.H.: Respiratory failure in disorders of the thoracic cage, Am. Rev. Respir. Dis. **119**:643-669, 1979.
10. Bernhard, W.N., and others: Adjustment of intracuff pressure to prevent aspiration, Anesthesiology **50**:363-366, 1979.
11. Birnbaum, M.L., and others: Effects of intermittent positive pressure breathing on emphysematous patients, Am. J. Med. **41**:552-561, 1966.
12. Bomalaski, J.S., and Phair, J.P.: Alcohol, immunosuppression, and the lung, Arch. Intern. Med. **142**:2073-2074, 1982.
13. Bone, R.C.: Acute respiratory failure and chronic obstructive lung disease: recent advances, Med. Clin. North Am. **65**:563-578, 1981.
14. Bone, R.C.: Treatment of respiratory failure due to chronic obstructive lung disease, Arch. Intern. Med. **140**:1018-1022, 1980.
15. Burnside, J.: Physical diagnosis: Physical diagnosis: an introduction to clinical medicine, ed. 16, Baltimore, 1981, The Williams & Wilkins Co.
16. Byrd, R.B., and Burns, J.R.: Cough dynamics in the post-thoracotomy state, Chest **67**:654-657, 1975.
17. Calvert, J.R., and others: Halothane as a depressant of cough reflex, Anesth. Analg. **45**:76-81, 1966.
18. Campbell, C.C.: Appreciation for advice, Phys. Ther. **60**:809-810, 1980. (Letter.)
19. Chopra, S.K., and others: Effects of hydration and physical therapy on tracheal transport velocity, Am. Rev. Respir. Dis. **115**:1009-1014, 1977.
20. Cherniack, R.M., and others: Respiration in health and disease, Philadelphia, 1972, W.B. Saunders Co.
21. Connors, A.F., and others: Chest physical therapy: the immediate effect on oxygenation in acutely ill patients, Chest **78**:559-564, 1980.
22. Connors, A.F., and others: The adult respiratory distress syndrome, Disease-a-Month **27**(4):10-75, 1981.
23. Corson, J.A.: Use of biofeedback in weaning paralyzed patients from respirators, Chest **76**:543-545, 1979.
24. Derenne, J., and others: The respiratory muscles: mechanics, control and pathophysiology, Part 1, Am. Rev. Respir. Dis. **118**:119-133, 1978.
25. Derenne, J.: The respiratory muscles: mechanics, control and pathophysiology, Part 3, Am. Rev. Respir. Dis. **118**:581-601, 1978.
26. Egbert, L.D., and others: The effect of site of operation and type of anesthesia upon the ability to cough in the postoperative period, Surg. Gynecol. Obstet. **115**:295-298, 1962.
27. Fareeduddin, K., and Abelmann, W.H.: Impaired orthostatic tolerance after bed rest in patients with myocardial infarction, N. Engl. J. Med. **280**:345-346, 1969.
28. Gross, D., and others: The effect of training on strength and endurance of the diaphragm in quadriplegia, Am. J. Med. **68**:27-35, 1980.
29. Guenter, C.A.: The role of diaphragm function in disease, Arch. Intern. Med. **139**:806-808, July 1979.
30. Guenter, C.A., and Buchan, K.A.: Acute infectious respiratory illnesses. In Guenter, C.A., and Welch, M.H., editors: Pulmonary medicine, Philadelphia, 1977, J.B. Lippincott Co.
31. Hammon, L.: Review of respiratory anatomy. In Frownfelter, D., editor: Chest physical therapy and pulmonary rehabilitation: an interdisciplinary approach, Chicago, 1978, Year Book Medical Publishers, Inc.
32. Hammon, W.E., and others: Cardiac arrhythmias associated with bronchial drainage, Phys. Ther. **61**:690, 1981. (Abstract.)
33. Hammon, W.E., and others: Effect on bronchial drainage on intracranial pressure in acute neurological injuries, Phys. Ther. **61**:735, 1981. (Abstract.)
34. Hammon, W.E., and Martin, R.J.: Chest physical therapy for acute atelectasis, Phys. Ther. **61**:217-220, 1981.
35. Hammon, W.E., and Martin, R.J.: Fatal pulmonary hemorrhage associated with chest physical therapy, Phys. Ther. **59**:1247-1248, 1979.
36. Hammon, W.E.: Pathophysiology of chronic pulmonary disease. In Frownfelter, D., editor: Chest physical therapy and pulmonary rehabilitation: an interdisciplinary approach, Chicago, 1979, Year Book Medical Publishers, Inc.
37. Hodgkin, J.E.: Chronic obstructive pulmonary disease: current concepts in diagnosis and comprehensive care, Park Ridge, Ill., 1979, American College of Chest Physicians.
38. Hogg, J.C.: The respiratory airways. In Guenter, C.A., and Welch, M.H., editors: Pulmonary medicine, Philadelphia, 1977, J.B. Lippincott Co.
39. Holland, J.C., and others: The ICU syndrome: fact or fancy, Psychiatry Med. **4**:241, 1973.
40. Holtackers, T.R., and others: The use of the chest cuirass in respiratory failure of neurologic origin, Respir. Care **27**:271-275, 1982.
41. Hopewell, P.C.: Adult respiratory distress syndrome, Basics Respir. Dis. **7**:1-6, 1979.
42. Huseby, J., and others: Oxygenation during chest physiotherapy, Chest **70**:430, 1975. (Abstract.)
43. Ibañez, J., and others: The effect of lateral positions on gas exchange

in patients with unilateral lung disease during mechanical ventilation, Intensive Care Med. **7:**231-234, 1981.

44. Irwin, R.S., and others: Cough: a comprehensive review, Arch. Intern Med. **137:**1186-1191, 1977.
45. Jacquette, G.: To reduce hazards of tracheal suctioning, Am. J. Nurs. **71:**2362-2364, 1971.
46. Johanson, W.G., Jr.: Lung defense mechanisms, Basics Respir. Dis. **6:**2, Nov. 1977.
47. Jung, R.C., and Gottlieb, L.S.: Comparison of tracheobronchial suction catheters in humans, Chest **69:**179-181, 1976.
48. Keens, T.G., and others: Ventilatory muscle endurance training in normal subjects and patients with cystic fibrosis, Am. Rev. Respir. Dis. **116:**853-860, 1977.
49. Kirby, N.A., and others: An evaluation of assisted cough in quadriparetic patients, Arch. Phys. Med. Rehabil. **47:**705-710, 1966.
50. Landa, J.F., and others: Effects of suctioning on mucociliary transport, Chest **77:**202-207, 1980.
51. Laurenzi, G.A., and others: Mucus flow in the mammalian trachea, Proceedings Tenth Aspen Ephysema Conference, U.S. Public Health Service, publ. 1787, pp. 27-40, 1967.
52. Laws, A.K., and McIntyre, R.W.: Chest physiotherapy: a physiological assessment during intermittent positive pressure ventilation in respiratory failure, Can. Anaesth. Soc. J. **16:**487-493, 1969.
53. Leith, D.E.: Cough, Phys. Ther. **48:**439-447, 1968.
54. Leith, D.E., and Bradley, M.: Ventilatory muscle strength and endurance training, J. Appl. Physiol. **41:**508-516, 1976.
55. Libby, D.M., and others: Acute respiratory failure in scoliosis or kyphosis: prolonged survival and treatment, Am. J. Med. **73:**532-538, 1982.
56. Loudon, R.G.: Cough, a symptom and a sign, Basics Respir. Dis. **9:**4, March 1981.
57. Loudon, R.G., and Shaw, G.B.: Mechanics of cough in normal subjects and in patients with obstructive respiratory disease, Am. Rev. Respir. Dis. **96:**666-667, 1967.
58. Mackenzie, C.F., and others: Chest physiotherapy in the intensive care unit, Baltimore, 1981, The Williams & Wilkins Co.
59. Macklem, P.T.: Respiratory muscles: the vital pump, Chest **78:**753-758, 1980.
60. Macklem, P.T.: Physiology of cough, Ann. Otol. **83:**761-768, 1974.
61. Macklem, P.T., and Wilson, J.J.: Measurement of intra-bronchial pressure in man, J. Appl. Physiol. **20:**653-663, 1965.
62. Marini, J.J., and others: Acute lobar atelectasis: a prospective comparison of fiberoptic bronchoscopy and respiratory therapy, Am. Rev. Respir. Dis. **119:**971-978, 1979.
63. McMichan, J.C., and others: Pulmonary dysfunction following traumatic quadriplegia. J.A.M.A. **243:**528-531, 1980.
64. Mead, J., and others: Significance of the relationship between lung recoil and maximum expiratory flow, J. Appl. Physiol. **22:**95-108, 1967.
65. Moss, E., and others: The effects of nitrous oxide, Athesin, and thiopentone on intracranial pressure during chest physiotherapy in patients with severe head injuries. In Shulman, K., and others, editors: Intracranial pressure, IV, New York, 1980, Springer-Verlag.
66. Mueller, R.E., and others: Ventilation and blood gas changes induced by pursed lips breathing, J. Appl. Physiol. **28:**784-789, 1970.
67. Murphy, R., and Holford, S.K.: Lung sounds, Basics Respir. Dis. **8:**1-6, 1980.
68. Murray, J.F.: The normal lung, Philadelphia, 1976, W.B. Saunders Co.
69. Neuhaus, A., and others: Pulmonary embolism in respiratory failure, Chest **73:**4, 1978.
70. Owens, G.R., and Rogers, R.M.: Managing respiratory failure in chronic airflow obstruction, J. Respir. Dis. **3:**24-37, 1982.
71. Remolina, C., and others: Positional hypoxemia in unilateral lung disease, N. Engl. J. Med. **304:**523-525, 1981.
72. Rogers, R.M.: Respiratory intensive care, Springfield, Ill., 1977, Charles C Thomas, Publisher.
73. Rochester, D.F., and Braun, M.T.: The respiratory muscles, Basics Respir. Dis. **6:**4, 1981.
74. Rochester, D.F.: Respiratory disease: attention turns to the air pump, Am. J. Med. **68:**803-805, 1980.
75. Sackner, M.A., and others: Pathogenesis and prevention of tracheobronchial damage with suction procedures, Chest **64:**284-290, 1973.
76. Sackner, M.A., and others: Effect of oxygen in graded concentrations upon tracheal mucous velocity, Chest **69:**164-166, 1976.
77. Sackner, M.A., and others: Effect of cuffed endotracheal tubes on tracheal mucous velocity, Chest **68:**774-777, 1975.
78. Saltin, B., and others: Response to exercise after bed rest and training, Circulation **37-38**(Suppl. 7):1-55, 1968.
79. Schoenfeld, M.R.: Terror in the ICU, Forum on Medicine, pp. 14-17, Sept. 1978.
80. Shaffer, T.H., and others: Respiratory muscle function, assessment, and training, Phys. Ther. **61:**1711-1723, 1981.
81. Shannon, D.C.: Respiratory care in the newborn, Crit. Care Med. **5:**10-17, 1977.
82. Shapiro, B.A., and others: Clinical application of respiratory care, Chicago, 1975, Year Book Medical Publishers, Inc.
83. Shim, C., and others: Cardiac arrhythmias resulting from tracheal suctioning, Ann. Intern. Med. **71:**1149-1153, 1969.
84. Siebens, A.A., and others: Cough following transection of spinal cord at C-6, Arch. Phys. Med. Rehabil. **45:**1-8, 1964.
85. Sonne, L.J., and Davis, J.A.: Increased exercise performance in patients with severe COPD following inspiratory resistive training, Chest **81:**436-439, 1982.
86. Staub, N.C.: Lung structure and function, Basics Respir. Dis. **10**(4):1-6, March 1982.
87. Strain, J.J.: Psychological reactions to acute medical illness and critical care, Crit. Care Med. **6:**39-44, 1978.
88. Thurlbeck, W.M.: Chronic bronchitis and emphysema: the pathophysiology of chronic obstructive lung disease, Basics Respir. Dis. **3:**1, Sept. 1974.
89. Thoman, R.L., and others: The efficacy of pursed-lips breathing in patients with chronic obstructive pulmonary disease, Am. Rev. Respir. Dis. **93:**100-106, 1966.
90. Tomlin, P.J.: Psychological problems in intensive care, Br. Med. J. **2:**441-443, 1977.
91. Wang, K., and Berman, D.A.: Artifacts simulating serious ventricular arrhythmia, Postgrad. Med. **69:**98-99, 1981.
92. Wanner, A.: Alteration of tracheal mucociliary transport in airway disease: effect of pharmacologic agents, Chest **80**(Suppl):867-869, 1981.
93. Wanner, A.: Clinical aspects of mucociliary transport, Am. Rev. Respir. Dis. **116:**73-125, 1977.
94. Wenger, N.K.: Rehabilitation after myocardial infarction, J.A.M.A. **424:**2879-2881, 1979.
95. Wong, J.W., and others: Effects of gravity on tracheal mucus transport rates in normal subjects and in patients with cystic fibrosis, Pediatrics **60:**146-152, 1977.
96. Zadai, C.C.: Physical therapy for the acutely ill medical patient, Phys. Ther. **61:**1746-1754, 1981.

SUGGESTED READINGS

1. Belman, M.S., and Sieck, G.C.: The ventilatory muscles: fatigue, endurance and training, Chest **82:**751-766, 1982.
2. Bergofsky, E.H.: Respiratory failure in disorders of the thoracic cage, Am. Rev. Respir. Dis. **119:**643-669, 1979.
3. Bone, R.C.: Acute respiratory failure and chronic obstructive lung disease: recent advances, Med. Clin. North Am. **65:**563-578, 1981.
4. Cherniack, R.M., and others: Respiration in health and disease, Philadelphia, 1972, W.B. Saunders Co.

5. Frownfelter, D., editor: Chest physical therapy and pulmonary rehabilitation: an interdisciplinary approach, Chicago, 1978, Year Book Medical Publishers, Inc.

6. Guenter, C.A., and Welch, M.H., editors: Pulmonary medicine, Philadelphia, 1977, J.B. Lippincott Co.

7. Irwin, R.S., and others: Cough: a comprehensive review, Arch. Intern. Med. **137**:1186-1191, 1977.

8. MacKenzie, C.F., and others: Chest physiotherapy in the intensive care unit, Baltimore, 1981, The Williams & Wilkins Co.

9. Macklem, P.T.: Respiratory muscles: the vital pump, Chest **78**:753-758, 1980.

10. Petty, T.L., editor: Intensive and rehabilitative respiratory care, ed. 3, Philadelphia, 1982, Lea & Febiger.

11. Rogers, R.M.: Respiratory intensive care, Springfield, Ill., 1977, Charles C Thomas, Publisher.

12. Shapiro, B.A., and others: Clinical application of respiratory care, Chicago, 1975, Year Book Medical Publishers, Inc.

13. Tyler, M.L.: Complications of positioning and chest physiotherapy, Respir. Care **27**:458-466, 1982.

14. Zadai, C.C.: Physical therapy for the acutely ill medical patient, Phys. Ther. **61**:1746-1754, 1981.

16

THOMAS R. HOLTACKERS

Physical rehabilitation of the ventilator-dependent patient

Ventilator dependency is a result of respiratory failure, which results from the patient's inability to maintain spontaneous ventilation for normal lung function. Primary causes of respiratory failure include complications of neuromuscular disease, trauma, and cardiopulmonary disease. Rehabilitation of ventilator-dependent patients often is tedious and limited, particularly during the acute stages of respiratory failure. However, rehabilitation programs should be based on the patient's condition and not on the equipment being used. Limited knowledge and understanding of the equipment may restrict the therapist's involvement with the patient receiving mechanical ventilation. This chapter provides the basis for developing a rehabilitation program for the ventilator-dependent patient.

Patients requiring mechanical ventilation because of respiratory failure are extremely vulnerable to complications. Mechanical ventilation itself may have serious side effects including an increased risk of pulmonary infection and tracheal damage. Positive-pressure ventilation may cause lung tissue damage (barotrauma) and, in the presence of hypovolemia, may decrease the blood pressure and cardiac output.[2] Other complications may result from multiple system failure, poor nutrition, psychological depression, poor patient motivation, lack of restful sleep, and lack of mobility.[1] These complications may further compromise the patient's already tenuous condition. A cyclic progression of respiratory failure, mechanical ventilation, complications, and further progression of respiratory failure may occur (Fig. 16-1). This cycle produces a frustrating, difficult situation for the patient and the health care practitioners.

Patients are often mechanically ventilated after trauma or surgery, but most are rapidly weaned from the ventilator and extubated. Although many of these patients require some degree of rehabilitation, the intent of this chapter is

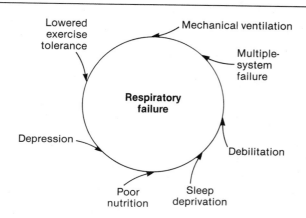

Fig. 16-1. A cyclic reaction of acute respiratory failure and mechanical ventilation.

to focus on those who require prolonged ventilatory support.

It is often difficult to identify those ventilator patients who will benefit from aggressive rehabilitation. Delays in identification may contribute to the development of complications that inhibit effective rehabilitation.

GOALS OF REHABILITATION

The ultimate goal of rehabilitation of ventilator-dependent patients is weaning from mechanical ventilation. Since this is not always possible, an alternative goal is to prepare the family to live with the patient who is dependent on the ventilator. Patients who cannot be weaned may require long-term institutional care, though some can be managed while on mechanical ventilators at home. Family and patient motivation, financial support, disease severity and complications, and the patient's level of physical function are variables that may determine long-term management.

Some patients are not entirely dependent on mechanical ventilation. They breathe spontaneously during the day when awake but need nocturnal mechanical ventilation. Such patients are more easily managed at home than those requiring continuous ventilation.

THE REHABILITATION TEAM

Rehabilitation is always a multidisciplinary endeavor. Rehabilitation of the ventilator-dependent patient is no exception. The team may be composed of physical therapists, nurses, occupational and recreational therapists, respiratory therapists, dietitians, social workers, and physicians. The physicians may include critical care specialists, pulmonologists, neurologists, and surgeons during the acute phases of care. Community medicine specialists, pediatricians, psychiatrists, and physiatrists may be involved during the chronic stages. Roles may be specific and structured in some institutions but quite flexible in others. In all cases, the roles should overlap to provide comprehensive teamwork for maximum patient care (Fig. 16-2).

PATIENT EVALUATION

The physical therapist's evaluation of the ventilator-dependent patient should include a thorough functional assessment of the patient's cardiac, pulmonary, neurological, and musculoskeletal systems. The therapist must also note possible multiple system involvement. It is imperative to evaluate each system independently and all systems collectively.[5]

Pulmonary assessment

Arterial blood gas analysis, respiratory muscle function testing, chest radiographs, and auscultation are the major tools for evaluating the respiratory system. Assessment of cough reflex, sputum culture and production, swallowing function, and shoulder girdle–chest wall mobility supplement the evaluation. The patient's respiratory rate and breathing pattern are also important but are dependent on the mode of mechanical ventilation.

Arterial blood gases. Analysis of the partial pressures of arterial oxygen (PaO_2) and carbon dioxide ($PaCO_2$) provides an expression of the ability of the lung to deliver oxygen to and remove carbon dioxide from the blood. PaO_2 indicates oxygen dissolved in the blood plasma but reflects the potential for the amount of oxygen combined with hemoglobin, the main carrier of oxygen to the tissues. The percentage of hemoglobin saturated with oxygen (SaO_2) is directly proportional to PaO_2 and is described by the oxyhemoglobin dissociation curve. PaO_2 is dependent partially on the concentration of inspired oxygen (FIO_2) and the barometric pressure (Pb). The partial pressure of

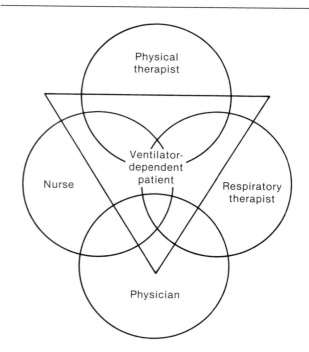

Fig. 16-2. Role overlap of health care team caring for the ventilator-dependent patient.

carbon dioxide ($PaCO_2$) is directly proportional to alveolar ventilation. An increase in $PaCO_2$ represents hypoventilation, and a decrease in $PaCO_2$ represents hyperventilation. Hypoventilation produces respiratory acidosis, and hyperventilation produces alkalosis. Changes in pH can also be produced with fluctuations of bicarbonate ion (HCO_3^-) levels in the arterial blood.[3,8]

There are several methods by which the lungs' ability to add oxygen to arterial blood (PaO_2) can be compared to the FIO_2. The alveolar-to-arterial (A-a) oxygen gradient reflects the difference in partial pressures of alveolar oxygen (PAO_2) and arterial oxygen (PaO_2). The normal A-a gradient when room air is breathed is less than 10 and less than 100 when 100% oxygen is breathed. The A-a oxygen ratio is another expression that compares the PAO_2 to PaO_2. The PaO_2/FIO_2 ratio, or P/F ratio, is also used as a comparison but is a less accurate value than the A-a gradient or ratio. The advantage of the P/F ratio is its simplicity of calculation. Increases in the A-a oxygen gradient and decreases in the A-a and P/F ratios indicate the lungs' inability to supply oxygen to the arterial blood.[3,8]

Respiratory muscle function. Respiratory muscle strength, endurance, and coordination are three elements of function. Evaluation of respiratory muscle function gives the therapist an indication of the patient's ability to breathe spontaneously.

The ability to produce maximum negative intrathoracic

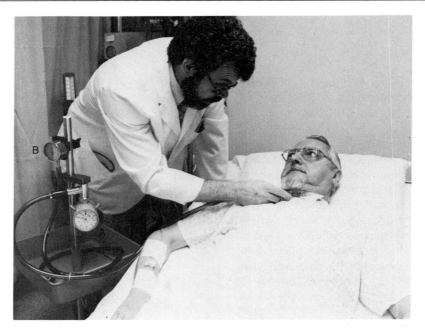

Fig. 16-3. Forced vital capacity (FVC) and maximum inspiratory and expiratory pressure measurements can be made with a portable spirometer, *A,* and manometer, *B.*

pressure (PI_{max}) and maximum positive intrathoracic pressure (PE_{max}) reflects inspiratory muscle and expiratory muscle strength, respectively. The PI_{max} and PE_{max} can be measured at the bedside with a portable static pressure manometer (Fig. 16-3, *B*). The manometer is easily attached to the endotracheal or tracheostomy tube. The patient is instructed to perform a maximal inspiratory effort from end expiration for PI_{max} measurements and an expiratory effort at the end of full inspiratory volume for a PE_{max} measurement. The maneuvers are repeated three or four times, and the best value is recorded. Both measurements are dependent on patient cooperation and effort.[2]

Forced vital capacity (FVC) measures the patient's ability to move the maximum amount of gas into or out of the lungs. Tidal volume (V_t) is the measurement of the patient's "normal" inspiratory or expiratory volume. FVC and V_t can be measured at the patient's bedside with a portable spirometer (Fig. 16-3, *A*). The spirometer is attached to the endotracheal or tracheostomy tube, and the patient is instructed to breathe normally. After 10 breaths, the total expired volume is recorded and divided by 10 to establish the tidal volume. The patient is then instructed to breathe in as deeply as possible and to exhale as fully as possible to determine vital capacity. Because of the time and effort needed to measure FVC and V_t, the patient may need to be reconnected to the ventilator for short periods of time to prevent fatigue.

Graphs of the patient's PI_{max}, PE_{max}, FVC, and V_t can indicate trends of improvement or deterioration of respiratory muscle function. When appropriate, these graphs can be an incentive to the patient.

One can evaluate respiratory muscle endurance by having the patient breathe spontaneously or with low ventilator settings that permit spontaneous breathing such as that occurring with intermittent mandatory ventilation (IMV). The length of time the patient can maintain spontaneous breathing without undue distress is one indication of respiratory muscle endurance. Respiratory rate, pulse rate, ECG response, and arterial blood gases should be monitored during these trials.

Respiratory muscle coordination can be subjectively assessed during spontaneous breathing. Paradoxical chest and abdominal wall movements indicate respiratory muscle dyskinesis or, in the presence of normal accessory muscle function, diaphragm paralysis.

Respiratory muscle function is examined more fully elsewhere in this text.

Chest radiographs. Chest radiographs are an important clinical tool for the therapist. During the acute stages of respiratory failure, chest radiographs may be taken daily. Atelectasis, effusions, infiltrates, and pneumothorax can be identified from a radiograph and must be considered in the design and redesign of the physical therapy program.

Chest assessment. Auscultation, palpation, and inspection should be performed before each physical therapy session for assessment of the patient's pulmonary status. Changes in breath sounds, adventitious sounds, and chest-wall movement or configuration may indicate acute changes in the lung and may necessitate changes in the physical therapy program. Diminished or absent breath sounds may indicate atelectasis, but they should be corroborated with chest radiograph findings. Rales and rhonchi usually indicate retained secretions. Wheezes commonly indicate bronchospasm of distal airways and may necessitate bronchodilators. Retention of secretions is often accompanied by decreases in PaO_2 and increases in $PaCO_2$,[5] and postural drainage with manual techniques is indicated.

Cardiovascular assessment

Assessment of the patient's cardiovascular status includes determination or estimation of heart rate, arterial blood pressure, electrocardiogram (ECG), pulmonary artery and pulmonary artery wedge pressures, cardiac output, and peripheral circulation. The patient's heart rate, blood pressure, and ECG status should be monitored before, during, and after physical therapy. Abnormalities during or after certain therapeutic procedures may preclude the use of those procedures. For example, a severe cardiac arrhythmia may prevent the patient from assuming certain postural drainage positions, changes in blood pressure may occur during ambulation, and tachycardia may occur after vigorous exercises. Physiological responses to therapeutic exercise must be monitored and well documented. Pulmonary artery catheters, which measure pulmonary vascular dynamics and cardiac output, are used primarily during the acute stages of respiratory failure to monitor body fluid balance and peripheral vascular perfusion. Patients with poor peripheral circulation, for example, those with atherosclerosis obliterans or diabetes, may have difficulty with ambulatory activities.

Neuromusculoskeletal evaluation

A thorough assessment of the patient's neurological status, muscular function and strength, and skeletal integrity is an important consideration when one is designing a rehabilitation program and should be included in the care of the ventilator-dependent patient. Emphasis is frequently placed on cardiopulmonary status, but because respiratory failure commonly results from neuromuscular disease, skeletal deformity, and trauma, the neuromusculoskeletal evaluation is imperative. Physical therapists' skills in evaluating and treating these systems should be utilized. The patient's sensory function, including proprioception, reflexes, coordination, and balance should be assessed when one is developing a therapeutic regimen. Muscle strength and joint range of motion should also be assessed though the patient's limited physical condition makes this task difficult and sometimes impossible to complete.

PHYSICAL THERAPY TREATMENT PROGRAM

Weaning from mechanical ventilation and restoration to a maximal functional level of activity is the general goal of the physical therapy program for the ventilator-dependent patient. Specific objectives of the program include maintaining or improving muscle strength and endurance, joint range of motion, chest-wall compliance, cardiovascular endurance, and secretion clearance. Other goals may include prevention and treatment of atelectasis and skin breakdown and maintenance of homeostasis. Psychological support and education of the patient and family in self-care and home activities is an additional treatment consideration. The treatment program should be dynamic and flexible depending on the patient's needs as ascertained through a thorough and continuing evaluation. Specific physical therapy procedures may include but are not limited to breathing-retraining exercises, postural drainage and manual techniques, range-of-motion and strengthening exercises, and ambulatory activities.

Breathing-retraining exercises

The purpose of breathing-retraining exercises for the ventilator-dependent patient is to maintain or improve respiratory muscle endurance, strength, coordination, and rhythmicity. Although breathing-retraining exercises cannot be performed by all patients being mechanically ventilated, it is possible with many. The type and appropriateness of breathing exercise depends on the patient's degree of respiratory failure, associated complications, and the mode of mechanical ventilation.

Coordination of breathing exercises and mechanical ventilation. For a better understanding of how breathing-retraining exercises can be utilized during mechanical ventilation, the types or categories of ventilators, the modes of ventilation, and use of positive end-expiratory pressure (PEEP) should be explained.[4,7,]

Following are several ways of categorizing ventilators:
1. Means of power
   a. Electrically driven
   b. Pneumatically driven
2. Mode of pressure delivered
   a. Negative
   b. Postive
3. Method of cycling or limiting breaths
   a. Pressure
   b. Volume
   c. Time

The form of pressure delivered to the patient by the ventilator may be positive as with most modern ventilators or negative as with earlier forms of ventilators such as iron lungs and cuirass ventilators. The method of powering the ventilator may be either electric or pneumatic. The means of cycling or limiting mechanical breaths may be with either time, pressure, or volume.[7] For example, a ventilator may be categorized as an electrically powered, time-

Table 16-1. Modes of mechanical ventilation	
Control	The patient is "guaranteed" a predetermined number of mechanical breaths but is unable or not permitted to initiate a mechanical breath or breathe spontaneously.
Assist	The patient is permitted to initiate a mechanical breath but is not guaranteed a predetermined number of mechanical breaths.
Assist-control	The patient is guaranteed a predetermined number of mechanical breaths and is permitted to initiate additional mechanical breaths.
Intermittent mandatory ventilation (IMV)	The patient is guaranteed a predetermined number of mechanical breaths and permitted to initiate spontaneous breaths through the ventilator.

cycled, volume-limited, positive-pressure ventilator. Ventilators can almost be compared to automobiles: they can be powered by several means, they look different and have different features, but they have basically the same function.

There are four modes of mechanical ventilation: control, assist-control, assist, and intermittent mandatory ventilation (IMV) (Table 16-1). The control mode simply does not "permit" the patient to initiate a ventilator breath, and all the breaths the patient receives are predetermined mechanical breaths. The type of ventilator used will determine the amount of tidal volume the patient receives during control ventilation. Volume-limited ventilators deliver a predetermined volume of gas. The volume of the pressure-limited ventilator's breath is established by a predetermined pressure limit. Basically, the ventilator "controls" the patient's ventilation. Patients requiring the control mode are often paralyzed or heavily sedated and are thus unable to breathe spontaneously.[4,7] Breathing-retraining exercises are usually not performed when this mode of ventilation is employed.

With the assist mode the patient "assists" the ventilator by inspiring to initiate a ventilator breath. Once the breath is initiated or "triggered," the ventilator will deliver a mechanical breath. This mode allows the patient to regulate his own respiratory rate. The volume of each breath is again determined by the type of ventilator being used.

The assist-control mode provides a preselected number of "control" breaths but permits the patient to "assist" the ventilator to receive additional mechanical breaths. The respiratory rate can vary with patient effort. Since the patient can trigger ventilator-supplied breaths, a lower limit of mechanical breaths is maintained with the control part of the mode.

Intermittent mandatory ventilation (IMV) is similar to the assist-control mode in that the ventilator provides a preselected number of breaths. Additional breaths that the patient initiates are spontaneous and not mechanical. The IMV mode provides an advantage over other modes by permitting the patient to breathe spontaneously during mechanical ventilation. The patient can maintain some degree of respiratory muscle endurance and coordination. When the IMV rate is lowered, the patient must initiate a greater number of spontaneous breaths to maintain minute ventilation.[4]

Diaphragmatic breathing. Diaphragmatic breathing exercises can be utilized with patients receiving assist, assist-control, and IMV modes. These exercises help maintain proprioception and rhythmicity of the diaphragm and foster abdominal wall relaxation. When patients receive progressively lower IMV rates, diaphragmatic breathing exercises become increasingly more important because of the patient's increased need for spontaneity of breathing. Diaphragmatic breathing exercises are performed when one has the patient protrude the abdomen during inspiration as the diaphragm descends. Simultaneously, the abdominal wall must relax to prevent resistance to the excursion of the diaphragm. The patient is instructed to concentrate on diaphragm contractions without accessory respiratory muscle contraction. Placing the patient's hand on the abdomen provides information to the patient about the depth and rate of diaphragm contractions and the degree of abdominal wall tension. The patient should be in a position that promotes abdominal wall relaxation and unrestricted diaphragm excursion. The semisitting or side-lying positions with the hips flexed are optimal positions for encouraging diaphragm contraction in the ventilator-dependent patient. Coaching by the therapist during these exercises is very important. The therapist should initially instruct the patient in diaphragm breathing, but because the patient may require continued coaching while receiving mechanical ventilation, continued reminders from nurses and other health care personnel are imperative. Patients can be instructed in diaphragm breathing for short periods of time while detached from the ventilator; however, most instruction occurs with patients receiving mechanical breaths. Therefore the therapist must coordinate the instruction with the mode of ventilation. Attempts at diaphragmatic breathing with the patient on the assist mode will result in mechanical breaths, but during IMV the attempt at a diaphragmatic breath will result in spontaneous breaths.

Deep breathing. Deep-breathing exercises are an attempt to utilize all the inspiratory muscles to produce a maximum sustained breath.[5,6] This type of breathing exercise can be performed during mechanical ventilation, but again it is dependent on the mode of ventilation or the patient's ability to tolerate spontaneous ventilation for short periods of time. The type of ventilator may also determine the effectiveness of deep-breathing exercises. A pressure-limited ventilator will permit the patient to take a deep breath because the breath is limited only by the preset pressure limit of the ventilator. With the volume- or time-limited ventilator, the breath is limited by the predetermined volume limit, inspiratory time, and flow rate. Patients receiving IMV can take deep breaths if the IMV rate is not too high. If the rate is high, the short time interval between mechanical breaths may not permit the patient to finish a deep breath before the next ventilator breath automatically occurs. However, some ventilators have synchronized IMV (SIMV), which may permit enough time for a deep breath. The therapist should again be instrumental in instructing and directing the deep-breathing exercises. Unlike diaphragm-breathing exercises, deep breathing need not be peformed continuously. A program of 5 to 10 deep breaths, two to three times a day can be utilized. Measurement of vital capacity with a spirometer at bedside provides a form of biofeedback for the patient and the therapist.

Segmental breathing. Segmental breathing emphasizes the expansion of a specific area of the chest wall during a deep breath.[5,6] The anterior-apical and lateral-basilar areas of the chest wall usually move freely with deep inspiratory efforts. The therapist's hands are placed over these areas, unilaterally or bilaterally, and the patient is instructed to inhale deeply, pushing the chest wall up against the pressure provided by the therapist's hands. This manual pressure is not sustained throughout the inspiratory effort but is released gradually as the patient continues with inspiration. A method of "quick release," however, utilizes constant pressure during inspiration with a rapid removal of the pressure at the end of the breath. This technique may facilitate a deeper breath and may locally alter the intrapleural pressure causing expansion of a lung segment. Another method of segmental breathing facilitation is the "quick stretch." A quick stretching of the chest wall at end expiration facilitates a stronger contraction of the accessory muscles in the area stretched, producing a deeper inspiratory effort. The effectiveness of these maneuvers requires excellent patient-therapist coordination. The mode of ventilation and the type of ventilator will also determine the efficacy of these techniques. A pressure-limited ventilator that cycles "off" when a predetermined pressure is reached is the most compatible with these facilitation techniques. The volume-limited or time-limited ventilator permits increased inspiratory efforts and chest wall excursion. However, the volume of each spontaneous breath is limited by the preset volume limit of the ventilator. Patients receiving the IMV mode of ventilation can achieve greater inspiratory volumes during the spontaneous phase of IMV. However, they can receive only the predetermined volume during the mechanical breaths, unless the ventilator is pressure limited. Whichever mode or type of ventilation the patient is receiving, segmental breathing should be attempted. Segmental breathing used with chest-wall stretching and inspiratory muscle facilitation techniques will help maintain chest-wall compliance and accessory respiratory muscle strength.

Abdominal breathing. Abdominal breathing emphasizes active expiration for patients who have paralyzed or extremely weak diaphragms, but with good accessory and abdominal muscle strength. Active expiration utilizes abdominal muscle contraction to increase intra-abdominal pressure. This increased pressure "pushes" the diaphragm to an unusually high position in the thorax. When the intra-abdominal pressure is reduced, the diaphragm passively "falls" to produce inspiration. The accessory mucles can assist with this inspiratory effort to produce a greater tidal volume. This type of breathing can be performed mechanically with a type of ventilator called a "pneumobelt." Two disadvantages of this type of breathing are that a conscious effort is necessary to breathe and the patient must be in an upright position to provide, using gravity, the maximum excursion of the diaphragm. Patients with paralyzed diaphragms who can effectively use abdominal breathing still require mechanical ventilation during recumbency and sleep.

Abdominal pursed-lip breathing is another form of abdominal breathing, more commonly used for patients with small airway disease, such as emphysema. This type of breathing permits the patient to maintain small airway patency during expiration by producing a controlled resistance at the lips. Pursed-lip breathing is not practical when the patient is intubated or tracheostomized but may be useful during weaning from the ventilator when the patient can breathe spontaneously through the mouth. Some ventilators can mimic pursed-lip breathing by retarding expiration. A valve to increase the resistance in the expiratory circuit of the ventilator can provide the pursed-lip effect.

Breathing retraining and the "weaning" process

During long-term mechanical ventilation the patient's respiratory muscles lose endurance and strength. These functional losses are attributable, in part, to poor nutrition and weight loss. These respiratory muscle problems occur most commonly in patients ventilated with control, assist, or assist-control modes. Because intermittent mandatory ventilation (IMV) permits the patient to breathe spontaneously between ventilator breaths, loss of respiratory muscle strength and endurance is delayed. Weaning from mechanical ventilation requires that the patient breathe spontaneously with increased respiratory muscle strength and endurance. To increase endurance, the patient receives lower rates with IMV or is removed from mechanical ventilation completely to breathe spontaneously for short periods of time three or four times a day. One should monitor these weaning sessions by arterial blood gas analysis to determine if the patient can maintain adequate ventilation, as indicated by the Pa_{CO_2}. Whichever method of weaning is used for breathing retraining, coaching and observation during weaning are important, both for breathing reeducation and psychological support. Breathing retraining and weaning must be coordinated with other rehabilitation activities. Suctioning and pulmonary hygiene should precede each breathing session to help reduce the amount of retained secretions and thereby reduce the work of breathing. Ambulation should be scheduled around the weaning sessions, but breathing retraining should be reinforced during both activities. Meals, nursing care, rest periods, and respiratory therapy have to be coordinated with weaning.

Weaning from mechanical ventilation can be tedious, time consuming, and frustrating for both the patient and the health care team. Weaning must be aproached cautiously with a controlled and coordinated effort particularly if the patient has been mechanically ventilated for a long time. Haphazard weaning with multiple, rapid attempts and failures produce patient anxiety, frustration, and discouragement.

Pulmonary hygiene

Pulmonary or bronchial hygiene is the process of removing secretions from the tracheobronchial tree. Cough, mucociliary transport, physical activity, and deep breathing normally provide secretion removal. Impairment of these normal mechanisms promotes the retention of secretions. The predisposition to secretion retention is escalated in the presence of pulmonary diseases that produce abnormally large amounts of mucus. Secretion retention impairs alveolar ventilation, promotes atelectasis, and results in reduced arterial oxygenation and increased arterial carbon dioxide. Secretion retention also increases in the work of breathing and decreases airway compliance.[3]

Respiratory failure with mechanical ventilation potentiates secretion retention, making pulmonary hygiene an important treatment for ventilator-dependent patients. A comprehensive program of pulmonary hygiene for these patients may include suctioning, postural drainage, manual techniques, aerosolized bronchodilators and mucolytics, ambulation, and adequate hydration.

Suctioning. Suctioning for intubated and tracheostomized patients requires sterile technique to prevent contamination of the tracheobronchial tree. To prevent hypoxemia and atelectasis the patient must be well oxygenated and ventilated before and after each pass of the suction catheter. A self-inflating bag with an oxygen source is usually used to hyperventilate the patient, but the ventilator can be adjusted to provide the same results. After the patient is well oxygenated, the sterile catheter is passed through the endotracheal or tracheostomy tube until either a cough reflex is elicited or firm resistance is met. Suction is then applied by placement of the thumb over the suction port of the catheter, and the catheter is gradually withdrawn. The patient is then reoxygenated and hyperventilated. Passing and removing the catheter should take no more than 12 seconds from the time the oxygen is removed until

Table 16-2. A guide to the frequency of postural drainage treatments

Daily or b.i.d.	General maintenance and prophylaxis
t.i.d. or q.i.d.	Moderate term care, i.e., postoperative linear atelectasis
q.i.d. or q4h	Moderately severe retained secretion or lobar atelectasis
q2h	Copious amounts of secretions or total lung collapse (this frequency should only be maintained for a short duration, i.e., 12 to 18 hours)

it is reattached. Instillation of 3 to 5 ml of normal saline solution followed by hyperventilation may be necessary if the secretions are thick and tenacious. The suctioning procedure is repeated until the secretions removed with suction are minimal. The frequency of suction depends on the amount of secretions. Suctioning should follow postural drainage and manual techniques and should precede ambulation and breathing retraining.

Postural (bronchial) drainage. Postural drainage is positioning of the patient to permit gravity to drain secretions from lung segments.[2,5,6] A specific position is used to drain each lung segment. Because of specific surgery, trauma, or patient intolerance, modification of the suggested drainage position may be necessary. Nursing procedures that include turning and repositioning the patient may help prevent retention of secretions. However, when focal atelectasis or lobar consolidation occur, a more specific program of postural drainage should be incorporated into the plan of care. Chest radiographs and auscultation are used to determine which lung segments have secretions. The appropriate drainage positions should then be used.

Postural drainage itself, in the absence of manual techniques, is a therapeutic entity. Although commonly accompanied by the manual techniques of chest percussion and vibration, postural drainage can be used alone to assist the drainage of pulmonary secretions. This fact is particularly important when patients cannot tolerate manual techniques or when there is limited access to persons who can provide manual techniques.

The frequency and length of time for postural drainage depends of the amount of secretions, the number of segments to be drained, and the patient's tolerance. A guideline for the frequency of postural drainage is listed in Table 16-2.

The order of drainage for secretions in multiple segments is determined by procedural considerations and the patient's tolerance of certain positions. One suggestion is to drain the most involved segment last and maintain the patient in that drainage position after the treatment session. Another suggestion is to treat the most involved segment first, especially if the patient can tolerate the treatment for only short periods of time. This would ensure that the most involved segment would be effectively treated even though the other segments would receive only minimal drainage during that session.

Patients receiving postural drainage must be monitored during treatment for changes in cardiac rhythm, pulse rate, blood pressure, and respiratory rate. Additional caution must be used with patients who have preexisting cardiac arrhythmias or vital-sign instability. Because several postural drainage positions involve placing the patient in a head-down position, caution must be used with patients who have recent head injuries, life-threatening cardiac arrhythmias, pulmonary hemorrhage, pulmonary edema, diaphragmatic and hiatal hernias, and gastrointestinal bleeding. When the patient is turned, care must also be taken to not dislodge or remove intravenous catheters, urinary catheters, or any other equipment or monitors attached to the patient.

Manual techniques. Chest percussion, vibration, and shaking are manual techniques applied to the chest wall during postural drainage to enhance the removal of pulmonary secretions.[2,5,6]

Chest percussion is performed by alternate striking of the thorax with cupped hands. This is done rapidly and as vigorously as the patient can tolerate to produce a mechanical force that is transmitted to the patient's airways. This force loosens mucus that has collected in the airways. The loosened mucus is drained proximally under the influence of gravity created by placement of the patient in a drainage position. Chest percussion is performed with caution over osteoporotic or fractured ribs, over hematomas, in the presence of bleeding disorders, and near incisions and chest tubes.

Vibration and shaking are performed on the thorax during expiration. Vibration is a finer, more rapid up-and-down motion, whereas shaking is coarser and slower. The same precautions are taken with vibration and shaking as with percussion, but vibration and shaking seem to be better tolerated. Vibration and shaking as facilitation techniques can supplement segmental breathing or can be used with other facilitation techniques such as ''quick stretching'' and ''quick release.'' A quick stretch of the thorax at the end of expiration after vibration or shaking may facilitate both a stronger contraction of the intercostal muscles and relaxation of their antagonists. In patients with spasticity, a quick stretch will facilitate a reflex contraction of the intercostal and diaphragm muscles thereby producing a greater inspiratory effort. A quick release of manual pressure on the thorax at the end of inspiration ''springs'' the chest wall, facilitating a deeper breath before the next vibration or shaking cycle. These techniques can be used with patients on volume-limited ventilators though quick stretch appears to be more effective for the patient on a pressure-limited ventilator.

The major indications for postural drainage and manual techniques are secretions and atelectasis. Patients with impaired mucociliary transport, such as smokers, patients with cystic fibrosis or chronic obstructive lung disease, and patients who have received a general anesthetic, are predisposed to retain secretions and develop atelectasis, particularly if their cough is impaired. Ineffective cough can result from inspiratory-expiratory muscle weakness, and pain can result from thoracic or abdominal surgery or trauma. Respiratory failure may result from any of these problems. Although intubated or tracheostomized and mechanically ventilated, the patient should be encouraged to cough to assist in the mobilization of secretions during suctioning and postural drainage.

Joint range-of-motion exercise. Maintaining joint range of motion (ROM) to prevent contractures is important for any immobilized or paralyzed patient, including those who are ventilator dependent. Joint and muscle contractures that develop could reduce functional activities and ambulation. Proper bed positioning, frequent turning and repositioning, use of splints and footboards, and encouragement of self-care activities supplement ROM exercises in preventing contractures. If contractures exist, it is imperative to stretch the involved joint or muscle.

One of the most difficult problems encountered with ROM exercises for ventilator-dependent patients, especially during the acute stages in intensive care, is the limitation of exercise on extremities with monitoring or life-support equipment attached. Restriction of specific joint movement occurs when intravenous or arterial lines, central venous pressure and pulmonary artery catheters, temporary cardiac pacemakers, traction devices, and renal dialysis cannulas are placed in arteries or veins close to or in a joint (Fig. 16-4). In most situations ROM exercises are not recommended for that joint. ROM exercises for other joints are not prohibited unless they change the position of another catheter or line. For example, shoulder elevation beyond 90 degrees may change the position of a transvenous pacemaker or pulmonary artery catheter placed in the basilic vein. Before initiation of ROM exercise a careful inspection and assessment of the equipment attached to the patient is imperative.

Since active and active-assistive ROM exercises not only maintain or improve joint mobility, but also help maintain or improve muscle strength, these exercises should be employed whenever possible.

Strengthening exercises. Maintaining or improving the strength of the ventilator-dependent patient is often a focal point of rehabilitation, particularly during the acute stages of respiratory failure. The effects of immobility are paramount and potentiate a multitude of complications, including muscle weakness. With immobility, loss of strength is rapid, but return of strength is slow. Prevention therefore is the best strategy for muscle weakness, and active exercises should be initiated as soon as possible. Manual resis-

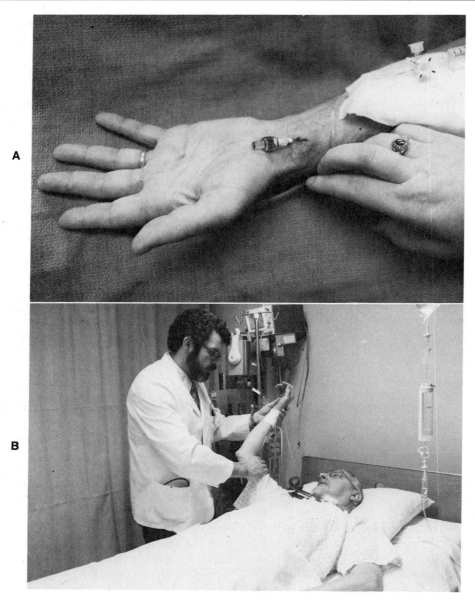

Fig. 16-4. An arterial line placed in the left radial artery, **A,** inhibits left-wrist range of motion (ROM) but not ROM of other joints, **B.**

tance, isometric, and progressive resistance exercises (PRE) are three methods of maintaining and increasing strength.[6] These exercises are no different for the ventilator patient from what they are for other patients, with one exception. Because most patients being mechanically ventilated are intubated or tracheostomized, they are unable to perform a Valsalva maneuver. The Valsalva maneuver, expiration against a closed glottis, increases intrathoracic pressure, which stabilizes the thorax during resistive exercise. Although not recommended for extended periods be-

cause of a decrease in blood pressure, the maneuver provides additional support during initiation of the resisted movement. The patent airway provided by the endotracheal or tracheostomy tube prevents the ventilator patient from closing the glottis, thereby preventing the increase in intrathoracic pressure. Patients may try to reproduce the effect by exhaling against the inspiratory cycle of the ventilator. However, this attempt interferes with the ventilator's normal inspiratory cycle by triggering the high-pressure alarm and "pop-off" valve of the ventilator. This

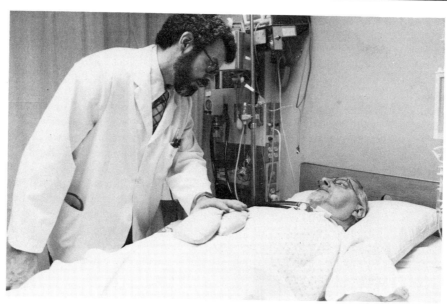

Fig. 16-5. Sand bags placed on the abdomen is one method of diaphragm-strengthening exercises for ventilator-dependent patients.

sequence of events may limit the tidal volume delivered to the patient and may precipitously and dangerously increase intrathoracic pressure. This pressure increase is not recommended, and the physical therapist should encourage relaxation of abdominal and thoracic muscles during exercises and must provide longer rest periods between repetitions.

Strengthening the respiratory muscles, especially the diaphragm, may be of particular benefit for the ventilator-dependent patient. The ventilator provides much of the work of breathing previously provided by the respiratory muscles. Prolonged mechanical ventilation combined with weight loss will weaken and diminish the endurance of the diaphragm and other inspiratory muscles. Strengthening of the respiratory muscles must be incorporated into a rehabilitation program when the patient is capable of breathing spontaneously. The same principles of strengthening for skeletal muscles can be applied to respiratory muscles. This means that the respiratory muscles must be resisted during contraction. This has traditionally been accomplished with manual resistance to diaphragmatic excursion, or placement of weights on the abdomen, or having the patient breathe with an inspiratory pressure restriction. The therapist can provide resistance by placing his or her hand on the patient's abdomen and manually resisting the excursion of the diaphragm during inspiration. The patient is asked to protrude the abdomen during inspiration, and the therapist can gradually increase the amount of resistance applied to the diaphragm as the patient begins to coordi-

nate breathing with the ventilator's cycle. Abdominal weights can be used in place of manual resistance with increases in weight administered as the patient gains strength (Fig. 16-5). Resistance to inspiration provided by the ventilator using its inspiratory triggering sensitivity can also be used but requires a thorough understanding of the ventilator. Each method requires much coaching by the therapist. The frequency, number of repetitions, and the amount of resistance must be carefully monitored by the physical therapist. A daily, or twice daily, inspiratory exercise session with three sets of 10 repetitions might be a starting or target regimen for manual resistance or abdominal weight training. Periodic testing of FVC, V_t, and PI_{max} provides an objective assessment of the patient's progress (p. 294).

Using the ventilator's inspiratory resistance offers a different regimen of exercise. By decreasing the ventilator's "triggering" sensitivity to inspiration, the patient must create a greater negative pressure to initiate a ventilator breath during the assist or assist-control mode. This increased inspiratory effort can serve as a strengthening exercise. The number of repetitions is initially between 4 and 8, but may be increased as the patient progresses. The pressure needed to trigger the ventilator should also be kept low initially—between 3 and 10 cm H_2O of negative pressure. With assist and assist-control modes of ventilation, this technique provides resistance to the initial excursion of the diaphragm. Once the ventilator is triggered, the remaining work of the breath is provided by the ventilator.

There is no evidence indicating which method of respiratory muscle strengthening is the most successful. Therefore the method of respiratory muscle strengthening used for the ventilator-dependent patient is determined largely by the clinical judgment of the physical therapist, with the condition of the patient and the mode of ventilation influencing the therapist's decision.

Ambulatory activities. The effects on patients of immobilization can be devastating. Pulmonary emboli, decubitus ulcers, orthostatic hypotension, and atelectasis are major complications of prolonged bed rest, which is often employed for treatment of acute respiratory failure. However, attempts to improve the patient's mobility should start early in the treatment program for acute respiratory failure. Frequent turning, ROM exercises, and progressive ambulation can help maintain or improve mobility.

The patient should not be permitted to remain in one position for more than 2 hours. Although turning patients is primarily a nursing responsibility, the physical therapist should provide recommendations about the positioning of patients, particularly those with paralysis. Proper positioning will prevent contractures and joint trauma. Proper placement of pillows to support flaccid extremities and to align the spine is a necessary part of the positioning procedure. For patients who are obtunded, paralyzed, or in traction, or are difficult to turn for other reasons, several types of turning beds may be utilized. The Stryker Frame, Foster Frame, and CircOlectric beds permit safe turning but limit the position of the patient to prone and supine. The Roto-Rest bed permits gradual turning from side to side in a continuous, slow motion.

Progression from sitting to standing to walking is an important aspect in mobilizing ventilator-dependent patients. Despite being mechanically ventilated, patients who are medically and physically able to increase their level of physical activity should have the opportunity to progress at their own rate during rehabilitative activities. The equipment used to support vital functions should not limit the patient's ambulation, but meticulous care is necessary to prevent dislodgment or accidental removal of therapeutic or monitoring machinery. In some cases it takes longer to arrange the equipment to permit ambulation than the time needed to actually have the patient ambulate! Assistance from nurses and respiratory therapists may be necessary to prepare the equipment. The therapist must remember that the equipment does not restrict mobility under most circumstances, but it is the patient's severely debilitated condition that becomes the inhibiting factor in rehabilitation.

The schedule for ambulation sessions must be coordinated with other activities or procedures the patient may need to receive. Generally, pulmonary hygiene, bronchodilator therapy, and endotracheal suction, if needed, should precede the ambulation session. Pulmonary hygiene, especially when provided before ambulation, helps remove secretions from the airways and reduces the work of breathing. Another consideration during ambulation sessions is allowing sitting time. The patient should have an opportunity to sit and rest after each attempt at ambulation. In addition, a "cooling-down" period after the physical therapy treatment may be necessary to permit the patient to recover from the fatigue caused by the physical demands of treatment.

Careful monitoring of the patient's pulse rate, respiratory rate, and blood pressure is imperative before, during, and after each ambulation session. The most likely time of critical changes in respiratory and hemodynamic status is when progressing from one stage of ambulation to another, such as walker to cane. Although there may be many pressures to have the patient walk, the therapist must control the progression of ambulation to ensure the tolerance of one stage before one advances to the next; for example, if the patient cannot tolerate sitting with good balance and stable vital signs, it is doubtful the patient will tolerate standing or walking.

When the patient begins to progress toward walking, a different method of mechanical ventilation must be provided. A portable, lightweight, pneumatically driven ventilator provides a degree of freedom for ambulation. A ventilator such as the Bird Mark VII can be attached to an E-sized cylinder of oxygen. The ventilator and attached oxygen source can be mounted on a walker with wheels (Fig. 16-6) or on a podium type of walker (Fig. 16-7). Intravenous lines and other equipment can be attached to the walker or placed on a portable intravenous-line pole. If the patient is receiving positive end-expiratory pressure (PEEP), portable PEEP valves can be attached to the walker and connected to the expiratory valve of the ventilator. If the patient has chronic obstructive pulmonary disease (COPD) and premature airway collapse, an expiratory retard cap can be added to the expiratory valve of the Bird ventilator. The expiratory retard cap acts similarly to pursed-lip breathing, which may enhance the patient's ability to tolerate the added physical stress of ambulation without becoming dyspneic. A self-inflating anesthesia or breathing bag is another method of ventilatory support while the patient is walking. These bags can also be attached to the E-sized oxygen cylinder on the walker, and the patient can be manually ventilated while walking. This can be a cumbersome task for the therapist, especially if the patient has difficulty ambulating because of weakness, instability, or the amount of equipment necessary. However, it is an alternative method that can be used when portable ventilators are not available.

One can also increase exercise tolerance by having the patient work with a bicycle ergometer at the bedside. The ergometer enables the patient to exercise in the hospital room while attached to the ventilator. The patient may have some difficulty getting on and off the ergometer, which may necessitate the presence of a therapist to supervise the patient's safety.

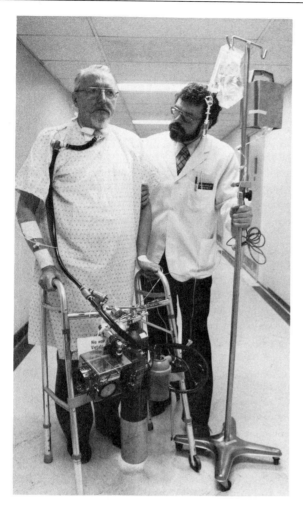

Fig. 16-6. Bird Mark VII ventilator attached to an orthopaedic walker permits more mobility for the ventilator-dependent patient.

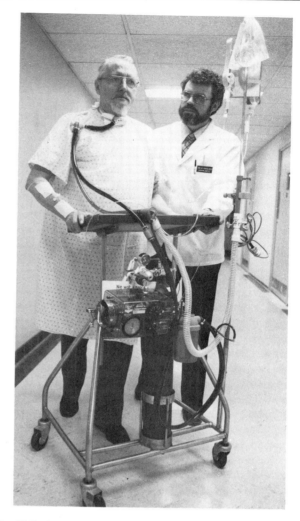

Fig. 16-7. A podium type of walker permits more mobility than the orthopaedic walker, but it gives less patient support. Arterial line equipment and intravenous tubes, **A,** are easily attached to the walker's intravenous tubing pole and with modification of the ventilator positive end-expiratory pressure (PEEP) can also be utilized during ambulation.

Ambulation must be well controlled and coordinated with other patient-care activities to prevent conflicts. Careful interdisciplinary coordination and communication are vital for the patient's well-being, for professional rapport, and for prevention of one activity from interfering with another. The patient's schedule must be flexible to provide for special activities or procedures the patient may receive from time to time. One or two specific activities, such as renal dialysis, ambulation, or ventilator weaning trials, should receive priority depending on the emphasis at that stage of rehabilitation. Some combination activities may be incongruous and injurious when attempted too soon. For instance, ambulation may be sufficiently fatiguing to interfere with subsequent trials of weaning from a ventilator. Decisions must be made to determine which activity

should take priority. It may be necessary to temporarily inhibit one effort to permit the progression of another. It is my opinion that patients tolerate ventilator weaning better if they are able to tolerate walking. Hence ambulation should take priority over weaning if there is a conflict or intolerance between the two. However, if the patient is unable to walk but seems to be progressing well with ventilator weaning, the weaning should take priority over ambulation *if* there is a conflict between the two.

Self-care activities. Patients in intensive care units receive intensive nursing care that provides all aspects of body hygiene and nutrition. Patients who are capable of providing some self-care are often not given the opportunity. These patients will become complacent and dependent on those who are providing their personal care. This dependency may be difficult to overcome despite an improvement in the patient's physical condition. Allowing patients to increase their self-care helps them develop a feeling of self-worth and provides some control over their personal environment. Undoubtedly some patients are physically unable to do anything for themselves. However, it is common to see patients being shaved or having their teeth brushed when they are capable of doing those tasks independently. Patients should be encouraged to perform independently, whenever possible, activities of daily living.

Awareness of environment. An intensive care unit (ICU) can be an overwhelming and threatening environment for the patient and family. The patient, in a situation of extraordinary need, is removed from the normal home environment, separated from family, and placed in the care of strangers, using strange equipment. Intensive care emphasizes a multidisciplinary approach that inundates the patient with different medical and paramedical services. Patients may become confused regarding who is responsible for different phases of their care. To reduce their confusion, one must keep the patient and family informed of the reasons for and goals of the various therapies and equipment being used.

As procedures and equipment are changed, the reasons for the changes must be explained. Open and frank communication helps develop a trusting, honest relationship with the patient. Without good communication the patient and family may develop resentment and mistrust, which can undermine the therapeutic effect.

DISCHARGE PLANNING

Continued mechanical ventilation is occasionally required by the patient after discharge from the hospital. It is imperative that the patient and family thoroughly understand and demonstrate proficiency in all techniques and skills necessary for safe and effective mechanical ventilation in the home. It is difficult to decide when to begin preparing the patient for discharge. This preparation includes teaching the patient and family to maintain and clean the equipment, such as the ventilator, tracheostomy tubes, and wheelchair. Instruction must include the many different kinds of therapy the patient may require. If patients and families are motivated and reasonably skillful

and have good financial support, it may be feasible for the patient to be maintained at home. The needs of the patient are many, and if the needs cannot be adequately met at home, arrangements should be made for discharge to a skilled nursing facility.

If there was good communication among the patient, family, and health care team during the acute illness, planning for discharge often becomes less problematic. Reinforcement of and instruction in activities demonstrated and explained while the patient was in the ICU becomes less threatening. The family members must provide pulmonary hygiene including postural drainage, manual techniques, and suctioning, and they must care for the ventilator, tracheostomy tube, and suctioning equipment. Depending on the status of the patient, family members may have to provide ROM exercises, personal hygiene, and ambulatory activities. Community-based support agencies can help provide some of these procedures. Home nursing care, physical therapy, and respiratory therapy are available in most geographical areas to assist the patient in the home environment. Social-service agencies can arrange to have equipment in the home to coincide with the patient's discharge from the hospital. The family can purchase or rent the equipment needed; however, medical-equipment companies usually provide for repair of rented equipment more readily than of purchased equipment. Many rental agencies strongly recommend the availability of back-up equipment in the home, which increases the expense of renting. An important aspect of care after discharge is to provide the opportunity for follow-up visits to the hospital. Periodically, the patient should return to the hospital or clinic for reinforcement of and reinstruction in those procedures taught to the patient and family before discharge.

REFERENCES

1. Burton, G., and others: Respiratory care, Philadelphia, 1977, J.B. Lippincott Co.
2. Bushnell, S.S.: Respiratory intensive care nursing, Boston, 1973, Little, Brown & Co. (Morrison, M.L, editor: ed. 2, 1979.)
3. Cherniack, R., and others: Respiration in health and disease, Philadelphia, 1972, W.B. Saunders Co.
4. Egan, D.: Fundamentals of respiratory therapy, ed. 3, St. Louis, 1977, The C.V. Mosby Co.
5. Frownfelter, D.: Chest physical therapy and pulmonary rehabilitation, Chicago, 1978, Year Book Medical Publishers, Inc.
6. Kottke, F., and others: Krusen's handbook of physical medicine and rehabilitation, Philadelphia, 1982, W.B. Saunders Co.
7. McPherson, S.: Respiratory therapy equipment, St. Louis, 1981, The C.V. Mosby Co.
8. West, J.: Respiratory physiology, Baltimore, 1979, The Williams & Wilkins Co.

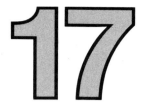

LINDA CRANE

Physical therapy for the neonate with respiratory disease

It is not uncommon for physical therapists to assess and treat pediatric patients or patients with cardiopulmonary dysfunction. However, when the patient is less than 16 inches long, weighs under 1200 grams, is receiving mechanical ventilation, and is attached to an ECG monitor (among other things), there appears to be a sudden unwillingness and discomfort among many physical therapists to be involved. The neonatal intensive care unit (NICU) seems to be one step beyond adult and pediatric intensive care units, which often, when first encountered, strike fear and trepidation in the hearts of health care workers. Actually, the technology, care delivered, and patient problems are not very different in a neonatal ICU (as compared to other ICU's) except for the size of the average patient (Figs. 17-1 and 17-2).

Physical therapists have a role in the NICU. We have a responsibility to recognize both the neonate's physical problems and the potential contribution of physical therapy to this evolving and very exciting area of health care. Infants have special problems related to their age and size, however, many of the same principles of physical therapy management employed for children and adults can be applied to this patient group.

This chapter discusses physical therapy management of the neonate with cardiopulmonary dysfunction. Pulmonary problems related to immaturity, neonatal distress and asphyxia, infection, and medical and surgical procedures are described. The chapter then presents guidelines for assessment and treatment of infants with cardiopulmonary dysfunction with special emphasis on a specific rationale for treatment procedures as they relate to physiology and pathophysiology. This chapter finally provides guidelines for discharge planning and home programs with emphasis on parent education.

Consider the following examples of "typical" patients

in the NICU who may be referred to a physical therapist. The case examples presented in this chapter are hypothetical and are not intended to refer to any actual patient but to represent infants with problems commonly encountered in the NICU setting.

CASE A

B.L. is a 2-day-old black male, admitted to the regional neonatal ICU 30 minutes after birth. B.L. is approximately 30 weeks of gestation by dates and 28 weeks by Dubowitz.[18] B.L.'s mother is 28 years old and has miscarried twice (2 and 5 years ago). Labor was precipitated by premature rupture of the membranes (PROM) 20 hours before B.L.'s birth. Apgar scores were reported as 5 at 1 minute and 8 at 5 minutes. B.L. breathed spontaneously once his mouth and nose were suctioned and almost immediately showed signs of respiratory distress manifested by subcostal retractions, expiratory grunts, and nasal flaring.

B.L.'s condition deteriorated rapidly, and when his arterial blood gases indicated a Pao_2 of 30 and $Paco_2$ of 70, he was intubated and placed on continuous positive airway pressure (CPAP) with an Fio_2 of 0.4. At 48 hours a ductal murmur, secondary to patient ductus arteriosus (PDA), was detected on auscultation.

CASE B

A.C. is a 4200 gm female born 24 hours previously. She is the product of 43 weeks of gestation, and her Apgar scores were 3 at 1 minute and 9 at 5 minutes. A.C. was meconium stained at birth but gasped before she could be suctioned. Several milliliters of meconium-stained fluid were eventually suctioned from the nose, mouth, pharynx, and trachea. A.C. demonstrated severe substernal and intercostal retractions within 12 hours of birth. Her Pao_2 was 28 mm Hg, $Paco_2$ 22 mm Hg, and respiratory rate 72. A.C. was placed under an oxygen hood and received 50% oxygen. A.C.'s chest radiograph at 24 hours showed hyperinflation and streaky atelectasis. A.C. developed hypercapnia and required intubation and mechanical ventilation with high positive pressures (30 cm H_2O). At 36 hours A.C. developed a left pneumothorax requiring surgical insertion of a chest tube.

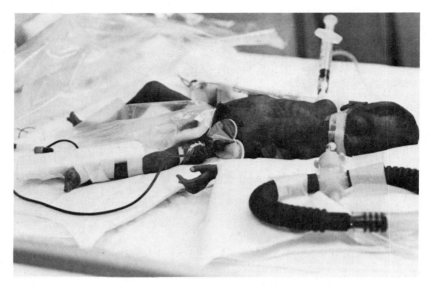

Fig. 17-1. Tiny neonate in NICU (neonatal intensive care unit).

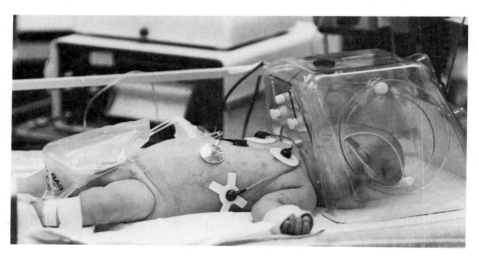

Fig. 17-2. Infant in NICU.

ANATOMIC AND PHYSIOLOGICAL DIFFERENCES OF NEONATES

Many anatomic and physiological differences exist between infants and older children and adults. These differences increase the infant's vulnerability to respiratory distress, airway obstruction, and respiratory failure.[8,27,39] Furthermore the structural and functional differences of premature infants exaggerate their susceptibility to cardiopulmonary problems and medical complications.[27] Some differences are protective and functional in a normal healthy baby but may contribute to problems in a sick or compromised infant.[8,26,30]

Anatomic differences that affect cardiopulmonary function in neonates include the following:

1. A *high larynx,* which enables the newborn to breathe and swallow simultaneously up to approximately 3 to 4 months of age.[30] The high laryngeal position along with the relatively low resistance of the nasal air passage make newborns and young infants *obligatory nose breathers.* Any compromise of the dimen-

sion of the nasal airway will significantly increase the work of breathing in an obligate nose breather.

2. Lymphatic tissue may be enlarged in the small infant and may contribute to upper airway obstruction.[26]

3. The full-term infant has approximately one twentieth the alveolar surface area of an adult.[26] Alveolar multiplication is rapid during the first year of life and continues to approximately 8 years of age.[52] The capacity of infants to increase alveoli is *protective*. In contrast to this postnatal alveolar growth, the formation of conducting airways is complete by 16 weeks of gestation.[40] Airway diameter and structural support are reduced in infants and children, and so the chances of airway obstruction and collapse are increased.

4. Channels for collateral ventilation in the lungs (pores of Kohn and Lambert's canals) are found in small numbers in the lungs of newborns.[40] Although little is known about these structures, an observation that the right middle and upper lobes (RML and RUL) have less collateral channels may be associated with the increased incidence of RML and RUL atelectasis in neonates.

5. Rib-cage configuration is circular in the horizontal plane in the infant. The diaphragm's angle of insertion is horizontal so that when it is combined with the horizontal and more cartilaginous rib cage, there is less efficiency of ventilation and more distortion in the chest-wall shape.[39]

Physiological differences affecting cardiopulmonary function include the following:

1. Decreased compliance (or distensibility) of the neonate's lungs. Normal full-term infants demonstrate increases in lung compliance in the first week of life.[47] Low compliance means that greater inflation pressures must be generated to maintain lung volume and infants must work harder to ventilate their lungs. This problem is exacerbated when surfactant is deficient and alveoli are maintained at lower volumes (decreased functional residual capacity, FRC), as commonly occurs in several neonatal diseases.

2. Neonates normally exhibit irregular respiratory patterns (the more immature the infant, the more irregular the breathing pattern).[47] Apnea, occurring for long enough periods of time to produce bradycardia (probably secondary to hypoxemia), is considered serious.[48] Apnea is commonly seen in infants distressed by intraventricular cerebral hemorrhage and sepsis. Reduced apnea in the *prone* position in premature infants may result from greater ventilation and improved oxygenation.[13,34,56]

3. Neonates compensate for respiratory difficulties by increasing the rate rather than the depth of ventilation.[15]

4. Newborns sleep up to 20 hours per day and may spend up to 80% of sleep in rapid eye movement (REM) sleep (as compared to 20% REM sleep in adults).[39] There is greatly increased work of breathing during REM sleep secondary to decreased postural muscle (and therefore intercostal muscle) tone, which causes the upper rib cage to move inward as the diaphragm contracts.[39] Work of breathing is further increased because of a 30% reduction in FRC during REM sleep.[25]

5. The diaphragm of the neonate has a reduced percentage (approximately 25% as compared with 50% in an adult) of type I, red, slow-twitch, fatigue-resistant, and high oxidative muscle fibers.[39] The diaphragm of a premature infant may have as little as 10% type I muscle fibers. The lack of oxidative fibers in the diaphragm increases the susceptibility of infants to respiratory muscle fatigue.

PATIENT PROBLEMS

Newborns in a neonatal intensive care unit present with and develop a myriad of problems related to immaturity, postmaturity, adverse prenatal or postnatal events, congenital defects, and iatrogenic complications. Although many problems of the neonate are interrelated, this section briefly addresses only those problems that primarily or secondarily affect the cardiopulmonary systems. Medical complications of cardiopulmonary problems and their management, which are important for the physical therapist to recognize and incorporate in a problem-solving approach to managing sick neonates, are also discussed.

Pulmonary problems secondary to immaturity

The premature infant and small-for-gestational-age (SGA) baby often develop pulmonary problems. Factors contributing to the normal newborn's susceptibility to airway obstruction and respiratory failure have been discussed. The tiny premature baby's vulnerability is compounded by the addition of several anatomic and physiological factors (Table 17-1).

The most common pulmonary disorder of the newborn is called the "idiopathic respiratory distress syndrome" (IRDS). IRDS, also called "hyaline membrane disease" (HMD), is characterized by alveolar collapse because of a deficiency of surfactant. Surfactant, composed of phospholipids and protein, is produced by type II alveolar epithelial cells and reduces surface tension of the fluid lining of alveoli.[21,26,57] Maturity of the surfactant system occurs at about 35 weeks of gestation. Therefore the risk of IRDS increases as the gestational age of the premature baby decreases. IRDS is also associated with several other factors that decrease surfactant production including (1) cesarean section, (2) maternal diabetes, (3) perinatal asphyxia, and (4) being the second born of twins.[18,48] Although the mechanisms are not completely understood, hypoxia and acidosis also contribute to surfactant deficiency.

Table 17-1. Factors contributing to pulmonary dysfunction in the premature infant

Anatomic	Physiological
Capillary beds not well developed before 26 weeks gestation.	Increased pulmonary vascular resistance leading to right-to-left shunting
Type II alveolar cells and surfactant production not mature until 35 weeks of gestation. Elastic properties of lung not well developed Lung "space" decreased by relative size of the heart and abdominal distention	Decreased lung compliance
Type I, high-oxidative fibers compose only 10% to 20% of diaphragm muscle	Diaphragmatic fatigue; respiratory failure
Highly vascular subependymal germinal matrix not resorbed until 35 weeks of gestation increasing the vulnerability of the infant to hemorrhage	Decreased or absent cough and gag reflexes; apnea
Lack of fatty insulation and high surface area to body-weight ratio	Hypothermia and increased oxygen consumption

Clinical signs and symptoms including tachypnea, intercostal and sternal retractions, flaring of nasal alae, and expiratory grunting usually appear within 2 to 3 hours after birth.[21] Pulmonary status deteriorates with 24 to 48 hours. Mortality usually occurs within, and recovery occurs after, 72 hours from birth.[18] If mechanical ventilation is required, the course of the disease is often prolonged and the incidence of complications is increased because of both the severity of the disease and the consequences of intubation and assisted ventilation.[42]

Treatment of infants with IRDS is supportive and generally includes adequate oxygenation, (to maintain cell metabolism), nutrition, thermal regulation, and often some type of continuous positive airway pressure.[18,48,57]

Bronchial drainage techniques are advocated in the literature for infants with IRDS.[10,15,20,36] Bronchial drainage is appropriate for treatment of airway clearance problems and prevention of pneumonia, atelectasis, and other complications of IRDS and its management.[10,45]

Pulmonary problems secondary to neonatal distress and asphyxia

The *meconium-aspiration syndrome* (MAS) occurs in approximately 10% to 30%[2] of infants who are meconium stained at birth. Meconium, the dark, "sticky," fecal material that accumulates in utero, is passed in approximately 10% to 20% of all deliveries,[31] especially when the fetus is at term or past term.[2] Once meconium is passed, the neonate is at risk for aspirating this substance, which can cause symptoms of chemical pneumonitis and airway obstruction within 12 to 24 hours after birth.[48] Passage of meconium and its aspiration are almost invariably associated with fetal hypoxia and often fetal distress and intrapartum asphyxia.[2,24,31,48] Gregory and co-workers[24] found that the presence of meconium in the trachea does not nec-

essarily result in MAS. It appears that meconium-stained infants suctioned with a catheter[22] (not a bulb syringe) *before* they took their first breath had decreased mortality and morbidity from MAS.[2,51] MAS characteristically causes partial airway obstruction with a "ball-valve" effect which causes hyperaeration of the lungs. Hyperaeration may result in pneumothorax or pneumomediastinum. Airway obstruction also contributes to right to left cardiopulmonary shunting, with resultant hypoxemia and hypercapnia (increased $PaCO_2$). Persistence of fetal circulation (PFC) is also occasionally associated with MAS.[48]

Once respiratory distress is manifested secondary to MAS, the treatment is supportive. Gregory and co-workers[24] advocated postural drainage and "thoracic physical therapy" for the first 8 hours of life if the infant was born through particulate, "pea-soup" meconium and meconium was suctioned from the trachea, or if the chest radiograph was consistent with meconium aspiration.

Central nervous system damage secondary to perinatal asphyxia can result in severe pulmonary problems often characterized by hypoventilation and poor airway clearance. Perinatal asphyxia may be caused by a variety of circumstances and events including but not limited to umbilical cord compression, maternal placenta previa and abruptio placentae, placental insufficiency, excessive maternal anesthesia and analgesia, bilateral choanal atresia (imperforate nares), tracheal web, and diaphragmatic hernia. The infant's failure to breathe at birth is attributable to suppression of intrinsic central nervous system mechanisms secondary to acidemia, hypoxemia, and drugs.[48]

Indicators of fetal distress (rapid fetal heart rate and fetal scalp blood gases) may be monitored during labor and delivery. Approximately 1% to 2% of all deliveries result in an infant with severe resuscitation problems. Low Apgar scores are useful in documenting a problem at 1 minute and are predictive of possible neurological damage at 5 minutes. The kidneys and brain may be damaged as a result of shock and hypoxemia secondary to asphyxia. Severe hypoglycemia and hypocalcemia are frequently associated with perinatal asphyxia. Initial muscular flaccidity with subsequent seizures and respiratory depression are most likely the result of significant central nervous system damage.[48] IRDS and aspiration syndromes are common complications in asphyxiated newborns. Other common complications of neonatal asphyxia include depressed cough, gag, and sneeze reflexes and defective swallowing mechanisms. These deficits along with frequent episodes of hypoventilation put the infant at great risk of developing pulmonary infection, atelectasis, airway obstruction, and respiratory failure.

Pulmonary problems secondary to surgery

Respiratory complications of general anesthesia and incisions in the thorax or upper abdomen are well documented.[3,5] Infants are believed to have decreased sensitivity to pain or decreased nervous system irritability.[49] This postulated imperception of pain may help prevent postoperative pulmonary complication in infants *if* there are no other complicating factors. A literature search revealed no studies that measured the incidence of postoperative pulmonary complications in this age group. Clinically my experience is that if the infant requires prolonged intubation and mechanical ventilation (greater than 24 hours) and is compromised by either preexisting lung lesions, central nervous system depression, general immobility, or other factors the infant is very susceptible to pulmonary complications after surgery. The addition of chest physical therapy to the care of these infants may reduce the incidence of postoperative pulmonary complications.[23]

The mechanisms of postoperative pulmonary complications are described in detail in Chapter 14. Some common congenital abnormalities requiring surgical repair are discussed below:

Diaphragmatic hernia is a defect of the posterior diaphragm where abdominal contents may herniate into the chest cavity.[29,48] The result is a hypoplastic lung on the affected side (usually the left).[29] A neonate with this defect exhibits respiratory distress at birth and requires immediate surgical intervention, usually by an abdominal approach.[29] Because the abdomen may be too small to contain the gut, closure of the abdominal wall may be delayed to avoid tension on the diaphragm.[48]

Esophageal atresia and tracheoesophageal (TE) fistulas are suspected in infants whose feeding results in excessive saliva, respiratory distress, and choking.[29,48] There are several variations in these anomalies, with the most common being esophageal atresia and a fistula between the distal esophagus and the trachea at a point above the carina. Surgical repair of these anomalies is commonly accom-

plished retropleurally through a right thoracotomy incision.[48] Aspiration pneumonia is common in infants with esophageal atresia and TE fistula. The survival rate in uncomplicated cases is 90%. Surgical repair in infants at risk may be in a staged approach starting with a gastrostomy to provide for adequate nutrition.[48] Swallowing may be impaired in infants who have had these surgical procedures. Dyskinesia of the distal esophagus, uncoordinated peristalsis, and gastroesophageal reflux may occur.[48]

Many other surgical procedures involving the thorax and abdomen may be necessary in neonates with specific abnormalities. Some of the more common abnormalities are congenital lobar emphysema, necrotizing enterocolitis, Hirschsprung's enterocolitis, meconium ileus, and congenital heart defects.

Respiratory problems consequent to neonatal ICU management

Bronchopulmonary dysplasia (BPD) is commonly associated with the use of mechanical ventilation with positive pressure and oxygen therapy in premature infants with IRDS.[28,42,48,59] Bronchopulmonary dysplasia is a form of chronic obstructive lung disease and was first described by Northway and others[42] in 1967. There is controversy regarding the exact cause of BPD[28]; however, all descriptions indicate that this syndrome is iatrogenic and may be minimized or prevented in the future.

The disease progresses from an acute stage, in which the pathological condition is indistinguishable from IRDS, through three additional stages to a chronic stage with atelectasis, emphysema, and cystic changes.[42] Onset of bronchopulmonary dysplasia often starts within the first few days of life with symptomatic and pathological progression continuing until approximately 1 month. Survivors of this disease usually require long-term follow-up care because of both the slow process of weaning from supplemental oxygen and the high incidence of recurrent pulmonary infection.[23,28,55] Lengthy hospitalizations during the critical first months of life and complex programs of home care are often necessary for infants with bronchopulmonary dysplasia (Fig. 17-3)

Some common complications and consequences of bronchopulmonary dysplasia include pulmonary hypertension and right-sided heart failure, frequent lower respiratory tract infections, poor growth, increased oxygen consumption, and complex emotional and behavioral problems.[54,55,58]

Mikity-Wilson syndrome (MW), or pulmonary dysmaturity, and bronchopulmonary dysplasia are often confused, since their radiographic and clinical courses are comparable.[28] The Mikity-Wilson syndrome is a separate entity of unknown cause that occurs in very premature infants and has not been directly associated with oxygen or ventilator therapy.[28,42] The pathogenesis of the Mikity-Wilson syndrome is now believed to be associated with unequal dis-

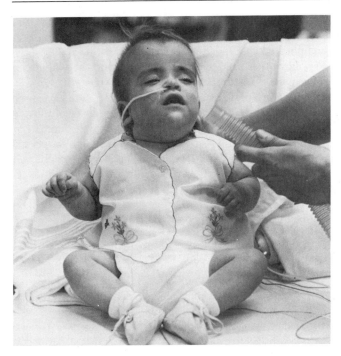

Fig. 17-3. Eighteen-month-old infant with BPD (bronchopulmonary dysplasia).

tribution of ventilation in the immature lung.[28,59] The problem with this hypothesis is that not every premature neonate develops this syndrome.

Subglottic and bronchial stenosis is associated with prolonged intubation and frequent endotracheal suctioning in some infants.[41,48] Subglottic narrowing can result in mild or pronounced upper airway obstruction. This problem often results in inspiratory stridor and may require tracheostomy until the infant grows. Once the diameter of the upper airway increases sufficiently to allow for adequate ventilation, the tracheostomy will be removed.

Patient problems that complicate management

Neonates and premature infants are prone to develop respiratory distress and pulmonary dysfunction. These infants are also susceptible to other complications of immaturity and neonatal ICU management. Many of these complications affect the subsequent management of the infant, especially chest physical therapy.

The most common of these problematic complications are described briefly below. How these problems affect physical therapy assessment and treatment is discussed later in this chapter.

Pneumothorax, pneumomediastinum, and *pneumopericardium* occur frequently in tiny infants, with poorly compliant lungs, who require positive-pressure ventilation.

Pneumomediastinum is often inconsequential and requires no specific therapy.[48] Pneumopericardium often occurs in association with pneumothorax and pneumomediastinum and can be serious if sufficient air collects in the pericardial sac to cause cardiac tamponade (pressure on the major vessels entering and leaving the heart). Tension pneumothoraces increase pressure in the intrapleural space resulting in decreased cardiac output, mediastinal shift to the contralateral hemithorax, and rapid clinical deterioration of the infant. Emergency treatment usually consists in insertion of a sterile needle into the pleural space to remove air. When the infant's condition improves, one or more chest tubes are surgically inserted to remove the pleural air.[28]

Hypothermia is a common problem of premature and sick neonates. Thermal regulation of the infant is extremely important because infants have a high surface area–to–body weight ratio, poor vasomotor control, and poor fat insulation to help protect them against hypothermia.[48] The neutral thermal temperature zone (NTTZ) is the environmental temperature at which oxygen consumption is minimized. Temperatures above and below the neutral thermal temperature zone increase oxygen consumption.[48] Incubators and radiant warmers with servoregulation are used to help maintain a constant thermal environment. Insensible water loss and convective heat loss can be reduced by use of a head shield[48] (inside an incubator) or transparent plastic wrap.[23]

Congestive heart failure (CHF) and cor pulmonale (right-sided heart failure) may occur in neonates secondary to patent ductus arteriosus (PDA), increased pulmonary vascular resistance, right-to-left shunting and other associated problems and congenital anomalies. Diuretics and digitalis are used to treat the peripheral and pulmonary edema that may result from heart failure.

Persistent fetal circulation (PFC) is characterized by pulmonary hypertension, probably caused by pulmonary vasoconstriction (vasospasm), increased pulmonary vascular smooth muscle, and decreased pulmonary vascular bed cross-sectional area.[28,46] A persistent fetal circulation results in increased hypoxemia and hypoxia because of right-to-left shunting of blood flow (usually through the foramen ovale or ductus arteriosus). Infants with persistent fetal circulation usually require high concentrations of oxygen and minimal handling.

Intraventricular hemorrhage (IVH), or more appropriately subependymal hemorrhage/intraventricular hemorrhage (SEH/IVH), is the most common neuropathological finding in premature infants.[23] SEH/IVH is most closely correlated with vaginal delivery (versus cesarean), gender (males more than females), and hypoxemia (PaO_2 less than 45 mm Hg).[4] Other associations have been made between SEH/IVH and gestational age, positive-pressure ventilation, idiopathic respiratory distress symptom, continuous positive airway pressure (CPAP), pulmonary air leaks, pa-

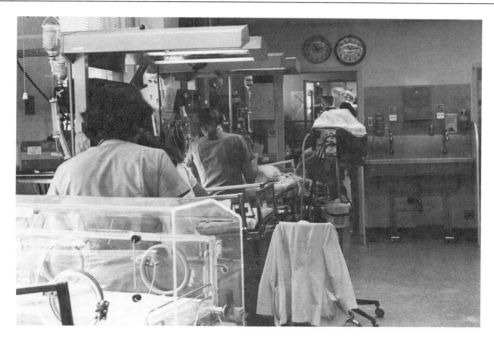

Fig. 17-4. Typical scene in NICU.

tent ductus arteriosus, administration of bicarbonate, and others.[4] The incidence of SEH/IVH is not clear. Because intraventricular hemorrhage is asymptomatic in most cases, noninvasive diagnostic tests such as computed tomography (CT) and high-frequency real-time ultrasound (RTU) scanning are invaluable. Intraventricular hemorrhage is graded I to IV according to the extent of bleeding.[23] Mortality with intraventricular hemorrhage is higher with grade IV lesions. Little is known about SEH/IVH. Important questions include the predictive morbidity according to the grade of the lesion and the relationship between common treatment techniques (e.g., endotracheal suctioning[43]) and the incidence of IVH. Bejar and associates[4] state that hemorrhage does not continue beyond the first week of life, and Ahmann and co-workers[1] found progressive hydrocephalus in only 23% of survivors of SEH/IVH.

ASSESSMENT AND PREPARATION

As mentioned earlier, entering a NICU can be an overwhelming experience for a therapist until the patients and the equipment are more familiar (Fig. 17-4). Table 17-2 describes some of the common equipment found in the NICU (also Fig. 17-5 to 17-11). One of the first tasks of a therapist when assessing an infant in a NICU is to become familiar with the monitors, equipment, and supplies on and around the baby (Fig. 17-12). Do this even before looking at the patient.

Preliminary activities of the therapist, before assessing the infant, include reviewing the medical record and chest radiographs (when available) and discussing the infant with the nurse and physician. In *reviewing the chart,* be sure to review:

1. Complete history of labor and delivery
2. Assessment of infant including:
   a. Apgar scores
   b. Dubowitz gestational age scores
3. Clinical course of infant from birth to present
4. History of respiratory distress and oxygen and ventilation assistance provided since birth
5. Arterial blood gas history
6. Report on previous chest radiographs (CXR)
7. Mode and frequency of nutrition and feedings
8. Physician orders (i.e., special tests, double-check the order for physical therapy, etc.)

The chest radiographs can be very helpful in identifying or locating a pulmonary pathological condition, indicating specific areas of the lung that may be involved and assisting the therapist to identify anatomical landmarks on a very tiny baby. In many NICU's the chest radiographs are readily available in the unit. The therapist will most likely need assistance interpreting these films.

Talking with the physician and the nurse taking care of the infant can provide the therapist with invaluable current information, some of which may not yet have been placed

Text continued on p. 317.

Table 17-2. Equipment commonly encountered in the neonatal intensive care unit

Equipment	Description
Radiant warmer (Fig. 17-5)	Unit composed of mattress on an adjustable table top covered by a radiant heat source controlled manually and by servo-control mode. Unit has adjustable side panels. *Advantage:* provides open space for tubes and equipment and easier access to the infant. *Disadvantage:* open bed may lead to convective heat loss and insensible fluid loss.
Self-contained incubator (Isolette) (Fig. 17-6)	Enclosed unit of transparent material providing a heated and humidified environment with a servo system of temperature monitoring. Access to infant through side portholes or opening side of unit. *Advantage:* less convective heat and insensible water loss. *Disadvantage:* infection control; more difficult to get to baby; not practical for a very acutely ill neonate.
Thermal shield	Plexiglass dome placed over the trunk and legs of an infant in an Isolette to reduce radiant heat loss.
Oxygen hood (Fig. 17-12)	Plexiglass hood that fits over the infant's head; provides environment for controlled oxygen and humidification delivery.
Mechanical ventilator: Pressure ventilator (Fig. 17-7)	Delivers positive-pressure ventilation; pressure-limited with volume delivered dependent on the stiffness of the lung.
Volume ventilator	Delivers positive-pressure ventilation; volume-limited delivering same tidal volume with each breath.
Negative-pressure ventilator	Ventilator that creates a relative negative pressure around the thorax and abdomen thereby assisting ventilation without endotracheal tube. NOTE: Difficult to use in infants weighing less than 1500 grams.[12]
Nasal and nasopharyngeal prongs	Simple system for providing continuous positive airway pressure (CPAP) consisting of nasal prongs of varying lengths and adaptor to pressure-source tubing.
Resuscitation bag	Usually a self-inflating bag with a reservoir (so high concentrations of oxygen may be delivered at a rapid rate) attached to an oxygen flowmeter and a pressure manometer.
ECG, heart rate, respiratory rate, and blood pressure monitor (Fig. 17-8)	Usually one unit will display one or more vital signs on oscilloscope and digital display. High and low limits may be set, and alarm sounds when limits exceeded.
Transcutaneous oxygen monitor (Fig. 17-9 to 17-11)	Noninvasive method of monitoring partial pressure of oxygen from arterialized capillaries through the skin. The electrode is heated, placed on an area of thin epidermis (usually abdomen or thorax). The monitor has capability of providing both a digital display and a continuous recording of $TcPo_2$ values.
Intravenous infusion pump (Fig. 17-12)	Used to pump intravenous fluids, intralipids, and transpyloric feedings at a specified rate. Pump has alarm system and capacity to monitor volume delivered, obstruction of flow, and other parameters.

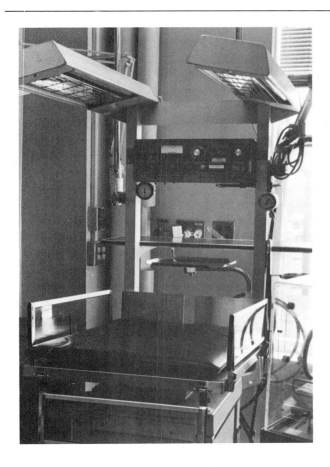

Fig. 17-5. Example of a radiant warmer.

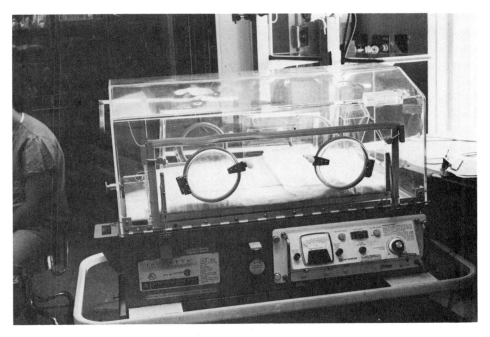

Fig. 17-6. Example of incubator (Isolette).

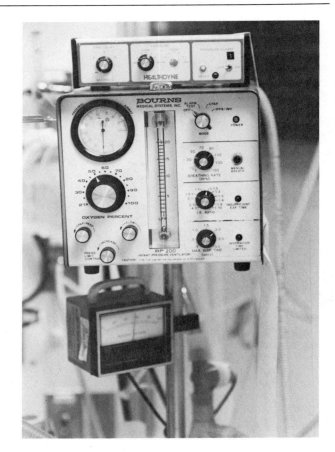

Fig. 17-7. Example of pressure-limited mechanical ventilator.

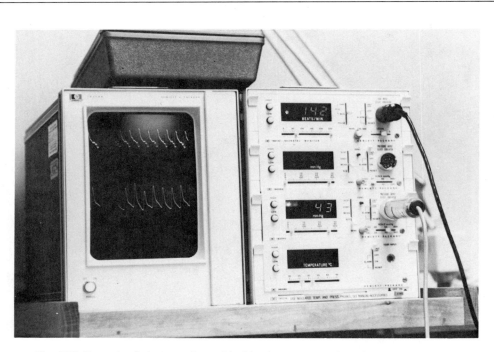

Fig. 17-8. Example of electrocardiographic, blood pressure, and respiratory rate monitor.

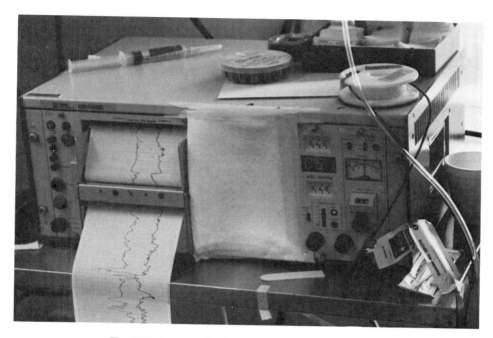

Fig. 17-9. An example of transcutaneous oxygen monitor.

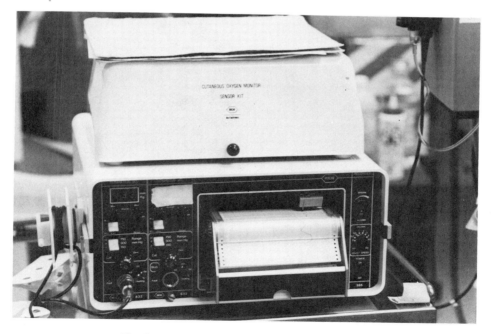

Fig. 17-10. Another transcutaneous oxygen monitor.

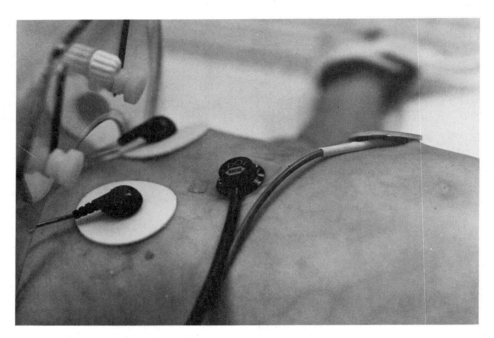

Fig. 17-11. Transcutaneous oxygen electrode *(center of photograph in black).*

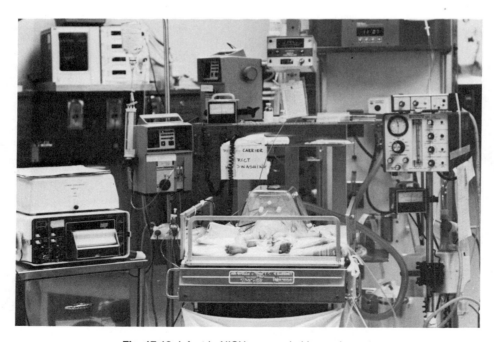

Fig. 17-12. Infant in NICU surrounded by equipment.

in the chart. Some common questions the physical therapist may ask include the following:

1. What kind of day (or afternoon, evening, night depending on when assessment is done) has the baby had?
2. Is the baby being fed orally or orogastrically, and when was the last feeding?
3. How does the baby respond to handling: i.e., does transcutaneous oxygen (TcPO₂) drop or does the baby have apnea and bradycardia?

CHEST EVALUATION

Once this preliminary information is gathered, the therapist assesses the infant. The evaluation of an infant's chest incorporates the four major skills used to assess any patient with pulmonary disease: observation and inspection, auscultation, palpation, and, rarely, mediate (i.e., indirect) percussion. *Observation* and *inspection* of a neonate includes:

1. Signs of respiratory distress (These signs may not be evident in infants who are intubated and receiving mechanical ventilation.)
   a. *Retractions* can be suprasternal, subcostal, substernal, or intercostal. Retractions occur because of the infant's very compliant chest wall, which is pulled inward by the high negative pressures generated in making greater than normal respiratory efforts. Severe retraction limits anteroposterior expansion of the chest and limits effective ventilation.[8,44] Mild retractions may be normal.
   b. *Nasal flaring* is a reflex dilatation of the dilatores naris muscles. The resulting widening of the nares is believed to decrease airway resistance in the nasal passages and is most likely a primitive response.[8]
   c. *Expiratory grunting* is an effort to increase functional residual capacity and improve both the distribution of ventilation and the ventilation-to-perfusion relationships by retarding expiration. The sound is produced by either expiration against a partially closed glottis or reflectory approximation of the vocal cords.[8,44]
   d. *Stridor* on inspiration occurs with obstruction or collapse of the upper airway (upper two thirds of the trachea and larynx). The intensity of stridor may change with the position of the infant, especially the degree of neck extension (NOTE: extending the neck of an infant tends to collapse the trachea).
   e. *Head bobbing* occurs in infants who are attempting to use accessory respiratory muscles (sternocleidomastoid, scaleni) to assist in ventilation. Because neck extensor muscles of infants are not strong enough to stabilize the head, accessory-muscle use often produces head bobbing.
   f. *Bulging* of the intercostal muscles occurs when obstruction to expiration creates high pleural pressures during expiration.[48]

2. Chest configuration: Some abnormal findings in sick neonates include *barrel-shaped chest* (indicating overinflation of air-trapping within the lungs) and *pectus excavatum* (funnel chest), a depression of the sternum, which may be acquired secondary to prolonged periods of sternal retractions in the first months of life.

3. Skin color:
   a. *Cyanosis,* if apparent in the mucous membranes and around the lips and mouth, is a significant sign of hypoxemia. Cyanosis is a *very unreliable* clinical sign because it depends on both the relative amount of hemoglobin in the blood and the adequacy of peripheral circulation.
   b. *Plethora,* or redness that may be noticed in a newborn with polycythemia.
   c. *Pallor* is commonly seen in distressed infants and may be associated with hypoxemia, sepsis, intraventricular hemorrhage, and other problems. Pallor in an infant is also considered a sign of respiratory distress and a sign of anemia.

4. Breathing pattern:
   a. *Tachypnea* is considered a sign of respiratory distress in infants. A normal newborn breathes most efficiently at approximately 40 breaths per minute.[44,47]
   b. *Irregularity* of respiration is *normal* in a newborn. Therefore one must count respiratory rates over a long period of time (i.e., 60 seconds) to account for the irregularity. Premature infants often have a breathing pattern called *"periodic breathing."* Periodic breathing is characterized by respirations of irregular rate and depth interrupted by apneic pauses of 5 to 10 seconds.[47]
   c. *Apnea* is also considered a clinical sign of respiratory distress, sepsis, intraventricular hemorrhage, and other stresses of the premature baby. Apnea is commonly differentiated from periodic breathing by the length of the nonbreathing episode. Most authors consider an apneic pause of 20 seconds or longer to be true apnea. Apnea is also commonly associated with bradycardia. Increasing environmental oxygen may be helpful in decreasing apneic episodes. Other techniques used to decrease apnea and bradycardia in neonates include cutaneous stimulation, nasal continuous positive airway pressure, administration of theophylline (a central nervous system stimulant) and placement of an alternating pressure cushion (sometimes referred to as a "whoopee cushion") under the infant.

5. Coughing and sneezing: Sneezing occurs more fre-

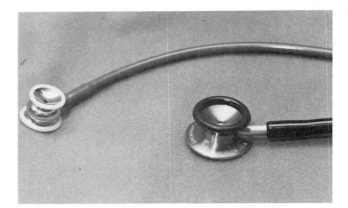

Fig. 17-13. Two sizes of pediatric stethoscopes.

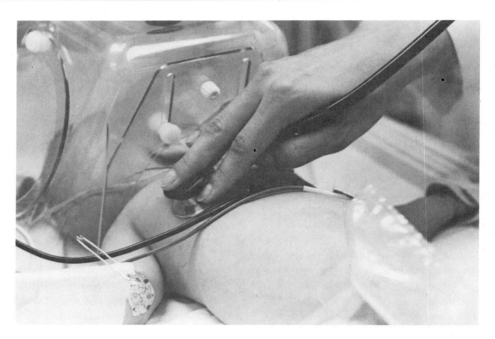

Fig. 17-14. Auscultation of the infant's lungs with larger stethoscope.

quently in neonates than coughing does probably because of a better developed neural pathway.[44] The gag reflex and sneeze seem to be more important protective mechanisms for the infant's airways than coughing is. It will be helpful for the physical therapist to determine if a cough can be stimulated or if the infant coughs or sneezes spontaneously.

AUSCULTATION

Auscultation of an infant or child is a gross assessment, at best, because of the thin chest wall, proximity of structures, and easy transmission of sounds. These problems

are even more confounding when one is auscultating the chest of a premature infant or an infant who is being mechanically ventilated.

The *stethoscope* used may vary according to the size of the infant or the personal preference of the therapist. Fig. 17-13 shows two sizes of stethoscopes commonly used for auscultation. The stethoscope should have both a bell and a diaphragm because it is often helpful to use both portions when listening to a neonate's chest.

Before attempting to auscultate an infant who is intubated or has a tracheostomy, be sure to empty the corrugated ventilator tubing of all water. Water will precipitate

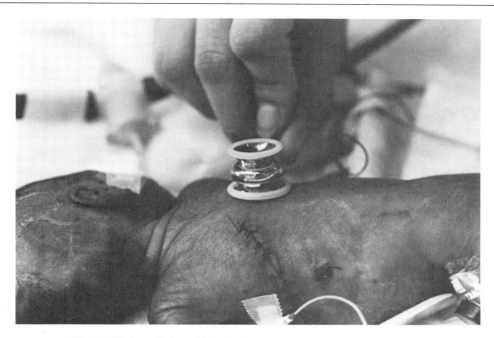

Fig. 17-15. Auscultation of infant's lungs with small, neonatal stethoscope.

in the tubing from the humid water vapor delivered with inspired gases. Water bubbling in ventilator tubing can mask breath sounds and mimic adventitious sounds. A baby who is receiving intermittent mandatory ventilation (IMV) may be receiving as little as two breaths per minute from the ventilator. It may be very difficult to hear breath sounds when the infant is breathing spontaneously. However, the mechanical breath will often enhance breath sounds.

The therapist listens for normal and abnormal breath sounds and adventitious sounds (Figs. 17-14 and 17-15). Abnormal sounds can be distinguished from normal sounds by thorough and careful auscultation.

Whenever possible auscultate with the infant's head in the midline position, since turning the head to the side may cause decreased breath sounds in the opposite side.[8] In infants, the specific location of the sound does not necessarily correspond with the underlying lung segment. It is extremely important to correlate physical signs, such as auscultation, with radiographic evidence of a pathological condition. The anteroposterior (AP) and lateral chest radiographs help to localize areas of atelectasis, infiltrate, and pneumothorax, but these abnormalities are not always present. The therapist must often rely on auscultatory findings to indicate areas for treatment emphasis and to describe the results of bronchial drainage techniques. Auscultation is therefore an *essential* component of the chest evaluation of neonates.

PALPATION

Chest palpation for a neonate is limited to palpating for the position of the mediastinum (position of trachea in suprasternal notch), for subcutaneous emphysema, edema, or rib fracture (Fig. 17-16). Symmetry of chest-wall motion is generally not palpable because the chest wall in a tiny baby moves very little. Paradoxical motion of the chest can be palpated in a neonate.

MEDIATE PERCUSSION

Mediate (or indirect) percussion is seldom appropriate for a small infant. Exceptions may include percussing for the presence of pneumothoraces, diaphragmatic hernia, enlarged liver, and masses. Percussion in an infant's chest is performed by one finger directly on the chest (direct percussion).

OTHER SYSTEMS

Assessment of systems other than the pulmonary system, particularly as they relate to physical therapy intervention, is extremely important in sick neonates.

The *cardiovascular system* is interrelated with the pulmonary system both anatomically and physiologically. Many patient problems affecting one system eventually affect the other. An example of this interrelationship would be the pulmonary vascular constriction caused by hypoxia and hypercapnia in neonates secondary to pulmonary dysfunction. Pulmonary hypertension, or increased pulmonary

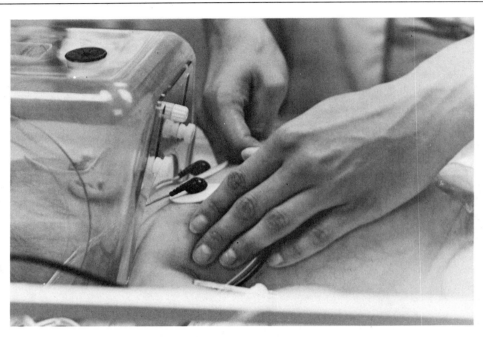

Fig. 17-16. Palpation of chest wall of infant.

vascular resistance, increases the pressure in the right ventricle, which may lead to shunting of blood through the ductus arteriosus or foramen ovale and possibly right-sided heart failure (cor pulmonale).

Vital signs, such as heart rate (HR) and blood pressure (BP), must be monitored carefully in the infant. These signs indicate cardiovascular status and reflect the infant's response to assessment and treatment techniques. The autonomic nervous system is well developed in the neonate, and vasomotor regulatory mechanisms are present in the premature and term infant.[38] The sympathetic tone of the myocardium is incompletely developed in the premature and newborn infant who may therefore not respond to stress, postural changes, or other situations in the same way as the adult.[28,61]

Detection of murmurs by auscultation of the heart may be important to the physical therapist. The murmur of a patent ductus arteriosus is usually characterized by a short ejection murmur with maximal impact along the left sternal border.[48]

Signs of poor peripheral circulation include pallor, cyanosis, weblike markings of the extremities, cool extremities, and poor correlation of transcutaneous oxygen ($TcPO_2$) values with arterial oxygen (PaO_2) values.

Arterial blood gas (ABG) values are extremely important indicators of adequacy of ventilation and oxygenation. So-called normal ABG values for preterm and term infants vary greatly according to age, size, and pathological condition. $TcPO_2$ values (which correlate with PaO_2) are generally 5 to 20 mm Hg less than PaO_2. Because $TcPO_2$ monitoring is noninvasive and continuous, it provides invaluable information to a physical therapist treating an infant with pulmonary dysfunction.

In a physical therapy assessment of the *skeletal* status of the infant the therapist uses radiographic and blood chemistry data. Hypocalcemia, hypophosphatemia, and vitamin-deficiency syndromes can result in acquired rickets or osteoporosis.

The *skin* should be assessed for signs of breakdown and bruising. Recent incisions should also be noted.

The therapist should be aware of the mode of *nutritional support* for the infant. Infants with respiratory distress are seldom fed orally. Gavage or orogastric (OG) feeding is as common as transpyloric nutrition (TPN) or nasojejunal feeding. With transpyloric feeding, vomiting and aspiration is not common. Infants fed orally or orogastrally are often placed on their right sides for 20 to 30 minutes to assist with gastric emptying.[23] Abdominal distention should be noticed because it may interfere with ventilation, especially with the baby in a head-down position.

The *neuromuscular* system is often affected by prematurity, hypoxia, and various prenatal, intranatal, and postnatal problems. The most common causes of central nervous system abnormalities in neonates are hypoxia and hemorrhage. Physical therapy assessment of the neurological and neuromuscular status of a neonate includes but is not limited to the following:

1. Primitive reflexes
2. Muscle tone
3. Limb movements and postures
4. Sucking and swallowing
5. Deep tendon reflexes
6. Behavioral assessment
7. State of quiet alertness
8. Joint range of motion

CASE EXAMPLES: ASSESSMENT

Consider the two cases presented earlier in this chapter with physical therapy assessment information included.

CASE A

B.L. was evaluated on his third day of life by the physical therapist. B.L. had a patent ductus arteriosus ligated 24 hours before the assessment and was being weaned from the mechanical ventilator and supplemental oxygenation. B.L.'s pulmonary diagnosis is idiopathic respiratory distress syndrome (IRDS).

Before assessment of the infant's physical signs and symptoms, the following data were collected:

B.L. is intubated with an orotracheal tube and is receiving 28% oxygen at an intermittent mandatory ventilation (IMV) of 12 breaths per minute. Positive end expiratory pressure (PEEP) is +2 cm H_2O.

Arterial blood gases: pH 7.41; $Paco_2$ 36; Pao_2 68; $TcPo_2$ reading in the low 60s; chest radiograph (today) shows reticulogranular pattern infiltrate and air bronchograms consistent with IRDS. Right upper lobe and left lower lobe atelectasis were apparent.

B.L. had a transpyloric tube in place and was receiving continuous infusion of formula.

An umbilical arterial catheter (UAC) was inserted.

B.L. is on a radiant warmer and has ECG leads, temperature servocontrol probe, and $TcPo_2$ electrode attached to his chest, back, and abdomen, respectively.

B.L. had a real-time ultrasound scan, which revealed a grade II SEH/IVH (subependymal hemorrhage/intraventricular hemorrhage).

The nurse caring for B.L. reports only one episode of apnea and bradycardia since surgery. Once his endotracheal tube was suctioned he had no further problem. She reports having suctioned B.L. 3 hours ago with the return of a moderate amount of yellow secretions. She reports B.L. does not exhibit a cough reflex when suctioned.

Chest evaluation revealed the following:

A tiny infant with a left thoracotomy incision (after patent ductus arteriosus ligation).

B.L.'s respiratory rate was 52 with mild retractions during his spontaneous ventilatory efforts.

On auscultation B.L. had harsh vesicular breath sounds, slightly decreased on the left. Rales were noticed over the left anterior chest, and occasional rhonchi were heard bilaterally on expiration.

B.L.'s trachea was palpated in the midline and mild rhonchal fremitus was felt over the anterior chest wall.

Heart rate was 160 beats per minute.

Blood pressure was 82/39.

B.L.'s skin was fragile and bruised. Blood studies demonstrated normal values for coagulation.

B.L. exhibited general hypotonia but could weakly suck a small nipple when stimulated.

B.L. was easily irritated with quick and noxious tactile stimuli. There was a decrease in his $TcPo_2$ during suctioning, during drawing of blood samples, and with turning, though the $TcPo_2$ returned to base-line value within 2 to 3 minutes after he was turned with no additional oxygen required.

CASE B

A.C. was 36 hours old when a physical therapy consultation was requested. Her pulmonary diagnosis was MAS (meconium-aspiration syndrome). She was extubated and was receiving 50% O_2 by oxygen hood when evaluated.

The following data were collected before the chest evaluation:

Arterial blood gases: Fio_2 50%; pH 7.29; $Paco_2$ 51; Pao_2 70; base excess (BE) +4.

Chest radiograph: hyperinflated lungs with patchy atelectasis bilaterally; infiltrate noted in right middle lobe; no sign of pneumothorax; right chest tube in place.

A.C. has ECG leads, temperature probe, and urine collection bag attached to her; an intravenous line was inserted into the left wrist.

A.C. has a transpyloric tube for nutritional support.

The nurse reported A.C. has been somewhat agitated. She reported suctioning meconium-stained secretions from A.C.'s mouth and nose every 3 to 4 hours. A.C. coughs when stimulated with a catheter. There was some concern about A.C. developing persistent fetal circulation (PFC), but so far this has not occurred.

Chest evaluation revealed the following:

A large infant; very pale; head under an oxygen hood.

A chest tube was sutured in place on the right anterior hemithorax and connected to suction by an underwater seal.

A.C. exhibited the following signs of respiratory distress: mild substernal retractions, nasal flaring, and tachypnea (respiratory rate is 60).

On auscultation A.C. had decreased breath sounds in the right lung fields and coarse rales were heard diffusely throughout the chest.

Heart rate was 152.

Blood pressure was 98/56.

CHEST PHYSICAL THERAPY

Chest physical therapy (CPT) appropriate for an infant is limited to the bronchial drainage techniques of positioning for gravity-assisted drainage, chest percussion, vibration, and airway suctioning. The techniques listed above are few, and therefore one might assume CPT for the neonate is relatively simple and straightforward. Unfortunately, the application of CPT techniques to tiny infants is more involved than it sounds.

The first complicating factor involves careful and appropriate determination of *need*. Sick neonates, especially prematures, often do not tolerate handling well, even with routine procedures.[50] Investigators have found that many procedures (i.e., heel sticks, intravenous insertion, position changes, feedings, diaper changes, chest percussion, and suctioning) result in hypoxemia and increased oxygen consumption.[32,50,60] It is therefore very important that CPT procedures be performed only when clearly indicated for an existing problem or when a potential problem in an infant at risk is to be prevented.

Another complicating factor involves selection of the safest and most appropriate combination of CPT procedures for this population. There are many precautions and contraindications for various positions, chest percussion, vibration, and suctioning. The most appropriate and safest treatment program must be individually designed for each infant.

The third complicating factor is related to the size of the baby. The infant who weighs less than 1000 grams is extremely tiny and manual techniques (chest percussion and vibration) are more difficult to administer and can be injurious.

POSITIONING

Positioning for postural drainage (PD) traditionally employs 12 classical positions to drain the bronchopulmonary segments. The 12 postural drainage positions vary from 45 degrees sitting to 45 degrees head down and prone to side-lying to supine. A neonate's conducting airways are completely developed, and therefore the classical positions are appropriately applied for postural drainage. Fig. 17-17 demonstrates the 12 positions for a neonate.

Many precautions and a few contraindications (Table 17-3) for some of the positions in some infants may necessitate modification. As a general rule, a modified postural drainage position should be as close as possible to the classical position. In many cases a position within one-fourth turn and 10 to 20 degrees from the classical position is well tolerated, safe, and effective. The intensive care setting and special problems of neonates often dictates some form of modified postural drainage, especially for head-down positions. Crane and associates[11] found significant increases in heart rate and blood pressure in a group of neonates with hyaline membrane disease in response to a 20-degree head-down position for chest physical therapy. These changes, however, were all well within normal ranges for those vital signs, and they returned to pretreatment levels within 30 minutes.

Positioning may also be helpful to patients with pulmonary dysfunction because of the effects of some positions on ventilation-perfusion relationships and lung volumes and capacities.[37] The *prone position,* in particular, has been shown to affect oxygenation, lung compliance, state of alertness, vital signs, and other factors.[34,56] (Table 17-4 and Fig. 17-18). Semierect positions as described by Ennis and Harris[16] may also improve oxygenation as compared to flat positions.

MANUAL PERCUSSION AND VIBRATION

Percussion and vibration are techniques used to accelerate the loosening and movement of secretions and mucus plugs in the conducting airways. Either or both techniques,

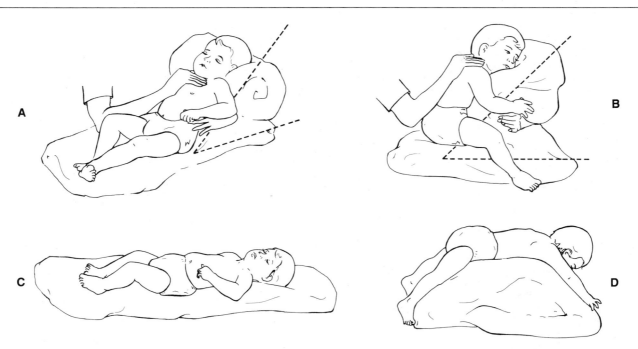

Fig. 17-17. Twelve positions for postural drainage (with **H** and **I** lying on right and left sides).

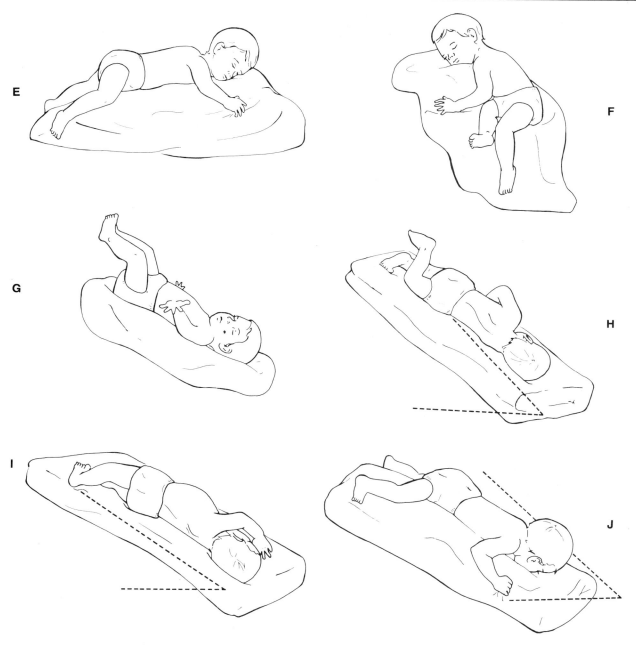

Fig. 17-17, cont'd. For legend see opposite page.

Table 17-3. Precautions and contraindications for postural drainage in a neonate

Position	Precaution	Contraindication
Prone	Umbilical arterial catheter Continuous positive airway pressure in nose Excessive abdominal distention Abdominal incision Anterior chest tube	Untreated tension pneumothorax
Trendelenburg position (head down)	Distended abdomen SEH/IVH* (grades I and II) Chronic congestive heart failure or cor pulmonale Persistent fetal circulation Cardiac arrhythmias Apnea and bradycardia Infant exhibiting signs of acute respiratory distress Hydrocephalus	Untreated tension pneumothorax Recent tracheoesophageal fistula repair Recent eye or intracranial surgery Intraventricular hemorrhage (grades III and IV) Acute congestive heart failure or cor pulmonale

*Subependymal hemorrhage/intraventricular hemorrhage.

Table 17-4. Effects of the prone versus supine position on the neonate

Effect when prone	Reference	Significance
More quiet sleep	Brackbill, Douhitt and West[6] (30 full-term neonates)	<0.05
More active sleep		<0.05
Less crying		<0.01
Less motor activity		<0.01
More regular respirations		NS
Slower heart rates		NS
Increased arterial oxygen tension	Martin and co-workers[34] (16 premature infants)	<0.001
Decreased chest wall asynchrony		<0.001
Increased arterial oxygen tension	Wagaman and co-workers[56] (14 neonates; mean gestational age, 34.5 weeks)	<0.05
Increased lung compliance		<0.05
Increased tidal volume		<0.05
Decreased number of apnea episodes	Dhande, Kattwinkel, and Darnall[13] (5 premature infants)	<0.001
Higher $TcPo_2$ values		<0.005

NS, Not significant.

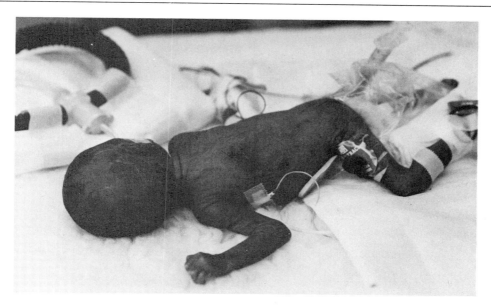

Fig. 17-18. Infant placed in prone position despite mechanical ventilation and artificial airway.

Table 17-5. Precautions and contraindications for chest percussion of a neonate

Precautions	Contraindications
Poor condition of skin	Intolerance to treatment as
Coagulopathy	indicated by low $TcPo_2$
Presence of a chest tube	values
Healing thoracic incision	Rib fracture
Osteoporosis and rickets	Hemoptysis
Persistent fetal circulation	
Cardiac arrythmias	
Apnea and bradycardia	
Signs of acute respiratory	
distress	
Increased irritability during	
treatment	
Subcutaneous emphysema	
Bronchospasm, wheezing,	
rhonchi	
Subependymal hemor-	
rhage/intraventricular	
hemorrhage (SEH/IVH)	

Table 17-6. Precautions and contraindications for vibration of a neonate

Precautions	Contraindications
Increased irritability	Untreated tension pneumothorax
during treatment	Intolerance to treatment as indi-
Persistent fetal cir-	cated by low $TcPo_2$ values
culation	Hemoptysis
Apnea and brady-	
cardia	

when combined with postural drainage, have been shown to improve oxygenation, decrease the incidence of postextubation atelectasis, and increase the amount of secretions removed in newborn infants with pulmonary disease.[17,19,20]

There are many precautions and contraindications for using these techniques (Tables 17-5 and 17-6) with neo-nates (especially percussion). It is therefore very important to consider percussion and vibration *separately* and use them individually or together as appropriate for each infant.

Percussion for a small infant can be administered manually or with one of a variety of percussion "devices" (Fig. 17-19). Manual percussion may be performed with the full-cupped hand, four fingers cupped, three fingers with the middle finger "tented," or the thenar and hypothenar surfaces of the hand (Figs. 17-20 to 17-24). The therapist's choice of hand position is personal and depends on the size of the hand, the baby, and the shape of the area to be percussed. Most percussion techniques include a larger area of the chest wall than the surface adjacent to the affected lung area segment. The therapist should avoid percussing over the liver, spleen, kidneys, or other struc-

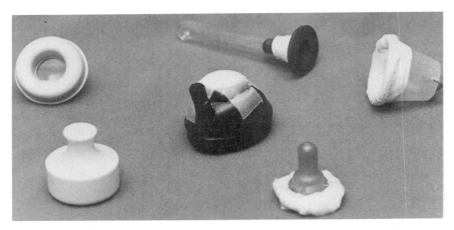

Fig. 17-19. Commercially available and adapted devices for percussion.

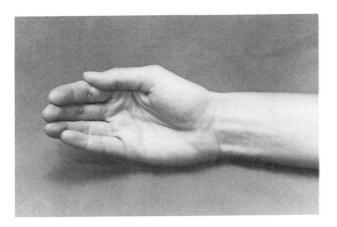

Fig. 17-20. Fully cupped hand for percussion.

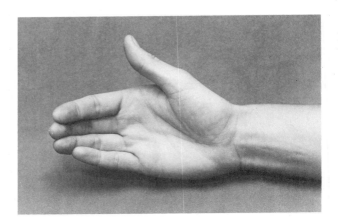

Fig. 17-21. Four fingers cupped for percussion.

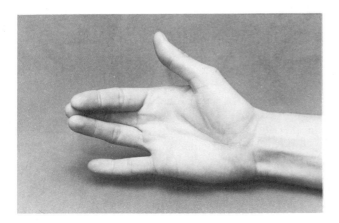

Fig. 17-22. Three fingers cupped for percussion with middle finger "tented"—anterior view.

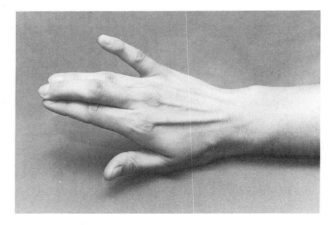

Fig. 17-23. Three fingers cupped for percussion with middle finger "tented"—posterior view.

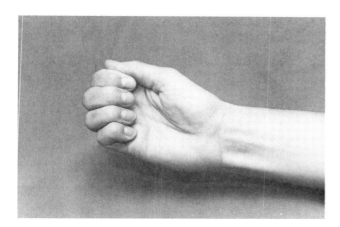

Fig. 17-24. Thenar and hypothenar surfaces for percussion.

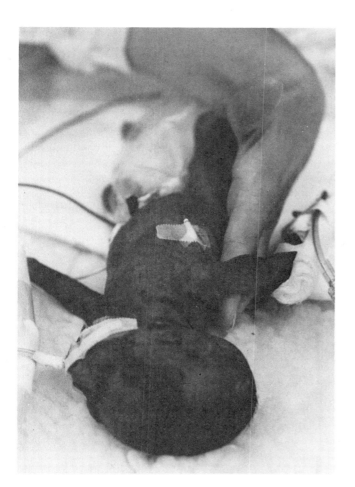

Fig. 17-25. Manual support to chest wall during percussion.

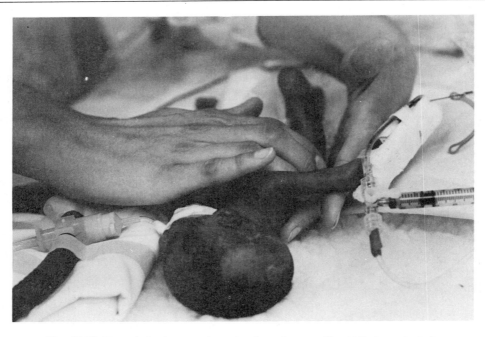

Fig. 17-26. Manual chest percussion using three fingers with middle finger tented.

tures by paying close attention to the borders of the lungs and surface anatomy.

Percussion is often well tolerated by infants and its rhythmic, nonpainful stimulus seems to soothe some babies to sleep. Regardless of the method used for percussion, a cupping effect should be maintained. When percussion is administered manually, the motion should come primarily from the therapist's wrist with firm support applied to the opposite side of the chest wall (Figs. 17-25 and 17-26). In most cases a thin blanket, sheet, or article of clothing should cover the area being treated (Fig. 17-27). In some premature infants, it is important to continually observe the chest wall for anatomical landmarks and to watch for signs of respiratory distress; therefore percussion is administered directly over the skin.

Vibration can be administered manually or with a mechanical vibrator. There are fewer precautions and contraindications for vibration (Table 17-6), and so vibration can often be used in place of manual percussion in a chest physical therapy treatment (Fig. 17-28). Curran and Kachoyeanos[12] advocate the use of a padded electric toothbrush for vibration. The mechanical vibrator (of which the electric toothbrush is one form) has not been conclusively demonstrated to be more effective or safer than other manual chest physical therapy techniques in infants. Be cautious that no electric motor capable of producing a spark is used around high concentrations of oxygen in which a spark could trigger an explosion.

One performs manual vibration by placing the palmar surface of the fingers over the chest-wall surface to be vibrated and isometrically contracting the muscles of the hand and arm to create a fine tremulous vibration. Very little pressure should be applied when one is vibrating the chest wall of a neonate. Vibration is traditionally done during the expiratory phase of breathing. That coordination may be impossible when an infant is breathing above 40 to 50 breaths per minute. If the baby is receiving mechanical ventilation with intermittent mandatory ventilation (IMV), vibration can easily be coordinated with the expiratory phases of the ventilator-assisted breaths.

Postural drainage, percussion, and vibration should be administered for at least 3 to 5 minutes per position in order to be effective. If postural drainage is used alone, the time for drainage in each position must be longer, at least 20 to 30 minutes. I strongly recommend that the therapist not attempt to employ all the positions necessary for a baby during one treatment session if it means significantly decreasing the time in each position. Rather, first treat the areas showing the signs of the pathological condition the most, and then treat the less-involved segments using short frequent treatments. In this manner all areas of the lung requiring drainage will be adequately treated.

Airway suctioning is usually required to help the infant clear the secretions loosened by the bronchial drainage treatment. Suctioning may also be considered an emer-

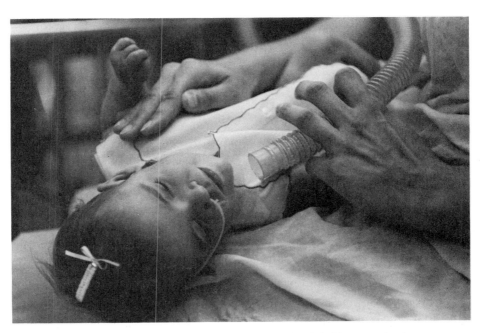

Fig. 17-27. Manual percussion with light article of clothing over chest.

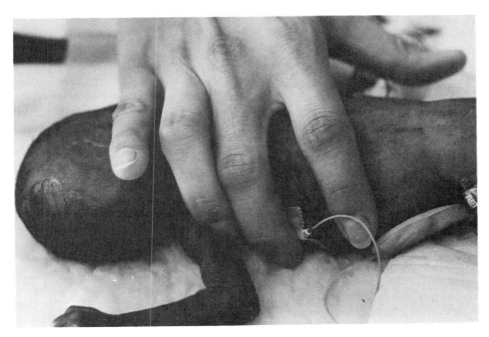

Fig. 17-28. Manual chest vibration on an infant with a thoracotomy incision.

gency procedure if a large airway or tube becomes obstructed by secretions. Suctioning is always potentially dangerous for the infant.[7,9,32] The risks can be reduced if suggested procedures are carefully followed and precautions are taken.

As a general rule, unless the situation is an emergency, nasotracheal suctioning should not be attempted without an endotracheal (ET) or tracheostomy tube. Deep tracheal suctioning is most effectively and more safely performed through an artificial airway. The therapist can suction the nasal and oral pharynges and try to stimulate a cough in an infant without an ET tube or tracheostomy. If the infant has an adequate cough and suctioning can be deferred, it is better not to perform the procedures.

When suctioning is necessary, the following procedure is suggested:[10,35]

1. *Preparation:* Place the infant supine, preferably with the head positioned in the midline. Be sure the suction apparatus is working properly and is connected, the suction is turned on, and the vacuum level is set between 60 and 80 cm H_2O. Make sure the oxygen flow is turned on and attached to the self-inflating breathing bag and the pressure manometer is connected. Check to see what pressures the ventilator is delivering to the baby or what pressure is required to properly ventilate the infant.

2. *Hyperventilation:* With a self-inflating bag and artificial airway connector, hyperventilate the infant at approximately 20 breaths per minute above the rate delivered by the ventilator up to a maximum of 60 breaths per minute at the pressure noted in step 1. Hyperoxygenate the infant by delivering an oxygen concentration 10% to 20% higher than the inspired concentration (FIO_2) the infant was receiving.

   If the FIO_2 is 0.5 or higher, deliver 100% oxygen. Hyperventilation and hyperoxygenation should precede and follow each pass of the suction catheter.

3. *Lavage* (OPTIONAL): Instill 0.5 to 1 ml, or 2 or 3 drops, of sterile normal saline solution (NaCl) directly into the endotracheal or tracheostomy tube.

4. *Suction:* Using *sterile* procedure:
   a. Wet the catheter in sterile saline.
   b. Insert the catheter (with *no* suction applied) into the airway until resistance is met. Pull the catheter back slightly and then withdraw the catheter while applying intermittent suction and turning the catheter. Suction should not last longer than 10 seconds.
   c. Repeat if necessary.
   d. Suction the nasal and oral pharynges.

Hypoxemia and hyperoxemia can be *minimized* during chest physical therapy if the infant is monitored with a transcutaneous oxygen ($TcPO_2$) monitor.[32] $TcPO_2$ monitoring is noninvasive and provides a continuous record of the infant's oxygenation. If the $TcPO_2$ values correlate with

PaO_2 values, this form of monitoring is invaluable to the physical therapist when one is assessing and treating infants in a neonatal intensive care unit.

CASE EXAMPLES: TREATMENT

The cases presented earlier in the chapter will provide examples of chest physical therapy treatment of infants with pulmonary dysfunction. Notice the careful consideration of precautions and contraindications and individualized treatment plans.

CASE A

B.L. is almost ready to be extubated and the following treatment is planned:

Short, frequent (approximately every 2 or 3 hours) bronchial drainage treatments to begin at least 1 hour before extubation and to continue for at least 48 hours. As a result of the chest radiograph and auscultation, treatment emphasis is placed upon the left lower lobe. Also emphasized are the right upper lobe and right middle lobe, which are susceptible to postextubation atelectasis. A maximum of four positions will be used for each treatment with a maximum of 15 minutes of treatment time. Vibration will be used in lieu of percussion because of a thoracotomy, coagulopathy, bruised skin, and intraventricular hemorrhage. Modified postural drainage positions will be used because of the intraventricular hemorrhage to avoid greater than 15 degrees with the head down. Postural drainage and vibration will be followed by suctioning through the endotracheal tube. Once the extubation is done, suctioning will be limited to stimulation of a cough reflex with the catheter and suctioning of the mouth and nose.

Nursing personnel will perform the chest physical therapy treatments at night to provide for 24-hour continuity of treatment. Between chest physical therapy treatments, B.L. will be positioned for modified postural drainage of lung segments not treated during the formal treatment session. If B.L.'s $TcPO_2$ drops during treatment, the FIO_2 will be increased slightly to keep the $TcPO_2$ between 40 and 70 mm Hg.

B.L. was able to breathe without the mechanical ventilator for 72 hours, but the left lower lobe infiltrate did not respond to antibiotic therapy and the infant became progressively more hypoxemic and hypercapnic with increased episodes of apnea and bradycardia. B.L. was reintubated to receive mechanical ventilation for 1 week. He was 13 days old. His chest radiograph then began to exhibit signs of early bronchopulmonary dysplasia (BPD) and copious amounts of secretion were suctioned from his endotracheal tube.

PLAN: Continue bronchial drainage treatments for all lung segments as tolerated. As B.L.'s infiltrate improves, he will still have changes consistent with bronchopulmonary dysplasia and will therefore be extremely susceptible to respiratory infection, airway obstruction, and respiratory failure. Chest physical therapy should continue routinely for prophylaxis until discharge, and B.L.'s parents will be instructed in chest physical therapy techniques for use at home.

CASE B

The following treatment plan was recommended for A.C.:

BRONCHIAL DRAINAGE:
1. Position to drain the right middle lobe (one-fourth turn from supine, right side up) and the right lower lobe (15 to 20 degrees head down; modified because of respiratory distress) with percussion and vibration performed for 3 to 5 minutes every 4 hours.

2. Treat the remaining lung segments as tolerated with modified head-down positions for lower lobe segments.
3. Follow chest physical therapy with cough stimulation and suctioning. NOTE: If a good cough is not evident and lower airways remain obstructed, temporary intubation for direct suctioning may be considered by the neonatologist.

If A.C. is agitated by vibration, percussion alone should be performed except where the chest tube exits the chest. Agitation may be secondary to hypercapnia: Pco_2 51. One performs vibration around the chest tube site by slipping the index and middle fingers on either side of the tube and vibrating at regular intervals. As respiratory distress abates, postural drainage should be performed in the classical positions.

The therapist must observe for signs of increasing hypoxemia—increased respiratory distress, cyanosis, tachycardia, or bradycardia—and must observe for spontaneous pneumothorax—sudden clinical deterioration with bradycardia or tachycardia, cyanosis or pallor, increased respiratory distress, shift of the mediastinum away from the side of the pneumothorax, and decreased or absent breath sounds on the side of the pneumothorax.

DISCHARGE PLANNING

Preparing the parents of an infant in the neonatal intensive care unit (NICU) for their baby's discharge is almost as important as preparing the baby. Discharge planning and teaching must begin early. Parents of infants requiring long hospitalizations should become involved in the care of their baby long before discharge.

The transition from hospital to home can be a crisis for the parents of a baby who has spent a long time in a NICU.[33] The stresses of discharge are overshadowed by the benefits, which include decreasing the fatigue of travel, decreasing the financial burdens of prolonged hospitalization, and ending the separation of the parents from the child.

If the NICU is a regional newborn intensive care nursery, the parents may live a long distance from the hospital. This distance can present a problem when it becomes necessary for the parents to visit the hospital frequently to learn the infant's home care. It is imperative that planning for parent involvement with the infant's care and teaching in preparation for discharge be started early, as soon as it is evident that the baby *will* eventually go home.

In most NICU settings someone is designated as the discharge planner. Often it is a nurse who coordinates the efforts of the team to assure that the plans are carried out.

Team assessment of needs

In most cases several disciplines will be involved in the care of the baby. As the infant progresses and the time for discharge approaches, the team members must communicate their assessments and plans among each other. This process is extremely important for consolidation of plans and avoidance of inconsistencies and duplication of effort in dealing with the parents.

The *physical therapist* has much to contribute to the parents' knowledge and skills. The physical therapist can assist parents regarding an infant's pulmonary, neurological, or orthopaedic problems. This section is a discussion of only the discharge planning for an infant with chronic pulmonary problems.

Bronchial drainage at home

If the infant has an airway clearance problem secondary to some form of chronic lung disease, central nervous system dysfunction or infectious process, bronchial drainage should be continued at home. Requiring parents to perform these treatments may present some inconvenience and interruption of the normal family routine. One advantage, however, is that treatments provide a period of time for the infant and parent to interact and be in close physical contact. When viewed in this way, bronchial drainage may be considered mutually beneficial.

What to include in home program

Positioning can often be limited to six or less modified postural drainage positions for prophylaxis or emphasis on problem areas. The positions chosen depend on many factors including the following:

1. Location of the pathological condition in the lung
2. Condition or conditions requiring modification of positions
3. What positions the infant is likely to be in most of the time

When teaching parents bronchial drainage for an infant with diffuse chronic lung disease, I recommend the following six positions:

1. Sitting, leaning back 45 degrees from vertical
2. Sitting, leaning forward 45 degrees from vertical
3. Lying one-fourth turn from supine with the right side up and head and thorax tilted 30 degrees down from the horizontal
4. Lying on left side with the head and thorax tilted 45 degrees down from the horizontal
5. Lying on right side with the head and thorax tilted 45 degrees down from the horizontal
6. Lying prone with the head and thorax tilted 45 degrees down from the horizontal

The *manual technique* usually taught to parents is chest percussion. Vibration may also be taught if in the opinion of the therapist the baby will benefit *and* the parents can learn the technique. Urge and observe for adequate force of percussion. Parents are reluctant to use sufficient percussion force believing they might harm the baby. Percussion and vibration should be practiced several times by the parent with the therapist present to assure that good technique is used.

Parents may need to be instructed how to stimulate a cough. They also need to know that infants commonly swallow cleared secretions and may vomit if a large amount of mucus accumulates in the stomach. This vomiting is usually *normal*.

Suctioning at home

If an infant has a tracheostomy, airway suctioning may be necessary. Parents must learn sterile, or "clean," techniques of airway suctioning and should practice this procedure with supervision. It is helpful for parents and baby to "room in" in a regular hospital room to practice routine care with assistance and encouragement close at hand.

Be sure to caution parents to avoid bronchial drainage for at least 1 hour after feeding. Preferably, the treatment should be just before feedings. The frequency of treatment is variable and depends on the infant's needs. The therapist and physician should consider the socioemotional effects frequent chest physical therapy treatments may have on the family.

Parents must also recognize signs and symptoms of respiratory infection. Early intervention with antibiotics, more frequent bronchial drainage treatments, and other measures may help avoid rehospitalization when an infection occurs at home.

SUMMARY

As NICU technology improves and more neonates of lower gestational ages survive the perinatal period, the role of the physical therapist in the NICU increases in importance. Tiny babies are very susceptible to cardiopulmonary, neurological, and orthopaedic problems. The physical therapist assesses and treats a neonate to prevent and remediate physiological and functional problems. Chest physical therapy is often indicated for neonates with pulmonary dysfunction to improve airway clearance, enhance ventilation, and decrease the work of breathing. Determining the need for physical therapy and designing apropriate treatment programs is especially important for this patient population. A physical therapist in a NICU must be familiar with the unique problems of small, sick neonates. When applied conscientiously, chest physical therapy can be safely and effectively administered to the tiniest babies.

REFERENCES

1. Ahmann, P., and others: Intraventricular hemorrhage in the high risk preterm infant, Ann. Neurol. **7:**118, 1980.
2. Bacsik, R.D.: Meconium aspiration syndrome, Pediatr. Clin. North Am. **24:**463, 1977.
3. Bartlett, R.H., and others: Studies on the pathogenesis and prevention of postoperative pulmonary complications, Surg. Gynecol. Obstet. **137:**925, 1973.
4. Bejar, R., Coen, R.W., and Glock, L.: Hypoxic-ischemic and hemorrhagic brain injury in the newborn, Perinatol. Neonatol. **6:**69, 1982.
5. Bendixen, H.H., Bullwinkel, B., and Hedley-Whyte, J., and others: Atelectasis and shunting during spontaneous ventilation in anesthetized patients, Anesthesiology **25:**297, 1964.
6. Brackbill, Y., Douthitt, T.C., and West, H.: Psycho-physiologic effects in the neonate of prone versus supine placement, J. Pediatr. **82:**82, 1973.
7. Brandstater, B., and Muallem, M.: Atelectasis following tracheal suction in infants, Anesthesiology **31:**468, 1969.
8. Chrisman, M.K.: Respiratory nursing: continuing education review, Flushing, N.Y., 1975, Medical Examination Publishing Co., Inc.
9. Cordero, L., and Hon, E.H.: Neonatal bradycardia following nasopharyngeal stimulation, J. Pediatr. **78:**441, 1971.
10. Crane, L.: Physical therapy for neonates with respiratory dysfunction, Phys. Ther. **51:**17, 1981.
11. Crane, L.D., and others: Comparison of chest physiotherapy techniques in infants with HMD, Pediatr. Res. **12:**559, 1978. (Abstract.)
12. Curran, C.L., and Kachoyeanos, M.K.: The effects on neonates of two methods of chest physical therapy, Matern. Child Nurs. J. **4:**309, 1979.
13. Dhande, V.G., and others: Prone position reduces apnea in preterm infants, Pediatr. Res. **16:**285A, 1982, part 2 of 2 parts. (Abstract.)
14. Dubowitz, L., Dubowitz, V., and Goldberg, C.: Clinical assessment of gestational age in the newborn infant, J. Pediatr. **77:**1, 1970.
15. Dunn, D., and Lewis, A.T.: Some important aspects of neonatal nursing related to pulmonary disease and family involvement, Pediatr. Clin. North Am. **20:**481, 1973.
16. Ennis, S., and Harris, T.R.: Positioning infants with hyaline membrane disease, Am. J. Nurs. **78:**398, 1978.
17. Etches, P.C., and Scott, B.: Chest physiotherapy in the newborn: effect on secretions removed, Pediatrics **62:**713, 1978.
18. Farrell, P.M., and Avery, M.E.: State of the art: hyaline membrane disease, Am. Rev. Respir. Dis. **111:**657, 1975.
19. Finer, N.N., and others: Postextubation atelectasis: a retrospective review and a prospective controlled study, J. Pediatr. **94:**110, 1979.
20. Finer, N.N., and Boyd, J.: Chest physiotherapy in the neonate: a controlled study, Pediatrics **61:**282, 1978.
21. Frownfelter, D.L., editor: Chest physical therapy and pulmonary rehabilitation, Chicago, 1978, Year Book Medical Publishers, Inc.
22. Gage, J.E., and others: Suctioning of upper airway meconium in newborn infants, J.A.M.A. **246:**2590, 1981.
23. Goldsmith, J.P., and Karotkin, E.H.: Assisted ventilation of the newborn, Philadelphia, 1981, W.B. Saunders Co.
24. Gregory, G.A., and others: Meconium aspiration in infants: a prospective study, J. Pediatr. **85:**848, 1974.
25. Henderson-Smart, D.J., and Read, D.J.: Depression of respiratory muscles and defective responses to nasal obstruction during active sleep in the newborn, Aust. Paediatr. J. **21:**261, 1976.
26. Johnson, T.R., Moore, W.M., and Jeffries, J.E., editors: Children are different: developmental physiology, ed. 2., Columbus, Ohio, 1978, Ross Laboratories.
27. Kattan, M.: Long-term sequelae of respiratory illness in infancy and childhood, Pediatr. Clin. North Am. **26**(3):525, 1979.
28. Klaus, M.H., and Fanaroff, A.A.: Care of the high-risk neonate, ed. 2., Philadelphia, 1979, W.B. Saunders Co.
29. Kottmeier, P.K., and Klotz, D.: Surgical problems in the newborn, Pediatr. Ann. **8:**60, 1979.
30. Laitman, J.T., and Crelin, E.S.: Developmental change in the upper respiratory system of human infants, Perinatol. Neonatol. **4:**15, 1980.
31. Levine, M.I., and Mascia, A.V.: Pulmonary diseases and anomalies of infancy and childhood, New York, 1966, Hoeber Medical Division, Harper & Row, Publishers.
32. Long, J.G., Philip, A.G., and Lucey, J.F.: Excessive handling as a cause of hypoxemia, Pediatrics **65:**203, 1980.
33. Lund, C., and Lefrak, L.: Discharge planning for infants in the intensive care nursery, Perinatol. Neonatol. **6:**49, 1982.
34. Martin, R.J., and others: Effect of supine and prone positions on arterial oxygen tension in the preterm infant, Pediatrics **63:**528, 1979.
35. McFadden, R.: Decreasing respiratory compromise during infant suctioning, Am. J. Nurs. **81:**2158, 1981.

36. Mellins, R.B.: Pulmonary physiotherapy in the pediatric age group, Am. Rev. Respir. Dis. **110**(6 part 2):137, 1974.

37. Menkes, H., and Britt, J.: Physical therapy: rationale for physical therapy, Am. Rev. Respir. Dis. **122**:127, 1980.

38. Moss, A.J., Duffie, E.F., and Emmanouilides, G.: Blood pressure and vasomotor reflexes in the newborn infant, Pediatrics **32**:175, 1963.

39. Muller, N.L., and Bryan, A.C.: Chest wall mechanics and respirator muscles in infants, Pediatr. Clin. North Am. **26**:503, 1979.

40. Murray, J.F.: The normal lung, Philadelphia, 1976, W.B. Saunders Co.

41. Nagaraj, H.S., and others: Recurrent lobar atelectasis due to acquired bronchial stenosis in neonates, J. Pediatr. Surg. **15**:411, 1980.

42. Northway, W.H., and others: Pulmonary disease following respirator therapy of hyaline membrane disease: bronchopulmonary dysplasia, N. Engl. J. Med. **275**:357, 1967.

43. Perlman, J.M., and Volpe, J.J.: The effects of oral suctioning and endotracheal suctioning on cerebral blood flow velocity and intracranial pressure in the preterm infant, Pediatr. Res. **16**:303A, 1982. (Abstract.)

44. Polgar, G.: Practical pulmonary physiology, Pediatr. Clin. North Am. **20**:303, 1973.

45. Remondière, R., and others: Intérêt de la kinésithérapie respiratoire dans le traitement de la maladie des membranes hyalines du nouveau-né, Ann. Pédiat. **23**:617, 1976.

46. Rudolph, A.M.: High pulmonary vascular resistance after birth, Clin. Pediatr. **19**:585, 1980.

47. Scarpelli, E.M., editor: Pulmonary physiology of the fetus, newborn and child, Philadelphia, 1975, Lea & Febiger.

48. Scarpelli, E.M., Auld, P.A.M., and Goldman, H.S., editors: Pulmonary disease of the fetus, newborn and child, Philadelphia, 1978, Lea & Febiger.

49. Smith, R.M.: Anesthesia for infants and children, ed. 3, St. Louis, 1968, The C.V. Mosby Co.

50. Speidel, B.D.: Adverse effects of routine procedures on preterm infants, Lancet **1**:864, 1978.

51. Sun, S.C., and others: Meconium aspiration and tracheal suction, J. Med. Soc. N.J. **74**:542, 1977.

52. Thurlbeck, W.M.: Postnatal growth and development of the lung, Am. Rev. Respir. Dis. **111**:803, 1975.

53. Tisi, G.M.: State of the art: pre-operative evaluation of pulmonary function, Am. Rev. Respir. Dis. **119**:293, 1979.

54. Vohr, B.R., Bell, E.F., and OH, W.: Infants with bronchopulmonary dysplasia, Am. J. Dis. Child. **136**:443, 1982.

55. Voyles, J.B.: Pulmonary problems in infants and children: bronchopulmonary dysplasia, Am. J. Nurs. **81**:510, 1981.

56. Wagaman, M.J., and others: Improved oxygenation and long compliance with prone positioning of neonates, J. Pediatr. **94**:787, 1979.

57. Wallis, S., and Harvey, D.: Respiratory distress: its cause and management, Nurs. Times **75**:1264, 1979.

58. Weinstein, M.R., and Oh, W.: Oxygen consumption in infants with bronchopulmonary dysplasia, J. Pediatr. **99**:958, 1981.

59. Wesenberg, R.L.: The newborn chest, New York, 1973, Harper & Row, Publishers, Inc.

60. Yeh, T.F., and others: Changes of O_2 consumption (VO_2) in response to NICU care procedures in premature infants, Pediatr. Res. **16**:315A, 1982. (Abstract.)

61. Young, I.M., and Holland, W.W.: Some physiological responses of neonatal arterial blood pressure and pulse rate, Br. Med. J. **2**:276, 1958.

18

JEANNE DeCESARE

Physical therapy for the child with respiratory dysfunction

FRAME OF REFERENCE

Improved diagnostic, surgical, and medical techniques have had an impact on pediatric care. In 1967, at the Children's Hospital in Boston, the average length of stay for a medical patient was 14.0 days. In 1978, that number had been reduced to 8.3 days.[14] Patient days in the hospital for the over-21-years-of-age group has almost doubled from 1967 to 1981. These statistics probably reflect improved medical care, which has increased the life expectancy of patients with chronic life-limiting diseases such as cystic fibrosis. For example, the patients with cystic fibrosis born today have a much better chance of living into their twenties than those of previous years.[67] On the other end of the spectrum, premature infants who would have died in past years are now surviving the newborn period because of improved, intensive neonatal care. Chemotherapy and aggressive surgical intervention has helped improve the life expectancy for many pediatric patients with neoplasms. Some patients with bone marrow dysfunction such as acute leukemia and aplastic anemia can undergo bone marrow transplantation, which may cure their otherwise fatal disease.

Cardiac and thoracic surgical advances also account for earlier correction of abnormalities in newborns and infants and survival of those with previously uncorrectable anomalies.

A wider range of care extending from the premature infant to the young adult has evolved with medical advances and has redirected the pediatric clinician's focus. Physical therapy evaluation and treatment must therefore reflect this diversification in pediatric care.

The developing lung

It is an accepted fact that children are different from adults. Not only do their emotional responses and small stature set them apart, but anatomical and physiological differences are apparent. Total care of the pediatric patient means consideration of growing systems—cardiopulmonary, skeletal, neurological, and so on.

Lung growth is not complete at birth. Normal growth and remodeling of the lung continues until adulthood.[45] The bronchial tree is fully formed by approximately 16 weeks of gestation. After birth the conducting airways continue to increase in diameter and length but not in number. Primitive alveoli are present at birth, but mature alveolar growth and development take place after birth. There is some controversy as to when the development of new alveoli stops. It has been suggested that by 8 years of age the number of alveoli is the same as that in the adult.[45] However, there is some evidence that the number of alveoli increases until 12 years of age.[11] The alveoli are developing throughout most of childhood. Alveolar diameter also changes with age. The diameter of alveoli at 2 months is approximately 60 to 130 μm. This diameter increases to a range of 100 to 200 μm in older children, whereas the adult has alveoli of 200 to 300 μm in diameter.[11] Changes in morphology and size of the alveoli appear to parallel increases in the lateral chest wall dimension.[8] The contour of an infant's chest is more rounded than an adult's and grows into an elliptical shape in the adult.

Branching of the pulmonary artery at 19 weeks of fetal life is the same as the adult pattern. Alveolar capillaries multiply as rapidly after birth as the alveoli do.

I would like to thank biomedical photographer, James Koepfler, Department of Orthopedic Surgery, Children's Hospital, Boston, for his outstanding contribution to this chapter; Claire McCarthy, Michelina Cassella, and the Physical Therapy staff at Children's Hospital, Boston, for their support and expertise; Pearl Stephens for the typing of this manuscript; and the patients and parents who so willingly agreed to pose for photographs.

334

There appears to be a greater density of mucous glands in relationship to the size of the bronchial surface in the young child. Nearly twice the density of glands per unit surface are present in children less than 4 years old compared to the adult.[11] Goblet cells, which generally do not extend beyond the cartilaginous portion of the tracheobronchial tree, often migrate rapidly into the bronchioles and replace ciliated cells in disease. These findings may explain why the severity of obstructive pulmonary disease is more striking in infants and young children with small airways than in older patients.

Because of the lack of smooth muscle development, which occurs by about 3 to 4 years of age, there is weakness in the bronchioles of infants and young children. This weakness may contribute to airway collapse and air trapping. It has also been found that peripheral airway conductance, or the freedom with which air flows through an airway, increases substantially at about 5 years of age.[11] There is most likely increased resistance to airflow in the peripheral airways during the first 5 years of life.

In addition to the lack of structural support in the small airways in the early years, collateral ventilation offered by the pores of Kohn and Lambert's canals is limited. Development of the pores of Kohn may not occur until 12 to 13 years of age.[11] Lambert's canals may not exist until 6 to 8 years of age.[8] The young child is therefore at higher risk for development of atelectasis and infection.

Lung volume and surface area increase steadily through adolescence and most likely relate to an increase in alveolar size and number. When ill, the infant and young child have less pulmonary reserve to depend on than the adult does. This poor reserve is probably attributable to a child's increased resting oxygen consumption demand in relationship to the lung surface area.[11]

Some investigators have noticed that lung compliance and distensibility may be low in young children. Elastic tissue may not develop in the walls of the alveoli until after adolescence.[64] In addition to lung compliance being decreased in children, chest-wall compliance is increased. This disparity can lead to severe chest retractions and loss of mechanical advantage to the inspiratory musculature during respiratory distress.

It is apparent from what we know about lung growth and development that the infant and young child represent a high-risk population for pulmonary dysfunction. Improved pulmonary reserve, greater airway support and patency, and collateral ventilation occur with growth. Chest physical therapy for the pediatric patient is therefore a challenge in both the treatment and prevention of pulmonary complications.

Importance of the family

Years ago family participation was not encouraged in pediatric care; however, today it is enthusiastically welcomed. The family, primarily parents, is an excellent resource to health professionals. Parents are needed to construct a comprehensive medical history of their child. They can offer vital information regarding their child's personality and usual responses to the environment. It is essential to establish a good relationship with both family and patient.

Family participation and cooperation during the care of a hospitalized child can mean better understanding and compliance with a home care program. Poor communication and exclusion of parents from their child's care can result in noncompliance with a treatment regimen. Comprehensive parental education is paramount to ensure continued care for the pediatric patient at home. If the parents are unavailable or uninvolved, then whoever will be the primary caretaker must be included in home treatment planning.

PATIENT PROBLEMS
Physical considerations

Easy fatigue, disturbed schedules. The infant and child are experiencing growth and physiological changes, which must be considered by the physical therapist when planning treatment. As has been discussed, lung growth and remodeling is taking place throughout childhood and possibly adolescence. The previous discussion of the anatomical and physiological immaturity of the growing lung shows that such immaturity contributes to airway collapse and increased airway resistance, atelectasis, and lack of pulmonary reserve during stress. This decreased reserve leads to easy fatigability. The length of chest physical therapy treatment sessions may have to be reduced for an acutely ill infant or child. Shorter, more frequent treatments may be indicated. Use of frequent position changes is essential and should be a part of a bronchial hygiene program.

When caring for an acutely ill child, one must carry out many medical interventions throughout the day and night. Sleep cycles and schedules can easily be disturbed. Chest physical therapy may be needed every 2 to 3 hours. One approach to this rigorous routine of medical care is to place a child on "stress precautions." This is an attempt to protect the child from unnecessary disturbances by use of a strict intervention schedule, with structured periods of rest and minimal contact. Physical therapy should be coordinated within this synchronized approach to help reduce patient stress.

Fig. 18-1 shows the medical equipment needed for the care of an acutely ill infant. This elaborate technological armamentarium becomes part of the infant's environment.

Small chests. The size of an infant's or child's chest will alter treatment technique. Hand positioning for bronchial drainage and the force of percussion techniques will have to be modified. The use of one hand or three fingers in a tented position may be sufficient to cover the indicated area of the chest for percussion techniques (Fig. 18-2).

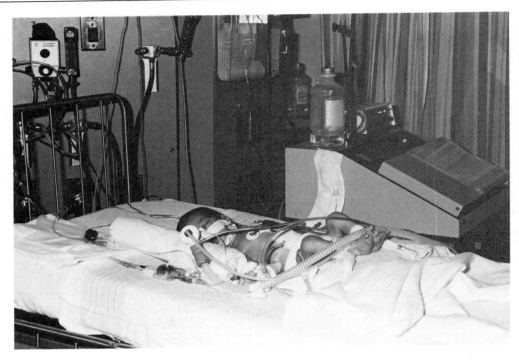

Fig. 18-1. Elaborate medical equipment becomes part of the environment of an acutely ill child.

Gastroesophageal reflux. A malfunction of the distal esophagus causing repeated return of stomach contents into the esophagus is known as "gastroesophageal reflux" (GER). If the stomach contents reach the pharynx, partially digested food may be aspirated into the lungs causing respiratory problems. A recent increased interest in gastroesophageal reflux has helped to identify it as a possible cause of recurrent pneumonias and pulmonary problems in children who repeatedly experience aspiration of refluxed gastric contents.[20] In the absence of vomiting, diagnosis of this problem becomes more difficult. It may be overlooked or misdiagnosed as bronchopulmonary dysplasia in the premature infant or allergic bronchitis or asthma in the older child. Many infants have mild gastroesophageal reflux that resolves when they begin to sit upright. The majority of cases (60%) will resolve by 18 months of age. However, about 30% will continue to have significant reflux until at least 4 years of age and sometimes longer.[20]

Conservative medical treatment may require that the child maintain an upright position after feedings or constantly when gastroesophageal reflux is severe. An upright prone position appears less favorable to reflux because the esophagogastric junction is located at the uppermost part of the stomach and the contents are less likely to be regurgitated[20] (Fig. 18-3). Prone positioning also encourages extensor muscle activity and strengthening, which is

a fringe benefit to the motor development of an infant. However, if bronchial drainage is necessary, the physician should be consulted regarding positioning especially if lower lobe secretions are present. The risks and benefits of head-down positioning for bronchial drainage must be considered. Bronchial drainage is always recommended before a meal or no earlier than 1 hour after meals. Treatment before a meal is preferred for any child suspected of having gastroesophageal reflux. If strict positional therapy must be maintained, bronchial drainage may have to be done in a modified position. Percussion and vibration techniques can be used without any precautionary measures.

Strict adherence to a pre-meal schedule for bronchial drainage is also recommended for the infant with feeding problems and the child with cystic fibrosis who has difficulty maintaining adequate nutritional intake and is likely to vomit when coughing. Always inquire if bronchial drainage has a tendency to cause vomiting.

Developmental delay. Developmental delay is another significant problem for a sick infant or child. Prolonged or frequent hospitalizations of a child or dependency on oxygen can create a limited environment (Fig. 18-3). There may be a lack of sensorimotor stimulation no matter how sensitive a hospital staff may be to this issue. Psychobiological deprivation studies clearly point out that a growing

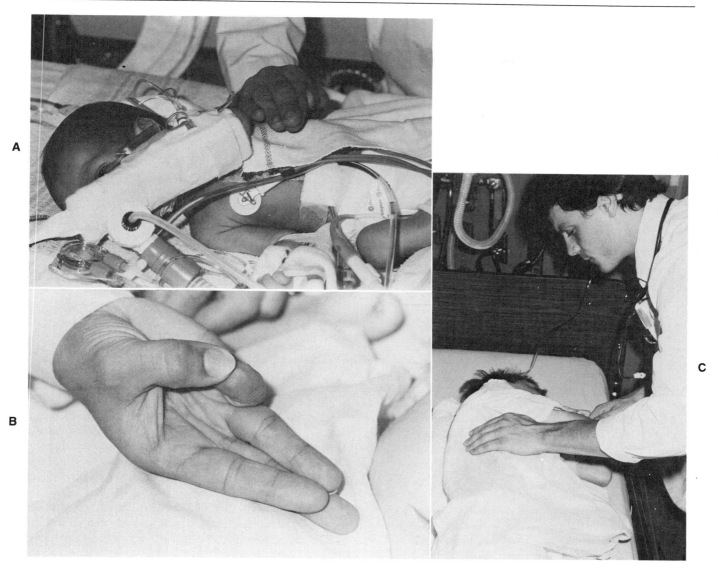

Fig. 18-2. A, "Tented" position of hand for percussion of small infant's chest. **B,** Underside view. **C,** Use of one hand for percussion on chest of small child.

neurological system needs appropriate stimulation to develop.[43]

The physical therapist working in pediatric chest care must realize that many patients requiring prolonged hospitalizations can experience secondary lung problems. These children will experience decreased environmental stimulation and be at risk for delays in sensorimotor development. The child with primary lung problems may also require extended hospitalizations and may be oxygen dependent. Increased secretions may interfere with feeding and normal oral motor development. Children with bronchopulmonary dysplasia may have constant oxygen re-

quirements, which, even though delivered at home, can restrict their ability to explore their environment. Physical therapists must be acutely aware of the developmental needs of their maturing patients regardless of the primary diagnosis.

Psychological considerations

It is essential when working in pediatrics to be aware of the emotional impact an illness has on a child. A large part of the problem is a child's inability to verbalize fears and concerns. Interpretation of the cries of an infant is not an easy task.

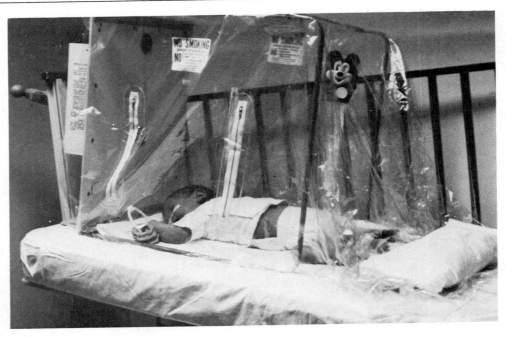

Fig. 18-3. Infant upright prone position to decrease chance of gastroesophageal reflux. The plastic oxygen tent is supplying necessary oxygen to the infant, but it provides a limited environment.

Illness can disrupt family security and unity. Anxiety regarding separation from parents and siblings may be paramount for the hospitalized child. Welcoming parents to stay during treatment may help alleviate some of this anxiety.

The fear of pain and invasive medical procedures can be overwhelming. Reassurance that chest physical therapy will not require use of a ''needle'' may help. Recognizing the fear and responding with concern and sensitivity can be the key to successful treatment. For example, the fear of dislodging a small intravenous needle in the arm or hand can prevent a child from moving or sleeping well. A therapist must respect these fears and assure the child that the intravenous line will be carefully watched and supported during treatment. A child's unwillingness to move may be caused by this anxiety and not uncooperative behavior.

Making treatment as comfortable and pleasant an experience as possible is very important. Utilizing games or songs to obtain therapeutic results will aid in capturing the child's attention and cooperation.

Frequent or prolonged illness may interfere with normal social development. The hospitalized infant or child may experience an overindulgence of attention by many different caretakers. There may also be interference with peer contact, which is important for the self-image of older children and adolescents. Respiratory illnesses especially may prevent participation in normal play and sports because of shortness of breath and fatigue.

Dealing with an illness can bring about stresses such as anger, guilt, and resentment in a child or adolescent who is often not emotionally mature. Acting out and inappropirate behavior may result. Feelings may be manifested through noncompliance with the medical regimen as is often seen in the adolescent.

Young patients grappling with a chronic disease may find that life-style changes, such as entry into college, require much planning and often compromise future goals and dreams.

Death and dying

Working with a dying patient is never easy and can be more difficult when the patient is a child. Several texts have been written about the topic.[32,51] Death brings to light our own personal death awareness and the fears we harbor regarding the loss of life. The physical therapist who works with children with respiratory illnesses cannot escape facing a dying child. Schowalter, who has written about the reactions of caregivers dealing with fatal illnesses in children, makes special mention of the physical therapist.[54] He believes that physical therapists may experience specialized stresses when working with patients who do not improve but, are maintained or deteriorate despite a rehabilitative approach. In the pediatric setting, therapists may personalize the loss of patients. Younger patients may be of similar age to a therapist's own children or siblings. For older patients, the age difference between patient and therapist may be small and may create in the therapist a heightened sense of personal vulnerability. In view of this, an emotional bond may be established between patient and therapist. This creates a significant impact upon the therapist when faced with the death of that patient.

We recommend that regular sessions with a staff psychologist, psychiatrist, or other trained professional be arranged for physical therapists who are faced with the stress of working with dying patients. It is not unusual for a therapist working in a major center for patients with cystic fibrosis to face several patient deaths in a short period of time.

An understanding of our own feelings and reactions toward loss of life can often help when working with a patient who is facing a terminal illness. In pediatrics, one deals with dying patients of all ages and with different conceptions of death. It is probably easiest to respond as naturally as possible and to continue to foster a therapeutic and personal relationship despite the grave prognosis. Finding the right words to say to a patient facing the end of life is the most difficult. Depend on the relationship you have already developed to ease the difficulty.

It is important to continue treatment for a dying patient with whom you have developed a relationship. The treatment components may change because of a lack of patient tolerance, but continued contact is essential. A child who expects daily physical therapy should believe it is being continued, even though modified, despite his or her deterioration. We are fortunate as therapists to have our manual skills to offer comfort and express our closeness and concern for the dying patient. Massage can be a soothing experience for a distressed, breathless patient. Parents or family members can be taught simple massage strokes to use in the therapist's absence. This technique may give parents an opportunity to offer comfort and remain physically close to their child. The therapist may discover that opportunities to offer comfort through massage or other manual techniques can replace the need to "find the right words."

Diseases
Chronic obstructive lung diseases

Chronic obstruction of the airways can be caused by increased secretions, bronchospasm, inflammation or destruction of the bronchial walls, or a combination of the above. There is an interference of the normal flow of air within the lung. Some reversibility of the obstructive components can be achieved through the use of bronchodilator or anti-inflammatory drugs (steroids) and chest physical therapy. For example, the airway obstruction in asthma is often reversible.

Lung changes attributable to structural damage as seen in cystic fibrosis are irreversible, but chest physical therapy continues to be extremely important in clearing airways of excessive secretions.

Asthma. Asthma is a condition characterized by in-creased irritability or hyperactivity of the tracheobronchial tree caused by an assortment of stimulants. Recurrent episodes of wheezing or dyspnea that are reversed with medication or spontaneously constitute the clinical picture of asthma. Asthma has been classified into two types. Extrinsic asthma is caused by allergens or environmental factors, whereas intrinsic asthma is caused by nonallergic factors including psychosomatic components. Childhood asthma is primarily of the extrinsic type, though a mixture of the two types may occur.

The primary clinical signs of an asthma "attack" include an increased respiratory rate, spasmodic cough, prolonged expiration with wheezing, and pulmonary hyperinflation. Initially the cough may be dry, but as secretions increase, the cough may become productive. If symptoms progress, severe bronchial obstruction may occur. The patient becomes so "tight" that little air is moving in the lungs and the patient becomes fatigued. Respiratory failure can ensue.

Standard medical treatment consists of drug therapy, primarily with bronchodilators and in severe cases corticosteroids. Environmental controls can minimize dust and other offending allergens, and reduction of emotional stress can help. Sudden cold or strenuous exercise may precipitate an attack. Hyposensitization through injection of gradually increasing doses of the offending allergens may offer some relief.

The physical therapist has much to offer the child with asthma. Outpatient treatment programs should include relaxation and controlled breathing techniques, exercises for thoracic mobility, and general conditioning exercises. Included also is parental and patient education with an emphasis on how to minimize attacks.[35,55] Treatment during an acute attack should focus on relaxation and controlled diaphragmatic breathing. Once bronchodilatation has taken place, bronchial drainage with percussion and vibration may help clear secretions. If the patient has difficulty with excessive secretions, instruction of parents or patient in bronchial drainage techniques for home care may be indicated.

Cystic fibrosis. Cystic fibrosis is the most common life-limiting genetic disease among white children.[67] It is characterized by generalized exocrine gland dysfunction. It affects many organ systems, but an elevated salt content in the sweat, chronic pulmonary disease, and pancreatic insufficiency resulting in nutritional compromise are the primary manifestations. Increased awareness of the disease and a valid diagnostic test, the sweat test, have aided in earlier recognition of symptoms and diagnosis. The clinical course of the disease is variable. However, with medical advances including appropriate antibiotic therapy and chest physical therapy to control lung infection, the life expectancy with cystic fibrosis has improved significantly, with many patients living into adulthood.[57]

Cystic fibrosis accounts for much of the chronic lung disease seen in children. Possible impairment of mucociliary transport, production of copious mucus secretions, mucus plugging of peripheral airways, recurrent infections, and eventual bronchial wall destruction all contribute to the obstructive lung disease. As the pulmonary involvement progresses, habitual coughing, abnormal distribution of ventilation, decreased pulmonary function, and weight loss compromise exercise tolerance.

Complications of the pulmonary disease include atelectasis, recurrent infection, pneumothorax, hemoptysis, and cor pulmonale.[21] Hospitalization and intensive therapy are generally indicated for control of exacerbations of pulmonary infections or other complications such as pneumothorax or massive hemoptysis.

Nutritional, pulmonary, and psychosocial needs of patients with cystic fibrosis are met through care at nationally recognized and supported cystic fibrosis centers. The physical therapist is an integral part of the medical team caring for the patient with cystic fibrosis.[60] Bronchial drainage with percussion, rib shaking, and vibration to all bronchopulmonary segments, breathing exercises and retraining, and postural and general conditioning exercise are the primary techniques incorporated into a person's treatment program. Family instruction of the various chest physical therapy techniques is essential for care at home. Normal physical activity and play should also be encouraged to promote mobilization and expectoration of secretions.

Psychosocial support needed by patients and families facing a genetically inherited and lethal disease cannot be underestimated.[42] The autosomal recessive pattern of inheritance in cystic fibrosis results in a one-in-four chance of two carriers producing a child with the disease and dictates the need for genetic counseling. With an increased number of patients living into adulthood, career and marital counseling should also be available. Finally, and most importantly, a hospital staff should be trained and prepared to offer support, care, and concern when a patient is facing deteriorating pulmonary status and terminal hospital admission or death at home.

Restrictive lung diseases

Restrictive lung disease is characterized by a reduction of lung volume caused by extrapulmonary or pulmonary factors.[18] Chest-wall stiffness, deformity, and respiratory muscle weakness can cause decreased thoracic excursion resulting in decreased lung volumes including vital capacity and total lung capacity. Loss of lung tissue caused by tumor or surgical removal, atelectasis, and pneumonia are also causes of restrictive pulmonary problems.

Some primary causes of extrapulmonary restrictive lung disease are seen in the pediatric population. The following section is a discussion of those particular disease entities.

Muscular weakness. Respiratory muscle weakness can lead to respiratory insufficiency with subsequent respiratory failure, which can be fatal especially in patients with progressive muscular diseases such as muscular dystrophy.

Inability to take deep breaths because of weak respiratory muscles can result in patchy areas of atelectasis.[39] The cough musculature can be weak, and effective removal of secretions is reduced. Patients with muscular weakness are at risk for aspiration pneumonia because of poor coordination of the muscles involved in swallowing. A hyperactive gag reflex, as seen in cerebral palsy, may cause frequent choking and aspiration.

Even when a neuromuscular disease is not progressive, skeletal and soft-tissue deformities resulting from inactivity and poor positioning can be progressive and can alter respiratory function. Decreased pulmonary reserve and the likelihood of confinement to bed or wheelchair adds to the risk of pulmonary infection for children with neuromuscular disease.

Intercostal and diaphragmatic muscle weakness, ventilatory insufficiency, chronic alveolar hypoventilation, and ventilatory failure are potential complications of muscular and neurological diseases.[39]

Many muscle diseases involve the diaphragm and the intercostals. Diaphragmatic weakness is much more disabling than intercostal weakness because of the primary inspiratory function of the diaphragm. Fortunately, in Duchenne muscular dystrophy, weakness of the diaphragm is not apparent until the end stage of the illness. In cerebral palsy, lack of neuromotor control and coordination and weakness of respiratory muscles may both be a factor in respiratory dysfunction.[49] Increasing intolerance of the supine posture is an indication of progressive diaphragmatic weakness. With a weakened diaphragm the vital capacity will decrease in the supine position and improve in the upright position.[39] These clinical signs may aid the therapist when assessing diaphragmatic function.

The volume of a voluntary deep breath and the force of a cough will be diminished with ventilatory insufficiency caused by muscular weakness. This may result in small atelectatic areas, which may reduce lung compliance.[16] Dyspnea upon exertion and accessory muscle use during inspiration are likely clinical signs.

Hypoventilation during sleep, in addition to diaphragmatic muscle weakness, can result in chronic alveolar hypoventilation. Increased $PaCO_2$ and decreased PaO_2 with evidence of cyanosis occur during sleep, with some correction obtained through conscious hyperventilation. A decrease in nocturnal hypoventilation can result in elevation of daytime arterial oxygenation and improved function.[39]

Ventilatory failure marks a serious decline in the patient's respiratory status and usually occurs in the end stage of progressive muscular diseases. The patient may be restless and confused with noticeable cyanosis and respiratory distress. Prolonged carbon dioxide retention may lead to coma and death.

Patients with muscular weakness have many physical therapy needs. Emphasis in the early stages of treatment is on improving muscle tone, maintaining strength and range of motion (including thoracic and spinal flexibility), and promoting physical function at an optimum level.

Emphasis on proper body alignment especially in sitting and recumbent positions is essential. Proper alignment may prevent deformities of the extremities, thorax, and vertebral column, which can alter respiratory function. Effective coughing and breathing exercises facilitate and maintain ventilation, chest mobility, and intercostal and diaphragmatic function. As physical function declines or confinement to a wheelchair occurs, close observation of respiratory status is important. As abdominal strength decreases, an abdominal binder or corset may help maintain a normal resting position of the diaphragm through external support.[1] The corset may also be helpful during coughing. A treatment priority is the maintenance of effective coughing through emphasis on abdominal muscle use and support and manually assisted coughing techniques. Manually assisted coughing is described in detail in Chapter 12. Parents should be taught this technique for use at home. If acute infection or chronic mucus retention occurs, a regimen of bronchial drainage with percussion and vibration must be incorporated into the treatment program.

Skeletal abnormalities

Scoliosis. Chest deformities may compromise lung function by restricting the space in which the lung must grow and function. Scoliosis can cause thoracic deformity and respiratory dysfunction in varying degrees depending on the severity of the malalignment. The size and shape of the lungs may be abnormal. Some lobes of the lung are involved more than others and the actual number of alveoli is reduced.[45] The lung in the convex hemithorax is generally the larger and most important to respiratory function.

Pulmonary function can range from normal for a patient with mild scoliosis to severely reduced in a patient with a severe rotational curve. In more advanced curves, lung volume can be affected with reductions in total lung, functional, residual, and vital capacities. In addition to reduced lung volume, decreased compliance of the lung and chest wall may occur. Bjure and others[4] believe that in patients of all ages with severe curves, premature airway closure may be a leading cause of respiratory problems.

The most common blood gas abnormality is a reduced PaO_2. Carbon dioxide tension is often normal, but it increases in older patients with scoliosis and in those with obstructive pulmonary disease.[25]

Scoliosis may be congenital, idiopathic, or associated with muscular weakness or spasticity. The patient with neuromuscular disease experiences the double insult of respiratory muscle weakness and the thoracic restriction from a scoliotic deformity.

Physical therapy in the nonsurgical management of scoliosis should always include exercises to improve deep breathing and thoracic mobility in the effort to improve ventilation and prevent atelectasis.

Operative correction of scoliosis is generally indicated for curves of 40 degrees or more in the growing child. Surgical access to the spine may be through a posterior vertebral approach or an anterior thoracotomy. Patients who undergo an anterior approach may be at higher risk for postoperative pulmonary complications because of the thoracotomy, diaphragm detachment, and lung manipulation necessary to gain access to the spine. Patients with neuromuscular disease or severe congenital curves are also at higher risk postoperatively than patients with idiopathic curves.

Patients without specific pulmonary problems postoperatively benefit from deep-breathing exercises and coughing to prevent atelectasis.[31] If secretion retention, atelectasis, or infection occurs, bronchial drainage with percussion and vibration may be indicated. Precautions should be taken when using Trendelenburg positioning. Depending on the operative procedure performed, stress on the spine must be avoided. The bottom of the bed may have to be raised on blocks to maintain straight spinal alignment. Incisional discomfort may necessitate modification of percussion or vibration.

Pectus excavatum. Pectus excavatum, or funnel chest, consists of an obvious depression of the sternum that does not appear to alter pulmonary function.[40] Surgical correction is generally done for cosmetic reasons or to alleviate cardiovascular complications when the deformity is severe. Postoperatively, the patient with a repaired pectus excavatum may need deep-breathing exercises and effective coughing to prevent atelectasis. If there is secretion retention, bronchial drainage techniques may be indicated. Patients may have an external metal strut in place to hold the sternum in the corrected position. Discussion should be held with the surgeon regarding precautions that should be observed around the operative site.

The immunosuppressed patient

Immunological deficiencies. There are several syndromes classified as immunological deficiencies. Hypogammaglobulinemia and agammaglobulinemia are two such deficiencies that the pediatric physical therapist may encounter. Patients with these disorders have increased susceptibility to infections, especially bacterial. This susceptibility is caused by a generalized or specific lack of immunoglobulins, which are important for immune function. Hypogammaglobulinemia can be transient when a young infant fails to synthesize his own immunoglobulins and is subject to recurrent infections in which the lungs are a common locus. These infants usually recover between 9 and 15 months of age.[3] However, recovery may not occur. In agammaglobulinemia, where there is a lack of all immunoglobulins, infections continue into childhood resulting in chronic otitis media, sinusitis, and bronchiectasis.

Treatment of these patients is focused primarily on prevention of infection. Physical therapy is directed toward bronchial hygiene for prophylaxis of lung infection. The resulting effects of chronic obstructive pulmonary problems, such as dyspnea, decreased exercise tolerance, and postural abnormalities must also be considered.

Bone marrow transplantation. Human bone marrow transplantation was first attempted in the late 1950s on radiation accident victims.[62] Historically, the technique has been used successfully for patients with varied immunological deficiencies, aplastic anemia, and acute leukemia. The treatment rationale is that engraftment of healthy marrow from a matched donor will provide normal marrow function to the recipient (patient) and eradication of the disease process.

In preparation for and again after bone marrow transplantation, a patient must be placed in a totally sterile atmosphere. The patient has heightened susceptibility to infection before and after transplantation until engraftment occurs. Laminar flow rooms have been designed for the purpose of isolation. The patients also undergo daily baths and bowel preparations to ensure skin and gut sterilization. Anyone entering a laminar flow room, including family, must scrub the hands and forearms with antibacterial soap and wear a surgical mask, gown, hat, and booties (Fig. 18-4). This creates a very alienating atmosphere, and it is not unusual for a patient to spend at least 2 to 3 months in a laminar flow room until successful bone marrow engraftment takes place. Rejection of the bone marrow graft and complications such as infection and graft versus host disease are the major problems of bone marrow transplantation and can result in death.[63]

Total suppression of the patient's own diseased bone marrow is required before one attempts transplantation of marrow from a matched donor. This suppression is accomplished through administration of an antilymphocyte serum and possible total body irradiation, especially if a malignant disorder exists and cancerous cells must be destroyed.

The most successful route for administration of the donor marrow to the patient is the intravenous one.[62] An intravenous or Thomas shunt is surgically inserted to connect the femoral artery to the femoral vein, which provides a route for the transplanted marrow.

The physical therapist is part of a team of medical personnel who address the complex needs of the patient having a bone marrow transplant.[68] The relationship between therapist and patient will entail weeks or months of hard work and understanding. A full physical therapy evaluation should precede the transplantation. The respiratory evaluation should be thorough, since patients with marrow diseases and a suppressed immunological system may have a history of recurrent pulmonary infections with possible chronic obstructive lung changes. A full functional evaluation of strength and range of motion should emphasize the extremity into which the shunt has been placed. The patient may protect that extremity with resultant loss of range of motion or strength. Hip movement of the shunted extremity may be restricted for 5 days after surgical inser-

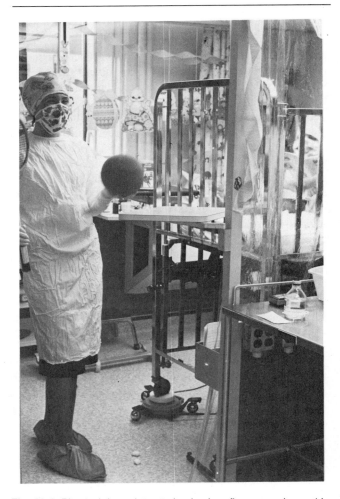

Fig. 18-4. Physical therapist entering laminar flow room dressed in surgical hat, mask, gown, gloves, and booties. She is holding a sterilized Nerf ball and badminton racket, which will be used as part of the therapeutic exercise program for a patient who has undergone bone marrow transplantation.

tion of the shunt, and guidelines regarding range of motion should be discussed with the surgeon.

The patient is at risk for infection from the point of total suppression of bone marrow in preparation for the transplant until total engraftment of donor marrow. Patients are particularly susceptible to viral illness. The most common infectious complication is interstitial pneumonia, which usually occurs after the marrow graft shows some function.[63] The most common pathogen associated with pneumonia is the cytomegalovirus. Chest physical therapy including bronchial hygiene, instruction in relaxed breathing patterns, and effective coughing are indicated. General mobility, maintenance of strength and range of motion, and encouragement of developmental milestones in the younger patient are all necessary in the rehabilitation of the restricted bone marrow transplant patient. Platelet counts will be compromised while the patient is immunosuppressed and should be considered before one institutes daily treatment. (See p. 358.)

Acute problems

Bronchiolitis. Bronchiolitis, which is commonly caused by the respiratory syncytial virus (RSV), is a leading cause of respiratory distress with wheezing in the young infant. The RSV infection usually occurs during November to March in infants under 2 years of age, with the majority being under 6 months.[46] The clinical picture is one of a preceding upper respiratory infection followed by an abrupt onset of dyspnea, retractions, tachypnea, and wheezing. A chest radiograph shows hyperinflation of the lungs with decreased lung markings. Histologically, there may be necrosis of bronchiolar epithelium with concurrent cilia destruction. Infiltration of lymphocytes into the peribronchial tissue, edema, and mucus plugging of the airways add to the problems. The poor development of collateral ventilation in the lungs of infants enhances the chance of atelectasis and decreased arterial oxygenation.

Treatment includes administration of oxygen and fluids as well as vigorous chest physical therapy. Bronchodilators are usually not effective.[46] Diminished cilia function compounded by increased necrotic tissue and mucus in the small airways dictate the need for frequent bronchial drainage with percussion and vibration as tolerated. If spontaneous coughing does not occur, nasotracheal suctioning is necessary. Wheezing should be evaluated before and after percussion techniques. If percussion causes an increase in wheezing or respiratory distress, positioning with only vibration may be effective.

There is increasing evidence that respiratory sequelae may continue through adulthood in children who have had bronchiolitis. Many of these children develop asthma, increased airway resistance, and abnormal arterial oxygen levels.[6,26,48]

Pertussis. Pertussis is an acute, contagious bacterial infection of the respiratory tract caused by *Bordetella pertussis*. The more serious respiratory manifestations are seen in children under 2 years of age.[12] It is also known as "whooping cough" because of the characteristic spasmodic cough followed by a high-pitched inspiratory "whoop." Cell infiltration and edema are present in the entire mucosal lining of the respiratory tract. Secondary pneumonia can occur causing an accumulation of pus and mucus within the alveoli. Obstruction of the airways caused by mucus, bronchospasm, and edema can cause paroxysmal coughing spells and cyanosis. The symptoms of pertussis last about 8 weeks. The paroxysmal stage, lasting 2 to 4 weeks, is the most severe. Fortunately, immunization against pertussis is available to infants and has greatly reduced the incidence of the infection.

Bronchial drainage with percussion and vibration is indicated to aid the removal of tenacious sputum and prevention of bronchial obstruction.

Aspiration. Aspiration involves inhalation of foreign matter into the lungs. The foreign material may cause local irritation and inflammation with the possibility of eventual infection. The right lower lobe is most prone to gastric aspiration, but in severe cases both lungs can be affected.[9] Neurological immaturity or insult may cause swallowing dysfunction, which can result in choking and aspiration of food or liquid. Aspiration can also accompany gastroesophageal reflux.

Mouthing objects is a means of exploration for the infant and young child, and these objects can be aspirated into the lungs. Improperly chewed food can result in choking and subsequent aspiration. Peanuts or other nuts are among the most common types of food that are aspirated.[10] The phenomenon of foreign-body aspiration and treatment has been examined over the years in many pediatric institutions.[5,10,33] The clinical manifestations are cough, wheezing, and cyanosis. Radiographic examination may show evidence of airway obstruction represented as air trapping or localized atelectasis. The small airways of children are easily blocked by foreign objects.

In the early 1970s, the usual treatment of immediate bronchoscopic removal of a foreign body was challenged by Cotton and Burrington.[5,10] They reported an 80% success rate of foreign-body removal using a combination of inhaled bronchodilator and bronchial drainage with chest percussion over a 24-hour period. In 1976, Law and Kosloske reported a study of 76 patients treated for foreign-body aspiration.[33] This later study did not confirm the high success rate of the bronchodilator inhalation and bronchial drainage regimen. Law and Kosloske suggested that a limited trial of 24 hours of bronchodilatation and bronchial drainage was of value only in the early management of foreign-body aspiration. If this early trial failed, they recommended bronchoscopy. In addition, they stated that long-standing aspiration of a month or more duration should be treated initially with bronchoscopy.

Bronchodilatation and bronchial drainage performed in the initial stage should be frequent, with vigorous percussion, vibration, and specific positioning for the affected lobe. Because of the anatomical configuration of the major airways, the majority of foreign bodies lodge in the right main bronchus and are found less frequently in the left main bronchus and trachea.

I strongly recommend bronchial drainage with percussion and vibration after bronchoscopic removal of a foreign body to clear any retained secretions or resultant acute pulmonary process.

Cotton and associates recorded cases of cardiorespiratory arrest during the therapy treatment.[10] Law and Kosloske postulated that a mobilized foreign body, especially in a main bronchus, could migrate. This migration could obstruct another bronchus or the glottis and may be accompanied by reflex bronchospasm.[33] We strongly recommend that the physical therapist carry out treatment where cardiac monitoring, oxygen, and resuscitation equipment are available.

Surgical problems

The benefits of chest physical therapy for the surgical patient have been well documented.[31] Surgical intervention in the pediatric population may result in postoperative pulmonary complications. The following discussion describes three conditions in which thoracic surgery is commonly indicated for the pediatric patient.

Cardiac anomalies. The physical therapist is an important part of the medical team caring for the infant or child who undergoes open-heart surgery for correction of cardiac anomalies. The types of anomalies and the corrective procedures are many and varied.[50]

Preoperative and postoperative physical therapy evaluation are essential.[47] Postoperative treatment should place emphasis on improving ventilation and mobilizing secretions if present. However, in some cardiac conditions, especially those involving pulmonary venous obstruction and hypertension, pulmonary congestion may be present preoperatively. These preoperative factors place the patient at a higher risk for postoperative pulmonary complications. In infants and children, pulmonary congestion may arise from valvular regurgitation, left ventricular outflow, or pulmonary venous obstruction or from any primary myocardial diseases.[58] Pulmonary venous hypertension can lead to engorgement of the pulmonary vessels with blood. Alveolar and airway mucosal edema can develop, resulting in bronchial compression, and obstruction to airflow, which leads to atelectasis and pulmonary infection. In addition to airway obstruction, pulmonary edema can lead to changes in lung surfactant and decreased lung compliance.[58] These alterations, when added to the risk of pulmonary infection and decreased lung volume because of an enlarged heart, can severely reduce pulmonary reserve. The result may be an increased work of breathing. The problems of pulmonary vascular overload can be surgically corrected. However, patients undergoing surgery may already have chronic lung changes and should be identified for vigorous treatment by the physical therapist.

Postoperative chest physical therapy for the pediatric cardiac patient should include frequent position change, breathing exercises, and instruction in effective coughing with incisional splinting or airway aspiration as necessary. Modified bronchial drainage techniques with consideration of the necessary postoperative precautions are performed only if there is secretion retention. Mobility exercises including range of motion, bed mobility, and progressive ambulation should also be part of the postoperative program.

Tracheoesophageal malformations. Malformations of the trachea or esophagus can cause respiratory distress in infancy. Tracheomalacia is a condition whereby the tracheal lumen is reduced because of absence or malformation of the cartilaginous rings of the trachea. Narrowing of the tracheal lumen becomes exaggerated during expiration because of this lack of structural support. Clinically the infant may have an increased respiratory rate, stridor, wheezing, cough, and possibly cyanosis. Increased pulmonary secretions may cause further distress and may interfere with feeding. Symptoms become exaggerated with crying. Conservative treatment is directed toward prevention of infection and management of secretions. If an infection occurs, bronchial hygiene is indicated to mobilize excessive secretions, especially before feeding. Recovery is promising as the infant grows and cartilaginous development occurs. Most clinical symptoms resolve by 6 months of age.[52]

Tracheoesophageal fistula (TEF) is a more difficult problem characterized by one or several interconnections between the trachea and esophagus. Overflow of food or liquids into the lung through these anatomical interconnections causes continued pulmonary injury and is a source for infection. This malformation comes in a variety of types and is often coincident with atresia, or absence, of part of the esophagus.

Presenting signs include significant coughing, choking, and cyanosis with the ingestion of fluids, or a history of recurrent pneumonia or upper lobe collapse. If the malformation is not diagnosed quickly, chronic pulmonary disease may occur because of continued irritation of the lungs by aspirated material.

Before and after surgical corrections through a lateral thoracotomy, many infants with tracheoesophageal fistual have lengthy hospitalizations. Upright positioning is necessary if gastroesophageal reflux is also present. After surgery, oral feeding is postponed, and deep endotracheal suctioning is contraindicated until suture healing occurs.

The physical therapist is often involved before diagnosis and after surgical correction. Pulmonary care is directed toward maintaining bronchial hygiene and resolving pulmonary infection. Developmental stimulation for gross motor and oral function also becomes a necessary part of the treatment.

Congenital lobar emphysema. Although uncommon, congenital lobar emphysema is one of the few reasons for a lobectomy in an infant.[59] The cause is unclear, and it appears that some infants are born with a larger than normal lobe of the lung. The lower lobes are rarely involved. The syndrome may represent a development abnormality of the alveoli or a multialveolar lobe where the number of alveoli is up to five times that of normal.[45] The emphysematous lobe will usually compress and displace the remaining lung causing varying degrees of atelectasis and diaphragmatic compression on the ipsilateral side. Mediastinal shift may also be present with atelectasis and compromise of the contralateral lung. The degree of respiratory distress will vary depending on the severity of the emphysema.

Immediate surgical correction is recommended. This involves thoracotomy and removal of the emphysematous lobe. The prognosis for these children is very good, and many are free of serious pulmonary problems or infections with recovery of normal lung volume and size postoperatively.[37]

PATIENT EVALUATION
Considerations

Approaching a sick infant or child is often a difficult task. As I have mentioned, children are often fearful of any procedures and may be overstimulated and stressed by the hospital environment. Evaluation and treatment of an infant or child must always include a thorough explanation to the family and patient of the physical therapy procedures. This explanation should be in clear, simple language. Capturing the cooperation and understanding of the family members and patient is important.

Techniques

The evaluation techniques of observation, inspection, palpation, auscultation, measurement, and interview are not only used for the adult respiratory patient, but are also applicable to the pediatric patient. However, depending on the age of the child, the therapist may have to rely more on acute observational skills to gather necessary information. Actual handling of an infant or child may increase anxiety and alter evaluative findings. Always be cognizant of the temperature of your hands and stethoscope. Cold hands on a warmly swaddled infant can begin a stress reaction of crying and increased respiratory rate. A pediatric patient may not be able to verbalize about the level of comfort or anxiety. Noting general posture and whether speech is even or gasping can help determine the level of comfort during an evaluation of respiratory status. A physical therapist can gather much information regarding the infant or child by observation without any manual contact.

Interviewing techniques also take on added importance during an evaluation of a pediatric patient. If the child is young, a therapist must depend on information from parents based upon their understanding and perception of their child's pulmonary problems. Questions should be asked that require several word answers not just yes or no. Phrase questions to avoid suggesting signs or symptoms. For example, do not say "Do you think your child experiences shortness of breath or tires easily with active play?" but rather "What are your child's favorite activities?" A response of "watching television" or "reading books" may indicate a limited activity level. More additional information, of course, would be necessary to confirm this suspicion. Good interviewing technique can be extremely beneficial in constructing a detailed patient profile.

A comprehensive evaluation

Before any chest physical therapy evaluation, it is important to obtain a complete medical and surgical history through chart review, interview, and physician communication. Emphasis should be placed on the history of the respiratory illness, arterial blood gases, chest radiograph findings, and pulmonary function tests. Pulmonary function tests are generally not done with a child under 6 years of age because of lack of cooperation and understanding of the procedures.[38]

If the patient is hospitalized, nursing progress notes and discussion with the patient's nurse provides current information about the child's status and vital signs over the previous 24 hours. Proper identification of all equipment and lines attached to and around the patient is important. If the patient is acutely ill, mechanical ventilator settings, electrocardiograph, and vital sign recordings must be noted.

Respiratory evaluation

Observation of the patient, without laying on hands, provides information regarding skin color, respiratory rate, nasal flaring, breathing pattern, chest symmetry, and general comfort. Observation of an infant can easily be done from the bedside. However, a toddler or older child may become anxious just by seeing someone approach the bed. Therefore comfort and posture, color, and breathing pattern and rate may be observed from a distance before one approaches the child.

Once contact is made with the patient, there should be a simple explanation of what is to be done. Initially, efforts to reduce fear and anxiety take precedence over therapeutic tasks.

The following summary of evaluative findings are specific to the pediatric patient and will aid the clinician:

Respiratory rate. The pulmonary mechanics of the infant and child are such that the resting respiratory rate is higher than in the adult. Respiratory rate is generally slower during sleep. This difference is more pronounced in the younger child.[53] The average respiratory rate for an awake, normal infant in the first year of life ranges between 30 and 40 breaths per minute. There will be a sharp decline in the rate during the second year to about 25 to 30 breaths per minute. A slow, steady fall in rate continues through childhood (20 to 25 per minute) and adolescence (15 to 20 per minute) when the rate approaches the adult level.[65]

Respiratory rate should be determined with the child relaxed and unaware of its being recorded. Respiratory rate can be observed at a distance from a child or while one is presumably taking a pulse. Observation of thoracic excursions is usually sufficient to obtain a respiratory rate, though the stethoscope may be used on the chest of a sleeping child. The rate should be taken for a full minute for accurate measurement.

Pulse rate. Pulse rate can vary among children and can be altered by activity level or stress. A newborn's heart rate is between 100 and 160 beats per minute. From 1 to 4 years of age the rate can range from 80 to 120 beats per minute. As the child approaches adolescence, the pulse rate becomes comparable to the adult range of 60 to 80 beats per minute.[53] It is most important to monitor any sudden change or irregularity in heart rate. If the heart rate rises or drops significantly in response to treatment, this change should be noted and reported. Modification or discontinuation of the treatment session may be appropriate.

Breathing pattern. Retractions are a sign of increased inspiratory effort. A common occurrence in infants, whose chests are more compliant than those of older children, is depression of the lower sternum accompanying a labored inspiration. Intercostal retractions, if present, may indicate decreased compliance or airway obstruction. Suprasternal retractions may indicate an upper airway obstruction such as croup. Subcostal retractions may indicate flattening of the diaphragm and diffuse lower airway obstruction.[19]

Intercostal bulging during expiration may be present when air trapping occurs because of airway narrowing as seen in asthma, cystic fibrosis, or bronchiolitis. This bulging represents increased expiratory effort.

During respiration the synchronization between the upper chest and abdomen should be observed. Normally, both areas should expand on inspiration. When an infant is distressed, a ''seesaw'' phenomenon occurs in which the upper chest expands during inspiration while the abdomen is pulled inward and the reverse occurs during expiration. Accessory muscles are recruited for use during a labored inspiration. The neck flexors, particularly the sternocleidomastoid, are commonly used to augment inspiration. The use of these muscles by an infant can be noticed by head bobbing. The child's head will bob forward during inspiration as the neck flexors contract. This action is particularly apparent when the child is held with the neck flexors placed in a shortened position. Nasal flaring is another indicator of increased work of breathing and is often present during accessory muscle use.

Disruption of normal breathing patterns, grunting, postural splinting, or agitation upon movement may accompany chest pain or discomfort in an infant or child.

Auscultation. Interpretation of breath sounds is the same for children as for adults. However, the ease with which auscultation can be accomplished may be altered by the child's respiratory rate or cooperation. Breath sounds often appear louder in an infant or child when compared to an adult's because of the proximity of the child's airways to the skin surface. The breath sounds of a child are often audible during both inspiration and expiration. Crying can alter the sound, allowing clearly heard inspiratory sounds but muffled expiratory sounds. Wheezing in an infant often originates in the major airways because of their small diameter compared to adult airways. Secretions

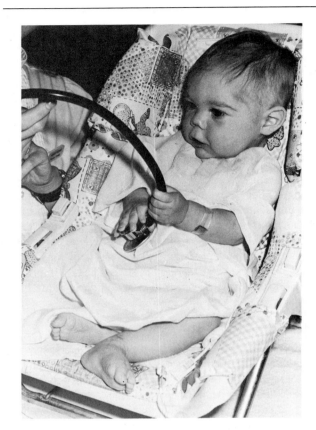

Fig. 18-5. This infant is given the opportunity to see and feel the stethoscope before it is used for auscultation.

in any part of the respiratory tree may be audible throughout the chest. The examiner must rule out upper airway sounds, which may be transmitted to other parts of the chest. Expiratory grunting can be heard either through the stethoscope or with the unaided ear.

The technique of auscultation of an infant or child's lungs is similar to that of an adult. The following suggestions should be kept in mind. Before placing the diaphragm or bell of the stethoscope on the child's chest, always make sure it is warm. Give the child the opportunity to see and feel the stethoscope (Fig. 18-5). Explain simply what you are going to do and that it will not hurt. Demonstrating auscultation on a doll or favorite toy may ease the child's fears. Stethoscopes designed specifically for pediatric patients are commercially available. Some believe that although small stethoscopes offer no acoustic superiority, they accommodate a small chest better.[53]

Functional and developmental assessment

Developmental assessments should always be part of the physical therapy evaluation of an infant or young child. Evaluation should be postponed until the child is free from stressful respiratory symptoms. Respiratory distress can al-

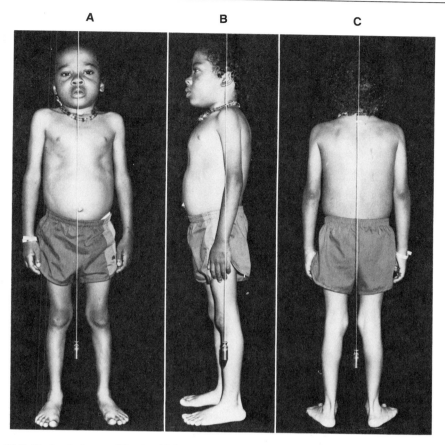

Fig. 18-6. Postural abnormalities in child with cystic fibrosis. **A,** *Anterior view.* Notice that the shoulders are held high especially on the right, a posture that appears to allow better mechanical advantage to the accessory muscles for breathing. The lower ribs are flared, and the thorax appears barreled and elongated because of the hyperinflation of the lungs. A full postural evaluation might reveal other less obvious abnormalities. **B,** *Lateral view.* The thoracic kyphosis and barreled chest seen here are common findings in children with obstructive pulmonary disease and hyperinflation of the lungs. **C,** *Posterior view.* The shoulders appear high with protraction of the scapulas. Notice the enlargement of the thorax in relation to the rest of this patient's body. Pronated feet are also noticeable.

ter muscle tone and the patient's normal activity level. Premature infants are often at risk for developmental delay and other subtle neurological manifestations. Consider the weeks of prematurity when determining the developmental age. Parents can provide helpful information about their child's developmental level before the illness.

A gross- and fine-motor assessment with evaluation of cognitive and social skills is important. Feeding and oral motor evaluations should also be performed on infants with respiratory problems. Respiratory illness and excessive secretions can make breathing while sucking or eating very difficult and may diminish nutritional intake. The child may appear to suck weakly or swallow poorly. Weak or spastic oral musculature and abnormal sucking, swallowing, or gag reflexes must be ruled out.

A functional assessment including an activities-of-daily-living (ADL) survey is important when one is evaluating

an older child or adolescent. These ADL surveys offer much insight into what extent the respiratory problem limits function. Specific questions regarding favorite play, sports activities, and hobbies can indicate a child's exercise tolerance. Children often lack the fear of becoming overfatigued that adult respiratory patients may harbor. A child with a respiratory problem will often function within his or her physical capability being limited only by overprotective parents.

Postural assessment

Postural alignment is often altered by an underlying respiratory disease. A postural evaluation should be carried out with any respiratory patient, especially a growing child. Muscle groups that are often tight or weak are the pectorals, scapular, neck, low back, and anterior hip, and the hamstring tendons. Hyperinflation of the lungs, often seen in the obstructive lung diseases, such as cystic fibrosis, can result in an increased anteroposterior thorax diameter and rigid barrel chest. The tight musculature in combination with a rigid, enlarged chest can greatly reduce thoracic excursion and spinal flexibility. Rigid deformities can result in thoracic spine kyphosis and functional or rotational scoliosis (Fig. 18-6). Postural abnormalities can further compromise pulmonary function. Discovering and treating these abnormalities before growth has ceased can possibly modify their progression.

Strength and range-of-motion assessment

Alterations in gross muscle strength and joint range of motion are seen in patients with chronic lung disease. Emphasis on evaluation of trunk musculature, especially the abdominal, back extensor, and scapular musculature, is indicated. Good abdominal strength is important for effective coughing. Back extensor and scapular musculature may be weak because of a kyphotic posture. Decreased range of motion from tight musculature may be evident in the neck and shoulders, especially in children with chronic pulmonary problems.

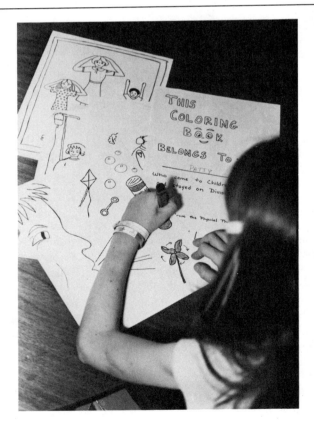

Fig. 18-7. Coloring book designed for use in preoperative teaching of the pediatric cardiac surgical patient.

Home program assessment

Evaluation of patient and family compliance with treatment is an important part of the home program assessment. Answers to specific questions regarding frequency and length of treatments provide insight into compliance and involvement of the family.

The following are examples of questions that should be asked:

1. Is any chest physical therapy done at home?
2. Can you describe the type of treatment?
3. How often is the treatment carried out? If it is daily, what time or times of the day?
4. How long does it take to do a treatment?
5. Does anyone help the patient with treatment, or does the patient do the treatment alone?
6. Is any special equipment used to aid in treatment? Describe the equipment.
7. Are any aerosol medications taken before or after treatment?
8. When was the last time a physical therapist reviewed the home program or therapy techniques?
9. Are there any specific problems with the home treatment program, i.e., with scheduling, performing treatment techniques, compliance, etc.?

Evaluation of the surgical patient

A preoperative physical therapy evaluation may be requested for a patient who is scheduled for major abdominal or thoracic surgery. Postoperative pulmonary complications are common, and the benefit of postoperative chest physical therapy are well documented.[31,47] A full respiratory, functional, and postural evaluation should be done. The therapist should understand the type of surgery to be performed, the surgical approach, the anticipated muscle or bone resections, and the respiratory and musculoskeletal limitations expected after surgical intervention. The evaluation session should also include an explanation to the parents and patient of the rationale for and demonstration of postoperative chest physical therapy. Preoperative explanation of postoperative procedures is extraordinarily important in pediatric care to help allay fears of the child or parents. A child, regardless of age, is entitled to explanations of the surgical experience. Fig. 18-7 is an example of a coloring book designed by Sylvia Dick, R.P.T., for preoperative instruction in chest physical therapy for the cardiac patients at Children's Hospital, Boston. This type of resource gives the child an opportunity to understand in a very nonthreatening way, the procedures he or she will experience.

PATIENT TREATMENT
Considerations

One of the challenges of chest physical therapy is capturing the cooperation of the pediatric patient. Imagination and patience are the keys to holding the attention of a child and obtaining the desired results. Once rapport is established, treating a child is both enjoyable and rewarding.

When one is treating children, many modifications and alternative treatment approaches have to be employed to accommodate small chests and bodies, alter behavior, allay fears, and respond to unpredictable changes in status. Treatment of the pediatric patient also presumes the importance of parents and family in the care of their child.

Techniques
Positions for breathlessness

Positions for the breathless patient should promote comfort and increase relaxation. The positioning should encourage mobility of the thorax and support of the spinal column. Hip flexion should be incorporated to relax the abdominal area and aid in increasing intra-abdominal pressure for coughing. Data suggest that postural relief for dyspnea may be related to an improved length-tension state of the diaphragm, which may increase its efficiency.[56] Some suggested positions for children who experience dyspnea are shown in Fig. 18-8. Diaphragmatic breathing with pursed-lips expiration combined with these illustrated positions should be taught to all patients who experience shortness of breath. Asthmatics, especially, can utilize these techniques during wheezing episodes to possibly avoid stressful attacks.

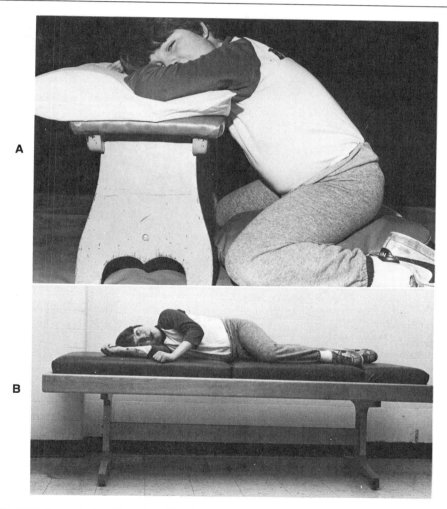

Fig. 18-8. Suggested positions for relief of dyspnea.
At home: **A,** Relaxed forward kneeling or sitting position with the upper chest supported on a pillow and the spine straight, allowing free excursion of the abdominal area for diaphragmatic breathing. **B,** Lying on one side either flat or propped up on three or four pillows. Hips and knees should be flexed with the top leg in front of the one underneath. Shoulders should be relaxed and spine straight.

Continued.

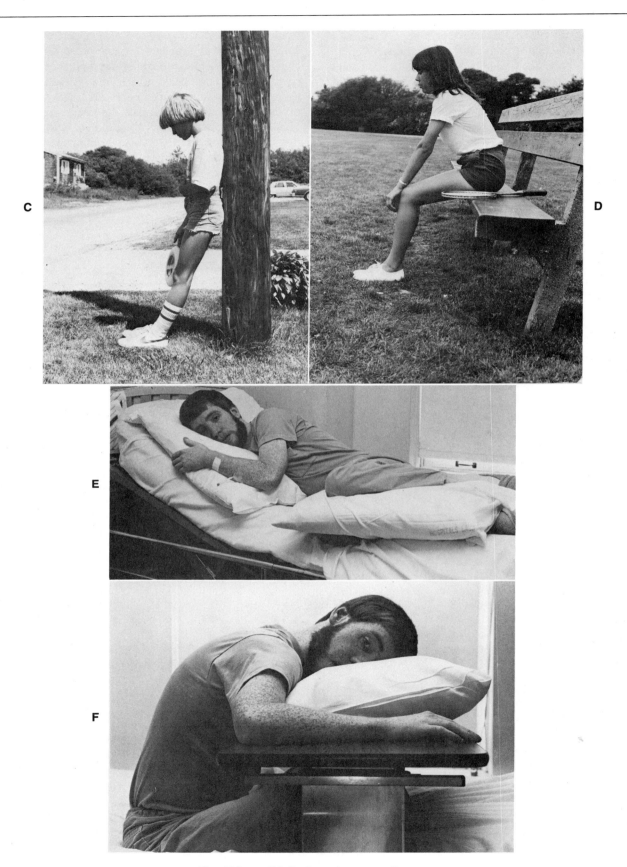

Fig. 18-8, cont'd. For legend see opposite page.

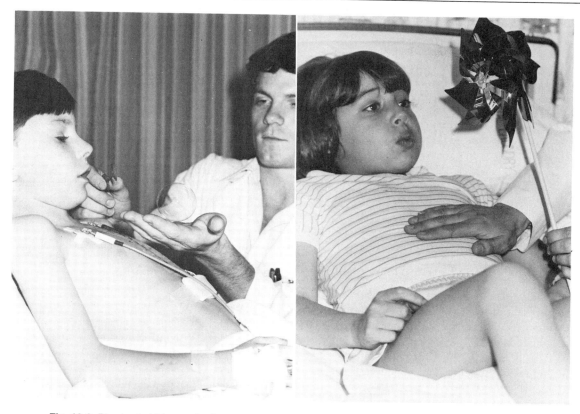

Fig. 18-9. Blowing bubbles or pinwheels can be fun for a child while also encouraging deep breathing.

Deep-breathing exercises and retraining

The cognitive level of a patient will dictate the ability to execute deep-breathing exercises. With infants, a therapist must rely on neurophysiological facilitation techniques such as quick stretching of the diaphragm and intercostals to obtain an increased contractile response of these muscles for inspiration.

Toddlers and young children may begin to participate in blowing games when they can imitate and voluntarily take a deep breath. This ability usually begins around 2 years of age. Some suggested blowing games are shown in Fig. 18-9.

Older children like adults can be taught deep-breathing exercises by using manual contact and verbal reinforcement. Before children are engaged in deep-breathing exercises it is useful to establish an understanding of their thoracic anatomy. Ask them to locate their lungs, ribs, and abdomen. If they are unsure, a simple explanation will enhance their understanding of deep breathing and augment their physical response to the exercises. Placing a small toy on the upper abdomen and asking the child to gently raise the toy up toward the ceiling on inspiration may promote use of the diaphragm. The therapist should be aware of any muscle substitutions for diaphragmatic contraction on inspiration. The child may attempt to raise the abdomen by thrusting the abdominal muscles outward by arching the lower back.

Fig. 18-8, cont'd. *During play or sports activities:* **C,** Leaning back against a telephone pole or wall, spine straight and supported with relaxed neck and shoulder muscles and slight hip flexion. **D,** Forward sitting position with a straight spine and relaxed neck and shoulder muscles, the wrists or forearms resting on the thighs.
In the hospital: **E,** High side-lying position with head elevated 45 degrees, hips and knees flexed with pillow between the knees, relaxed neck and shoulder muscles, small pillow under waist to straighten the spine. **F,** Forward leaning over bed tray, upper chest supported on a pillow, neck and shoulders relaxed, hips flexed.

Breathing retraining with utilization of paced breathing techniques should not be overlooked for the pediatric population. Patients with cystic fibrosis, especially those with advanced disease and dyspnea during functional activities, can benefit from breathing control techniques. First, carefully assess particular activities that cause breathlessness. The patient should be instructed in controlled and paced diaphragmatic breathing while lying, sitting, standing, walking, and stairclimbing. Once this sequence is mastered, the patient can practice combining paced breathing with simulated activities such as carrying a weighted load to imitate handling schoolbooks. Breathing control should be taught to the younger patient who complains of dyspnea during bike riding, play, or sports activities. Paced breathing techniques can be used with any patient old enough to understand the concept of regulating breathing rate and pattern with physical activity.

Bronchial drainage, percussion, vibration, and shaking

Modifications of these techniques will vary depending on the age and condition of the patient. Regardless of the size of the patient, adaptation of the therapist's hand position can accommodate any size of chest. A tented position of the fingers is recommended for small infants. One hand can accommodate a toddler and young child's chest (Fig. 18-2, *C*). The force of the percussion, vibration, and shaking will also vary with the age and condition of the patient. Since an infant's chest is more compliant than an adult's, the force of manual techniques should be of less magnitude. My opinion is that manual techniques, rather than adapted or mechanical equipment, are highly recommended with infants and young children. Use of the hands allows easier monitoring of the force of the technique. Rib shaking is generally reserved for an older child or patient with a rigid chest as is often seen with advanced cystic fibrosis. Coordinating manual vibration with the expiratory cycle of an infant who breathes at a rapid respiratory rate is difficult. Therefore short rapid bursts of vibration coordinated as well as possible with expiration is recommended.

Bronchial drainage positioning for the infant and toddler is often performed on the therapist's lap. Transition from the lap to a drainage table or bed is recommended when the child is approximately 2 years old or too large to handle comfortably and safely on the lap. Lap positioning with suggested hand positioning for the different lung segments is shown on infants in Chapter 17.

Frequent position changes (approximately every 2 hours) are recommended for the child or infant who is unable to move independently, or is being mechanically ventilated. Changing position not only promotes pulmonary drainage, but also alleviates skin pressure to prevent decubiti. The benefits of position changes for the bedridden patient have been reviewed by Kigin,[31] Zadai,[69] and Hyland.[23] Position changes that promote bronchial hygiene

are shown in Fig. 18-10. These positions are used in combination with percussion and vibration when modified bronchial drainage positioning is necessary.

Coughing techniques

Eliciting a voluntary cough from a pediatric patient can be a challenge. Refusal to cough may stem from fear, pain, or just not being in the mood. Much time may be spent trying to convince a strong-willed child that it is important to cough. Instead, success may come by making coughing a game. For example, a child can be motivated to cough by earning a colorful star on a "cough score sheet" for each good cough. The child can then proudly display these efforts to parents, doctors, and nurses. Children who enjoy drawing are told that each time they cough, they may draw part of a face or object. The therapist then guesses who or what has been drawn! Huffing techniques to promote coughing can be performed during the story of the big bad wolf who "huffed and puffed and blew the house down." Imaginative approaches often work when a more straightforward approach has failed.

To ease the discomfort or fear of coughing for surgical patients, have them splint their incision with a favorite stuffed animal or teach the parents to give a gentle hug with incisional support. Children will usually not welcome manual incisional support from the therapist (Fig. 18-11, *A*). Patients who have spasmodic coughing episodes or thickened secretions may benefit from manual compression or vibration over the midsternal area to facilitate sputum expectoration (Fig. 18-11, *B*).

The technique of tracheal stimulation or tickling can be used for young patients who do not understand the concept of coughing. It is recommended only if the therapist is trained in the technique and the child is not unduly distressed by the maneuver. The stimulation is performed by placement of the index finger or thumb on the anterior side of the neck against the trachea, just above the sternal notch. A gentle, but firm inward pressure in a circular pattern as the patient begins to exhale may elicit a reflex cough. Fig. 18-12 shows finger placement for tracheal tickling.

Endotracheal suctioning is often needed to stimulate coughing and raise secretions in the intubated and acutely ill infant or child. When large amounts of secretions are present, suctioning may be needed both during and after therapy.

General mobility

Whenever an ill infant's or toddler's status allows, bronchial drainage using the therapist's lap is preferable to treatment in bed. Regardless of lines or tubes attached to the child, holding a sick infant during therapy is encouraged. The tactile stimulation may be quite comforting.

Range-of-motion exercises to maintain joint mobility

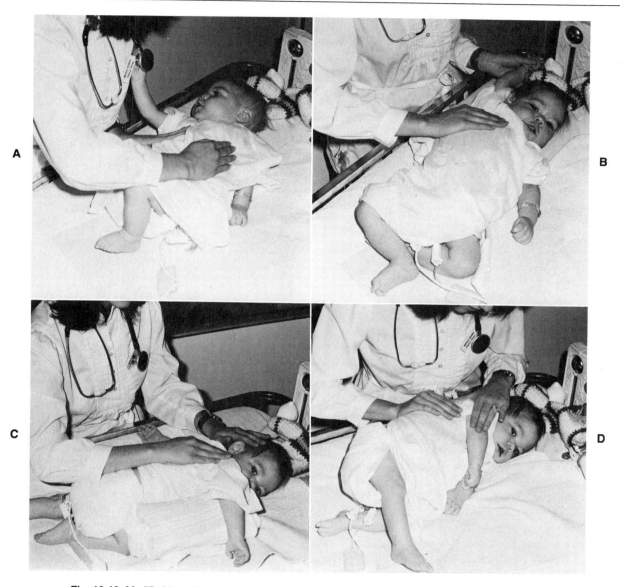

Fig. 18-10. Modified bronchial drainage positions. **A,** Anterior segments of the upper and lower lobes can be drained in a supine position. **B,** Right middle lobe or the lingula segment can be drained by positioning in a one-fourth turn from supine. **C,** The posterior segments of the upper and lower lobes can be drained in a three-fourth prone position. **D,** The lateral segments of the lower lobes can be drained in a side-lying position.

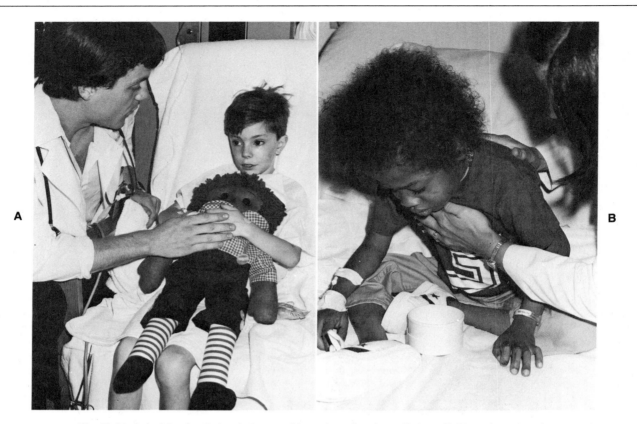

Fig. 18-11. A, Incisional splinting during coughing using a favorite stuffed toy. **B,** Manual compression over the midsternum to facilitate sputum expectoration.

should always be part of chest physical therapy when the patient is unconscious or bedridden.

Early mobility should be stressed for the postoperative patient. Emphasis is placed on mobility in bed immediately after surgery with ambulation when indicated (Fig. 18-13). Specific range-of-motion exercises of a joint near an incisional site is often necessary. Thoracic surgical patients especially need help with motion of the upper extremity on the side of the thoracotomy. Thoracic mobility exercises to prevent muscular tightness and enhance thoracic excursion for deep breathing are also a necessary part of the postoperative program. Children who are aware that they have had surgery often assume a rigid posture. During gait there is a lack of proper spinal alignment, hip and knee flexion, and arm swing. Infants and toddlers without postoperative anxieties often move more freely than older children.

Musculoskeletal mobility, particularly of the thorax and shoulder girdle, is important to the patient with respiratory dysfunction. Decreased range of motion and tight muscles in the shoulder and thorax can create ineffective patterns of ventilation and increased work of breathing. Exercises should emphasize mobility of the spine, thorax, and shoulder girdle in coordination with deep breathing. Making the exercising fun is very important in pediatrics. Games like "Simon Says" or songs like "The Itsy-Bitsy Spider" or "Bend and Stretch" can be quite appealing. Ball games can promote both upper extremity and thoracic mobility. Exercising to music geared toward the age level of the child or adolescent can also be quite successful.

Physical exercise and conditioning

Exercise intolerance is common in chronic respiratory diseases and is most likely related to decreased pulmonary function. This intolerance can be a source of frustration and sadness for children with lung disease who cannot physically emulate their peers. Increasing evidence indicates that physical exercise and conditioning can benefit children with chronic respiratory diseases. Limited evidence exists for similar benefit for those children with respiratory dysfunction attributable to primary neuromuscular diseases. These studies and programs have recently been reviewed.[28,61]

Swimming programs appear to be most successful with

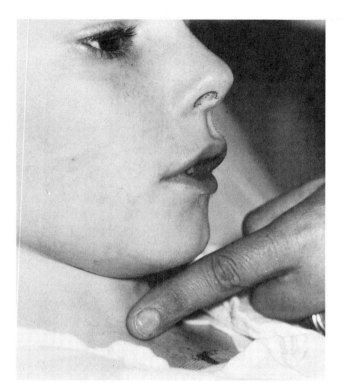

Fig. 18-12. Finger placement for tracheal "tickle" maneuver.

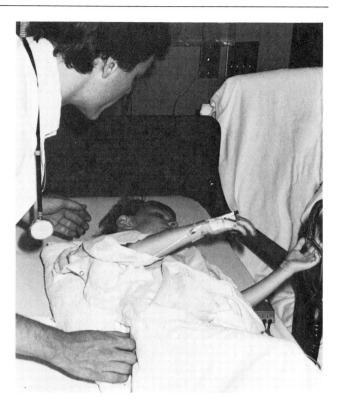

Fig. 18-13. Independent mobility in bed should be emphasized for the postoperative patient.

asthma patients, since swimming is less conducive to exercise-induced bronchospasm (EIB) than free running is. Mallinson and others reported improvements in general health and peak expiratory flow rates of children with asthma participating in a twice-weekly exercise and swim program.[35] The duration and intensity of the exercise is also a factor in exercise-induced bronchospasm (p. 358).

Orenstein and others recently demonstrated the effects of a 3-month running program on 21 patients with cystic fibrosis.[41] These patients, who trained three times a week, had improved exercise tolerance and peak oxygen consumption. In addition, heart rates were lower for submaximal work loads. A control group of 10 patients showed none of these improvements.

Recent evidence has shown that it is possible to specifically strengthen and increase endurance of the respiratory muscles.[34] A maneuver utilizing rapid and deep breathing known as the maximal sustainable ventilatory capacity (MSVC) can be used to train respiratory muscles.[29] The equipment necessary for this specific training is not currently available to the clinician. The traditional method of utilizing a series of weighted objects on the epigastric area to offer resistance to diaphragmatic excursion is often not an appealing form of exercise for a younger child. A study

by Keens and associates indicated that a group of patients with cystic fibrosis who participated in 4 weeks of daily physical activities such as rowing and swimming had more improvement in their MSVC than two control groups who did specific MSVC training.[29] Based on this limited work, upper extremity conditioning may offer respiratory muscle strengthening and endurance in addition to being more fun for a child than specific respiratory muscle training.

Planning a physical exercise program for a patient with respiratory problems can be based on the patient's physical needs and activity interests. Remind the patients that performing regular physical exercise will increase their ability to do more exercises. The vicious cycle of inactivity resulting in decreased endurance and greater inactivity can be broken. Patients will have, one would hope, more confidence in their physical abilities and improved endurance that will expand their daily activity level.

Before a general conditioning exercise program is planned for a patient, it would be ideal for the patient to undergo exercise and pulmonary function testing. Exercise testing should assess peak heart rate response to exercise. A target heart rate during exercise of 75% to 80% of the predicted peak heart rate is the goal for conditioning effects. If exercise testing is not available, a low-intensity program monitoring the pulse and respiratory rates before, immediately after, and 5 minutes after exercise will offer values by which the intensity of the exercise program can be varied. Generally, an increase in intensity of exercise should be in small increments. One to 2 minutes of additional exercise per session or per week is a reasonable increment depending on the patient's tolerance. Controlled breathing should always be emphasized during exercise. Improved physical conditioning will provide the pediatric patient with a better self-image to feel more socially acceptable. The patient's jogging shoes and bathing suits will have that look of regular use!

Before and after the conditioning exercises, a warm-up and cool-down phase of exercise must be done. The warm-up phase should emphasize stretching, flexibility, and deep breathing. The cool-down phase can include walking or slow stretching exercises. These exercises can be coordinated to music for more fun. Warm-ups for the younger population could include a ball-throwing game. Games that involve total body movements and are fun would appeal to the youngsters.

If it is difficult to include a patient in a structured exercise program, physical exercise can take a freer form with encouragement for daily physical activity such as walking. If the benefits of regular physical activity are carefully explained, a patient may be more compliant with the regimen.

Postural exercises

As discussed on p. 347, postural abnormalities are often present in patients with chronic respiratory disease. Thoracic surgical patients are also at risk for developing postural problems because of large thoracic incisions, muscle resections, and incisional splinting from pain. Postural exercises for the respiratory patient should emphasize stretching for the pectorals and anterior hip muscles and strengthening for the scapular, upper back extensor, and abdominal muscles. One can perform thoracic spine flexibility exercises sitting in front of a mirror to provide visual feedback and promotion of pelvic stability.

If scoliosis is suspected, an orthopaedic surgeon should be consulted to assess the severity of the curve and presence of a rotational component. An exercise program should be based on the surgeon's findings. Deep breathing is always coordinated with any exercises performed by a respiratory patient.

Treatment precautions

There are few absolute contraindications or reasons to discontinue chest physical therapy. The risks and benefits of modifying or discontinuing a treatment because of a precarious situation should be carefully weighed and discussed with the patient's physician. Certain modifications of treatment techniques and precautionary measures should be considered when the therapist encounters the following

nine situations. These guidelines will be helpful in making sound decisions.

Respiratory or cardiac instability

Respiratory or cardiac instability may require modification of positioning. Positioning to tolerance attempting to achieve a level horizontal position is recommended with careful monitoring of skin color, respiratory rate, and heart rate.

Severe gastroesophageal reflux

Supine and Trendelenburg positioning may enhance gastroesophageal reflux (GER) (p. 336). The severity of a child's GER and the need for flat or Trendelenburg positioning for therapeutic bronchial drainage must be carefully considered with the physician. Modified bronchial drainage in an upright position may be necessary for children with severe GER with treatments scheduled before feedings.

Hemoptysis

Hemoptysis, or coughing up blood, is one of the complications of chronic lung disease. It is often seen in older patients with advanced cystic fibrosis.[21] Fresh blood streaking of sputum is common in patients with cystic fibrosis because of inflammation of the bronchial mucosa with resultant venous bleeding with no further consequence. However, there is great concern when the patient coughs up larger volumes of blood with evidence of little or no sputum. The amount of hemoptysis can range from a teaspoonful to several cupsful, the latter being a medical emergency. Patients will often describe a feeling of "warmth" or "gurgling" in one area of the chest before the hemoptysis. Hemoptysis can occur anytime and is not always related to strenous activity or vigorous coughing. Some patients complain that they bleed when in a head-flat position, but are fine when upright.

Most modifications of treatment involve bronchial drainage techniques and vary with each patient based upon the amount of bleeding and precipitating factors. A patient who raises only 5 to 10 ml of blood but whose sputum is clear of blood with subsequent coughing may not need the treatment altered. However, if the bleeding continues, vigorous percussion and positions that appear to induce bleeding should be avoided. Depending on the amount of hemoptysis, breathing exercises, modified positions, vibration, and instruction in controlled, effective coughing may continue. A patient who is not receiving some form of chest physical therapy may find that coughing becomes difficult and strained, thereby, imposing added intrapulmonary pressures on inflamed and bleeding bronchial walls. Therapy will aid in mobilizing blood and secretions from the airways so that the effort of coughing is reduced. Full treatment may be resumed once the active bleeding has stopped and should emphasize clearance of retained

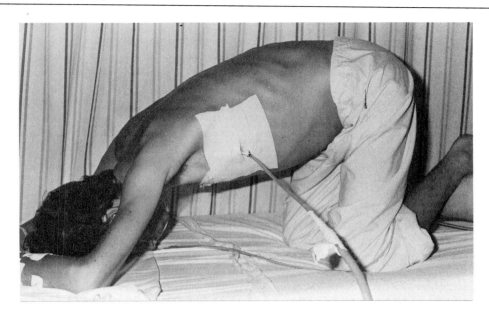

Fig. 18-14. Alternative position for the posterior segments of the lower lobes in a patient with a chest tube. This position would be particularly recommended for a patient who has anterior placement of a chest tube.

secretions and blood from the airways. It is crucial for the therapist to reassure the patient that continued, careful re-evaluation of the patient's status will occur during treatment, with necessary modifications made as indicated. Discussion and education of the physician regarding the chest physical therapy management of a patient who has experienced hemoptysis is important. Decisions should be based on individual situations, and the importance of modified, but continued, physical therapy should be stressed to the physician.

If the patient has a large hemoptysis, the therapist should help the patient into an upright position. A basin into which the patient can expectorate should be quickly provided. Above all, the patient should be encouraged to relax as much as possible with slow controlled breathing to avoid a rise in blood pressure. Never leave the patient, but notify the physician as soon as possible.

Pneumothorax

Pneumothorax can occur as a complication of cystic fibrosis, severe asthma, or any pulmonary problem necessitating mechanical ventilation with high inspiratory pressure. Chest physical therapy is contraindicated in the presence of an untreated, progressing, or tension pneumothorax. Treatment can continue with a small, stable pneumothorax and with a pneumothorax that has resolved through treatment with a thoracostomy and insertion of a chest tube for vacuum drainage of air.

A patient with a chest tube in place has some discomfort. Scheduling of treatment after pain medication is recommended. If bronchial hygiene is needed, percussion should not be performed directly over the chest-tube site, but percussion to tolerance is acceptable elsewhere on the thorax. If subcutaneous emphysema is present, percussion is often uncomfortable and vibration is recommended. Depending on the site of chest-tube placement, modification of some bronchial drainage positions may be necessary to ensure chest-tube patency at all times. Pressure on or kinking of the tube must be avoided (Fig. 18-14). An understanding of the negative-pressure treatment apparatus is important for recognition of the presence of air leaks.

Although dislodgment of a chest tube from the chest is a rare circumstance, if it should happen, apply immediate pressure to the thorax at the chest-tube site. If the tubing ever becomes disconnected from the negative-pressure apparatus, immediately clamp the portion of tubing inserted into the chest. All these measures will prevent the reaccumulation of air in the pleural space.

Bronchoconstriction

There has been some concern that manual chest techniques, particularly percussion, can increase bronchoconstriction during treatment.[7] However, Huber and associates studied 21 asthmatic children, 11 of whom received bronchial drainage including percussion and vibration. The treated group demonstrated a 40% increase in forced expiratory volume in 1 second at 30 minutes after treatment. The control group showed no improvement. Huber and associates concluded that bronchial drainage techniques were not detrimental for mildly to moderately obstructed asthmatic patients.[22] However, the use of percussion should be carefully considered during treatment of patients with asthma or others who have a bronchospastic component to their disease. These patients may benefit from an aerosol bronchodilator before and possibly during treatment to reduce the risk of increased bronchoconstriction. Auscultation of the chest before and immediately after percussion can be used to monitor increased wheezing. The patient may also complain of feeling "tighter." With evidence of increased bronchoconstriction, bronchial drainage and only vibration with controlled coughing may allow the safe continuation of treatment. Sound judgment in choosing the appropriate techniques and the use of a bronchodilator may help reduce the risk of increased bronchospasm.

Exercise-induced bronchospasm (EIB) is a recognized and common complication of asthma in childhood.[15,27] Kahn and Olson reviewed the subject in relationship to physical therapy in 1975.[30] Several studies have indicated that certain types of exercises are more likely to cause bronchospasm. The consensus is that activities involving running are more likely to cause EIB than cycling. Swimming may be the least likely cause of EIB.[17,24] The severity of EIB also appears to relate to the rate of work and duration of exercise.[15,17] Jones and co-workers found that short-term exercises of 1 to 2 minutes in duration caused bronchodilatation, but longer exercise of 4 to 12 minutes resulted in bronchoconstriction.[24] These factors should be considered when one is planning an exercise program for children with asthma or other bronchospastic problems. Exercises of short duration interspersed with relaxation should be planned for the asthmatic child.

Decreased platelet counts

Children who have decreased production of platelets (thrombocytopenia) are predisposed to bruising. Platelets are essential for the maintenance of the integrity of the capillary walls. Platelets also donate substances that aid in coagulation or clotting. The normal platelet count is approximately 259,000 platelets per cubic millimeter of blood. Patients with acute leukemia may have platelet counts of less than 50,000. A severely traumatized or ill patient may experience disseminated intravascular coagulation with a resultant drop in platelets. Vigorous techniques such as chest percussion could cause bruising in a pediatric patient with a significant decrease in platelets. Guidelines for percussion to be discontinued should be established for patients with low platelet counts. A guideline proposed at Children's Hospital, Boston, is as follows: if the platelet count is greater than 50,000, percussion is acceptable with caution; counts between 20,000 and 50,000 dictate the use of vibration and positioning for bronchial drainage only; below 20,000 only bronchial drainage is used. Breathing exercises and coughing may continue regardless of the platelet level.

Increased intracranial pressure

Position changes, especially placing the head downward, cause an increase in the intracranial pressure (ICP). Percussion techniques and suctioning may have the same effect on the intracranial pressure. In certain conditions, such as surgery or trauma to the head and Reye's syndrome, the control of intracranial pressure is essential.

Intracranial pressure can be recorded constantly through the placement of cranial monitoring bolts. Through discussion with the physician, the maximum intracranial pressure allowed during physical therapy interventions should be established. If the intracranial pressure becomes significantly elevated, limitations on positioning changes and percussion may have to be imposed.

Surgical precautions

Because of the size of pediatric patients, some postoperative precautions may be necessary. Percussion techniques used over thoracic incisions will cause the patient great discomfort. Because of the highly compliant developing thorax, percussion is also avoided over the anterior chest of a child having had a recent midsternal incision. This precaution is not only to reduce discomfort but also to prevent the seesaw effect of percussion on the incisional area. Vibration within the child's tolerance is acceptable if indicated. Percussion is also avoided on the anterior chest of any patient with an unstable open sternum caused by a wound infection. The sternal area, in this case, should be supported manually during treatment.

Physical therapy is usually not initiated in postoperative pediatric cardiac patients until after intracardiac monitoring lines have been removed. These delicately placed lines are inserted intraoperatively in the patient's left atrium, right atrium, and pulmonary artery to monitor hemodynamic values postoperatively. Because of the small size of the child's heart and importance of the monitoring lines, excessive external pressure on the chest should be avoided while the lines are in place. Treatment may be initiated after removal of the lines, unless a major pulmonary problem dictates earlier intervention.

Osteoporosis

Children with advanced or severe paralytic conditions may develop thin, osteoporotic bones. A lack of the normal muscular forces exerted on the bones can compromise the integrity and strength of the bony matrix. Osteoporosis or fragility of the ribs may occur in children with paralysis. With evidence of thoracic osteoporosis, caution should be employed with percussion or vigorous shaking techniques.

DISCHARGE AND HOME CARE
Discharge planning

In an acute care setting, a pediatric patient's status can change quickly, and many patients can substantially improve in a few days. Therapists working in an acute care facility know only too well that a decision for discharge can be made quickly and with little time for preparation and planning. Although this may sound premature, discharge planning should begin the first day of treatment, especially if a need for home care or follow-up physical therapy is anticipated. A specific plan of treatment cannot always be determined early in the hospitalization, but the process must begin so that with a quick decision for discharge, home treatment planning, and family instruction is possible. Always schedule a return appointment in 1 to 2 weeks for review of the home instructions.

Early contact between the therapist and family or other primary caretaker is ideal. Several sessions, if possible, should be scheduled for parental and patient instruction. Discharge planning and home instructions carried out under severe time constraints will be frustrating for both the therapist and family. Early planning is particularly important when the patient has been diagnosed to have a chronic illness such as cystic fibrosis. It is important to allow time for careful assessment of the family's abilities to carry out the necessary treatment. This assessment will help in determining a family's need for community support. Community physical therapists can help monitor a family's or patient's performance of the treatment at home and can direct care if necessary.

Part of discharge planning also involves good communication with other medical team members for the patient. Taking part in and offering necessary input at discharge planning meetings is essential.

Home care

A physical therapist's primary responsibility regarding home care is to plan a comprehensive and realistic program and to instruct and educate those involved.

When planning a home program of chest physical therapy for an infant or child, the therapist must remember that the treatment regimen will be in addition to daily routine child care. Parenting is a difficult task, and appreciation of the daily stresses for a family with a handicapped child provides an essential framework in which to plan appropriate treatment.

Practical suggestions regarding scheduling and duration of treatment are always greatly appreciated by the family. Involvement of both parents, responsible siblings, and relatives may help ease the treatment burden. If the patient is older, encouraging responsibility for self-care will diminish the dependency on parents.

A family may have the added burden of caring for more than one child with a respiratory dysfunction. Cystic fibrosis is an inherited disease, and often more than one child in a family is afflicted with the disease. Reviewing family histories of patients with asthma may also reveal other siblings who have the disease.

Although the ultimate responsibility of home respiratory care rests with the family, community support may help ease the stress on the family. Qualified physical therapists working for either a home health agency or privately can help evaluate a family's or patient's performance of the treatment or can offer direct care as necessary. Private insurance policies or state aid through crippled children's programs may pay for or supplement the cost of these treatments.

For patients with cystic fibrosis or other chronic lung diseases, daily chest physical therapy may be indicated from the time of diagnosis throughout the patient's life. As children grow, they face many critical stages of emotional development and life-style changes. It is no surprise then that a constant routine in one's life, such as chest physical therapy must also "weather the storm" of emotional crises. The physical therapist must be aware of these critical periods during which treatment schedules and components may have to be modified. Additional guidelines and support may be needed to promote family or patient compliance with treatment. The following discussion presents critical stages during which families or patients may need review of chest physical therapy skills as well as reevaluation and revision of treatment plans.

The resistant toddler

It is a difficult time for parents who are earnestly attempting to comply with treatment but are meeting great resistance from their small, but rebellious toddler. This is the appropriate time to make the transition from bronchial drainage on the lap to a bed or drainage table. This change will ease management of the child in different positions, and should add to the child's feelings of independence. The idea of having a special place to do therapy might be quite appealing. Treatment time may have to be altered to accommodate shorter attention spans. It is better to do a shorter, effective treatment than a lengthy, emotionally exhausting treatment on a crying, squirming child. The therapist should suggest dividing the bronchial drainage treatment into two or three shorter sessions rather than one long session. Simple effective methods to increase the attention span of the child during treatment may include reading or telling the child a favorite story, watching an appealing television show, or listening to a musical recording. A sibling can often be recruited to keep a brother or sister entertained during treatment.

The concept of coughing should be introduced early, between 2 and 3 years of age, and encouraged as a vital part of treatment. Blowing games can be used effectively in early childhood to aid in improving ventilation (Fig. 18-9).

The most important thing for young children with respiratory problems to learn is that therapy is a regular event in their lives. Consistency is important. As soon as the regularity or routine of the therapy is disturbed, cooperation of the child may be lost.

Issues regarding the school-aged child

When a child is ready for school, treatment schedules must be arranged accordingly. If treatment is needed before school, additional time for this must be provided. A therapist may be helpful in organizing a treatment session for the early morning that is more directed and focused upon problem areas of the lungs.

School absenteeism, which is often high in children with respiratory diseases, is another concern. The child may struggle to keep up with the class, adding to feelings of alienation. Children who fatigue easily or need chest physical therapy at midday may not be able to complete a full day of school and must attend part time. Efforts to teach a school nurse or other responsible adult bronchial drainage techniques could be useful in providing a midday treatment that might allow full attendance.

A child will often work hard to suppress coughing to avoid embarrassment and may return from school very congested and fatigued. Therapists should reinforce the importance of coughing when necessary. If a child is adamantly against coughing in the classroom, suggesting the lavatory as a private place for coughing may be helpful.

Activity and sports, within tolerance, should be encouraged. Parents can be reassured that physical exercise is good and aids in mobilizing secretions. Guidelines for the child with exercise-induced bronchospasm can be suggested.

The rebellious adolescent

Coping with a respiratory illness during the adolescent years can become challenging for all concerned. The emphasis on physical appearances in adolescence can create much stress for the teen-ager with lung problems. Adolescents with cystic fibrosis often experience weight loss from nutritional problems. Barrel chests and digital clubbing may be obvious in patients with more advanced chronic lung disease. These physical changes are hard to hide. A chronic cough and frequent illnesses can further alienate the adolescent from peers whose acceptance is so important.

It is no surprise that teen-agers frequently express anger about their disease. This anger may take the form of rebellion and noncompliance with the treatment regimen. Medications may not be taken. This noncompliance can be detrimental for the asthmatic who must maintain a therapeutic level of medication to control wheezing and a severe bronchospastic attack may result. Chest physical therapy is the treatment against which the child most often rebels. Treatments are time consuming and often re-

quire the participation of a parent or other authority figure. This reliance on others becomes a threat to independence.

The physical therapist must be acutely aware of how these issues affect compliance with therapy. Instruction in self-care techniques should begin when the patient is both interested in and responsible for carrying out self-care. Twelve or 13 years of age is often appropriate to begin teaching bronchial self-drainage techniques with either manual or mechanical percussion, as discussed in the next section. Self-drainage with percussion can be easily attained for all anterior and lateral bronchopulmonary segments. Percussion for posterior segments often requires the aid of another person. However, some mechanical percussors are designed to allow access to areas of the upper back. Parents must be reassured that instructing adolescents in self-care may help sustain compliance without compromising the effectiveness of treatment. Even though the adolescent may assume some responsibility for care, he or she may still need and seek out the encouragement that only a parent can offer. Adolescent patients may need both support and independence.

Emphasis should also be placed on designing an acceptable treatment program that encourages compliance and independence without compromising therapeutic goals. When discussing therapy with a teen-ager, the therapist should not lecture about the necessity of pulmonary care but should allow some compromise and decision making on the part of the patient. For example, an agreement may be reached whereby a trial period of 3 months of routine therapy is tried by the patient. If there is benefit noted from the regimen, the patient may take it upon himself to continue on a regular basis. It should be suggested that therapy can be done while the patient is watching television or listening to music. Headphones can allow appreciation of music while diminishing the sounds of chest percussion!

If an adolescent is totally opposed to the regimen of bronchial drainage, a regular program of physical exercise can aid sputum removal and improve conditioning.[66] This may be more socially acceptable to the adolescent. A firm commitment on the part of the therapist to therapeutic goals with sensitive consideration of the needs of the adolescent may spell success.

The college-bound or working young adult

As a teen-ager matures and grows toward college age and young adulthood, other issues surface. The patient faces a decision to leave the security of family life to begin living independently. The young adult living independently has the total responsibility of care. The demands of a college program can mean physically and mentally rigorous schedules. Patients with more advanced lung disease often experience a decline in their health because of the stress of school. Hospitalizations may interfere

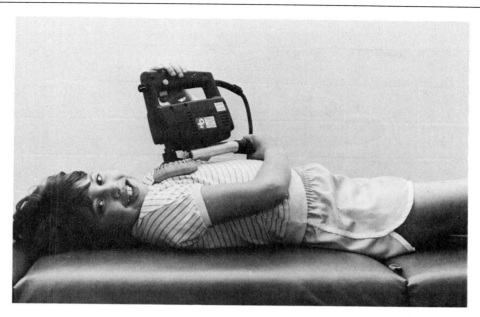

Fig. 18-15. Patient using mechanical percussor over anterior segment of right upper lobe.

with classes and exams. Keeping up with academic and social schedules of classmates can be difficult and can lead to dropping out of school temporarily or permanently.

The therapist may help by organizing a realistic treatment schedule and suggesting and demonstrating the use of a mechanical percussor to ease the stress of self-drainage. Arranging treatments through a hospital near campus, home health agency, or student health facility on campus may be helpful. An understanding roommate or college friend can be taught the skills of percussion and vibration. Many patients, however, do not want to burden friends or reveal the needs imposed upon them by their illness, and the latter suggestion may be rejected.

The young adult with lung disease often finds job hunting difficult. Describing a chronic illness to a prospective employer may be difficult, and many questions may be asked. Once a job is begun, the patient is faced with the stress of staying well to meet the responsibilities of the job. Therapy, which becomes even more important, may be more difficult to schedule into a busy day. Careful scheduling, organization of treatment time, and planning more directed treatment for involved areas of the lung may become necessary.

Friendship, dating, and marriage

Friendship, dating, and marriage bring another significant person into the life of a patient. This important person can offer much support and help and should be encouraged to take part in the care of the patient. A close

friend may be willing to learn various chest physical therapy techniques to help a patient who is living independently or refuses family support. A dating partner may also be willing to assist and encourage chest physical therapy. Instructing and educating a prospective spouse in therapy techniques is important to the future marital relationship when a patient needs pulmonary care at home. It is healthy for prospective spouses to understand and accept the daily demands of their partner's illness before the marriage. Spouses are often more enthusiastic about regular treatments than patients themselves and can make significant contributions to the maintenance of optimum health of their partner. Often it is the patient's reluctance to accept assistance rather than the partner's lack of enthusiasm to help that stands in the way of effective care.

Equipment suggestions
Mechanical percussors and vibrators

Mechanical devices that approximate chest percussion and vibration are available for home use. The most commonly used are mechanical percussors. These are designed with a small motor that drives a shaft onto which attaches a padded cupshaped head. Most percussors of this type weigh approximately 3 pounds. The padded head is placed on a designated area of the chest, and the motor will drive the shaft up and down. The head will then rhythmically strike the chest to provide percussion (Fig. 18-15). The speed of the shaft is variable creating diversified amounts of force on the chest. There are many types of percussors

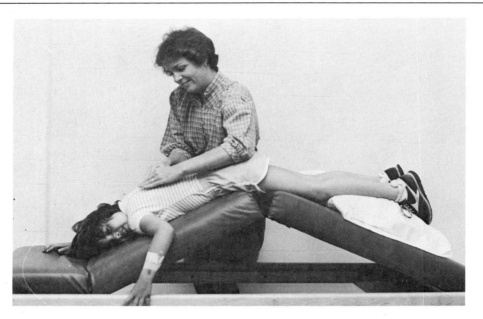

Fig. 18-16. Bronchial drainage table.

including smaller models that are accommodated to a child's chest.

There are some questions of the effectiveness of mechanical percussion versus manual percussion. Study results have been limited and variable.[13,36,44] I believe that manual techniques are preferable over mechanical means for providing chest percussion especially for the younger child. Manual percussion allows more sensitivity for the therapist regarding forces on the chest. Monitoring the force of percussion is very important when one is working with small, compliant chests. However, the mechanical percussor has its place in the care of patients requiring bronchial drainage. The percussor offers independence to some patients who, because of choice or circumstances, cannot employ manual percussion. Percussors are portable and can be taken on trips or to college. Parents may elect to use mechanical means to administer percussion and vibration because they lack the ability or physical dexterity to perform manual skills.

Mechanical vibrators are also commercially available. However, they can create sliding of the skin over the rib cage rather than the quick up and down force of manual vibration.

Before deciding to purchase a mechanical percussor or vibrator, the patient and parents should both see and try the machine to be sure it is sufficient. The device should be easy to use and should offer the desired results. Careful evaluation of the mechanics, effectiveness, and comfort of the apparatus during use is necessary before a machine is purchased.

Drainage tables

Bronchial drainage tables are commercially available and are designed to offer comfortable positioning for both the patient and the parent administering treatment. Various degrees of head-down positioning can be obtained with most tables. Examples of a type of table made expressly for the purpose of bronchial drainage is shown in Fig. 18-16. Many talented parents have been able to design and construct their own table once they understand the principles of bronchial drainage.

Money spent buying equipment such as mechanical percussors and bronchial drainage tables is often reimbursed, at least in part, by third-party payers. Justification by the physician for the equipment may be required before payment is approved.

Home positioning methods

Therapists must be prepared to offer suggestions on ways to accommodate Trendelenburg positioning for home drainage if a family is unable or chooses not to purchase a drainage table. Fig. 18-17 shows a few ideas that can be adapted for home use.

Follow-up

It is important to schedule a follow-up visit with patients and parents who have been instructed in a chest physical therapy home program. Reevaluation of the patient's status, compliance, and ability to carry out a home treatment program can take place at the follow-up visit.

Components of the treatment program can be reviewed

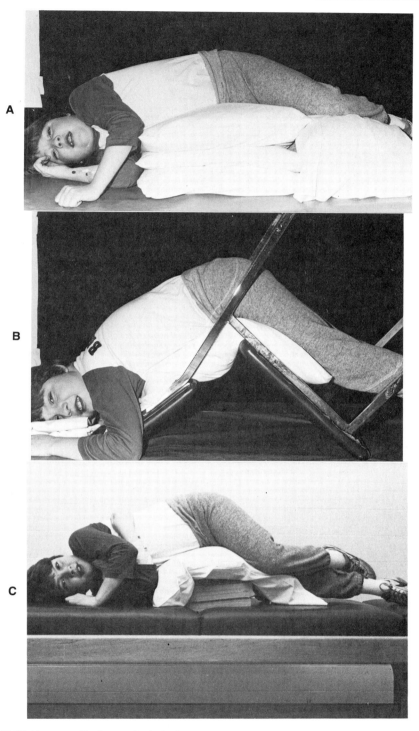

Fig. 18-17. Home positioning methods for bronchial drainage. **A,** Bed pillows. **B,** Desk chair. **C,** Stack of magazines with bed pillow.

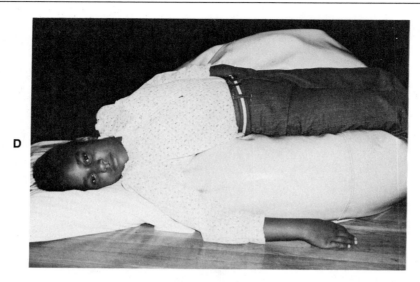

Fig. 18-17, cont'd. D, Bean-bag chair.

as needed. The follow-up visit also helps promote communication between the therapist, patient, and family. Additional outpatient appointments at established intervals may be indicated as the therapist deems necessary. The first follow-up appointment after discharge or initial instruction in the home program should be scheduled for 1 to 2 weeks later.

If distance or transportation prevents a return outpatient visit, follow-up can be arranged through a local facility or home health agency.

Role of physical therapist in the pediatric outpatient clinic

The role of the physical therapist in a cystic fibrosis or pulmonary specialties outpatient clinic is usually consultative. The physical therapist is part of the team made up of physicians, nurses, social workers, nutritionists, and psychologists.

Therapists who act as consultants to outpatient clinics should have specialized knowledge of the physical therapy management of pediatric patients with pulmonary disorders. They should demonstrate the ability to assist physicians in determining when chest physical therapy is indicated and then suggest appropriate referrals.

They should carry out interviews with patients and parents and introduce them to the role of chest physical therapy in the management of their child's specific lung problem. Therapists should be prepared to answer any questions regarding chest physical therapy.

The physical therapy consultant may be responsible for arranging physical therapy appointments for instruction or review of home programs. They should also have a comprehensive knowledge of chest physical therapy resources available in surrounding communities and coordinate follow-up or home care with outside agencies as necessary.

It is recommended that the physical therapist attend team conferences, offer input on total patient management, and teach the other medical professions about chest physical therapy.

REFERENCES

1. Alvarez, S.E., Peterson, M., and Lunsford, B.R.: Respiratory treatment of the adult patient with spinal cord injury, Phys. Ther. **61:**1737, 1981.
2. Anderson, S., and others: Comparison of bronchoconstriction induced by cycling and running, Thorax **26:**396, 1971.
3. August, S., and Elis, E.F.: Disorders of immune mechanisms. In Kempe, C.H., Silver, H.K., and O'Brien, D., editors: Current pediatric diagnosis and treatment, ed. 3, Los Altos, Calif., 1974, Lange Medical Publications.
4. Bjure, J., and others: Respiratory impairment and airway closure in patients with untreated idiopathic scoliosis, Thorax **25:**451, 1970.
5. Burrington, J.D., and Cotton, E.K.: Removal of foreign bodies from the tracheobronchial tree, J. Pediatr. Surg. **7:**119, 1972.
6. Burrows, B., Knudson, R.J., and Lebowitz, M.D.: The relationship of childhood respiratory illness to adult obstructive airway disease, Am. Rev. Respir. Dis. **115:**751, 1977.
7. Campbell, A.H., O'Connell, J.M., and Wilson, F.: The effect of chest physiotherapy upon the FEV_1 in chronic bronchitis, Med. J. Aust. **1:**33, 1975.
8. Charnock, E.L., Fischer, B.J., and Doershuk C.F.: Development of the respiratory system. In Lough, M.D., Doershuk, C.F., and Stern, R.C., editors: Pediatric respiratory therapy, ed. 2, Chicago, 1979, Year Book Medical Publishers, Inc.
9. Clutario, B.C., and Holzman, B.H.: Uncommon diseases, extrapulmonary diseases, system diseases, and toxins. In Scarpelli, E.M.,

Auld, P.A.M., and Goldman, H.S., editors: Pulmonary disease of the fetus, newborn and child, Philadelphia, 1978, Lea & Febiger.

10. Cotton, E.K., and others: Removal of aspirated foreign bodies by inhalation and postural drainage, Clin. Pediatr. **12:**271, 1973.

11. Doershuk, C.F., Fischer B.J., and Matthews, L.W.: Pulmonary physiology of the young child. In Scarpelli, E.M., editor: Pulmonary physiology of the fetus, newborn, and child, Philadelphia, 1975, Lea & Febiger.

12. Eller, J.J.: Infections: bacterial and spirochetal. In Kempe, C.H., Silver, H.K., and O'Brien, D., editors: Current pediatric diagnosis and treatment, ed. 3, Los Altos, Calif., 1974, Lange Medical Publications.

13. Flowers, K.A., and others: New mechanical aid to physiotherapy in cystic fibrosis, Br. Med. J. **2:**630, 1979.

14. Ford, T.: Personal communication, Boston, 1982.

15. Ghory, J.E.: Exercise and asthma: overview and clinical impact, Pediatrics **56**(suppl.):844, 1975.

16. Gibson, G.J., and others: Pulmonary mechanics in patients with respiratory muscle weakness, Am. Rev. Respir. Dis. **115**(3):389, 1977.

17. Godfrey, S., Silverman, M., and Anderson, S.: The use of treadmill for assessing exercise induced asthma and the effect of varying severity and duration of exercise, Pediatrics **56**(suppl.):893, 1975.

18. Gold, M.: Restrictive lung disease, Phys. Ther. **48:**455, 1968.

19. Gundy, G.H.: Physical examination. In Gundy, J.H.: Assessment of the child in primary health care, New York, 1981, McGraw-Hill Book Co., Inc.

20. Herbst, J.J.: Gastroesophageal reflux, J. Pediatr. **98:**859, 1981.

21. Holsclaw, D.S.: Common pulmonary complications of cystic fibrosis, Clin. Pediatr. **9:**346, 1970.

22. Huber, A.L., Eggleston, P.A., and Morgan, J.: Effect of physiotherapy on asthmatic children, J. Allergy Clin. Immunol. **53:**109, 1974. (Abstract.)

23. Hyland, J.: Neonatal and pediatric therapy. In Frownfelter, D., editor: Chest physical therapy and pulmonary rehabilitation, Chicago, 1978, Year Book Medical Publishers, Inc.

24. Jones, R.S., Wharton, J.J., and Bustong, O.H.: The effect of exercise on ventilatory function in the child with asthma, Br. J. Dis. Chest **56:**78, 1962.

25. Kafer, E.R.: Respiratory and cardiovascular functions in scoliosis and the principles of anesthetic management, Anesthesiology **52:**339, 1980.

26. Kattan, M., and others: Pulmonary function abnormalities in symptom free children after bronchiolitis, Pediatrics **59:**683, 1977.

27. Kattan, M., and others: The response to exercise in normal and asthmatic children, J. Pediatr. **92:**718, 1978.

28. Keens, T.G.: Exercise training programs for pediatric patients with chronic lung disease, Pediatr. Clin. North Am. **26:**517, 1979.

29. Keens, T.G., and others: Ventilatory muscle endurance training in normal subjects and patients with cystic fibrosis, Am. Rev. Respir. Dis. **116:**853, 1977.

30. Khan, A.V., and Olson, D.L.: Physical therapy and exercise induced bronchospasm, Phys. Ther. **55:**878, 1975.

31. Kigin, C.M.: Chest physical therapy for the postoperative or traumatic injury patient, Phys. Ther. **61:**1724, 1981.

32. Kübler-Ross, E.: On death and dying, New York, 1969, The Macmillan Publishing Co., Inc.

33. Law, D., and Kosloske, A.M.: Management of tracheobronchial foreign bodies in children: a reevaluation of postural drainage and bronchoscopy, Pediatrics **58:**362, 1976.

34. Leith, D.L., and Bradley, M.: Ventilatory muscle strength and endurance training, J. Appl. Physiol. **41:**508, 1976.

35. Mallinson, B.M., and others: Exercise training for children with asthma, Physiotherapy **67:**106, 1981.

36. Maxwell, M., and Redmond, A.: Comparative trial of manual and mechanical percussion technique with gravity-assisted bronchial drainage in patients with cystic fibrosis, Arch. Dis. Child. **54:**542, 1979.

37. McBride, J.T., and others: Lung growth and airway function after lobectomy in infancy for congenital lobar emphysema, J. Clin. Invest. **66:**962, 1980.

38. McBride, J.T., and Wohl, M.E.B.: Pulmonary function tests, Pediatr. Clin. North Am. **26:**537, 1979.

39. Newsom-Davis, J.: The respiratory system in muscular dystrophy, Br. Med. J. **36:**135, 1980.

40. Nolan, S.P., and others: Letter: Does pectus excavatum cause functional disability? J. Thorac. Cardiovasc. Surg. **71:**148, 1976.

41. Orenstein, D.M., and others: Exercise conditioning and cardiopulmonary fitness in cystic fibrosis, Chest **80:**392, 1981.

42. Patterson, P.R., Denning, C., and Kutscher, A.: Psychological aspects of cystic fibrosis: a model for chronic lung disease, New York, 1973, Columbia University Press.

43. Proceedings of the special session of the fourth meeting of the PAHO Advisory Committee on Medical Research, 1965: Deprivation in psychobiological development, Pub. No. 134, Washington, D.C., 1966, Pan American Health Organization–World Health Organization.

44. Pryor, J.A., Parker, R.A., and Webber, B.A.: A comparison of mechanical and manual percussion as adjuncts to postural drainage in treatment of cystic fibrosis in adolescents and adults, Physiotherapy **67:**140, 1981.

45. Reid, L.: The lung: its growth and remodeling in health and disease, Am. J. Roentgenol. **129:**777, 1977.

46. Reynolds, E.O.R.: Bronchiolitis. In Kendig, E.L., editor: Pulmonary disorders, vol. 1, Philadelphia, 1972, W.B. Saunders Co.

47. Rockwell, G.M., and Campbell, S.K.: Physical therapy program for the pediatric cardiac surgical patient, Phys. Ther. **56:**670, 1976.

48. Rooney, J.C., and Williams, H.E.: The relationship between proved viral bronchiolitis and subsequent wheezing, J. Pediatr. **79:**744, 1971.

49. Rothman, J.G.: Effects of respiratory exercises on the vital capacity and forced expiratory volume in children with cerebral palsy, Phys. Ther. **58:**421, 1978.

50. Sade, R.M., Cosgrove, D.M., and Casteneda, A.R.: Infant and child care in heart surgery, Chicago, 1977, Year Book Medical Publishers.

51. Sahler, O.J.Z., editor: The child and death, St. Louis, 1978, The C.V. Mosby Co.

52. Salzberg, A.M.: Congenital malformations of the lower respiratory tract. In Kendig, E.L., editor: Pulmonary disorders, vol. 1, Philadelphia, 1972, W.B. Saunders Co.

53. Scarpelli, E.M.: Examination of the lung. In Scarpelli, E.M., Auld, P.A.M., and Goldman, H., editors: Pulmonary diseases of the fetus, newborn and child, Philadelphia, 1978, Lea & Febiger.

54. Schowalter, J.E.: The reaction of caregivers dealing with fatally ill children and their families. In Sahler, O.J.Z., editor: The child and death, St. Louis, 1978, The C.V. Mosby Co.

55. Seligman, T., Randel, H.O., and Stevens, J.J.: Conditioning program for children with asthma, Phys. Ther. **50:**641, 1970.

56. Sharp, J.T., and others: Postural relief of dyspnea in severe chronic obstructive pulmonary disease, Am. Rev. Respir. Dis. **122:**201, 1980.

57. Shwachman, H., Kowalski, M., and Khaw, K.T.: Cystic fibrosis: a new outlook, Medicine **56:**129, 1977.

58. Talner, N.S.: Congestive heart failure. In Moss, A.J., editor: Heart disease in infants, children, and adolescents, Baltimore, 1968, The Williams & Wilkins Co.

59. Tapper, D., and others: Polyalveolar lobe: anatomic and physiologic parameters and their relationship to congenital lobar emphysema, J. Pediatr. Surg. **15:**931, 1980.

60. Tecklin, J.S., and Holsclaw, D.S.: Cystic fibrosis and the role of the physical therapist in its management, Phys. Ther. **53:**386, 1973.

61. Tecklin, J.S.: Physical therapy for children with chronic lung disease, Phys. Ther. **61:**1774, 1981.

62. Thomas, E.D., and others: Bone marrow transplantation (part 1), N. Engl. J. Med. **292:**832, 1975.

63. Thomas, E.D., and others: Bone marrow transplantation (part 2), N. Engl. J. Med. **292:**895, 1975.

64. Turner, J.M., and others: Elasticity of human lungs in relation to age, J. Appl. Physiol. **25:**664, 1968.

65. Waring, W.: The history and physical examination. In Kendig, E.L., editor: Pulmonary disorders, vol. 1, Philadelphia, 1972, W.B. Saunders Co.

66. Wilbourn, K.: The lung distance runners, Runner's World, p. 62, Aug. 1978.

67. Wood, R.E., Boat, T.F., and Doershuk, C.F.: State of the art: cystic fibrosis, Am. Rev. Respir. Dis. **113:**833, 1976.

68. Young, C.: Physiotherapy in bone marrow grafting, Physiotherapy **64:**274, 1978.

69. Zadai, C.C.: Physical therapy for the acutely ill medical patient, Phys. Ther. **61:**1746, 1981.

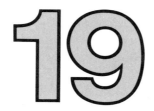

CYNTHIA COFFIN ZADAI

Rehabilitation of the patient with chronic obstructive pulmonary disease

PULMONARY REHABILITATION

Chronic obstructive pulmonary disease (COPD) is one of the major health problems in this country today. The disease is found in up to 20% of American adults over 40 years of age. Its financial impact was estimated in the 6-billion-dollar range in 1976.[51] Additionally, cystic fibrosis is the most prevalent congenital inherited disease in this country today. It affects one in every 2000 live births in the U.S.A. Morbidity and mortality associated with this disease is exclusively related to pulmonary complications.[49] Pulmonary disease is both prevalent and expensive because it affects the pediatric, adult, and geriatric populations.

Treatment for persons with disease that compromises the pulmonary system has historically been directed toward correction of the acute complications that frequently hospitalize these patients. Pneumonia and respiratory failure are often the admitting diagnoses when medical therapy is sought. Both acute and long-term therapy have focused on prevention and treatment of these acute exacerbations with medication and adequate rest. Once the acute episode was resolved, the patients were commonly left on their own to "stay healthy." Rehabilitation programs for pulmonary patients were random, inconsistent and varied. Over the last 100 years therapeutic measures have included such treatments as diathermy, various forms of mechanical assists to breathing, and "total rehabilitation programs" including breathing exercises, bronchial hygiene, and exercise in an effort to cure, correct, or control the underlying physiological abnormalities of COPD.[17,18,54] As early as 1901, breathing exercises were used in treatment programs for patients with bronchiectasis and bronchial affections.[16] In 1915, health care workers used exercise as a therapeutic mode for soldiers with pulmonary complications of war injury.[33] From the 1930s through the 1960s physical therapists treating pulmonary patients employed various

breathing exercises and physical conditioning programs in an attempt to reverse or stabilize the chronic progressive debilitation of COPD.[17,23,52] Nonetheless, this population of patients with COPD remained a depressingly debilitated group destined to a sedentary existence. As recently as the mid-1970s researchers could document only an improved feeling of well-being as the major gain in a pulmonary rehabilitation program that included exercise.[28] In 1974, the American College of Chest Physicians' Committee on Pulmonary Rehabilitation met, discussed the total care of this patient group, and adopted the following:

Pulmonary rehabilitation may be defined as an art of medical practice wherein an individually tailored, multidisciplinary program is formulated which through accurate diagnosis, therapy, emotional support and education, stabilizes or reverses both the physio- and psychopathology of pulmonary diseases and attempts to return the patient to the highest functional capacity allowed by his pulmonary handicap and overall life situation.[41]

This perspective acknowledges pulmonary disease as an entity that requires comprehensive medical management. This definition includes emotional support and education in addition to stating the long-term goal of highest possible functional capacity. It assumes that although research findings of the past may not have been able to document measurable physiological change with various rehabilitation programs these patients are entitled to comprehensive care and the resultant functional improvements.[10,38,53] This perspective is distinctly different from the expectation that pulmonary function will change with rehabilitation or that the disease process will be arrested.

In 1981, the American Thoracic Society incorporated that definition into their official statement on pulmonary rehabilitation.[41] This statement specifies the two objectives of pulmonary rehabilitation as follows:

1. To control and alleviate as possible the symptoms

and pathophysiological complications of respiratory impairment

2. To teach the patient how to achieve his or her optimum potential to carry out activities of daily living.

Here medicine acknowledges both the concept of intervention and the treatment to alleviate acute problems and decrease symptoms as well as the need to follow up with teaching to help the patient adapt to a chronic disease and attain that highest functional capacity. This progressive defining and study of the components of pulmonary rehabilitation programs has brought us to the point at which we treat not only the acute complications of pulmonary disease, but attempt to maintain the patients at an optimal functional level. This is usually done with multidisciplinary intervention before total lung destruction occurs. Rehabilitation brings the patient to the highest functional level thereby preventing deterioration and decreasing morbidity and mortality in the population.[50] This chapter initially is an examination of the patient population that could be included or benefit from a pulmonary rehabilitation program. Second, evaluation and treatment techniques are discussed including case studies to illustrate possible patient problems and various programs. The chapter concludes with discharge planning considerations and suggestions for clinical study.

PATIENT POPULATION

Chronic obstructive pulmonary disease (COPD) has become a clinical catch phrase that includes several pathologically separate diseases. Emphysema, chronic bronchitis, asthma, and even cystic fibrosis have been included under this single, clinical description. The pathological and clinical aspects of these diseases are described in an attempt to clarify each. The summary discussion then describes the pathological and clinical picture of the patient with COPD incorporating as appropriate, all four entities. Rarely is the patient examined who does not display combined symptoms in the clinical picture of COPD.

Emphysema

"Emphysema is characterized by abnormal enlargement of the terminal air spaces. In part, the condition is an expression of normal pulmonary senescence, a loss of elastic tissue from the lung leading to expiratory collapse of the larger air passages, difficulty in expiration and dilatation of the terminal airways."[14] The emphysematous patient has been described clinically as the "pink puffer." Traditionally, they are very thin in appearance, using their accessory muscles to accomplish inspiration and breathing out through pursed lips. They have increases in their residual volume (RV), subcostal angle, and anteroposterior diameter. Because of the low, inefficient position of their diaphragm, these patients frequently depend on a fixed elevated shoulder girdle to cope with the work of breathing (Fig. 19-1).

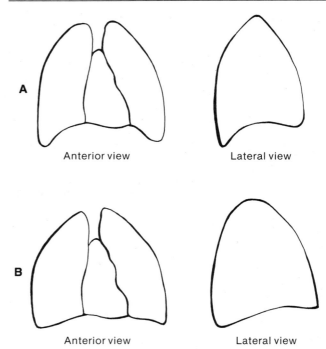

Anterior view   Lateral view

Fig. 19-1. Relative position of diaphragm and chest wall in normal persons, **A,** and in patients with chronic obstructive pulmonary disease, **B.**

Chronic bronchitis

Chronic bronchitis is defined clinically based on its symptoms. "If the subject has a chronic or recurrent productive cough on most days for a minimum of three months per year in not less than two successive years,"[2] he is considered to have chronic bronchitis. These patients are known as "blue bloaters." Typically they are overweight and cyanotic with edematous feet and ankles. Chronic bronchitics have frequent bouts of upper respiratory tract infections complicated by right ventricular heart failure, pulmonary hypertension, hypoxia, and hypercapnia.

Asthma

Although asthma or reactive airway disease is frequently included in the COPD category, it is more accurately termed "reversible airway disease." The asthmatic state is characterized by increased bronchial reactivity to multiple physical, chemical, and pharmacological stimuli.[46] Diagnosis is based on history, results of physical examination, and airway response to exercise or an inhaled noxious stimulus, such as cold or methacholine, in the laboratory setting.[46] Patients with an exacerbation of asthma will characteristically be wheezing, using accessory muscles of respiration to breathe, and have a cough productive of stringy, clear secretions. When not in an asthmatic state, these patients have little or no evidence of airway obstruction by either pulmonary function test or physical exam.

Cystic fibrosis

Cystic fibrosis is a genetically determined systemic disease of the exocrine glands. It can be diagnosed in infancy, or it can go undetected until symptoms become more severe during childhood or the teen-age years. The severity, range, and degree of symptoms varies. Pulmonary symptoms and complications include chronic cough, persistent respiratory infections, obstructive lung disease, and finally cor pulmonale.[49]

Combinations

Patients with COPD may exhibit any combination of the previously described symptoms. Their physiological abnormality is one of airways obstructed or collapsed by bronchospasm and secretions because of hyperplasia of mucus-secreting structures within the airways. Obstructed airways result in decreased expiratory flow and an increase in residual volume. This increase in retained volume shortens the diaphragm, the muscle responsible for the major work of inspiration, placing it in a low, flat, mechanically inefficient position (Fig. 19-1). Collapsed, destroyed airways result in a loss of surface area available for gas diffusion. Decreased diffusion reduces both oxygen delivery into pulmonary capillaries and carbon dioxide elimination from pulmonary capillaries. This combination of impaired ventilation caused by an inefficient thoracic pump (the diaphragm) and decreased gas transfer through loss of surface area decreases the efficiency of both gas delivery and transport and increases the work of breathing. Patients with COPD share the problem of increased energy resources being utilized for breathing with little energy remaining for activities of daily living. A multifaceted pulmonary rehabilitation program directed toward the specific problems of each patient can provide comprehensive care to this pulmonary impaired population.

PATIENT EVALUATION

An accurate patient history is essential before the routine steps of observation, palpation, and auscultation. Frequently the onset of emphysema and chronic bronchitis is insidious. Persons who smoke for many years often cough on awakening and with activity, yet deny the presence of a cough because it is integral and habitual in their daily routine. Occupational disease can also be masked because its slow onset and gradual debilitation is sometimes assumed to be related to the aging process. Frequently family members are useful and informative during evaluation because they notice symptoms and change with greater objectivity than the patients themselves. Asthma, particularly when exercise induced, is frequently more dramatic in onset, and patients can relate the tightening in their chest to

a specific event. An accurate medical history includes questions related to the following topics:

Medical history
> Onset of symptoms: original date, time, frequency, precipitating factors
> Dyspnea: functional level, walking distance, stairs
> Orthopnea: sleep habits
> Allergies
> Medication usage
> Other medical problems and complications

Family history
> Parents: disease, death
> Siblings: disease, death
> Children

Social history
> Occupation: present and past
> Habits: smoking, alcohol, exercise
> Living location: present and past
> Avocations

Observation

Observation begins with pulmonary patients as they enter the room. Pattern of respiration, use of musculature, posture, and ease of ambulation are noted mentally and taken into account throughout the patient interview. A patient will commonly walk into the examination area breathing through pursed lips with the arms placed stiffly on the hips to elevate the shoulder girdle. If this patient states that only a minor problem exists with shortness of breath, the therapist must question the reliability of the patient in presenting an accurate or realistic history.

To observe the thorax, seat the patient on a level surface with hips and knees flexed and the thoracic surface as exposed as possible (Fig. 19-2). Position of the shoulders and head are noted for symmetry. Scoliosis and kyphosis both limit thoracic mobility and produce restrictive lung disease. The neck musculature is observed for hypertrophy of the accessory muscles. Supraclavicular retraction, a frequent sign of COPD, may also be observed (Fig. 19-3). Observation includes notation of the patient's rate, rhythm, and pattern of breathing. The respiratory rate will frequently be greater than 25 to 30 after ambulation but may slow to 20 or less after rest. The inspiratory to expiratory time ratio is normally 1:2 and becomes progressively greater with advancing expiratory obstruction. Many patients use pursed-lips breathing automatically as their routine pattern of breathing. Notice whether the pursed-lips technique is employed with activity, at rest, or both. Use of the ventilatory musculature is also significant. Patients with COPD frequently use their abdominal muscles to breathe at rest after bracing the upper thorax with the extremities. The abdomen will protrude on inspiration and will recede on expiration. With an increase in stress the accessory muscles will frequently contract with the abdominal protrusion. Severely limited patients may display a pattern of discoordinated breathing where the abdomen

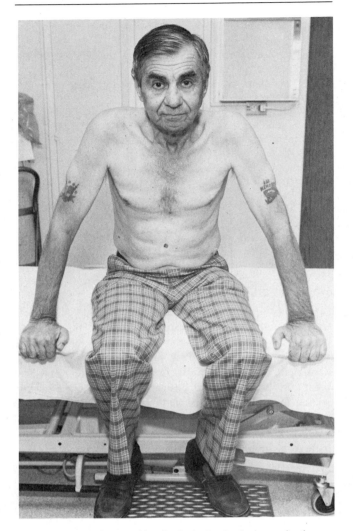

Fig. 19-2. Patient position for thoracic physical examination.

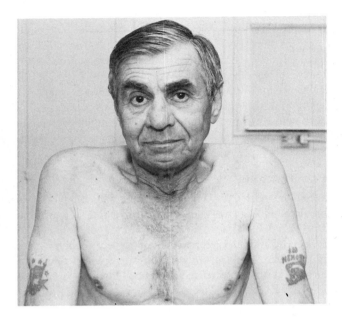

Fig. 19-3. Hypertrophy of the accessory muscles of respiration; supraclavicular retraction.

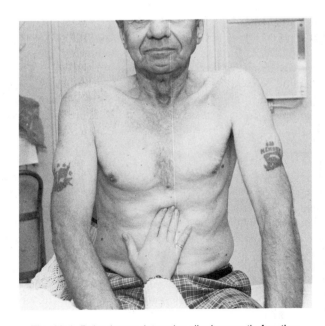

Fig. 19-4. Palpation to determine diaphragmatic function.

is drawn in on inspiration as the accessory muscles pull up, technically termed "respiratory paradox." This is not always easily observed but can be confirmed by palpation[32] (Fig. 19-4).

Palpation

After observation of the patient, palpation is useful to both confirm suspicions formed during observation and elicit further information. Assessment of the subcostal angle and determination of the ratio of anteroposterior (AP) to lateral thoracic (LAT) diameter determines the degree the thorax has progressed into the position of inspiration because of an increased residual volume (Fig. 19-5). The normal subcostal angle is 90 degrees, and the AP:LAT ratio is 1:2. Patients with COPD frequently exhibit a subcostal angle of greater than 100 degrees and a 1:1 ratio

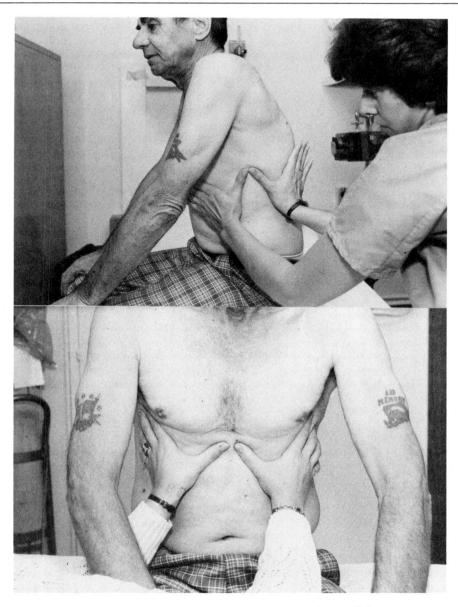

Fig. 19-5. Comparison of the anteroposterior-to-lateral chest wall diameter.

commonly termed a "barrel chest" (Fig. 19-6). This thoracic fixation limits excursion and can be assessed by palpation both anteriorly and posteriorly (Fig. 19-7).

Percussion

Mediate percussion is particularly useful in the assessment of patients with COPD to determine the location of the bases of the lungs. Hyperinflation and the resultant low, flattened diaphragm places the base of the lung tissue below its normal level of the tenth rib. Percussion also locates areas of increased density as occurs with consoli-

dation or collapse. Hyperresonance, which can be attributable to hyperinflation and destruction of underlying lung tissue or pneumothorax, can also be located with percussion.

Auscultation

The art and science of listening to breath sounds is both a useful and a necessary portion of the physical examination of patients with pulmonary impairment. The initial examination establishes a base line because treatment is often based upon the presence or absence of normal, abnormal,

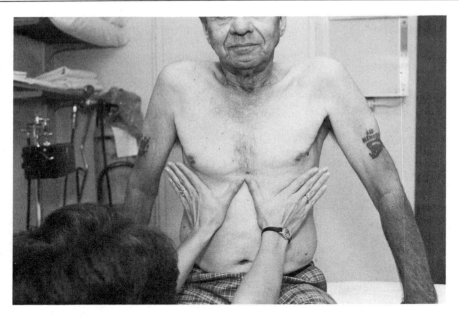

Fig. 19-6. Palpation of the subcostal angle.

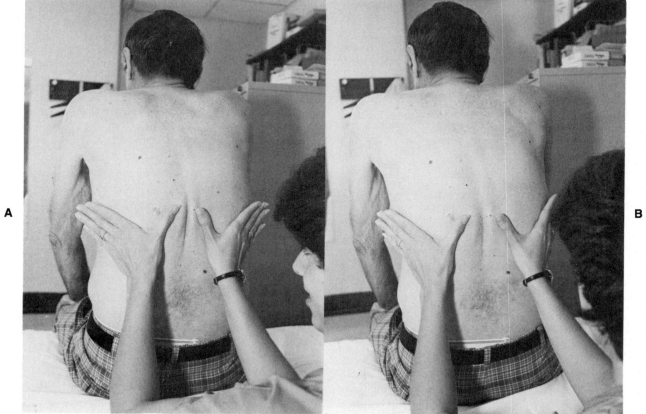

Fig. 19-7. Palpation of posterior thoracic excursion. **A,** Expiration. **B,** Inspiration.

or adventitious breath sounds. The terms "normal," "abnormal," and "adventitious" specifically apply to the breath sounds described in Chapter 12. However, "normal" breath sounds for any given pulmonary patient will be those heard at the base-line examination. A patient with COPD and severe emphysema will have decreased, distant, or inaudible breath sounds at the lung bases. Patients with chronic bronchitis or cystic fibrosis will routinely have adventitious sounds because of secretions obstructing their airways. Changes in these base-line breath sounds become clinically significant, for example, when the emphysematous patient develops adventitious sounds not routinely heard, or the chronic bronchitic patient develops the fine fluid rales of congestive heart failure.

FUNCTIONAL EXAMINATION

Based on the cumulative findings of the patient's history and physical exam, a clinical picture of each patient begins to develop. The COPD patient with a long-term smoking history and signs of both emphysema and chronic bronchitis will separate from the patient with cystic fibrosis who has only recently noted pulmonary impairment with exercise. For futher assessment of the patient and determination of functional abilities a stress test is performed. The goals of stress testing are twofold—an objective assessment of the patient's symptoms and a quantification of the impaired function. Although pulmonary abnormalities at rest may be minimal, exercise is used as a tool to provoke and then assess the severity of the condition.[24]

Indications for stress testing

Because of the massive reserve capabilities of the pulmonary system and the insidious nature of many pulmonary diseases, compromise of the patient's functional abilities may occur over a long period of time without arousing the patient's awareness. There are often great discrepancies between the pulmonary patient's perception of limitations and actual functional abilities. Therefore stress testing can serve as an objective documentation of a patient's functional limitations as related to symptoms. Patients who complain of dyspnea, dizziness, or nausea related to activity can be monitored during that activity to assess the level of onset and severity of symptoms. Assessment of a patient's work disability and documentation of increased oxygen requirements are two other practical uses of stress testing. Disability compensation requires the objective classification of patients into disability categories based on their functional level.[25] Stress testing is also used diagnostically for the pulmonary population. Jones and Campbell conservatively list: chronic bronchitis, pulmonary emphysema, pulmonary infiltration, alveolitis and fibrosis, and pulmonary thromboembolism in hypertension in a list of conditions for which stress testing might be diagnostically useful.[25] Diagnosis as used here relates to assessment of functional impairment. Patients with reactive airways are also good candidates for stress testing to determine the onset, nature, and severity of their symptoms and to analyze the effectiveness of varied forms of therapy as well. Additionally, a stress test sets a base line for functional performance from which both progress or deterioration can be evaluated. Therefore stress testing is useful as a safe and effective method of evaluating pulmonary patient symptoms and functional impairment.

Methods of stress testing

Protocols for stress testing of pulmonary patients are as numerous and varied as those for the cardiac population. The key to selecting an appropriate protocol is directly related to both the patient's level of function and the symptoms under investigation. A severely compromised patient with COPD whose functional limitations keep him housebound is appropriately tested by an intermittent walking protocol such as the one described in the top chart on p. 374. Less severely impaired patients may require higher levels of activity to elicit symptoms. Those with orthopaedic or neurological disabilities in addition to their pulmonary condition may be tested best with bicycle or arm ergometry. The bottom chart on p. 374 lists a few protocols and their advantages and disadvantages for pulmonary patients. In a setting where there is little testing equipment, a 12-minute walk test can be simply and safely administered to these patients.[36] During this test both pulse and blood pressure are monitored, and if dyspnea occurs, patients can rest at their discretion. The addition of an ear oximeter to record oxygen saturation makes this an extremely attractive method of assessment in terms of practicality, safety, and usefulness. Regardless of the protocol chosen, the essential procedure and values monitored are similar.

Initially the process and its aims and goals are described for the patient, whose cooperation, understanding of the procedure, and confidence in the therapist can enhance the accuracy of the results. The initial portion of test time is used for patient and equipment preparation. Stress testing, which involves monitoring ventilation and arterial blood gases in addition to the standard electrocardiogram, blood pressure, and heart rate, is more time consuming and can provoke anxiety in the patient. Adequate time and attention is allotted to the patient to ensure accuracy of the patient's understanding and participation in the testing process. To best administer a pulmonary stress test that includes monitoring of arterial blood gases, one needs three knowledgeable persons. The traditional two-person team can adequately attend to the patient and the monitoring equipment. The third person analyzes the blood gases either on site or in the lab to provide direct feedback as the test progresses. Parameters that are useful for monitoring and assessment both at rest and during the stress test include heart rate, blood pressure, electrocardiogram, respiratory rate, pulmonary function tests, arterial oxygen, ar-

EXERCISE TEST PROTOCOL
Beth Israel Hospital, Pulmonary Medicine Department

Collect resting data (supine and sitting):	ECG, blood pressure, Pao_2, $Paco_2$, pH, A-aDo_2,* A-aDco_2, oxygen consumption ($\dot{V}o_2$), respiratory quotient (RQ), expired ventilation (V_E), respiratory rate (RR), heart rate (HR), dead-space ventilation (V_D), dead-space ventilation/tidal volume (V_D/V_T)
Stage I:	Assessment of dyspnea: treadmill set at 2 mph, 0% grade Walk 6 min = 4 min stabilization + 2 min gas collection Rest: Patient returns to base-line HR, RR, and ABG's†
Stage II:	Occupational assessment: treadmill set at speed and incline to equal functional work capacity Walk 6 min = 4 min stabilization + 2 min gas collection Rest: Patient returns to base-line HR, RR, and ABG's
Stage III:	Exercise tolerance: treadmill set to produce HR of 70% to 85% maximum Walk 6 min = 4 min stabilization + 2 min gas collection Rest: Patient returns to base-line HR, RR, and ABG's
Nitrogen washout:	Patient receives 100% O_2; draw ABG; calculate right-to-left shunt
Criteria to terminate test:	85% predicted maximum heart rate, development of metabolic acidosis, fall in Pao_2 of 20 torr from resting, reaching a ventilatory maximum (35 × FEV_1‡), CO_2 retention of more than 10 torr from base line, development of cardiac arrhythmias, or development of significant symptoms

*A-aD, Alveolar-arterial gas-pressure difference.
†ABG, Arterial blood gases.
‡FEV_1, Forced expiratory (or expired) volume in 1 second.

SAMPLE: STRESS-TESTING PROTOCOLS

PROTOCOL	METHOD	COMMENTS
Twelve-minute walk*	Level walking for 12 minutes, distance recorded	No equipment necessary yet correlates well with study results of more complex tests; can be used for patients who cannot accomplish either treadmill walking or bike riding because of dyspnea
Modified Naughton†	Treadmill speed constant at 2.0 mph; grade initially 0%, increased by 3.5% every 2 min	Slow speed allows patient with pulmonary impairment to be stressed without walking fast
Beth Israel Hospital protocol	(See preceding box)	Intermittent walk test for use with severely impaired patients; allows flexibility of work-load assignment and establishes an accurate base line
Balke test†	Treadmill speed constant at 3.0 mph; grade initially 0%, increased by 3.5% every 2 min	Slight increase in speed for patient with less impairment allows pulmonary and cardiovascular stress to come before leg fatigue
Bruce†	Treadmill speed initially 1.7 mph; grade initially 10%, both increased every 3 min in a specified manner	Can be used with relatively fit persons to stress accurately all systems' response to exercise; good to assess exercise-induced bronchospasm in fit persons
Bicycle test‡	Specific work load, i.e., watts or kg/min; patient rides for a preset time; next work load determined by patient response	Intermittent subjective test based on patient response; requires lower extremity strength and endurance to reach high metabolic response level

*McGavin, C.R., Gupta, S.P., and McHardy, G.J.R.: Br. Med. J. 1:822, 1976.
†From Physician's handbook for evaluation of cardiovascular and physical fitness, Nashville, 1972, Tennessee Heart Association (now called American Heart Association–Tennessee Affiliate).
‡Ellestad, N.H.: Stress testing: principles and practice, Philadelphia, 1979, F.A. Davis Co.

terial carbon dioxide, oxygen saturation, and expired-gas concentrations. The analysis of these values will provide information regarding the patient's ventilatory capacity and work of breathing with exercise, adequacy of pulmonary blood flow, indications of pulmonary gas exchange, and factors that limit functional performance.

Throughout each stage of the stress test subjective data regarding the patient's performance are recorded in addition to the physiological values. The person observing and communicating with the patient asks appropriate questions, such as ''Is your breathing tighter?'' ''Are you dizzy?'' and gives verbal cues and encouragement. Patients are instructed to give simple hand signals should they be unable to continue, since they cannot speak with the ventilatory monitoring equipment in place.

Criteria to stop a pulmonary stress test relate more directly to the pulmonary system and are more subjective than those used with cardiac patients (see top chart on p. 374). Specific criteria include reaching 85% maximum heart rate, development of metabolic acidosis, fall in PaO_2 of 20 torr from resting, reaching a ventilatory maximum, CO_2 retention of over 10 torr from resting, or development of cardiac arrhythmias. In the pulmonary population dyspnea is frequently described as the limiting factor in exercise when the ventilatory capacity is unable to meet the increased ventilatory demand of exercise.[25] Dyspnea from hypoxia may be accompanied by higher heart rates in patients with COPD than would normally be seen with similar low levels of stress in normals or cardiac patients.[8] The upper limit of a pulmonary stress test is commonly symptom limited or is an arterial desaturation below 80%, rather than the traditional upper limit of maximal heart rate as that seen in cardiac testing.[22] Some examples of symptom limitations are extreme dyspnea, wheezing, dizziness, nausea, weakness, and cramping or pain in the extremities. When criteria to stop are met, the test is terminated, the level achieved is recorded, and the patient is noted as having reached 85% maximum heart rate or a ''symptom-limited maximum.''

TREATMENT PROGRAM
Accepting candidates, setting goals

After comprehensive evaluation, a determination is made regarding the patient's rehabilitation potential. Individualized short-term and long-term goals can both focus and direct the rehabilitative process. The University of Nebraska has been collecting data on patients in their pulmonary rehabilitation program for several years.[48] They have detected several statistical trends among their successful patients compared to those who have been unsuccessful. Data have been collected for both physiological and psychological parameters. Their data show that physical indicators are more reliable than psychosocial indicators in predicting the success of a patient receiving pulmonary rehabilitation. Patients with a forced expiratory

volume in the first second (FEV_1) of greater than 50% of predicted and a maximum voluntary ventilation (MVV) of greater than 40% show greater improvements and have more success with rehabilitation than those with lower FEV_1 and MVV values. However, highly motivated persons with a specific profession and those with the capacity to modify their job to accomodate their disease have proved to be successful candidates despite less than acceptable physical predictors. On the other hand, patients with multiple physiological or psychological problems, such as patients having chronic bronchitis with heart failure or chronic pulmonary edema with recurrent infection, patients with recent life-style changes that result in rapid clinical deterioration, and patients with an inability to mobilize their psychosocial support systems, do not have the same positive results or success rate.[48] Patients who both thoroughly understand their rehabilitation and are willing to take responsibility for their progress have a good chance to benefit from a comprehensive program.

Setting goals is an individual process once the patient begins the program. For example, patients with mild to moderate COPD and minimal limitations to functional performance may aspire to improve exercise capacity with a jogging program (see case study 1, p. 378). Persons with severe COPD characterized by frequent infections, hospital admissions, and functional limitation may focus on stabilization of their medical condition and set walking and stair climbing as long-term goals (see case study 2, p. 379). The importance of individual assessment is to determine reasonable, realistic, achievable goals toward which patients can work, document their progress, and note their improvement. Achieving personal goals increases patient compliance with the program and provides long-term benefit.[50]

Bronchopulmonary hygiene

The techniques of bronchopulmonary hygiene include positioning or postural drainage, percussion, vibration, shaking, and cough facilitation. Historically, techniques such as breathing exercises, intermittent positive-pressure breathing (IPPB), and the use of humidity and bronchodilators have also been considered techniques of bronchopulmonary hygiene. Breathing exercises and patterning are discussed with exercise conditioning. Humidity and other forms of therapy are discussed as adjuncts to physical therapy techniques.

Members of the population with COPD as previously described repeatedly complain of dyspnea because of excess secretions and reactive airways. Success in a pulmonary rehabilitation program depends on attention to all components of the disease process. Before an exercise program is begun, efforts are made to improve airway clearance. Postural drainage and positioning to clear the airways of excess secretions are particularly useful for patients with chronic bronchitis, bronchiectasis, and cystic fibrosis.[13,34,56] Manual techniques of percussion and shaking have been successful at clearing secretions from central, mid-, and peripheral lung regions in the stable COPD population.[7] Once secretions are loosened, patients are instructed in proper airway clearance techniques including coughing and huffing. Huffing is useful because it may provide stabilization of the airways thereby enhancing effective secretion clearance in this patient population.[47,55] The optimal program or combination of techniques to successfully clear secretions will vary from patient to patient. Information related to the amount and consistency of secretions and the patient's perception of the ability to clear the airways gathered during patient evaluation will be useful in treatment planning. A simple program of positioning, vigorous percussion, deep breathing, and shaking delivered bilaterally for 10 minutes may adequately clear the airways for effective ventilation during exercise yet does not tire the patient or render him unable to walk or cycle. In some patients, coughing during exercise will be all that is required to clear the airways.

Adjuncts to physical therapy

Humidity and bronchodilators are an integral part of many COPD patients' treatment programs. The routine use of bronchodilating drugs for patients with COPD continues to be an area of discussion and controversy within the medical community.[11,28,35] If a patient demonstrates a significant airflow improvement with administration of a bronchodilator, its use is recommended before an exercise program. Additionally, patients with only small functional changes at the time of drug administration may actually find greater therapeutic benefit during exercise and throughout the course of the drug's effectiveness.[28,35] A therapeutic trial both with and without bronchodilators is an effective method for assessment of those patients with equivocal results from bronchodilators. Aerosol sympathomimetics are generally the drugs of choice because they have been shown to improve ventilatory function and exercise tolerance.[28,30]

Humidity delivered during an inpatient admission generally requires an equipment setup, including either a nebulizer or a bubble humidifier. When prescribed for an outpatient, more simplified equipment is recommended. Patients can simply spend extra time in the shower or steam-filled bathroom to aid in the clearance of morning or evening secretions. An effective way of assuring mobile, liquid secretions is the daily consumption of fluids. Patients without restricted fluid volumes are encouraged to keep a quart of water in the refrigerator and drink it on a daily basis. Home humidifiers are recommended only to be used with great caution and careful sterilizing instruction because they easily become a source of infection.

Oxygen therapy

The use of either long-term oxygen therapy or oxygen-supplemented exercise continues to be an area of discussion and controversy among persons working with patients with COPD. Proponents of oxygen administration during exercise have demonstrated that greater amounts of exercise are performed with a lower respiratory rate, exercise minute ventilation, and oxygen uptake when one is using supplemental oxygen.[15] Other studies do not demonstrate these improvements.[29] Some clinicians argue that participants whose oxygen saturation levels are not dangerously low should train while breathing room air to allow them to accommodate to their dyspnea.[22] There is general agreement that desaturation below the 85% level is neither safe nor desirable for the patient with COPD; therefore supplemental oxygen is commonly used during exercise to keep oxygen saturation above 85%.[48]

Exercise

Exercise both for the ventilatory muscles and for the total body has become the mainstay of pulmonary rehabilitation programs. Historically this has not been true, as demonstrated by Haas and Luczak in 1971.[20] Their "pulmonary rehabilitation program" was composed of breathing exercises, positioning, percussion, vibration, shaking, and cough facilitation. Changes have also occurred in the type of exercises recommended. The emphasis was originally on total body exercise. The concept of actually "training" the ventilatory muscles developed as recently as 1976.[27] The current concept in pulmonary rehabilitation, as previously described, encourages a comprehensive, multidisciplinary program comprising all therapeutic measures beneficial to pulmonary patients.[41] The exercise component is then a portion of the total program and directed toward an individual patient's performance on exercise tests and medical evaluation.

Breathing exercises. Techniques associated with breathing exercises or breathing retraining have been varied during the last 50 years, but the objectives have remained relatively unchanged. The goals of maximizing ventilatory performance and decreasing the work of breathing are standard.[23] During the 1930s, Winnifred Linton described breathing retraining to accompany the techniques of bronchopulmonary hygiene and aid in the treatment of patients with COPD.[17] During the 1960s, Innocenti noted an "inspiratory bounce" or discoordinated breathing pattern in patients with COPD. This pattern was corrected with breathing exercises before patients could participate and progress in the exercise program.[23] Pursed-lips breathing exercises were studied throughout the 1960s and 1970s and were agreed upon as a technique that slowed the respiratory rate and improved gas mixing and oxygenation for benefit both at rest and during exercise.[19,40,43,45] Breathing exercises today incorporate many of the techniques developed by earlier researchers and clinicians to improve functional performance.[5,23,27]

Training principles for the ventilatory muscles are in many ways similar to those developed for training all skeletal muscles. Ventilatory muscles can be trained for either strength, endurance, or both. Techniques that have been proved successful are those originally developed by Leith and Bradley.[27] These are known as "hyperpnea and maximal resistance training" or the technique termed "inspiratory resistive training" or "inspiratory muscle training," which combines training for strength and endurance into one maneuver.[4,27] Inspiratory muscle training is done by performance of "training runs" or inspiration for a measured amount of time against an increased resistance or a narrowed airway. Investigators have used several equipment setups to attain the desired effect; however, all employ the same principle.[4,12] An external load is placed on the muscles (airway narrowing) to improve strength, and contractions are performed for set periods of time to increase endurance. The result of this training, as described by Leith and Bradley and others, is to improve both the strength and endurance of ventilatory muscles. The benefit or gains from improved strength and endurance are still being investigated. Asher and associates' group of patients who demonstrated improved strength and endurance of ventilatory muscles after inspiratory muscle training could not show similar improvement in mean exercise performance during either progressive or submaximal testing.[4] Casciari, however, examined two groups of patients with COPD in exercise conditioning programs—one group used inspiratory muscle training in addition to physical conditioning, and one did not. After a control period of training, inspiratory muscle training was added to the program of only one patient group. Significant differences between groups were noticed only after the addition of inspiratory muscle training. Changes were noticed in resting oxygen consumption, in decreased respiratory rate at rest, and during maximal exercise and increased arterial oxygenation during exercise.[12] The long-term significance of breathing retraining and exercise may eventually prove to be twofold. Patients may be able to improve functional performance by using trained ventilatory muscles during exercise to counter the increased work of breathing in COPD. Second, this functional improvement may decrease the frequency of exacerbations and decompensation in this chronically ill population.

Physical reconditioning. The addition of physical reconditioning to pulmonary rehabilitation programs is not new, yet the activity has not gained widespread acceptance until recently. In 1952, Barach noted that physically active patients functioned better than inactive patients and emphasized the importance of activity and ambulation for patients with COPD.[6] Although some programs employed exercise, researchers could not document improvement in lung function as measured by pulmonary function tests.[10,38,53] The most consistent finding in rehabilitation programs that employ exercise is an increased ability to exercise with a reduced oxygen consumption. The reasons postulated for this change include decreased sensitivity to dyspnea, decreased oxygen cost of breathing through a controlled coordinated ventilatory pattern, increased coordination and efficiency in movement, and increased peripheral oxygen utilization attributable to an increased peripheral blood flow.[10,26,30,42,57]

Exercise programs for the pulmonary patient are individually prescribed based on stress-test results and goals related to functional improvement. The training mode selected is consistent with both the patient's preference and the practicality or availability of equipment. Patients living in geographic areas that permit regular outdoor walking can participate in walking-jogging programs. Patients living in cold climates or in large cities may not have easy access to climate-controlled or safety-controlled areas for walking, and stationary bicycle programs are an alternative mode of training. Patient preference is of great significance, since compliance will be a problem if a patient dislikes the mode of exercise selected.

Three components—frequency, duration, and intensity—guide the exercise prescription. Guidelines developed for the normal population are made under the assumption that aerobic training occurs and the patient achieves a "central training effect" over a prescribed period of time.[1] The concept of a "training effect" is modified in the patient with COPD because there remains a question whether the patient with COPD is capable of aerobic training or ever reaches anaerobic threshold.[9] Therefore modifications may be necessary at the beginning of a program to allow the patient to increase exercise intensity gradually to a training level. Intensity is the most significant element in planning an exercise program.[21] Guidelines used for exercise prescription recommend training at a heart rate of 60% of maximum or greater.[1] Since pulmonary patients reach higher heart rates with much lower levels of exercise, a more appropriate guideline for intensity relates to the patient's symptom-limited maximum heart rate.[8] If dyspnea is a patient's limiting factor, an appropriate training level may be related to exertion that safely stresses the patient as measured by a guideline on the dyspnea index.[39] This training level can be correlated to the heart rate, thereby giving the patient two useful indices of intensity. Intensity can also be mingled with frequency and duration to produce a prescription whose sum total complies with the minimal criteria for training. Minimal criteria to achieve a central training effect for normal persons includes an intensity of 60% maximum heart rate or greater, a frequency of three times per week, and an exercise duration of 20 minutes.[1] For a pulmonary patient who can achieve only a 2-minute walk without stopping the above criteria are unrealistic. Consequently, modified prescriptions aim at a total effect. If 10 minutes of walking or cycling at the appropriate intensity is achievable, the frequency can be increased to twice a day. If only 5 minutes are possible, the frequency can be four times daily. Intermittent exercise with gradual lengthening of time periods is also useful. Two minutes of cycling and 2 minutes of rest intermittently over 40 minutes can be progressed to 3 minutes of cycling, 1 minute of rest, and so on. The initial goal of functional improvement can be gradually increased, as the patient improves, to a goal of training in the traditional sense.

Exercise periods are preceded and followed by warm-up and cool-down exercises. The pulmonary patient is directed particularly toward thoracic mobilization exercises that include the upper extremities and trunk rotation. These are coordinated with breathing exercises using the principles of controlled relaxation of the shoulder girdle, rhythmic swinging exercises, and maneuvers including inhalation with thoracic lifting and exhalation with effort. Reminders to employ pursed-lips breathing are also useful.

The length of formal training programs in or out of medical facilities greatly varies.[37] The important component to any rehabilitation program is the patient's commitment. Beneficial effects of exercise have been demonstrated to last only as long as training is continued.[3] To increase exercise compliance, the patient should understand both the disease process and the effects of exercise. Patients can keep a log or diary that documents their daily progress; distance walked, cycled, or swum; subjective feelings; and any problems or questions that occur.[44] In addition to their exercise program, patients can also chart their dietary program, questions about their medical problems, and subjective feelings about their condition.

Nutrition, education, and psychosocial support

Other components of the rehabilitation program, sometimes overlooked yet equally important, are the patient's eating habits, his or her understanding of the disease process, and psychosocial support. These aspects are often managed by nursing, dietary, and social service, yet all members of the team must recognize the importance of all portions of the rehabilitation program and support its concepts. Patients with emphysema, chronic bronchitis, and cystic fibrosis commonly have nutritional problems concomitant with the pulmonary disease. Emphysematous patients are typically cachectic because of the difficulty of eating and chewing when they are severely dyspneic. Patients with chronic bronchitis are frequently overweight, and the pancreatic enzyme deficiency of patients with cystic fibrosis prevents them from properly digesting fats and proteins. A complete nutritional assessment is necessary to develop a nutritional enhancement program to provide the additional calories required for exercise. Education is often required to ensure patient compliance with the entire program.[28] If the patient can participate in making decisions regarding medications, exercise, nutrition, and so on, there is a significant increase in their program success rate.[44] Family involvement is also useful, since patients who can mobilize psychosocial support systems are commonly successful program participants.[48]

DISCHARGE PLANNING

Discharge planning for patients with COPD should include a review of their goals and program components. Patients leaving the hospital after an acute pulmonary exacerbation require a review of their medications and bronchopulmonary hygiene, and a modification of their activity level is often necessary. They can be scheduled to return within 6 weeks for an exercise test and prescription.

Patients who complete a 4-week, outpatient exercise program will usually be discharged with more emphasis placed on all components of the home program. This includes reminders about medications, nutrition, self-monitoring during exercise, and specific instructions for maintenance of their log. The return visit after discharge from a comprehensive program will vary, but 4 weeks is generally an acceptable period of time for the initial check. If all continues well, a 3- or 4-month checkup is appropriate. Initial retesting of pulmonary patients can be delayed for at least 6 months because gains in this population are small and slow. This group of patients can also be discouraging to treat because of frequent setbacks.[31] Upper respiratory infections and exacerbations of asthma will often reduce a patient to a less functional level. Continuous rehabilitation programs, however, have demonstrated a decrease in the frequency of hospitalization over a 10-year period.[50]

Many questions in the therapeutic area of pulmonary rehabilitation remain unanswered. If patients could be identified and treated earlier in their disease progression, would this early treatment change the course of the disease? What is the optimal combination of therapeutic modalities? Should all patients train with inspiratory muscle training and exercise or would one of the two be enough, and which one? These and other questions keep this area of care a positive, stimulating, progressive, and challenging arena in which to practice.

CASE STUDY 1
Recent medical history

R.F. is a 55-year-old retired welder with a 7-year history of increasing dyspnea on exertion. He was admitted to the hospital 14 days previously with a temperature of 101.6 and a cough productive of copious amounts of yellow-green secretions. Although he has a 30-pack-per-year history of cigarette smoking, he admits only to an occasional morning cough. His upper respiratory infection has now resolved, and he has been referred to the pulmonary rehabilitation program because he complains of inability to play nine holes of golf without experiencing shortness of breath.

Thoracic physical exam
At rest

Supine:	RR = 18	Standing:	RR = 20
	HR = 75		HR = 80
	BP = 125/85		BP = 125/85

Inspiration:expiration ratio = 1:4   Normal pattern/no pursed-lip breathing
Breath sounds: decreased bases bilaterally, otherwise clear
Head, neck, and shoulders: some hypertrophy of accessory muscles, minimum retraction on inspiration, no jugular venous distension
Subcostal angle: 100 degrees
Posterior excursion: 2 inches
No clubbing, no peripheral edema

Functional assessment

Height: 68 inches
Weight: 150 lb
Age: 55 years

Pulmonary function tests

	Actual	Predicted	% predicted
FVC (forced vital capacity)	4.5 L	4.7 L	96%
FEV$_1$ (forced expired volume)	2.5 L	3.4 L	74%
FEV$_1$/FVC%	55.5	72.3	77%
MMEF (maximum midexpiratory flow)	2.2 L/sec	3.3 L/sec	66%

Arterial blood gases:
  Pao$_2$ = 86
  Paco$_2$ = 43
  pH = 7.4
  Base excess (BE) = +1
  O$_2$ saturation = 94%
Chest radiograph: Lung fields clear, moderate hyperinflation
Pulmonary stress test:
  BIH protocol; treadmill test (see top chart on p. 374) progressed through all 3 stages
  Stage 3 maximum = 3 mph at 2% grade
  HR$_{max}$ during stage 3 = 142; no arrhythmias
  RR = 34; O$_2$ saturation = 91%
  BP$_{max}$ = 150/85
Stage 3 values:
  Pao$_2$ = 77   V̇o$_2$ = 1.571 L/0.04 ml/kg
  Paco$_2$ = 37   RQ = 0.975
  pH/BE = 7.38/0   V$_E$ = 68.0 L/min
  A-aDo$_2$ = 36.78

Assessment

Patient has mild to moderate obstructive lung disease and is able to safely exercise to approximately 4 MET's (metabolic equivalents) without significant hypoxia or arrhythmias. *Goals:* Walking program to improve functional capacity with bronchopulmonary hygiene to clear lungs in the morning.

Bronchopulmonary hygiene

Patient instructed in bilateral drainage positions with pillows. To drain in bed for 10 min per side each morning. Breathing exercises and cough to clear while draining. Instructed to watch for temperature or sputum change. Will consume four 8 oz glasses of water daily.

Exercise program

Patient begins with 5 min of rhythmic bend and stretch exercises, trunk twisting, side bends, and reach and stretch. Progresses to treadmill walking for 5 min at 1 mph, 0% grade. HR increases to 114, O$_2$ saturation 94%, BP 133/85. Increase treadmill to 2 mph, 1% grade. HR stabilizes at 124, O$_2$ saturation

93%, BP 133/85. Patient able to walk 15 min without arrhythmia or desaturation. Decrease treadmill grade, then speed throughout next minute, patient walks at 1 mph, 0% grade for another 3 min, completes program with 1 min rhythmic bend and stretch. HR returns to 78, RR to 18, BP to 125/85. Exercise sessions are scheduled three times a week.

CASE STUDY 2

Brief history

Patient is a 68-year-old man with severe COPD. Has been retired on disability insurance payments for 20 years. Has remained working by illegally driving a medical cab. The patient uses 2 liters of oxygen through nasal prongs while driving whenever he "has to." He has recently become concerned because he is no longer able to climb the stairs to his apartment. His doctor has requested a pulmonary stress test and rehabilitation program. The patient has no history of upper respiratory infections or chronic sputum production; he takes no bronchodilators.

Functional assessment

Pulmonary function report

  Height: 67 inches
  Weight: 142 lb
  Male
  Age: 68 years

Lung mechanics (liters)	Actual	Predicted	% predicted
Forced vital capacity (FVC)	1.41	3.98	35
Forced expired volume (FEV$_1$)	0.64	2.73	24
FEV$_1$/FVC × 100 (FEV$_1$%)	46	69	67
Maximum midexpiratory flow (L/sec)	0.24	2.60	9
Lung volumes (liters)			
Inspiratory capacity (IC)	1.13	2.76	41
Expiratory reserve volume (ERV)	1.10	1.22	90
Vital capacity (VC)	2.22	3.98	56
Functional residual capacity (FRC)	7.29	3.55	205
Total lung capacity (TLC)	8.41	6.31	133
Residual volume (RV)	6.19	2.33	265
(RV/TLC) × 100 (%)	74	37	200
Helium (He) mix time (min)	5	<3	
*Single-breath diffusing capacity (ml/min/mm Hg)**			
D$_{LCO}$ (predicted alveolar volume, V$_A$)	7.4	25.0	30
D$_{LCO}$ (actual V$_A$)	7.4	25.6	29
D$_{LCO}$ corrected for Hgb	0	25.6	0
Lung volume, L (STPD) (V$_A$)	4.28		
Lung volume (BTPS) (SBTLC)	5.11		
Mean of 1			

---

*BTPS, Body temperature, ambient pressure, saturated with water vapor; *D$_{LCO}$*, diffusing capacity of carbon monoxide in lung; *Hgb*, hemoglobin; *SBTLC*, single-breath total lung capacity; *STPD*, standard temperature, standard pressure, dry.

Pulmonary stress test

	Supine	Resting	Ex. 1	Ex. 2	Ex. 3
Speed (mph)				2	2	2
Incline (%)				0	0	0
PaO$_2$	80	75		66.3	73.8
PaCO$_2$	32.2	29.8		33.2	34.2
pH/BE	7.38/−6	7.44/−4		7.38/−5	7.38/−5
A-aDO$_2$					
A-aDCO$_2$ (calculated/ measured)					
V̇O$_2$ (O$_2$ consumption in liters)					
RQ					
V$_E$ (liters/min)					
Respiratory rate		9			
Heart rate		91		121	121
V$_D$ (liters)					
V$_D$/V$_T$					
Right to left shunt (on 100% O$_2$)					

Ex. 1 column note: Could not do on mouthpiece; had to stop after 55 sec

Ex. 2 column note: Stopped at 1 min, 55 sec

Ex. 3 column note: Stopped at 1 min, 45 sec on 2 L of O$_2$ by nasal prongs

Diagnosis. Emphysema

Clinical impression. Incomplete study because of patient's inability to use a mouthpiece while walking. He is extremely limited in exertion even at a very low level, but the small fall in PO$_2$ is insufficient to explain his limitation on a gas-exchange basis.

Exercise assessment. Because patient was too incapacitated to complete the stress test despite the small drop in PO$_2$, a determination was made to attempt a low-level functional program combined with inspiratory muscle training. Patient was given a tube with airway sufficiently narrowed to allow a 10 min training run to be accomplished three times a day. Patient was then set up on a bike-ergometer exercise program 3 times a week to strengthen lower extremities and improve functional performance climbing stairs. Wearing a nasal cannula delivering 2 liters of O$_2$, the patient spends 5 min warming up, alternating upper extremity exercises with walking in place. He then rides the bike for intervals of 2 min of pedaling followed by 1 min of rest, for a 20 min period twice a day. The bike is set at its lowest resistance, 1 kpm (kilopound meter). He cools down with 5 min of intermittent walking in place and arm circles. His saturation remains at 89% measured by ear oximeter and his heart rate is stable at 121 throughout the session.

After 6 weeks the patient was able to ride the bike for a solid 20 min exercise period at 1 kpm during the training session. His stair climbing had improved. Further functional goals were then determined.

REFERENCES

1. American College of Sports Medicine: Guidelines for graded exercise testing and exercise prescription, Philadelphia, 1975, Lea & Febiger.
2. American Thoracic Society: Chronic bronchitis, asthma and pulmonary emphysema, Am. Rev. Respir. Dis. **85**:762, 1962.
3. Amsterdam, E.A., Wilmore, J.H., and DeMaria, A.N., editors: Exercise in cardiovascular health and disease, New York, 1977, Yorke Medical Books.
4. Asher, M.I., Pardy, R.L., Coates, A.L., and others: The effects of inspiratory muscle training in patients with cystic fibrosis, Am. Rev. Respir. Dis. **126**:855, 1982.
5. Ashutosh, K., Gilbert, R., Auchincloss, J.H., and others: Asynchronous breathing movements in patients with chronic obstructive pulmonary disease, Chest **67**(5):553, 1975.
6. Barach, A.L., Bickerman, H.A., and Beck, G.J.: Advances in the treatment of non-tuberculous pulmonary disease, Bull. N.Y. Acad. Med. **28**(6):353, 1952.
7. Bateman, J.R.M., Newman, S.P., Daunt, K.M., and others: Regional lung clearance of excessive bronchial secretions during chest physiotherapy in patients with stable chronic airways obstruction, Lancet **1**:294, 1979.
8. Belman, M.J., and Kendregan, B.A.: Exercise training fails to increase skeletal muscle enzymes in patients with chronic obstructive pulmonary disease, Am. Rev. Respir. Dis. **123**:256, 1981.
9. Belman, M.J., and Wasserman, K.: Exercise training and testing in patients with chronic obstructive pulmonary disease, A.T.S. News **10**(2):38, 1982 (American Thoracic Society).
10. Brundin, A.: Physical training in severe chronic obstructive lung disease: I. Clinical course, physical working capacity and ventilation, Scand. J. Respir. Dis. **15**:25, 1974.
11. Carasso, B.: Therapeutic options in COPD, Geriatrics **37**(5):99, 1982.
12. Casciari, R.J., Fairshter, R.D., Harrison, A., and others: Effects of breathing retraining in patients with chronic obstructive pulmonary disease, Chest **79**(4):393, 1981.
13. Cochrane, G.M., Webber, B.A., and Clarke, S.W.: Effects of sputum on pulmonary function, Br. Med. J. **2**:1181, 1977.
14. Cumming, G., and Semple, S.G.: Disorders of the respiratory system, Oxford, 1973, Blackwell.
15. Editorial: Br. Med. J. **2**:1909, 1981.
16. Ewart, W.: Treatment of bronchiectasis and chronic bronchial affections by posture and respiratory exercise, Lancet **2**:70, 1901.
17. Gaskell, D.V.: Physiotherapy for medical and surgical thoracic conditions, London, England, 1960, Brompton Hospital.
18. Gray, F.D., and Field, A.S.: The use of mechanical assistance in treating cardiopulmonary diseases, Am. J. Med. Sci. **8**:146, 1959.
19. Guthrie, A., and Petty, T.: Improved exercise tolerance in patients with chronic airway obstruction, Phys. Ther. **50**(9):1333, 1970.
20. Haas, A., and Luczak, A.: The importance of rehabilitation in the treatment of chronic pulmonary emphysema, Arch. Phys. Med. Rehab. **54**:315, 1972.
21. Hellerstein, H.K.: Principles of exercise prescription. In Naughton, J.P., and Hellerstein, J.K., editors: Exercise testing and exercise training in coronary heart disease, New York, 1973, Academic Press, Inc.
22. Hodgkin, J.E.: Pulmonary rehabilitation. In Simmons, D.H., editor: Current pulmonology, vol. 3. New York, 1981, John Wiley & Sons, Inc.
23. Innocenti, D.: Breathing exercises in the treatment of emphysema, Physiotherapy **52**:437, 1966.
24. Jones, N.L., and Goodwin, J.F.: Respiratory function in pulmonary thromboembolic disorders, Br. Med. J. **1**:1089, 1965.
25. Jones, N.L., and Campbell, E.J.M.: Clinical exercise testing, Philadelphia, 1982, W.B. Saunders Co.
26. Laros, C.D., and Swierenga, J.: Rehabilitation program in patients with obstructive lung disease: proposition for the selection of the most promising candidates, Respiration **29**:344, 1972.
27. Leith, D., and Bradley, M.: Ventilatory muscle strength and endurance training, J. Appl. Physiol. **41**(4):508, 1976.
28. Lertzman, M.M., and Cherniack, R.M.: Rehabilitation of patients with chronic obstructive pulmonary disease, Am. Rev. Respir. Dis. **114**:1145, 1976.

29. Longo, A.N., Moser, K.M., and Luchsinger, P.C.: The role of oxygen therapy in the rehabilitation of patients with chronic obstructive lung disease, Am. Rev. Respir. Dis. **103**:690, 1971.

30. Luce, J.M., and Culver, B.H.: Respiratory muscle function in health and disease, Chest **81**(1):82, 1982.

31. MacDougall, J.D., Elder, G.C.G., Sale, D.G., and others: Effects of strength training and immobilization on human muscle fibers, Eur. J. Appl. Physiol. Occup. Physiol. **43**:25, 1980.

32. Macklem, P.T.: The diaphragm in health and disease, J. Lab. Clin. Med. **99**:601, 1982.

33. MacMahon, C.: Breathing and physical exercises for use in case of wounds in the pleura, lung and diaphragm, Lancet, p. 769, 1915.

34. May, D.B., and Munt, P.W.: Physiologic effects of chest percussion and postural drainage in patients with stable chronic bronchitis, Chest **75**(1):29, 1979.

35. McDonald, G.L., and Hudson, L.D.: Important aspects of pulmonary rehabilitation, Geriatrics **37**(3):127, 1982.

36. McGavin, C.R., Gupta, S.P., and McHardy, G.J.R.: Twelve minute walking test for assessing disability in chronic bronchitis, Br. Med. J. **1**:822, 1976.

37. Miller, W.F., Taylor, H.F., and Jasper, L.: Exercise training in the rehabilitation of patients with severe respiratory insufficiency due to pulmonary emphysema: the role of oxygen breathing, Southern Med. J. **55**:1216, 1962.

38. Miller, W.F., Taylor, H.F., and Pierce, A.K.: Rehabilitation of the disabled patient with chronic bronchitis and pulmonary emphysema, Am. J. Pub. Health. **53**(3, suppl.):18, 1963.

39. Moser, K.M., Bokinsky, G.E., Savage, R.T., and others: Results of a comprehensive rehabilitation program, Arch. Intern. Med. **140**:1956, 1980.

40. Motley, H.: The effects of slow deep breathing and blood gas exchange in emphysema, Am. Rev. Respir. Dis. **88**:485, 1963.

41. Official American Thoracic Society statement: Pulmonary rehabilitation, Am. Rev. Respir. Dis. **124**:663, 1981.

42. Paez, P.N., Phillipson, E.A., Masangkay, M., and others: The physiologic basis of training patients with emphysema, Am. Rev. Respir. Dis. **95**:944, 1967.

43. Paul, G., and others: Some effects of slowing respiration rate in chronic emphysema and bronchitis, J. Appl. Physiol. **21**(3):877, 1966.

44. Perry, J.A.: Effectiveness of teaching in the rehabilitation of patients with chronic bronchitis and emphysema, Nurs. Res. **30**(4):219, 1981.

45. Pfeiffer, V.R., Wilson, N.L., and Wilson, R.H.: Breathing patterns and gas mixing, Phys. Ther. **44**(5):331, 1964.

46. Pratter, M.R., Hingston, D.M., and Irwin, R.S.: Diagnosis of bronchial asthma by clinical evaluation: an unreliable method, Chest **84**(1):42, 1983.

47. Pryor, J.A., and Webber, B.A.: An evaluation of the forced expiration technique as an adjunct to postural drainage, Physiotherapy **65**(10):304, 1979.

48. Pulmonary rehabilitation medical manual, Lincoln, Nebraska, 1977, University of Nebraska Medical Center, Publisher.

49. Robbins, S.L., and Angell, M.: Basic pathology, ed. 2, Philadelphia, 1976, W.B. Saunders Co.

50. Sahn, S.A., Nett, L.M., Petty, T.L.: Ten year follow-up of a comprehensive rehabilitation program for severe COPD, Chest **77**(2 suppl.):311, 1980.

51. Schwartzstein, R.M.: Extrapulmonary effects of chronic obstructive lung disease, Cardiopulmonary Q. **4**(3):2, 1983.

52. Shutz, K.: Muscular exercise in the treatment of bronchial asthma, N.Y. State J. Med. **42**:79, 1955.

53. Smodlaka, V.R., and Adamovich, D.R.: Reconditioning of emphysema patients using interval training, N.Y. State J. Med. **6**:951, 1974.

54. Stewart, H.E.: Diathermy in pneumonia, Physiotherapy News Bull. **3**(5):7, 1925.

55. Thompson, B., and Thompson, H.T.: Forced expiratory exercises in asthma and their effect on FEV_1, N.Z. J. Physiother. **3**(15):19, 1968.

56. Wong, J.W., Keens, T.G., Wannamaker, E.M., and others: Effects of gravity on tracheal transport rates in normal subjects and in patients with cystic fibrosis, Pediatrics **60**(2):146, 1977.

57. Woolf, C.R., and Suero, J.T.: Alterations in lung mechanics and gas exchange following training in chronic obstructive lung disease, Dis. Chest **55**(1):37, 1969.

20

MARLA R. WOLFSON
VINOD K. BHUTANI
THOMAS H. SHAFFER

Respiratory muscles

The respiratory muscles, like the heart, form an organ system that acts as a pump.[40] The movement of air in and out of the gas-exchange units of the lung is accomplished by the action of the respiratory pump. Because of the vital importance of the respiratory muscles, the scope of this chapter is to provide a synthesis of what is currently known of respiratory muscle function, which may be of direct help or interest to the student of pulmonary physical therapy. Of course, it includes a section on muscle mechanics, but this is placed in proper perspective for understanding how the respiratory muscles move and how airflow ensues. Furthermore, we have described the most recent techniques for assessment of respiratory muscle function and training methods and assessment of the effect of lung and neuromuscular disease and musculoskeletal dysfunction on respiratory muscles. Finally, we present a current review of training studies and their effects on cardiopulmonary function on respiratory muscle strength, endurance, and fatigue, and on exercise tolerance.

RESPIRATORY MUSCLE MECHANICS
Description of muscle function

Most of the information on muscle function is summarized from the work of Campbell and co-workers.[13]

During quiet breathing, the primary muscle responsible for ventilation is the diaphragm. Although not essential for breathing, it is the principal muscle of inspiration. The diaphragm's contribution to tidal volume has been estimated to be two thirds in the sitting and standing positions and three fourths or greater in the supine position. This large thin sheet of skeletal muscle separates the thoracic from the abdominal cavity (Fig. 20-1). Its alpha motoneurons leave the spinal cord in the anterior roots of the third to fifth cervical segments and run downward in the phrenic nerve. Since the diaphragm is attached all around the circumference of the lower thoracic cage, contraction of the muscle pulls down mainly the central part. In addition, the diaphragm compresses the viscera, displaces the abdomen

outward, and lifts the rib cage. The inspiratory movement of the diaphragm decreases intrapleural pressure, which inflates the lungs, and increases intra-abdominal pressure, which displaces both the abdomen and rib cage.

Also active during inspiration, the external intercostal muscles elevate the anterior portion of the rib cage and pull it upward and outward (Fig. 20-1). The intercostal nerves, which innervate these muscles, leave the spinal cord from between the first through the eleventh thoracic segments. In addition, other accessory muscles come into play during vigorous breathing including the sternocleidomastoid and scalene muscles in the neck, the muscles of the shoulder region, and the pectoral muscles.

Expiration is a passive process during quiet breathing and occurs because of the elasticity of the lung and chest wall. As breathing becomes more vigorous, as in exercise, or labored, as in respiratory disease, expiration is no longer a passive process. The internal intercostal muscles and abdominal muscles contract to increase intrapleural and intra-abdominal pressure during expiration. The internal intercostal muscle group is, like the external intercostal muscles, innervated by the intercostal nerves. The abdominal muscles are innervated by nerve fibers that originate in the lower six thoracic and first lumbar segments of the spinal cord. Normally, the abdominal muscles are regarded as powerful expiratory muscles whose action increases the intra-abdominal pressure to force the diaphragm cephalad. However, Grimby and associates[22] have demonstrated the role of the abdominal muscles in certain inspiratory maneuvers.

Intrinsic properties of the respiratory pump

As previously discussed, the respiratory pump is composed of numerous skeletal muscle groups. Like other skeletal muscle, respiratory muscle force is dependent on muscle length and velocity of shortening. In the respiratory system, force-length relationships can be expressed indirectly as pressure-volume curves, whereas force-velocity

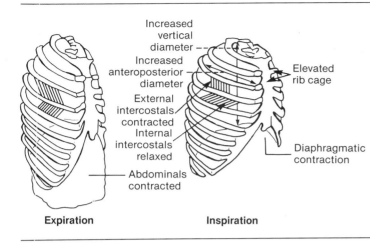

Fig. 20-1. Illustration of diaphragmatic contraction, elevation of the rib cage, and function of the intercostals. (From Guyton, A.C.: Textbook of medical physiology, Philadelphia, 1971, W.B. Saunders Co.)

Table 20-1. Properties of muscle fibers

Naked eye	Microscopic	Histochemical	Contractile properties
Red	High myoglobin content Rich in sarcoplasm Many mitochondria	High oxidative activity Low phosphorylase	Slow
White	Lower myoglobin content Less sarcoplasm Fewer mitochondria	Low oxidative activity High phosphorylase	Fast

Modified from Campbell, E.J.M., Agostoni, E., and Davis, J.N.: The respiratory muscles, Philadelphia, 1970, W.B. Saunders Co.

relationships are described in terms of pressure-flow curves. Such curves describe the overall behavior of the respiratory pump yet do not provide direct information concerning the intrinsic properties of individual respiratory muscle groups.[18]

As predicted by these principles, Rohrer[48] and Rahn and associates[47] have experimentally demonstrated that maximal inspiratory pressure diminishes as lung volume increases whereas maximal expiratory pressure increases. Furthermore, studies involving maximal flow efforts have shown that the maximal pressure developed by the respiratory system decreases as flow increases.

Morphology and properties of the respiratory muscles

The respiratory muscles are striated and microscopically classified into two muscle fiber groups. In general, fast muscle fibers are white and slow muscle fibers are red. The description of skeletal muscle as slow-twitch or fast-twitch is a relative designation only applicable within a single species. For example, muscles of smaller animals are usually faster than similar muscles of larger animals.[13] Table 20-1 shows a simplified classification of muscle-fiber properties. Precise correlation of microscopic, histochemical, and contractile characteristics has not been established. Recent studies of the histochemical properties of muscle fibers have demonstrated that the oxidative capacity and therefore the resistance to fatigue of the ventilatory muscles increases greatly from midgestation to early childhood.[31] Premature infants have less than 10% high-oxidative, slow-twitch fibers in the diaphragm as compared to 55% found in the adult diaphragm. It has been suggested that the ventilatory muscles of newborns are more susceptible to fatigue than those of older subjects and may contribute to the respiratory problems of preterm neonates.

EVALUATION AND CLINICAL DIAGNOSIS OF RESPIRATORY MUSCLE PERFORMANCE

Performance of any muscle can be assessed by its strength, endurance, and inherent ability to resist fatigue. Determination of these characteristics provide sensitive indices to respiratory muscle function.

Respiratory muscle strength

The strength of the respiratory muscle contraction is directly related to the intrinsic muscle properties. The pressures generated within the respiratory system are dependent on the forces generated during muscle contraction and on the elastic properties of the lung and chest wall. Thus respiratory muscle strength has been defined as the maximum or minimum pressure developed within the respiratory system at a specific lung volume.[12,16]

Inspiratory and expiratory muscle strength are determined by measurement of the maximum static inspiratory (MSIP) and expiratory (MSEP) pressures. Both MSIP and MSEP are measured as the static pressures developed at the mouth at a given lung volume. The subject's lung volumes are determined by a volume plethysmograph. The subject breathes through a mouthpiece attached to a pressure tap and a shutter. The maximum static pressures are generated against a closed shutter during inspiratory and expiratory maneuvers. These measurements are made commonly over the range of the vital capacity at intervals of 20% of total lung capacity. Each maneuver is sustained for 3 to 5 seconds and both MSIP and MSEP are correlated to the particular lung volume.[37] A typical relationship is shown in Fig. 20-2. These pressures are reduced with muscular weakness and fatigue and are increased with strength training.

Diaphragmatic strength can be estimated by measurement of the transdiaphragmatic pressure (P_{di}). Maximal P_{di} is measured during maximal diaphragmatic contraction.[51] The ratio of $P_{di}/P_{di\ max}$ at various lung volumes or maneuvers can be used to assess the strength of diaphragmatic contractions. Similarly, the ratio of inspiratory mouth pressure (P_m) to $P_{m\ max}$ (maximal inspiratory mouth pressure) can be utilized to quantitate the combined strength of the inspiratory muscle groups.[50]

Respiratory muscle endurance

The endurance capacity of the respiratory muscles is dependent on the mechanics of the respiratory system and the energy availability of the muscles. The endurance of these muscle groups is defined as the capacity to maintain maximal or submaximal levels of ventilation under isocapnic conditions.[20,37] The endurance capacity is standardized by (1) maximal ventilation for a specific duration of time, (2) ventilation against a known resistance, or (3) sustained ventilation at a given lung volume.[24,37]

The endurance of ventilatory muscles as a group is determined with respect to a specific ventilatory target (tidal volume × respiratory rate) and the time to exhaustion.[37] During this procedure of hyperpnea, a partial rebreathing system is used to maintain oxygen and carbon dioxide levels relatively constant. Fig. 20-3, *A*, details one such system; simpler modifications of this system have been used for purposes of training (Fig. 20-3, *B*). A sequence of maximal ventilatory targets and the time to exhaustion are

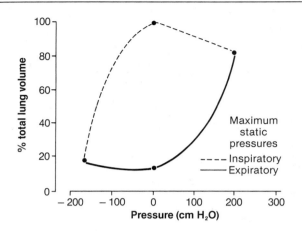

Fig. 20-2. Maximum inspiratory and expiratory pressures as a function of lung volumes. (Modified from Leith, D.E., and Bradley M.: J. Appl. Physiol. **41**:508-516, 1976).

measured and correlated (Fig. 20-4). This relationship is geometric, and its asymptote has been defined as the sustainable ventilatory capacity (SVC). This value is one criterion of ventilatory muscle endurance but may be further standardized as a fraction of the 15-second maximal voluntary ventilation.

Inspiratory muscle endurance is measured when one breathes against inspiratory resistive loads, such as a narrow-bore tube, and gauged by the pressures generated at the mouth ($P_m/P_{m\ max}$) or across the diaphragm ($P_{di}/P_{di\ max}$).[50,51] The subject is instructed to breathe through a known, usually large, resistance and generate a constant, target P_m but allowed to choose his own tidal volume or frequency. The endurance time is determined at the point of exhaustion or inability to generate the target P_m. Likewise, the measurement of P_{di} during these maneuvers allows assessment of diaphragmatic endurance. Roussos and Macklem[51] (Fig. 20-5) have shown that a $P_m/P_{m\ max}$ of 60% or less can support indefinite cyclical ventilation and that the diaphragm can generate 40% of its maximum pressure indefinitely. At these levels fatigue is prevented, and complete recovery from the inspiratory effort occurs during expiration.

Respiratory muscle fatigue

The respiratory muscles, like any other skeletal muscle, fatigue when the rate of energy consumption exceeds the rate of energy supplied to the muscle. Depletion of the energy stores within the muscle subsequently leads to its failure as a force generator.[18] Diaphragmatic and other inspiratory muscle fatigue is an important potential clinical problem because it is the final common pathway toward respiratory failure. The psychological and physiological

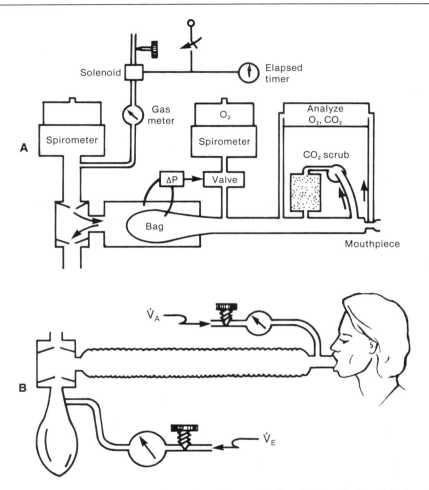

Fig. 20-3. A, Partial rebreathing system for endurance testing. **B,** Simplified partial rebreathing system for endurance training. (Modified from Leith, D.E., and Bradley, M.: J. Appl. Physiol. **41**:508-516, 1976.)

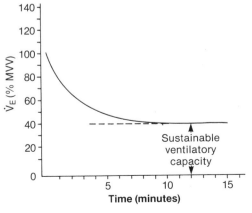

Fig. 20-4. Sustainable ventilatory capacity (SVC) defined as asymptote of the relationship between maximal ventilation performance ($\dot{V}_E$), expressed as a percentage of maximum voluntary ventilation (MVV), and the time to exhaustion. (Modified from Leith, D.E., and Bradley, M.: J. Appl. Physiol. **41**:508-516, 1976.)

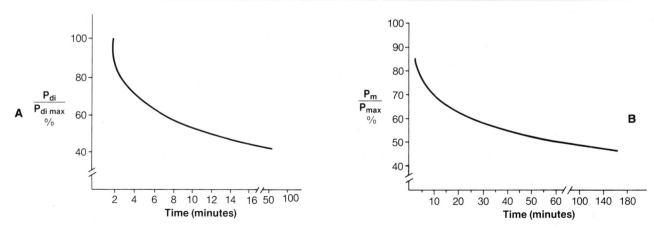

Fig. 20-5. Diagram of, **A,** transdiaphragmatic pressure (P_{di}) expressed as a fraction of maximum inspiratory pressure at functional residual capacity (FRC) ($P_{di}/P_{di\ max\ \%}$) as a function of time and, **B,** mouth pressure (P_m) as a percentage of maximum inspiratory pressure at FRC ($P_{max\ \%}$) plotted as a function of time. (Modified from Roussos, C., and others: J. Appl. Physiol. **46**(5):897-904, 1979.)

factors[54] contributing to respiratory muscle fatigue are depicted in Fig. 20-6. Muscle fatigue also accounts for exercise intolerance, which is increased in patients with lung disease, in those with neuromuscular and musculoskeletal disorders, and in those being weaned from mechanical ventilators. Decreased muscle strength, endurance, or both, in these patients may lead to premature onset of respiratory muscle fatigue. Abnormal chest wall and lung mechanics, as well as abnormal lung volumes, compromise the pressure-generating capabilities of the inspiratory muscles.[47]

The diagnosis of the onset of respiratory muscle fatigue assumes critical importance, since it is this end point that measures strength, endurance, and response to training programs. Ventilatory muscle fatigue may be assessed clinically. Though histochemical and biochemical changes also provide indices of fatigue, these are not used clinically because of the accompanying difficulties and potential complications when inspiratory muscle tissue samples are obtained.

Clinical evaluation of respiratory muscle fatigue

Inspection and palpation. Inspection of the thoracic cage may reveal out-of-phase and incoordinated chest-wall movements, which produce combined or alternating diaphragmatic and intercostal breathing patterns. An inward movement of the costal margins (Hoover's sign) is observed in fatiguing patients with chronic obstructive pulmonary disease (COPD). Inward inspiratory motions of the abdomen may often predict severe respiratory failure. Palpation of the chest wall and neck allows evaluation of increased activity of the accessory respiratory muscles. Although these are important clinical signs and are

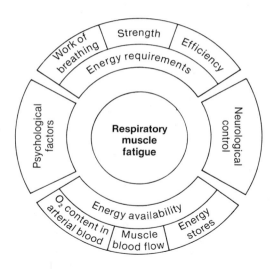

Fig. 20-6. Factors associated with respiratory muscle fatigue. (From Shaffer, T.H., Wolfson, M.R., and Bhutani, V.K.: Phys. Ther. **61**:12, 1711-1723, 1981.)

commonly associated with an increased respiratory load, these signs are difficult to measure and are neither specific nor sensitive indicators of fatigue.

Lung volumes. The values of total lung capacity (TLC) and residual volume (RV) are governed by elastic recoil of the lung chest wall and the respiratory muscle force. Thus, at total lung capacity the inspiratory muscle forces are most active, whereas at residual volume the expiratory muscle groups are predominant.

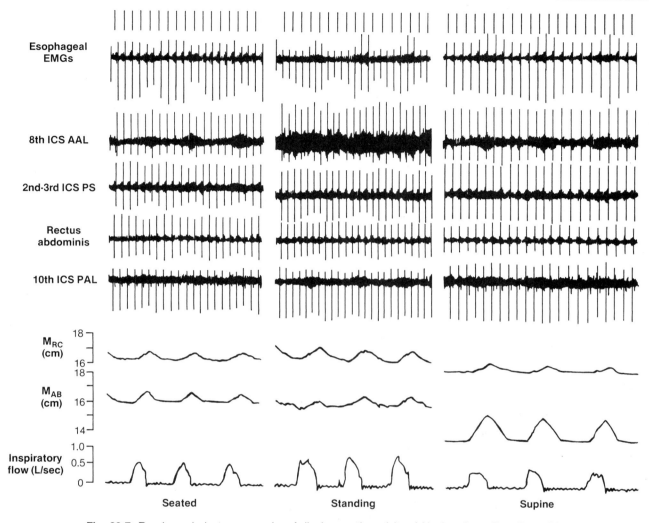

Fig. 20-7. Esophageal electromyographs of diaphragmatic activity. *AAL,* Anterior axillary line; *ICS,* intercostal space; M_{AB}, abdominal displacement; M_{RC}, rib cage displacement; *PAL,* posterior axillary line; *PS,* posterior scapular. (Courtesy Dr. Sanford Levine, Philadelphia, Pa.)

Magnetometry. The dimensional changes of the rib cage and abdomen are measured with magnetometers and are useful for coordination of clinical observations.[36] These data may be used to infer lung volume displacements rather than respiratory muscle group activity. The subtle, mechanical signs of fatigue include (1) rapid, shallow respiratory cycles, (2) paradoxical abdominal movements, and (3) alternation between predominantly abdominal movement and rib-cage movement during inspiration. However, it is erroneous to attribute abdominal motion solely to the diaphragm and to attribute the rib cage motion solely to the intercostal muscles. Thus this mode of evaluation is not a specific indicator of fatigue.

Pressures. The pressures generated at the mouth (P_m), esophagus (P_{es}), stomach (P_g), and the difference between P_{es} and P_g, which is P_{di} can be measured during ventilatory maneuvers. Although useful, these pressure measurements require that the patient swallow an esophageal balloon. This may be an uncomfortable, or impossible procedure for an person with severe dyspnea. These maneuvers have been described earlier and when repeated at intervals may be utilized to predict fatigue.

Electromyography. The electromyograph (EMG) presents an exceedingly complicated signal of motor-unit behavior during muscle contractions.[6] However, it has been recognized as a valuable predictor of muscle activity, timing, and fatigue.[23,44] As shown in Fig. 20-7, EMG activity of individual respiratory muscles can be associated with specific respiratory maneuvers and body positioning. Diaphragmatic EMG is obtained by electrode placement at

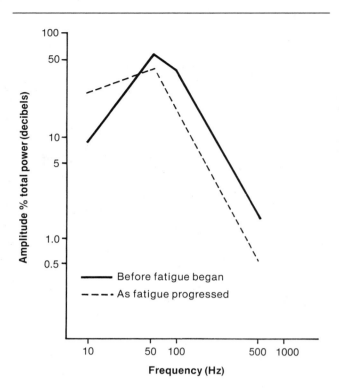

Fig. 20-8. Changes in high- and low-frequency components of EMG activity during diaphragmatic muscle fatigue. (Modfied from Derenne, J.-P.H., Macklem, D.T., and Roussos, C.H.: Am. Rev. Respir. Dis. **118**(1-3):119, 373, 581, 1978.)

creased amplitude of high-frequency (150 to 350 Hz) components, and (3) decreased ratio of high to low (H:L ratio) frequency components. The H:L ratio is independent of respiratory muscle force and begins to decrease long before the muscle reaches its limit of endurance.[35]

The other aspects of EMG power spectrum also need to be considered for the evaluation of fatigue. These include (1) the maximum amplitude of the power spectrum, (2) the area under the amplitude-frequency curve, (3) the first movement of inertia, and (4) the centroid frequency. The role of these factors as the best predictor of respiratory muscle fatigue still needs to be evaluated.

RESPIRATORY MUSCLE FUNCTION IN DISEASE

One of the major problems associated with respiratory management is the maintenance of adequate alveolar ventilation. Patients with primary pulmonary, neuromuscular, or musculoskeletal disease are at risk for respiratory failure. Respiratory muscle strength may be normal or increased in patients with primary pulmonary disease (Table 20-2) yet insufficient to overcome increased respiratory loads. In patients with neuromuscular or musculoskeletal disease (Table 20-3), inadequate respiration results from primary muscle dysfunction, immobility, or respiratory center abnormalities. Regardless of the predisposing factors, respiratory muscle fatigue ensues, and although the clinical course may differ (Fig. 20-9), respiratory failure can result.

Although patients can usually be classified as having either primary pulmonary, neuromuscular, or musculoskeletal disease, mixed problems are frequently seen; for example, immobility and bulbar involvement associated with neuromuscular or musculoskeletal disease (typically leading to restrictive lung disease) may cause ineffective coughing, aspiration syndrome, or mucus plugging; airway obstruction results and so obstructive lung disease is diagnosed.[27] This further increases the demand on the respiratory muscles, which are already insufficient.

TRAINING PROGRAMS AND PHYSIOLOGICAL RESPONSES
General considerations and categories

Exercise programs have long been advocated as a therapeutic procedure for patients with respiratory dysfunction. Assessment of the efficacy of these programs have typically reported on changes in spirometric variables of lung function or on psychological advantages of rehabilitation training programs. However, unlike training programs for the physically healthy population, limited quantitative physiological data are available for assessment of programs for the respiratory impaired. This dearth of information may be a function of several variables including complicating health factors, ambiguous programming and assessment methods, and patient and personnel logistics within a predominantly outpatient population.

sites with minimal or poor intercostal activity during inspiration. These sites are (1) the tenth intercostal space in the midaxillary line by needle electrodes, (2) the seventh, eighth, and ninth intercostal spaces in the midclavicular line by surface electrodes, and (3) the esophagus.[23] Diaphragmatic and intercostal muscle EMG activity are observable primarily during inspiration as indicated by inspiratory flow and by chest-wall and abdominal displacement. Inasmuch as quiet expiration is passive, there is no expiratory muscle EMG activity.

More recently, investigators have studied the frequency of respiratory muscle EMG activity.[53] Power-density spectral analysis of the frequency components has been used for assessment of the power of the myoelectric signal. Studies have shown that the diaphragmatic EMG spectrum is concentrated in the bandwidth of 25 to 250 Hz. Analysis of these EMG's have been used to make an early diagnosis of the onset of diaphragmatic fatigue. Characteristic patterns of electrical activity have been observed on the EMG of a fatiguing skeletal muscle. Similar shifts in the power spectrum of the EMG have been observed during diaphragmatic fatigue.[23] These observations (Fig. 20-8) document the onset of fatigue through (1) increased amplitude of low-frequency (20 to 46.7 Hz) components, (2) de-

Table 20-2. Primary pulmonary diseases affecting respiratory muscle function

Adult	Pediatric
Obstructive diseases	
Asthma	Asthma
Bronchitis	Meconium aspiration
Emphysema	Amniotic fluid aspiration
Aspiration syndrome	Bronchiolitis
Bronchiolitis	Cystic fibrosis
Tumor	Congenital disorders of larynx and trachea
Restrictive diseases	
Alveolar	
Pneumonia	Hyaline membrane disease
Pulmonary edema	Atelectasis
Adult respiratory distress syndrome	Pneumonia
Interstitial	
Interstitial fibrosis	Bronchopulmonary dysplasias
Connective tissue disorders	Connective tissue disorders
	Cystic fibrosis
Vascular	
Thromboembolic disease	Persistent pulmonary hypertension of newborn
Pulmonary hypertension	
Pleural	
Pleural effusion	Pleural effusion
Mesothelioma	Chylothorax

From Shaffer, T.H., Wolfson, M.R., and Bhutani, V.K.: Phys. Ther. **61**(12):1711-1723, 1981.

Table 20-3. Neuromuscular and musculoskeletal dysfunction affecting respiratory muscle function

Acute	Chronic
Neuromuscular	
Cord Transection	Spastic quadriplegia
Guillain-Barré syndrome	Hemiplegia
Botulism	Cerebral palsy
Cholinergic poisoning	Parkinsonism
Poliomyelitis	Multiple sclerosis
Tetanus	Spina bifida
Diaphragmatic paralysis	Myasthenia gravis
Congenital diaphragmatic paralysis	Muscular dystrophy
	Diaphragmatic fatigue of prematurity
Musculoskeletal	
Crush injury of chest	Kyphoscoliosis
Postcardiothoracic surgery	Ankylosing spondylitis
	Pectus excavatum

Modified from Shaffer T.H., Wolfson, M.R., and Bhutani, V.K.: Phys. Ther. **61**(12):1711-1723, 1981.

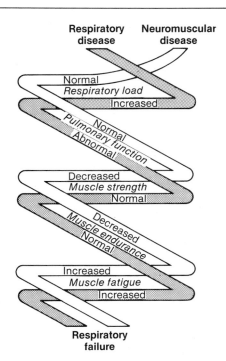

Fig. 20-9. The interrelationship between respiratory muscles and pulmonary function in the pathogenesis of respiratory failure. (From Shaffer, T.H., Wolfson, M.R., and Bhutani, V.K.: Phys. Ther. **61**:12, 1711-1723, 1981.)

Nonetheless, exercise is a critical component in the care plan of the respiratory impaired. If the long-term goal of rehabilitation is to return or maintain maximum functional level, the student of pulmonary physical therapy should be capable of designing, administering, and reevaluating a rehabilitation program and assessing the efficacy of this program for the population toward which it is intended.

To this end, the purposes of this section are as follows:

1. Compare and contrast effects of exercise in the normal and respiratory-impaired populations.
2. Highlight assessed rehabilitation programs with respect to pulmonary function, hemodynamics, cardiovascular function, respiratory muscle strength, fatigue, endurance, and exercise tolerance.

Exercise programs take on many forms, but for convenience they can be divided into two groups: general (systemic) and specific (localized training of respiratory muscles). General programs include activities using extremity muscles in addition to respiratory musculature with or without supplemental oxygen.[11,14,15,17,34,61] Almost all combinations of exercise have been studied: general conditioning, including treadmill and bicycling, breathing exercises, and psychological support; bicycling and treadmill or treadmill alone[2,7,26,45,47,62]; treadmill and breathing exercises, calisthenics-gymnastics-swimming, and patient

education for children[28]; jogging for adolescents[60]; and walking.[57,59] These programs have been designed to improve the physiological factors of pulmonary function, strength, endurance, cardiac function, and exercise tolerance as well as nonphysiological factors such as cooperation and psychological well-being.

Alternatively, specific training refers to exercises primarily involving and emphasizing ventilatory muscle groups. Diaphragmatic training alone or with incentive spirometry has been recommended in patients with chronic obstructive pulmonary disease.[4] In these patients, a flattened, depressed diaphragm was observed to have limited respiratory excursions and consequently minimal contribution to ventilation. Use of a Gordon-Barach belt and diaphragmatic breathing with active abdominal contraction during expiration is directed at causing a cephalic displacement of the diaphragm.[4] As the diaphragm lengthens, the abdominal and inspiratory rib-cage musculature shortens. Length-tension relationships are optimized providing increased contraction and pressure change for improved diaphragmatic respiration.[21] However, substantial data are scant and of questionable support of this modality as an independent means to enhance respiration.[14] Pursed-lips breathing, the pattern of exhaling through the mouth against the pressure of pursed lips, is used spontaneously by some patients and often is taught to other patients as one facet of breathing retraining.[1,29,43] Pursed-lips breathing is believed to prevent airway closure and provide relief to some patients from unpleasant sensations associated with breathing.

Ventilatory muscle strength training (VMST) has been shown to increase isometric pressures generated by inspiratory and expiratory muscles.[37] For example, maximum static inspiratory and expiratory pressures (MSIP and MSEP) are performed on the spirometer against a closed shutter at 20% intervals over the range of vital capacity. Each maneuver is sustained for 3 to 5 seconds, and the performance is repeated so that the exercise lasts one-half hour a day.

Ventilatory muscle endurance training (VMET) results in the capacity for sustaining higher levels of ventilation for relatively long periods of time, approximately 15 minutes. Leith and Bradley[37] described VMET as sustained ventilation achieved three to five times, until exhaustion, interspersed with recovery intervals of unspecified duration. Each episode lasted 12 to 15 minutes; the duration of the session was 45 to 60 minutes, 5 days a week. Normocapnic hyperpnea was achieved with a partial rebreathing system. Use of a breathing bag provided visual biofeedback to the patient, and the CO_2 scrubber was adjusted to maintain a normal end tidal CO_2. Both VMST and VMET are current approaches in exercise programs and areas of active research in pulmonary rehabilitation.

Other unique collaborative therapeutic approaches to training may be required when respiratory problems are caused or complicated by nonrespiratory disabilities. For example, children with cerebral palsy are extremely vulnerable to respiratory disease because of shallow, irregular respirations and ineffectual cough.[10,49] Although respiratory functions are impaired in these children, concomitant decreased efficiency and poor coordination of the breathing mechanisms further jeopardize ventilatory capacity.[9] In addition, impaired neuromotor control is often coupled with reduced physical activity, which by itself is another respiratory disease risk factor.

Effect of training programs on pulmonary function

Respiratory muscles, like other skeletal muscles in the normal population, improve their efficiency after training. This improvement is reflected in improved breathing function. Training effects on pulmonary ventilation are associated with a decrease in rate and an increase in depth of breathing.[30] In the trained subject these changes are noticed at rest and during heavy exercise as well.

Pulmonary function response to general training programs for patients with COPD is reviewed by Shaffer and co-workers.[54] In general, no significant change was seen in most pulmonary function variables. A decreased respiratory rate with a deeper breathing pattern was noted.[42,59,61] One investigator suggested that a more efficient breathing pattern resulted, whereas others described a task-specific improvement in ventilation. A few studies found an increase in forced vital capacity (FVC), which may have reflected a reduction in air trapping[57]; additionally, improvements in maximal voluntary ventilation and inspiratory capacity are reported.[7] High pretraining values for specific and static lung compliance decreased (though not significantly) toward normal after training.[2] In addition, a trend toward improved dynamic compliance and reduced respiratory work are reported as a result of training.[62]

Less information is available about the effects of specific training programs on pulmonary function. Furthermore, conflicting results are reported such that some studies report improvement in lung volumes and maneuvers[8,37,49] whereas others report no significant change after training.[33,41] Mechanisms for pulmonary function improvement after specific training programs have been suggested. Postural compensation, forward leaning upon respiratory stress, compresses the abdomen. Because of mechanical relationships, the diaphragm is stretched upwards, and this stretching facilitates the length-tension relationship, thereby increasing the capacity of the diaphragm to generate tension. Alternatively, research on animals possibly indicates a neurophysiological mechanism by which costovertebral joint mobilization may stimulate joint mechanoreceptors. This information may be processed through the medullary-pontine ''rhythm generator'' to influence the respiratory pattern.[55]

Effect of training programs on hemodynamics and cardiopulmonary function

Training programs improve certain hemodynamic and cardiopulmonary functions in the normal population[4,52] Maximal oxygen consumption ($\dot{V}O_{2\,max}$), oxygen extraction (a-$\bar{v}O_2$), cardiac output, and stroke volume increase, whereas resting heart rate is found to decrease after training. In general, oxygen consumption ($\dot{V}O_2$) and $\dot{V}O_{2\,max}$ are used to evaluate the effectiveness and intensity of training, since they reflect a change in cardiac output and oxygen extraction by the tissues.

Oxygen consumption increases linearly as a function of escalating work loads and becomes stable with maximal work, the point of $\dot{V}O_{2\,max}$. Thereafter, the oxygen needs of the muscle are not met by the cardiovascular-respiratory system, and the energy for increased work is derived from anaerobic metabolism. Lactic acid accumulation results. Therefore a higher $\dot{V}O_{2\,max}$ implies increased oxygen use by the peripheral musculature at maximal loads with associated increments in a-$\bar{v}O_2$ and decrements in exercise blood lactate levels. As such, an objective indication of a training effect is an increase in $\dot{V}O_{2\,max}$. Furthermore, in the normal population, the rate of change of $\dot{V}O_2$ at each level of exercise is not physiologically altered by mild training once the exercise is learned, whereas $\dot{V}O_{2\,max}$ increases. General training programs are known to produce slower heart rates regardless of the exercise employed. The reasons for this are unclear; however, it has been suggested that general muscle training may alter autonomic control, levels of circulating catecholamines, stroke volume, or the integrating ability of the central nervous system. Increases in stroke volume are also associated with training. These increases are related to increased ventricular volume or bradycardia. Finally, cardiac output increases parallel the increase in $\dot{V}O_{2\,max}$ in response to training.[52]

Research of general training programs in patients with COPD report changes in some of the aforementioned parameters. Several studies demonstrated a decrease in $\dot{V}O_2$ at each level of exercise relating this finding to improved coordination and exercise efficiency.[2,45] One group of investigators reported that the greater the initial exercise load (higher $\dot{V}O_2$), the greater the decrease in $\dot{V}O_2$ at a given exercise level after training.[59] They suggest that this relationship emphasizes the importance of beginning exercises at the highest safe level. Increases in $\dot{V}O_{2\,max}$ and a-$\bar{v}O_2$ values are also reported.[17,45] These findings are most probably related to improved oxygen extraction capacity of the muscles or oxygen delivery to the muscle (i.e., elevated myoglobin concentration or increased number of capillaries per skeletal muscle fiber).

Conflicting data are reported as to changes in heart rate and cardiac output after general training. Some studies report decreases in heart rate, whereas others found no significant change in either parameter. It may be that severely disabled pulmonary patients are unable to reach the level of activity needed to induce a training effect.[15] This has been related to the low level of peripheral activity because of the high oxygen cost of breathing, at rest, for patients with COPD. This reason might also explain why no increase in stroke volume was found as a result of a general training program in the COPD population. These findings seem to support the possibility that increased work tolerance in these patients is most probably attributable to improved oxygen extraction by exercising muscles.

Finally, little is known about general training program effects on gas transport in the respiratory-impaired population. One study reports smaller alveolar-arterial oxygen gradients and improved venous admixtures, implying improved ventilation-perfusion relationships.[62] Oxygen-assisted exercise increased arterial oxygen (PO_2) values while the pH remained stable because of the supplemental oxygen, which reduced exercise-induced lactic acidosis.[11] Furthermore, blood lactate levels have been reported to decrease in another study.[62] This decrease may demonstrate the training effects of producing a more efficient capillary blood supply, providing additional oxygen to the muscle, and thereby reducing anaerobic metabolism.

In contrast to the data for general training programs, relatively little is known about the effects of specific training programs on hemodynamic and cardiopulmonary parameters in the population with COPD. Reports include increases in $\dot{V}O_{2 \text{ max}}$ and maximal exercise heart rate and are associated with the higher exercise levels that were attained.[8] Recruitment of low-oxidative, high-glycolytic, fast-twitch muscle fibers at higher levels of exercise may explain reported increases in postexercise blood lactate levels.[8] Other studies propose improvement in aerobic capacities yet report insignificant changes.[33] This dearth of information is not surprising because specific training techniques are relatively new. This is an area of active investigation, and one would expect more definitive forthcoming data.

Effect of training programs on respiratory muscle strength, endurance, fatigue, and exercise tolerance

The training response of respiratory muscle is similar to that of skeletal muscle. Muscles respond differently to exercises oriented to improving strength as compared to improving endurance. One important difference is that strengthening exercises produce mostly muscle hypertrophy whereas endurance exercises increase the vascularity of muscle fibers.[30] The reason for this difference is not as yet fully understood.

As mentioned previously, respiratory muscle strength is defined as the maximum and minimum static pressures measured at the mouth attributable to the muscular effort needed to produce the change, whereas ventilatory muscle endurance may be defined and measured as the capacity

for sustaining high levels of ventilation under isocapnic conditions for relatively long periods. Diaphragmatic fatigue is defined as the point at which the diaphragm is unable to sustain a predetermined level of transdiaphragmatic pressure. Exercise tolerance is the ability to exercise without discomfort. Strength, endurance, fatigue, and dyspnea play a role in determining an exercise tolerance level.

Limited quantitative data are available on respiratory muscle strength and endurance response to a general exercise program in the population with COPD. Some studies attribute an increase in exercise tolerance to psychological components of improved motivation and a sense of well-being and confidence.[1,34,39,42,61] Several studies allude to improved neuromuscular coordination as the causative factor.[15,45,49] Reported stride-length increments and improvements in specific exercises used in general training programs may demonstrate improved neuromuscular coordination and efficiency of movement. Recent studies demonstrate that nonspecific upper-body exercise, such as swimming and canoeing, is effective in improving respiratory muscle endurance in children with cystic fibrosis.[33]

Specific training programs are reported to affect respiratory muscle strength and endurance, as well as exercise tolerance. Leith and Bradley[37] trained normal volunteers according to the VMET and VMST methods previously described. They concluded that VMST improved strength whereas VMET improved endurance. A similar study of children with cystic fibrosis reports increased endurance and exercise tolerance after 4 weeks of training.[33] After training with inspiratory flow–resistive loads, quadriplegic patients with respiratory muscle dysfunction are reported to demonstrate improvement in ventilatory muscle strength and endurance[24]; in addition, dyspnea in other patients disappeared during routine daily activities.[3,46] Specific weight training in healthy subjects such as use of weights placed on the abdomen, does not increase maximal shortening, velocity of shortening, or strength of the diaphragm.[41] Postural compensation, such as forward leaning, provides relief of dyspnea in patients with COPD.[56] This modality may be an effective means to increase exercise tolerance by maximizing the diaphragmatic length-tension relationship and enhancing full synergistic cooperation of the inspiratory muscles.

Respiratory muscle fatigue has not been assessed after a general training program. Several studies suggest that dyspnea curtails activity levels of patients with COPD before respiratory muscle fatigue occurs. It is unclear whether the physiological or psychological components of dyspnea or general debilitation characterized by early extremity skeletal muscle fatigue limit exercise tolerance.

A few studies indicate that specific training programs increase respiratory resistance to fatigue. Reported improvements in endurance after VMET suggest that fatigue is delayed.[33] Animal studies demonstrate delayed onset of fatigue with strength and endurance training associated with increases in cellular oxidative capacity, mitochondrial enzymes, and capacity for fatty acid oxidation.[32,38] Recruitment of other inspiratory muscles is suggested to prevent fatigue when one is breathing against a resistive load. By monitoring the abdominal pressure, investigators noticed that the diaphragm and intercostal muscles contributed alternately in time.[50] Recovery may occur during the alternate rest periods, possibly postponing the onset of fatigue. Although reduced accessory inspiratory muscle EMG activity is noted during forward leaning, patients utilizing this form of postural compensation experience relief of dyspnea.[56] It seems that the force generated by these muscles may be more effectively applied to the rib cage in this position. It is suggested that by stabilization of the upper extremities and use of the reverse action of the muscle, synergy of the inspiratory muscle may be enhanced, and overall respiratory muscle fatigue may thereby be reduced. Hyperinflation through intermittent positive-pressure mechanical ventilation is often recommended as a therapeutic modality in primary pulmonary disease and respiratory dysfunction secondary to neuromuscular and musculoskeletal disease.[19,58] This technique is reported to improve ventilation and gas exchange either by improving pulmonary compliance or by preventing atelectasis. When intermittent positive-pressure ventilation is used in patients with respiratory muscle weakness, the work of breathing required to overcome the elastic forces of the lung is reduced, and therefore oxygen consumption is decreased. Ultimately, respiratory muscle fatigue may be prevented.

REFERENCES

1. Agle, D.P., Baum, G.L., Chester, E.H., and Wendt, M.: Multidiscipline treatment of chronic pulmonary insufficiency. I. Psychologic aspects of rehabilitation, Psychosom. Med. **35**:41-49, 1973.
2. Alpert, J.S., Bass, H., Szucs, M.M., and others: Effects of physical training on hemodynamics and pulmonary function at rest and during exercise in patients with chronic obstructive pulmonary disease, Chest **66**:647-651, 1974.
3. Anderson, J.B., Dragsted, L., Kann, S., and others: Resistive breathing in severe chronic obstructive pulmonary disease: a pilot study, Scand. J. Respir. Dis. **60**:151-156, 1979.
4. Åstrand, P.O., and Rodahl, K.: Textbook of work physiology, New York, 1977, McGraw-Hill Book Co.
5. Barach, A.L., and Seaman, W.: Role of diagram in chronic pulmonary emphysema, N.Y. State J. Med. **63**:415-417, 1963.
6. Basmajian, J.V.: Muscles alive. Baltimore, 1978, The Williams & Wilkins Co.
7. Bass, H., Whitcomb, J.F., and Forman, R.: Exercise training: therapy for patients with chronic obstructive pulmonary disease, Chest **57**:116-121, 1970.
8. Belman, M.J., and Mittman, C.: Ventilatory muscle training improves exercise capacity in chronic obstructive pulmonary disease patients, Am. Rev. Respir. Dis. **121**:273-280, 1980.
9. Bjure, J., and Berg, K.: Dynamic and static-lung volumes of school children with cerebral palsy, Acta Paediatr. Scand. **204**(suppl.):35-41, 1970.
10. Blumberg, M.: Respiration and speech in the cerebral palsied child, Am. J. Dis. Child. **89**:48-53, 1955.
11. Bradley, B.L., Garner, A.E., Biliu, D., and others: Oxygen-assisted excercise in chronic obstructive lung disease, Am. Rev. Respir. Dis. **118**:239-243, 1978.
12. Byrd, R.B., and Hyatt, R.E.: Maximal respiratory pressures in obstructive lung disease, Am. Rev. Respir. Dis. **98**:848-856, 1968.
13. Campbell, E.J.M., Agostoni, E., and Davis, J.N.: The respiratory muscles, Philadelphia, 1970, W.B. Saunders Co.
14. Casciari, R.J., Fairshter, R.D., and Morrison, J.T.: Effects of breathing retraining in patients with chronic obstructive pulmonary disease, Chest **79**:393-398, 1981.
15. Chester, E.H., Belman, M.J., Bahler, R.C., and others: Multidisciplinary treatment of chronic insufficiency. III. The effect of physical training on cardiopulmonary performance in patients with chronic obstructive pulmonary disease, Chest **72**:695-702, 1977.
16. Cook, C.D., Mead, J., and Orzalesi, M.M.: Static volume-pressure characteristics of the respiratory system during maximal efforts, J. Appl. Physiol. **19**:1016-1022, 1964.
17. Degre, S., Sergysels, S., Mession, R., and others: Hemodynamic responses to physical training in patients with chronic lung disease, Am. Rev. Respir. Dis. **110**:395-402, 1974.
18. Derenne, J.-P.H., Macklem, P.T., and Roussos, C.H.: The respiratory muscles: Mechanics, control, and pathophysiology, Am. Rev. Respir. Dis. **118**(1-3): 119-131, 373-390, 581-601, 1978.
19. DeTroyer, A., and Drisser, P.: The effects of intermittent positive pressure breathing on patients with respiratory muscle weakness, Am. Rev. Respir. Dis. **124**:132-137, 1982.
20. Freedman, S.: Sustained maximum voluntary ventilation, Respir. Physiol. **8**:230, 1970.
21. Goldman, M., and Mead, J.: Mechanical interaction between diaphragm and rib cage, J. Appl. Physiol. **35**:197-204, 1973.
22. Grimby, G., Goldman, M., and Mead, J.: Respiratory muscle action inferred from rib cage and abdominal V-P partitioning, J. Appl. Physiol. **41**:739, 1976.
23. Gross, D., Grassino, A., Ross, W.R.D., and Macklem, P.T.: Electromyogram pattern of diaphragmatic fatigue, J. Appl. Physiol. **46**(1):1-7, 1979.
24. Gross, D., Ladd, H.W., Riley, E.J., and others: The effect of training on strength and endurance of the diaphragm in quadriplegia, Am. J. Med. **68**:27-35, 1980.
25. Guyton, A.C.: Textbook of medical physiology, Philadelphia, 1971, W.B. Saunders Co.
26. Hale, T., Spriggs, J., and Hamley, E.J.: The effects of an exercise regime on patients with lung malfunction, Br. J. Sports Med. **11**:181, 1977.
27. Harrison, B.D.W., Collins, J.V., Brown, K.G.E., and Clark, T.J.H.: Respiratory failure in neuromuscular diseases, Thorax **26**:579-584, 1971.
28. Heimlich, D.: Evaluation of a breathing program for children, Respiratory Care **20**:64-68, 1975.
29. Ingram, R.H., and Schilder, D.P.: Effect of pursed lips expiration on the pulmonary pressure-flow relationship in obstructive lung disease, Am. Rev. Respir. Dis. **96**:381-388, 1967.
30. Johnson, W.R., and Buskirk, E.R.: Science and medicine of exercise and sport, ed. 2, New York, 1974, Harper & Row.
31. Keens, T.G., Bryan, A.C., Levison, H., and Ianuzzo, C.D.: Developmental pattern of muscle fibers types in human ventilatory muscles, J. Appl. Physiol. **44**:909-913, 1978.
32. Keens, T.G., Chen, V., Patel, P., and others: Cellular adaptations of the ventilatory muscles to a chronic increased respiratory load, J. Appl. Physiol. **44**(6):905-908, 1978.
33. Keens, T.G., Inese, R.B., Krastins, I.R., and others: Ventilatory muscle endurance training in normal subjects and patients with cystic fibrosis, Am. Rev. Respir. Dis. **116**:853-860, 1977.
34. Kimbel, P., Kaplan, A.S., Alkalay, I., Lester, D.: An in-hospital program for rehabilitation of patients with chronic obstructive pulmonary disease, Bull. Am. Coll. Chest Physicians **60**:6-105, 1971.
35. Kogi, K., and Hakamada, T.: Slowing of surface electromyogram and muscle strength in muscle fatigue, Rep. Instit. Sci. Labour **60**:27, 1962.

36. Konno, K., and Mead, J.: Measurement of the separate volume changes of rib cage and abdomen during breathing, J. Appl. Physiol. **22**:407-422, 1967.

37. Leith, D.E., and Bradley, M.: Ventilatory muscle strength and endurance training, J. Appl. Physiol. **41**:508-516, 1976.

38. Lieberman, D.A., Maxwell, L.C., and Faulkner, J.A.: Adaptation of guinea pig diaphragm muscle to aging and endurance training, Am. J. Physiol. **222**(3):556-560, 1972.

39. Lustig, F.M., Haas, A., and Castillo, R.: Clinical and rehabilitation regime in patients with chronic obstructive pulmonary disease, Arch. Phys. Med. Rehabil. **53**:315-322, 1972.

40. Macklem, P.T.: Respiratory muscles: the vital pump, Chest **78**:753-758, 1980.

41. Merrick, J., and Axen, K.: Inspiratory muscles function following abdomen weight exercises in healthy subjects, Phys. Ther. **61**:651-656, 1981.

42. Moser, K.M., Bokinsky, G.E., Savage, R.T., and others: Results of a comprehensive rehabilitation program, Arch. Intern. Med. **140**:1597-1601, 1980.

43. Mueller, R.E., Petty, T.L., and Filley, G.F.: Ventilation and arterial blood gas changes induced by pursed lips breathing, J. Appl. Physiol. **28**:784-789, 1970.

44. Muller, N., Gulston, G., Cade, D., Whitton, J., and others: Respiratory muscle fatigue in infants, Clin. Res. **25**:714A, 1977.

45. Paez, P.N., Phillipson, E.A., Masangkay, M., and Sproule, H.J.: The physiologic basis of training patients with emphysema, Am. Rev. Respir. Dis. **95**:944-953, 1967.

46. Pardy, R.L., Rivington, R.N., Despas, P.J., and Macklem, P.T.: The effects of inspiratory muscle training on exercise performance in chronic airflow obstruction, Am. Rev. Respir. Dis. **123**:426-433, 1981.

47. Rahn, H., Otis, A.B., Chadwick, L.E., and Fear, W.D.: The pressure volume diagram of the thorax and lung, Am. J. Physiol. **146**:161, 1946.

48. Rohrer, F.: Der Zusammenhang der Atemkräfte und ihre Abhängigkeit von Dehnungzustand der Atmungsorgane, Pflugers Arch. Ges. Physiol. **165**:419, 1916.

49. Rothman, J.G.: Effects of respiratory exercises on the vital capacity and forced expiratory volume in children with cerebral palsy, Phys. Ther. **58**:421-425, 1978.

50. Roussos, C., Fixley, M., Gross, D., and Macklem, P.T.: Fatigue of inspiratory muscles and their synergistic behavior, J. Appl. Physiol. **46**(5):897-904, 1979.

51. Roussos, C.S., and Macklem, P.T.: Diaphragmatic fatigue in man, J. Appl. Physiol. Respirat. **43**:189-197, 1977.

52. Scheuer, J., and Tipton, C.M.: Cardiovascular adaptations to physical training, Ann. Rev. Physiol. **39**:221-251, 1977.

53. Schweitzer, T.W., Fitzgerald, J.W., Bowden, J., and others: Spectral analysis of human inspiratory diaphragmatic electromyograms, J. Appl. Physiol. **41**:152-165, 1979.

54. Shaffer, T.H., Wolfson, M.R., and Bhutani, V.K.: Respiratory muscle function, assessment, and training, Phys. Ther. **61**:12, 1711-1723, 1981.

55. Shannon, R.: Respiratory pattern changes during costovertebral joint movement, J. Appl. Physiol. **48**:862-867, 1980.

56. Sharp, J.T., Drutz, W.S., Moisan, T., and others: Postural relief of dyspnea in severe chronic obstructive pulmonary disease, Am. Rev. Respir. Dis. **122**:201-211, 1980.

57. Sinclair, D.J.M., and Ingram, C.G.: Controlled trial of supervised exercise training in chronic bronchitis, Br. Med. J. **280**(6213):519-521, 1980.

58. Sinha, R., and Bergofsky, E.H.: Prolonged alteration of lung mechanics in kyphoscoliosis by positive pressure hyperinflation, Am. Rev. Respir. Dis. **106**:47-55, 1972.

59. Unger, K.M., Moser, K.M., and Glansen, P.: Selection of an exercise program for patients with chronic obstructive pulmonary disease Heart Lung **9**:68-76, 1980.

60. Wilbourn, K.: The long distance runners, Runner's World, Aug. 1978.

61. Woolf, C.R.: A rehabilitation program for improving exercise tolerance of patients with chronic lung disease, Can. Med. Assoc. J. **106**:1289-1292, 1972.

62. Woolf, C.R., and Suero, J.T.: Alterations in lung mechanics and gas exchange following training in chronic obstructive lung disease, Dis. Chest **55**:37-44, 1969.

21

JANE WETZEL
BRENDA RAE LUNSFORD
MARGERY J. PETERSON
SUSAN ENRIQUEZ ALVAREZ

Respiratory rehabilitation of the patient with a spinal cord injury

CLASSIFICATION OF PATIENTS AND THEIR PROBLEMS

Patients with an injury to the spinal cord vary in levels of breathing function as a result of the degree of neurological deficit. For patients with significant impairment, respiratory rehabilitation is an important determinant in achieving their maximum functional level. The problem of decreased ventilation occurs as a result of (1) decreased strength, (2) decreased thoracic mobility, and (3) inadequate bronchial hygiene.

Ventilation or the ability to circulate new air, is a result of inspiration and expiration.[15] In normal persons the muscles of inspiration are the diaphragm, neck accessory muscles, and external intercostals.[1,9,22] Expiration is passive. Forced expiration or coughing is produced primarily by contraction of the abdominal muscles.[19]

Mechanics of breathing

The diaphragm is a dome-shaped muscle, innervated by nerve roots C3 to C5, which originates from the dorsal aspect of the xiphoid process, the last six ribs, and the bodies and transverse processes of the upper thoracic vertebrae. The fibers insert onto a central tendon.[13] When the diaphragm contracts, it descends on the abdominal contents increasing intra-abdominal pressure. The descending action of the diaphragm and the contraction of external intercostal muscles cause an increase in vertical and horizontal dimensions of the thoracic cavity, thereby decreasing intrathoracic pressure. This change creates a pressure gradient and air moves into the lungs.[2,5,17] Although the diaphragm and external intercostals are responsible for this inspiratory action during normal quiet breathing, neck accessory muscles assist in elevation and stabilization of the ribs during stressful inspiration.[17]

To produce adequate ventilation the muscles of breathing must overcome the elasticity of the soft tissues of the thorax. According to Hooke's law, the property of a substance that deforms as a force is applied to it and returns to zero when the force is removed is that of elasticity. At the point of relaxed expiration the soft tissues are in a resting position. When the muscles of inspiration contract, they produce a force that causes the thorax to change shape primarily by elevating the ribs. The force that allows the thorax to return to its original shape is the elasticity of the tissues. The change in inspiratory volume relative to the quantity of force generated by the inspiratory muscles describes the phenomenon of compliance.

The importance of abdominal muscles in the upright position is to counter the increase in abdominal pressure created during the descent of the diaphragm.[9] Normal tone in the abdominal muscles maintains the intra-abdominal pressure necessary to allow the diaphragm to return to its elevated resting position. This elevated position is necessary to provide for full excursion of the diaphragm during inspiration. Forced expiration is produced by active contraction of abdominal muscles during high levels of activity. The active contraction forces the diaphragm further up into the thoracic cavity and thus increases the intrathoracic pressure forcing air out of the lungs. A cough is produced as a result of a deep inspiration and a quick forceful contraction of the abdominal muscles.[10]

Ventilatory reserve

There are two basic questions that need to be answered regarding the breathing ability of a patient with a spinal cord injury. First, is there adequate muscle strength for the patient to breathe without assistance from a mechanical ventilator? If the answer is yes, then what amount of ven-

395

tilatory reserve does the patient have for activity? Ventilatory reserve is defined as the amount of vital capacity greater than the resting tidal volume. It is logical that the lower the level of spinal injury the more muscles are active and therefore the greater the ventilatory reserve.

Given the segmental innervation to the muscles of breathing, patients can be grouped or classified according to the muscles that are perserved. For example, the patient who is neurologically intact at the level of C6 will have normal innervation and function of both the sternocleidomastoid and the diaphragm.[11,13,16] Patients in this group will have minimal ventilatory reserve for high levels of physical activity (Fig. 21-1). The concept of ventilatory reserve has become especially important today when many spinal cord–injured patients have a diagnosis of an incomplete injury. For example, the patient with a complete lesion at C6 will not have obvious ventilatory restrictions to activity because he has so little innervated skeletal muscle with which to challenge his respiratory system. On the other hand, the patient with an incomplete lesion at C6 who has skeletal muscles preserved that allow him to walk will have severe restrictions because of his ability to challenge a limited ventilatory reserve.

The muscles of ventilation work together to produce the most efficient method for moving air through the lungs. Each of the muscles in normal breathing is responsible for producing specific motions that contribute to the whole respiratory process. The paralysis of selected muscles causes deficiencies in ventilation, thoracic mobility, and cough function. The severity of these problems is best seen after a detailed evaluation is completed.

EVALUATION

The respiratory evaluation is an important phase of assessing the functional potential of the spinal cord–injured patient. The evaluation allows the physical therapist to determine any problems with ventilation, thoracic mobility, or cough. In addition to a thorough review of a patient's medical history, the following must be included in a clinical examination to assure a complete assessment:

Respiratory rate
Breathing pattern
Chest mobility
Vital capacity
Muscle strength
Cough effectiveness

Medical information

All available information regarding each patient's respiratory function must be thoroughly reviewed before you begin any physical evaluation. Interview the patient and consult with appropriate personnel to be sure facts are complete and sensible. A record of past medical history and a recent report of the physician's physical exam are primary sources of information. Information concerning

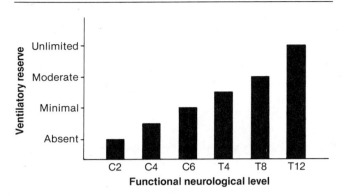

Fig. 21-1. Patient classification.

diagnosis, present symptoms, problems, and physical findings are assessed. The following areas are important:
1. Past history of lung disease (obstructive, restrictive?)
2. Present history of pulmonary complications
   a. Chest radiographs
   b. Thoracic surgeries
3. Laboratory findings
   a. Arterial blood gases
   b. Pulmonary function tests
4. Respiratory equipment
   a. Type of respirator
   b. Tracheostomy equipment
   c. Suctioning equipment
   d. Intermittent positive-pressure unit
5. Chest trauma
   a. Rib fractures
   b. Pleural effusion
   c. Pneumothorax-hemopneumothorax
   d. Contusions to lung or heart
   e. Trauma to diaphragm
6. Prior treatment for complications
   a. Medical
   b. Other (respiratory therapy, postural drainage, etc.)

Once a thorough review of the patient's medical history has been completed, a detailed evaluation can begin.

Respiratory rate

The importance of evaluating rate is to determine the efficiency of respiratory muscles to ventilate the patient.[2] The respiratory rate for normal adults is 12 to 16 cycles per minute.[22] One cycle is measured from the beginning of inspiration through the end of expiration. When assessing the respiratory rate, the therapist counts the number of cycles completed in 1 minute with the patient at rest, breathing quietly. The therapist begins counting when it is evident that the patient is not aware of any evaluation.

Results are accurate only when the patient does not know his breathing frequency is being monitored. Anxiety and attempts by the patient to "make an effort" will alter the rate.

If the diaphragm in the spinal cord–injured patient is normal and there are no other complications, there should be no change in respiratory rate related to muscle paralysis, since the diaphragm alone can maintain normal tidal volume. However, the patient with a high cervical lesion may have a diaphragm that functions less than normally. Here an increase in respiratory rate may be substituted to maintain adequate ventilation and prevent hypoventilation, which may occur because of inadequate respiratory muscle strength. Hypoventilation must be identified as soon as possible so that the patient can be properly managed. If muscle weakness is the problem, ventilatory assistance may be needed, as discussed in the next section.

Breathing pattern

Muscle groups in the neck, chest, abdomen, and the diaphragm contribute to normal breathing.[1,9] When the breathing pattern is assessed, a total of four points are used to describe the degree to which each muscle group is responsible for displacement of thoracic and epigastric regions during full inspiration. The normal breathing pattern consists of thoracic expansion and epigastric rise. Thoracic expansion results from the contraction of the external intercostal muscles, and the epigastric rise is the result of diaphragm contraction. With normal breathing the patient would be said to have a "2-diaphragm, 2-chest" pattern, since both thoracic and epigastric regions are moving equally.

Evaluation of the breathing pattern is an observational assessment of how the patient gets air into the lungs. When the therapist inspects the breathing pattern, the patient should be in the supine position, breathing quietly. The displacement of thoracic and epigastric areas at full inspiration should be compared to their position at the end of expiration (Fig. 21-2). Palpation is then used to complement the findings of observation. One hand is placed on the midthoracic region while the other hand rests on the epigastric region (Fig. 21-3). The dominance of one area or another may be palpated to confirm observational assessment.

When chest movement is questionable, the hands can assist in determining the amount of thoracic excursion. Place the hands, with the fingers spread and the thumbs together, over the middle of the sternum, 1 inch below the top of the rib cage. At full inspiration the therapist observes the amount of separation between the thumbs. The greater the distance between the thumbs, the more the chest muscles are acting to expand the chest.

The patient with a low cervical spinal cord lesion will have chest muscle paralysis and isolated diaphragm movement. The epigastric rise is dominant, and there is no chest expansion. Since the diaphragm is the only active muscle, the patient is considered a diaphragmatic breather. This pattern should be recorded as "4-diaphragm" to indicate the dominance of the diaphragm (Figure 21-4).

Patients with a high cervical spinal cord lesion will have chest muscle paralysis and diaphragmatic weakness. When the breathing pattern is observed, there will be an epigastric rise (diaphragm contraction) with no chest expansion. However, contraction of the neck muscles will be evident by their prominence. This breathing pattern is variable. It may be "1-neck, 3-diaphragm," or "2-neck, 2-diaphragm," or even "3-neck, 1-diaphragm" depending on the degree of displacement in the upper chest and epigastric region.

Patients with midthoracic lesions may show signs of active contraction of some intercostal muscles. The chest rises slightly along with the epigastric rise, which is still dominant. These patients are primarily diaphragmatic breathers but are assisting inspiration with chest muscles. Therefore the pattern is "3-diaphragm, 1-chest." The patients with lower thoracic injuries approach the normal breathing pattern because the intercostal muscles are working more effectively to raise the chest.

Chest mobility

During maximum inhalation, the thorax is enlarged in three diameters—transverse, anteroposterior, and vertical.[21] The movements of the thorax in the anteroposterior and transverse diameters are inseparable. The intercostal muscles lie between the ribs and consist of short parallel fibers that run oblique to the ribs. The external intercostals lift the ribs to increase the size of the thoracic cavity. The internal intercostals depress the ribs and decrease the size of the thoracic cavity. There are changes in both the transverse and anteroposterior diameters.[11,16,17] The vertical thoracic dimension is enlarged through diaphragm contraction. Chest expansion refers to the change in the transverse and anteroposterior dimensions and therefore relates to intercostal function.[21]

Chest expansion is defined as that circumferential change from full forced expiration to maximum inspiration.[6] With the patient supine, measurement of circumferences are taken with a soft flexible tape measure at both the xiphoid process and the axilla. The xiphoid process is easy to palpate and thus assures that measurements can be accurately reproduced (Fig. 21-5). A reading is also taken at the axilla to monitor the expansion of the upper thorax.

Normal chest expansion when measured at the axilla in 20- to 30-year-old persons is 3¼ inches ± ¼ inch.[6] The chest and the epigastric region rise simultaneously. The diaphragm and the intercostals work together to expand the chest by increasing the volume of air brought into the lungs.

Patients with low thoracic spinal cord lesions have initially decreased chest expansion. All muscles of respiration

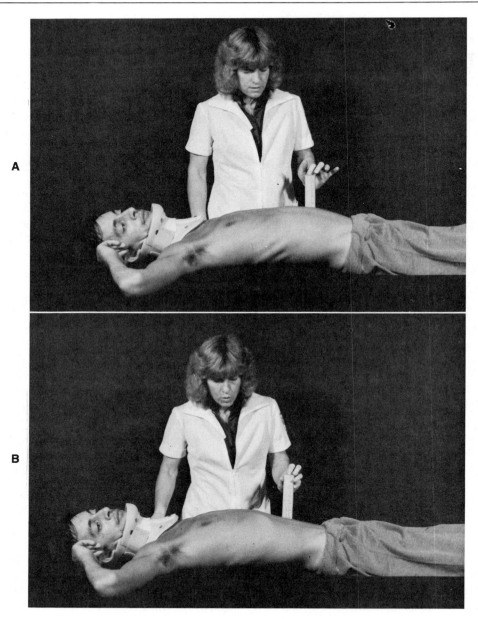

Fig. 21-2. A, Patient shown at maximum inspiratory effort. **B,** Same patient at his maximal expiration. Notice ruler, which shows 1½-inch change.

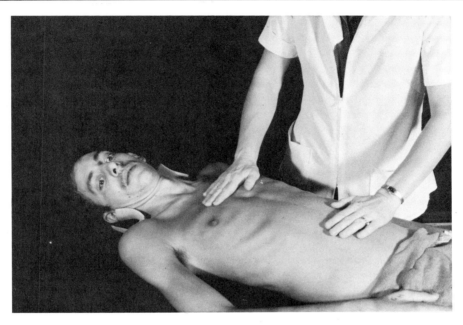

Fig. 21-3. Hand placement during resting-breathing evaluation.

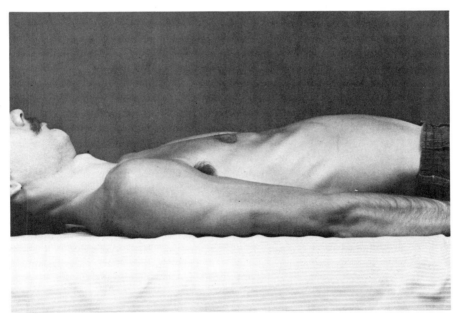

Fig. 21-4. Patient with "4-diaphragm" breathing pattern. (Reprinted from Alvarez, S.E., and others: Phys. Ther. **61:**1737-1745, 1980, with the permission of the American Physical Therapy Association.)

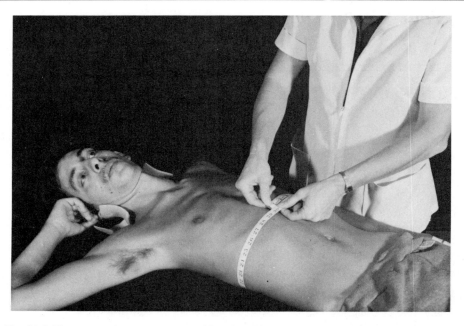

Fig. 21-5. Placement of tape measure and hand position when one measures chest expansion.

are fully innervated, but clinically the expansion measurements at the xiphoid level average 2 or 2½ inches. This decrease in inspiratory muscle activity shortly after the injury is transient, and normal values for chest expansion recur by the end of an intensive rehabilitation program.

Midthoracic injuries result in weakness of intercostal and abdominal muscles. This weakness contributes to a decrease in chest expansion. Since the abdominal muscles are weak or absent, forced expiration may not be complete. With intercostal muscle weakness, chest expansion is diminished.

The degree of epigastric rise increases as the diaphragm dominates inspiration. A patient with an upper thoracic spinal injury may have larger chest-expansion measurements at the axilla than at the xiphoid process because only the upper intercostal muscles are working. Patients with cervical spine injury breathe without the assistance of intercostal muscles and rely totally on the diaphragm. Their chest-expansion measurements are between ½ inch and −½ inch.

The negative values for chest expansion are attributable to contraction of the diaphragm without intercostal muscle opposition. The rib cage is retracted as the diaphragm descends during inspiration.[2,4,17] This is called "paradoxical movement," since the action works to decrease chest expansion. Anatomically, lung size increases, but only in the vertical dimension. The transverse and anteroposterior dimensions are not increased, and chest expansion values of −¼ inch to −½ inch are common.

Chest expansion should be measured throughout the respiratory program. Increases occur as intercostal muscle strength or chest mobility improve.

Vital capacity

Vital capacity is the total of the inspiratory reserve volume, the tidal volume, and the expiratory reserve volume.[10] Vital capacity is defined as the maximum amount of air that can be expelled from the lungs after peak inspiration.[5,10] The vital capacity is an objective and reproducible measurement that is used to monitor changes in respiratory muscle strength and chest mobility. Because of its ease of use and portability, a hand-held spirometer is a convenient instrument for measuring vital capacity within the clinical setting. The volume on most spirometers is recorded in cubic centimeters or milliliters. Each set of patient values is matched to predicted normal values in regard to sex and height.[5,9,18] The patient's volume is compared to the normal to establish a percentage. Shortly after the injury vital capacity measurements are commonly less than 25% of normal in high cervical injuries and as high as 80% for low thoracic injuries.[2]

Frequent vital capacity determinations throughout the treatment program are important to document progress. As strengthening and chest stretching techniques are employed, the ventilatory ability improves. Because the vital capacity is tested repeatedly, a standard method for its measurement is necessary. Testing should be done with the patient supine. The patient inhales maximally, places the

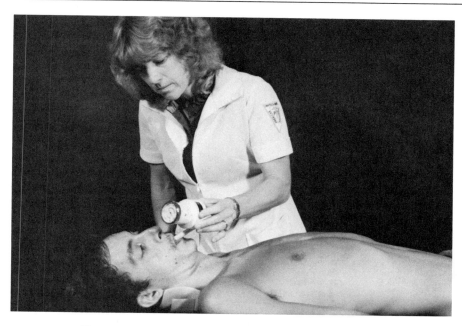

Fig. 21-6. Recording vital capacity using hand-held spirometer.

lips fully around the mouthpiece, and then exhales maximally. On exhalation there must be no leakage around the mouth or through the nose. The patient must leave the lips around the mouthpiece until having completely and forcefully exhaled one full breath (Fig. 21-6). This sequence is repeated three times, and the best value is recorded.

Caution must be taken when one is measuring vital capacity. Trunk spasticity, which does not reflect the volitional and functional ability of the respiratory muscles, may invalidate the testing procedure. Rib fractures, chest trauma, and other medical complications will also alter values.

The patient with an injury at the C3 to C5 levels may have a vital capacity equal to the tidal volume.[10] The patient tested in the supine position should be retested in the sitting position. The effects of gravity in the upright posture act to decrease vital capacity in the absence of abdominal support. The sternocleidomastoid muscles assist strongly with inspiration in patients who have no reserve volume; i.e., vital capacity equals tidal volume. Although these patients have adequate vital capacity for ventilation, the lack of reserve volume does not permit adequate ventilation during activity. While vital capacity is an important measure of breathing ability, the muscles that contribute to the breathing pattern and their strength ultimately determine a patient's breathing efficiency. For example, two patients with equal vital capacities may be using different muscles for ventilation. A patient who uses neck muscles will have less endurance than a patient using the

diaphragm because ventilation with the diaphragm uses less metabolic energy than ventilation with the neck muscles.[1]

Muscle evaluation

The purpose of evaluating the muscles of respiration is to identify specific areas of muscle weakness and to be aware of potential restriction of activity because of ventilation problems. This evaluation is best accomplished by specific muscle testing of the diaphragm, sternocleidomastoid, intercostal, and abdominal muscles. A grade should be separately designated for each group. The neck and truck muscles can be evaluated with standard muscle-testing procedures.[11,16] The strength evaluation of the diaphragm and intercostals involves interpretation of the total neurological picture, component respiratory evaluations, and observational techniques. These evaluations provide a measure of the contributions of each muscle to the total ventilatory effort.

Diaphragm. The strength of the diaphragm is best evaluated with the patient in the supine position. The epigastric rise should be examined first for visible action resulting from diaphragm movement. The patient is observed by placement of one's eyes level with the patient's trunk, which is then viewed from the side. Recall that the patient with normal chest and diaphragm movement has a 2-chest, 2-diaphragm breathing pattern. If the patient has no assistance from the intercostal muscles and has a 4-diaphragm breathing pattern, the epigastric rise should have full ex-

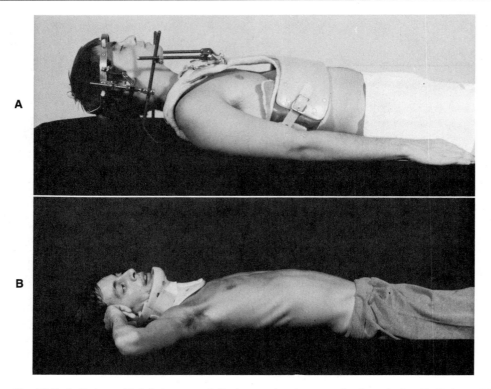

Fig. 21-7. A, Patient with fully innervated diaphragm showing normal epigastric rise. **B,** Patient with C$_5$ level of injury showing less than full epigastric rise.

cursion with maximum inspiration (Fig. 21-4). This response indicates at least a "fair" muscle grade for the diaphragm. Since the diaphragm is innervated by roots C3 to C5, a patient with an injury at the C6 level and lower is expected to have normal innervation to the diaphragm. The diaphragm in Fig. 21-7 is less than "fair," since it does not complete normal excursion. The sensory dermatomes and muscles in the C3 to C5 nerve distribution must be evaluated to assist in the interpretation of diaphragm strength. For example, the patient with C5 quadriplegia or higher may not have a full epigastric rise.

Once diaphragm strength is graded at least "fair," resistance is applied. This is done with the patient in the supine position. The therapist's hands are placed over the epigastric area with fingers spread. The patient is asked to inhale while maximal manual resistance is applied. If the patient has complete epigastric rise and holds the contraction firmly against this resistance, the diaphragm is "good" in grade. Remember, the presence of spasticity or volitional control of the abdominal muscles may invalidate this test.

Diaphragmatic weakness designated as "less than fair" must be studied critically because its contraction may be difficult to palpate. To help confirm an independent finding of a weak diaphragm, test the upper extremity muscles and the sensory dermatomes that are supplied by the same nerve roots as the diaphragm (sternocleidomastoid, C3; upper trapezius, C4; deltoid, C5). If weakness or sensory impairment is found, the suspicion of diaphragm weakness is reinforced. The patient with C4 quadriplegia who is able to breathe without continuous mechanical ventilation may be using the sternocleidomastoid muscles to assist with breathing. Observe the patient breathing quietly in the supine position. Active contraction of sternocleidomastoid will indicate a weak diaphragm. The patient should be reevaluated for the use of the sternocleidomastoid muscles for ventilation in the sitting position and again during activity. Active contraction of the sternocleidomastoid in C4 or C5 quadriplegics indicates that diaphragm function alone is too weak to maintain tidal volume. When the patient demonstrates neck breathing, the tidal volume and vital capacity are often found to be equal. Therefore the diaphragm is "poor."

The patient with a "poor" diaphragm may have additional diagnostic evaluations to document its excursion. Fluoroscopy or radiographs are used to provide an objective record of diaphragm excursion.[7,9,20]

Fluoroscopy is a cineradiograph of the patient's breathing. As the patient breathes quietly, the excursion of the

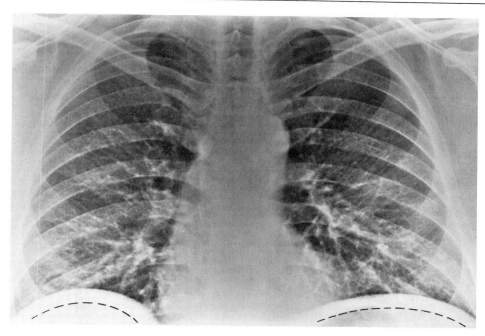

Fig. 21-8. Cineradiograph showing patient with a "poor" diaphragm. *Dotted line,* Position of diaphragm at maximum inspiratory effort. Excursion is less than one full intercostal space.

diaphragm is recorded on film. During quiet breathing the normal excursion should be at least one intercostal space (1.5 cm). During deep inspiration the diaphragm will descend at least three to four intercostal spaces (7 to 13 cm).[20,21] The diaphragm is dome-shaped on observation but is always higher on the right side because of displacement by the liver[7] (Fig. 21-8). A poor or less diaphragm is evident when the movement is the same for deep breathing and quiet breathing.

When no contraction of the diaphragm during quiet breathing is observed with fluoroscopy, ask the patient to sniff. This action will cause a contraction if the diaphragm is innervated. Fluoroscopy will also aid in determining an imbalance in diaphragm strength when right and left excursion is unequal.[7] Radiographs, used as an alternative to fluoroscopy, are less expensive and do not expose the patient to as much radiation. One radiograph is taken at full inhalation, and one is taken at full exhalation. One picture is superimposed on the other, the anatomical landmarks are matched, and the excursion of the diaphragm is determined by a count of the intercostal spaces as is done with fluoroscopy.

Patients with a high quadriplegia will have weak or paralyzed diaphragms and require ventilators. It is important to learn about the ventilator and emergency care procedures before evaluation of the condition of the diaphragm. The therapist must establish good rapport with the patient and become familiar with the hospital's phi-

losophy and protocol for phasing quadriplegic patients from the ventilator. Consult with the appropriate personnel and together determine the patient's tolerance to be detached from the ventilator. Initially the patient can usually tolerate 10 seconds comfortably. Tolerance is increased gradually to approximately 1 minute without ventilatory assistance.

Once the patient can be comfortable detached from the respirator, diaphragm strength can be assessed. Litten's sign is useful when one is confirming the presence of an extremely weak diaphragm. Litten's sign, which is more easily observed on thin patients, is a rippling action that may be seen between the intercostal spaces of the eighth, ninth, and tenth ribs.[2,9] Litten's sign can be seen only when there is total paralysis of the intercostal muscles. As the diaphragm contracts and pulls from its costal origins, there is a decrease in intrathoracic pressure causing the intercostal spaces to move inward so that this rippling action results (Fig. 21-9).

Sternocleidomastoid muscles. The sternocleidomastoid muscle is the primary muscle of substitution in patients with diaphragm weakness. This muscle assists with inspiration during quiet breathing when the tidal volume is inadequate. With the head fixed, either by its own weight or if the patient is in a halo vest, the bilateral action of the sternocleidomastoids is to pull the chest toward the head. It is important to have complete knowledge of the condition of the spine before muscle testing of the sternoclei-

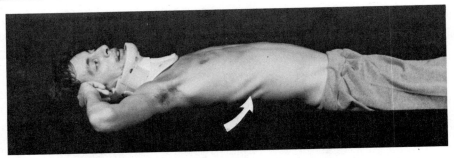

Fig. 21-9. Litten's sign demonstrated as patient initiates inspiratory effort.

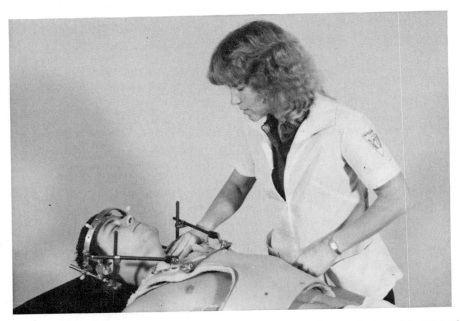

Fig. 21-10. Muscle testing can be done even when patient is in a halo vest. An isometric contraction gives information about presence and quality of muscle belly.

domastoids. Consult the physician regarding the stability of the spine and any contraindications to positioning or moving the head and neck for testing.

Initially the patient may be positioned supine in traction or in a halo vest, each restricting movement of the head and neck. In this case palpation of the sternocleidomastoid should be done. Ask the patient to perform an isometric contraction to determine the presence or absence of contraction of the muscle (Fig. 21-10).

After the patient has received medical clearance for active motion, muscle strength up to "fair" can be tested. It is not uncommon to find limitation in neck range of motion because of bony block, fusion, or wiring. After

the flexion range has been identified passively, ask the patient to produce the same movement actively. If pain at the fracture site occurs during motion, consult the physician. Once the patient is cleared for resistive testing, the strength of the sternocleidomastoid can be determined by standard muscle-testing procedures.

Abdominal and intercostal muscles. Standard muscle-testing techniques are used when one is evaluating trunk musculature.[11,16] Precautions should be discussed with the physician before testing. Because motion of the spine is often contraindicated, the evaluation of abdominal muscle strength may be limited to palpation. When no palpable contraction is obtained, one way to verify that the abdominal muscles are absent (0) is to ask the patient to cough.

Intercostal strength is evaluated indirectly by measurement of chest expansion. Taking measurements at both the axillary and xiphoid landmarks provides a comparison of upper and lower intercostal function. Remember that external intercostals lift the rib cage up and out during inspiration whereas the internal intercostals depress the ribs pulling down and in during forced expiration. Observation of these actions is important to confirm intercostal contraction.

Cough evaluation

In the normal person, forced expiration is accomplished primarily by the abdominal muscles, which are assisted by the internal intercostals.[19] These muscles function to clear secretions or foreign material adequately from the lungs. Initially, when one is evaluating a cough, it is best to have the patient in the supine position. Both hands of the evaluator are placed on the patient's abdominal muscles to palpate for their contraction. The patient is asked to cough.

The cough is graded as "functional," "weak-functional," or "nonfunctional." The degree of expulsive force is determined by sound and the ability to cough twice within one exhalation. A functional cough will be loud and vigorous. The patient will be able to repeat at least two vigorous expulsive forces in one exhalation. This patient can adequately clear secretions. A weak-functional cough is less vigorous, and the sound is soft. The patient is not able to repeat the cough effort more than once during exhalation. The weak-functional cough is adequate only for clearing the throat. A nonfunctional cough has no expulsive force and sounds like a sigh or clearing the throat.

Clinically, patients can change cough function by altering volume or by eliciting abdominal spasticity. Patients without abdominal muscles and vital capacities over 2000 cc generally have a weak-functional cough. These patients are able to compensate for the lack of abdominal muscles by using a quick volume release to generate force.

OBJECTIVES AND TREATMENT METHODS

The appropriate treatment plan is designed to increase ventilation by improving any or all of these three parameters:

Strength
Chest mobility
Bronchial hygiene

Attention to all of these parameters is critical. However, the interpretation of the respiratory evaluation may indicate one parameter contributing more significantly to the problem of decreased ventilation. The respiratory evaluation is integrated with the complete physical therapy evaluation and pertinent evaluations noted by other members of the medical team.

Once treatment priorities have been established the therapist must select the best mode to improve strength, chest

mobility, and bronchial hygiene. As various treatment programs are employed, the patient should be periodically reevaluated for changes in ventilation. As medical conditions change, the treatment program must also be altered to meet the patient's needs. This section on treatment method will provide guidelines for planning and progressing a patient through respiratory rehabilitation.

Diaphragm strengthening

Diaphragm strengthening can be beneficial to any patient with a less than normal vital capacity. Thus all patients with cervical and high thoracic injuries are candidates for intensive diaphragm strengthening. Patients with lower thoracic or lumbar injuries will have decreased vital capacity secondary to limited activity. These patients, until they are again fully active, will benefit from a daily routine of coughing, deep-breathing, and abdominal exercises. The strength of the diaphragm is used to determine which treatment technique to employ. Patients with fair+ strength of the diaphragm are candidates for progressive resistive exercise, whereas patients who have less strength must use active or active-assistive exercise techniques.

When beginning a strengthening program, examine the methods of resisting the movement of the diaphragm. The resistance should allow the diaphragm to contract through its full range so that ventilation in the normal breathing pattern for the patient is not altered. Some methods of progressive resistive exercise are (1) weights, (2) manual, (3) positioning, and (4) incentive inspiratory spirometry.

Progressive resistive exercise by use of weights is one method for diaphragm strengthening. To begin, the patient is placed in the supine position. The diaphragm weight pan is placed over the epigastric region.[1,12] To allow full excursion of the diaphragm, the weight pan should not rest on the ribs. The degree of epigastric rise should remain the same after weight is added (Fig. 21-11). The patient with a neurologically intact diaphragm can usually start comfortably with 5 pounds. The amount of weight used as resistance is appropriate when the patient can maintain a coordinated, unaltered breathing pattern for 15 minutes. Observe the degree of epigastric rise and the sternocleidomastoid muscles as well. If the patient begins to use the sternocleidomastoid muscles or noticeably alters his breathing pattern, the weight should be decreased.[1]

The benefits of progressive resistive exercise for strengthening the diaphragm are documented by increased weight and increased vital capacity. Progressive resistive exercise should continue with weights added* until the patient's strength reaches a plateau; that is, the vital capacity is the same from one evaluation to the next or the patient

---

*As weights are added there is an increased tendency for the weights to topple off the patient at full inspiration. Precaution should be taken to protect the patient's arms.

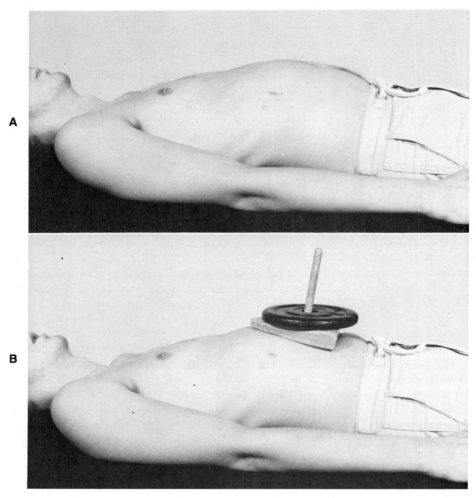

Fig. 21-11. A, Patient shown with full epigastric rise. **B,** Same patient still has full epigastric rise after diaphragm weights are added.

can tolerate the challenge of full activity without early signs of fatigue.

When the diaphragm is "fair," caution must be taken not to overchallenge and fatigue a muscle that must function throughout the day. Unlike other skeletal muscles, the diaphragm has no total rest period to recover after exercise. It is important to recognize that the abdominal contents provides resistance to the diaphragm. The force of the abdominal contents acting against the diaphragm increases in the head-down position. At a 15-degree head-down incline this force is equivalent to 10 pounds.[12] Resistive strengthening by altering patient position or by diaphragm weights must be done carefully so as not to fatigue the diaphragm. Inspiratory muscle training by resistive breathing is being investigated as a means of applying appropriate work loads that will challenge the diaphragm without causing fatigue.[14]

Incentive spirometers provide low-level resistive training while minimizing the potential of fatigue to the diaphragm.[3,14] Incentive spirometers are designed to provide the patient with visual input during a sustained maximal inspiration. These devices are commonly used in postoperative conditions. The major purpose of incentive spirometry is to prevent alveolar collapse. Its secondary goals of cough stimulation and strengthening of weakened respiratory muscles are important benefits to spinal cord–injured patients. The visual input of balls rising in chambers, colored lights, or dials reflect the degree of inspiratory effort.

The supine position for the patient is preferred when the patient is instructed in incentive spirometry. A patient with a fair + diaphragm will tolerate a level position, whereas a patient with only a fair diaphragm will do better in a 10- to 15-degree head-up incline. This incline will be adequate to relieve the resistance applied by the abdominal contents. Once positioned correctly, the patient should take four slow easy breaths letting the air out normally between the first three. After the fourth breath the air should flow out slowly until the patient cannot exhale any more. Have the patient place the spirometer mouthpiece in the mouth and form a tight seal. Instruct the patient to take a slow deep breath in through the mouthpiece to elicit the visual input, that is, balls rising, lights, and so on. The visual cue should be maintained as long as possible. The patient should remove the mouthpiece and relax. Repeat eight to ten times and three or four sessions per day.

Presently, commercially available incentive spirometers are used to increase inspiratory effort by increasing the volume of inspired air. As more volume is inspired, resistance is increased only minimally as a result of increased flow through the spirometer. Primarily this is an active inspiratory exercise. New incentive spirometers that measure mouth pressure are under development. Mouth pressure reflects the amount of force the respiratory muscles are able to generate. Resistive inspiratory muscle training studies have shown that muscular force passes a certain threshold beyond which fatigue will eventually result.[14] The advent of clinically practical mouth pressure–measuring devices should provide therapists with an objective means of monitoring appropriate low-level resistive training to inspiratory muscles.

The patient with "poor" diaphragm strength requires special consideration with regard to position and fatigue. As with any skeletal muscle when strength is "poor," the arc or motion is decreased and fatigue occurs rapidly. The patient with a poor diaphragm may breathe comfortably when resting supine. There is no epigastric rise, since the diaphragm cannot displace the abdominal contents. This patient rests comfortably when supine because the ventilatory requirement for resting supine is less than for upright. An active assistance device, that is, the pneumobelt (exhalation belt), must be used when this patient begins to sit.

Abdominal supports

Pneumobelt (exhalation belt). When a patient has a weak diaphragm, he will automatically use the sternocleidomastoid to assist in the breathing effort when breathing difficulty or distress is encountered. Since the patient with a high cervical injury (C3 and C4) gains function only through use of head and neck motions, that is, mouthstick, chin-controlled electric wheelchair, it is important to preserve use of the neck muscles for these activities. Therefore the following sequence and technique is recommended for the patient with a weak diaphragm that fatigues rapidly.

A patient with an initial vital capacity between 500 and 1000 cc, when upright, is a candidate for a pneumobelt. A pneumobelt is a corset with an inflatable bladder (Fig. 21-12). The pneumobelt corsets come in small, medium, and large sizes with an inserted inflatable bladder placed over the abdominal area. It is easy to modify most custom corsets to accommodate both the inflatable bladder and varying sizes of patients. The bladder is connected to a respirator by a hose. The respirator must be able to deliver positive pressure with an easily adjustable respiratory rate. The rate and pressure should be set according to the person's comfort. It may be necessary to increase the pressure setting when the activity level increases.

The mechanics of the pneumobelt depends on the passive descent of the abdominal contents; thus it must be used when the patient is sitting. Inflation of the bladder causes exhalation by pushing the abdominal contents in and up and thereby pushing the diaphragm into optimal ascended position within the thoracic cavity. Inspiration becomes active assistive, since the abdominal contents will passively descend as pressure is decreased in the bladder.

Fatigue of the diaphragm can occur even when a patient uses the pneumobelt. Monitoring the patient for fatigue is done by observation for contraction of the sternocleidomastoid muscles during inspiration. When these contractions occur, you should increase the pressure delivered to the bladder to see if the additional assistance to the diaphragm will decrease the patient's need for the sternocleidomastoids. If these neck muscles are still being used, put the patient back to bed. It is important to continue daily attempts to increase tolerance of the upright posture with the pneumobelt.

When the patient has been upright on an active program for 8 hours without signs of fatigue, begin phasing the patient off the pneumobelt. First, decrease the pressure in the bladder with the patient sitting but not active. If the sternocleidomastoid muscles are used, increase the pressure to the lowest level that will prevent their use. Once the patient can tolerate decreased pressure during inactive periods, begin decreasing pressure when the patient is active, that is, while using chin control or during mouthstick training. Continue to watch for signs of fatigue. Eventually, the patient will tolerate less pressure assistance from the bladder and should begin to wear the pneumobelt only for activity sessions but should wear a corset during quiet periods. The ability of the patient to breathe without a pneumobelt will always depend on fatigue.

Corsets. If the abdominal muscles are weak, that is, "less than fair," a patient will have a diaphragm that rests in the descended position because of the gravitational pull of the abdominal contents. The excursion of the diaphragm during contraction is therefore decreased (Fig. 21-13, *B*) A decrease in inspiratory reserve volume is the result of this decreased mechanical advantage of the diaphragm. A corset helps to compensate for weak or absent abdominal muscles by supporting the abdominal contents and displaces the diaphragm to a higher resting position in the thoracic cavity.[2,17] The range of diaphragm descent during

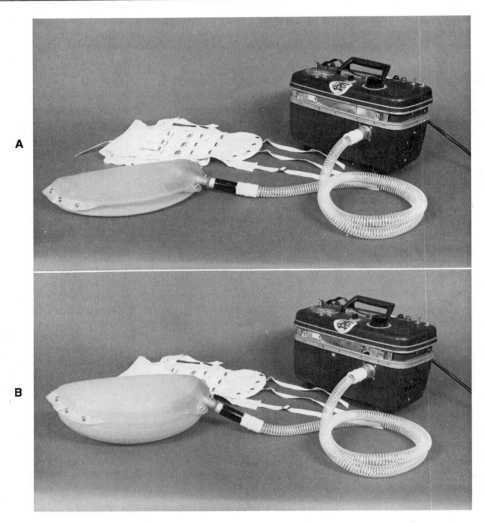

Fig. 21-12. **A,** Pneumobelt equipment shown: corset, inflatable bladder, and positive-pressure respirator. **B,** Pneumobelt equipment with bladder inflated. (Reprinted from Alvarez, S.E., and others: Phys. Ther. **61:**1737-1745, 1980, with the permission of the American Physical Therapy Association.)

contraction is therefore increased and inspiratory reserve volume also increases (Fig. 21-13, *C*).

The corset should lie just over the last two floating ribs and cover the iliac crest over the anterior superior iliac spines (ASIS) bilaterally. If the corset is applied too high, it will restrict chest mobility and will not support the abdomen. The lower buckles should be tighter than the upper ones. The appropriate fit is firm yet allows a hand to be slipped between the abdomen and the corset on the upper border (Fig. 21-14).

Corsets may be custom fit or stock sized. Patients with partial innervation to abdominal muscles may get sufficient support with a stock elastic binder. The elastic component must be evaluated for effective support of the abdominal

contents. Corsets with metal stays should be used with caution because skin pressure problems can result from them.

Another indication for using a corset is the patient who becomes hypotensive when sitting. When this happens, be sure to check the corset for snug fitting. Well-fitting elastic stockings are also necessary to prevent blood pooling.

Careful monitoring of blood pressure and heart rate will provide information to evaluate the effectiveness of the corset in prevention of blood pooling secondary to splanchnic nerve dysfunction.

The patient may discontinue use of the corset if the diaphragm strength improves or abdominal tone increases to adequately support the abdominal contents. Before discon-

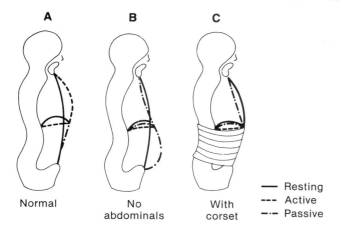

A   B   C

Normal   No   With
           abdominals corset

—— Resting
--- Active
-·- Passive

Fig. 21-13. A, Normal diaphragm positioning. **B,** Weak abdominal muscles allow diaphragm to rest in descended position because of gravitational pull. **C,** Corset application allows optimal positioning of the diaphragm. (Reprinted from Alvarez, S.E., and others: Phys. Ther. **61:**1737-1745, 1980, with the permission of the American Physical Therapy Association.)

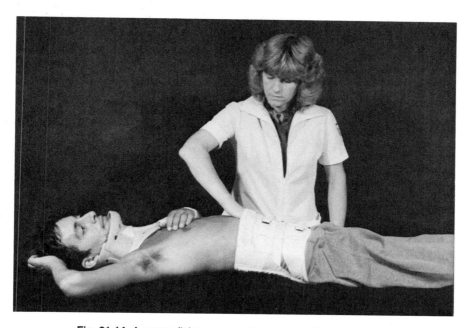

Fig. 21-14. A proper fitting corset will not restrict chest expansion.

tinuing the use of the corset, the patient should be tested in bed with and without the corset while positioned with the head up and the body inclined 45 degrees. Evaluate vital capacity and breathing pattern, and check the vital signs. When there is no difference without the corset in ease of breathing and vital signs, the patient may be progressed to more upright postures. Eventually the patient will tolerate the sitting position with legs down.

It is especially important to test the patient in the upright

position without a corset before he or she bathes. Bathing in any spinal cord–injured patient will alter blood pressure through changes in body temperature, which increase circulation to the periphery and increase splanchnic blood pooling. If the patient cannot tolerate 8 hours upright without a corset, an extra corset should be available to wear while bathing. The patient will ventilate better, and the body can more effectively adapt to temperature changes when the corset is worn.

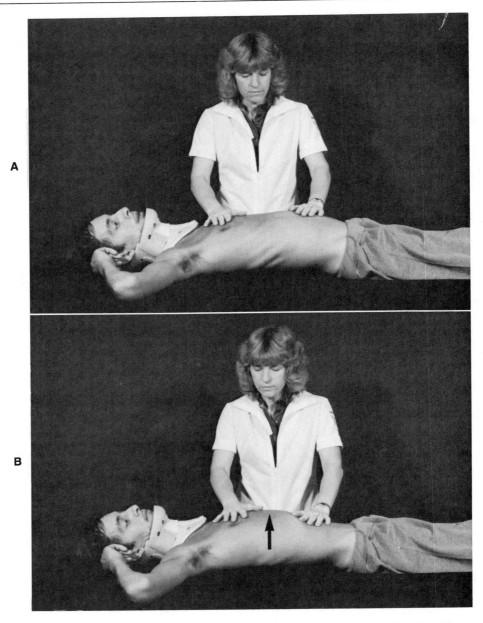

Fig. 21-15. A, Hand placement for air-shift instruction. Patient inhaling maximally before doing an air shift. **B,** Same patient having completed the air-shift maneuver. Notice increase in chest expansion.

Chest mobility

A strengthening program means little if joint mobility is not maintained. Just as a knee-flexion contracture can impair walking, so can chest-wall tightness prevent strong respiratory muscles from effectively ventilating the patient. The treatment technique selected will depend on the muscles the patient has functioning and any contraindications. Deep breathing, positive pressure, manual chest stretching, airshift manuever, and glossopharyngeal breathing are

methods for improving chest mobility. Specific chest mobilization treatment is indicated in patients whose chest-expansion range with deep breathing is less than 2 inches.

Deep breathing. Patients who have a voluntary chest-expansion range of greater than 2 inches should be encouraged to take a few deep breaths followed by a cough, every day they are confined to bed. Even though they may have no specific neurological deficit that affects their breathing, the effects of long-term bed rest are generally

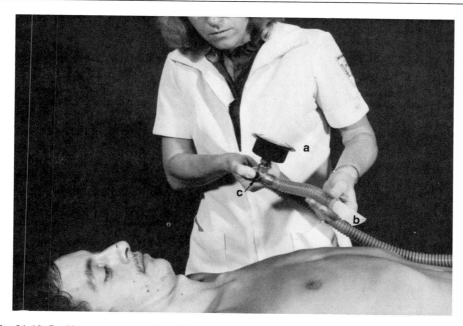

Fig. 21-16. Positive-pressure respirator hose with pressure gauge, *A;* air-delivery mouthpiece, *B;* and air-relief valve, *C.*

debilitating. Deep breathing is a good way to avoid possible complications later.

Airshifts. The patient is taught to maintain chest mobility by doing an airshift. Technically, an airshift is a maneuver in which a person inhales maximally, closes the glottis, and relaxes the diaphragm to allow the air to shift from the lower to upper part of the thorax. Once successfully mastered, airshifts can potentially expand the chest from ½ inch to 2 inches. To maintain chest mobility, patients are instructed to do airshifts every day.

To teach the patient an airshift, place one hand on the patient's epigastric area and one hand on the upper part of the chest. Ask the patient to take a deep breath and hold it. Tell the patient to suck the stomach in and move the air to the upper part of the chest (Fig. 21-15). If the technique is done correctly, you should see the top hand raise. Be aware that the patient may hyperventilate and become dizzy.

Not only is an airshift manuever beneficial to the range of motion to the rib cage, it is also a method of learning laryngeal control as a precursor to glossopharyngeal breathing. To be sure that the patient is closing the glottis and not holding air in the lips or cheeks, have the patient hold his breath with the mouth open. An airshift should be reproducible when the mouth is open.

Positive pressure. Routine intermittent positive pressure (RIPP) is a method of mobilizing the chest.[10] Unlike intermittent positive-pressure breathing (IPPB), there are no medications administered. For RIPP to be ad-

ministered the patient should wear a corset or cloth binder. The abdominal restriction will ensure that the volume of air expands the chest in the transverse plane. The rate and pressure of air delivered to the patient are controlled by the therapist. Initial treatment begins at 5 cm H_2O and progresses to a maximum of 40 cm H_2O pressure.

A positive-pressure respirator can be adapted to provide passive chest stretching. The respirator hose is attached to a tubular Y fitting. A sterilized mouthpiece tubing is inserted over one end of the Y. The therapist controls the air entering the lungs by moving a thumb over the air-relief valve. When the air-relief valve is completely closed off, the pressure, as set on the machine, is delivered to the patient (Fig. 21-16).

When beginning RIPP treatment, explain the purpose of the treatment to the patient. As the patient breathes normally, observe the respiratory rate and begin to move air into the lungs slowly at the same rate that the patient is breathing (Fig. 21-17). The treatment consists of 3 sets of 5 breaths, with an increase of the pressure, if tolerated, at each set. After each set, ask the patient if the pressure and rate are comfortable. Pressure is increased in 5 cm increments. Observe the pressure reading at the end of inspiration. If it does not reach the pressure dialed, there is a leak in the system. Either the patient is leaking air through the mouth or nose, the hoses are not connected completely, or the therapist does not have the thumb completely over the air-relief valve.

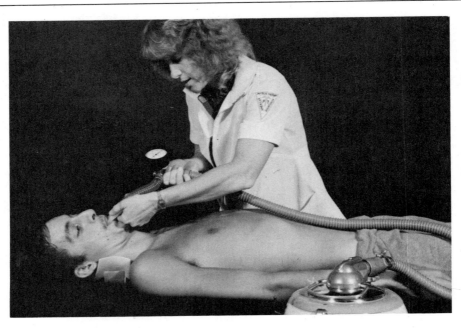

Fig. 21-17. Positive-pressure treatment being administered.

The RIPP treatment progresses from 1 week to 6 weeks depending on the patient. The patient is progressed to 40 cm H_2O, which has been found to be a safe limit for chest expansion.[10] The treatment is discontinued once the patient is active and has learned an airshift maneuver to maintain chest mobility. If for some reason the patient is placed on bed rest, positive pressure would be reinitiated.

RIPP is contraindicated in patients with chronic obstructive airway disease, since fragile airways may rupture under high pressure. RIPP is also contraindicated in patients who have respiratory infections producing secretions. Positive pressure only pushes secretions deeper into the lungs. Positive pressure delays healing in patients who have an unhealed tracheostoma. Patients with rib fractures may not tolerate RIPP though they may tolerate careful manual stretching to the opposite side.

Manual chest stretching. Manual chest stretching is done segmentally to lower, middle, and upper thoracic areas. The patient is supine while the therapist applies the treatment technique illustrated in Fig. 21-18.

Employ any technique that is safe and creates movement at the costal articulation. Stretch once a day to maintain the range of motion, or more often if attempting to increase the range.

Glossopharyngeal breathing (GPB). Glossopharyngeal breathing (GPB) is a substitute method of increasing the volume of air that is brought into the lungs.[8] It is indicated to increase chest expansion for any patient with intercostal muscle paralysis or weakness. Glossopharygneal breathing

is an alternate method of breathing for respirator-dependent patients. Also any patient with loss of abdominal muscles can use glossopharyngeal breathing to improve the force of coughing. The patient learns to force air into the lungs by using the mouth, tongue, and pharyngeal and laryngeal structures (Fig. 21-19). The use of glossopharyngeal breathing can increase lung volumes by as much as 1000 cc. The details of this technique are beyond the scope of this chapter.[8]

Bronchial hygiene

Clear airways must be maintained in all spinal cord–injured patients. Patients with cervical or high thoracic injuries can develop respiratory infections rapidly if bronchial hygiene is not adequate. Once respiratory complications develop they are difficult to clear. Thus these patients are taught bronchial hygiene as a preventive measure and as necessary to treat pulmonary infections. The patient depends on help from the family or attendant to provide manual cough assistance, postural drainage, and suctioning. A good preventive program will reduce the likelihood of respiratory complications, decrease the need for IPPB treatments, and diminish the possibility of mechanical ventilation.

Coughing. A patient with absent or weak abdominal muscles can attain adequate coughing power for clearing secretions. The following techniques may be employed—manual cough, self-manual cough, glossopharyngeal breathing, or, for patients with very low vital capacities,

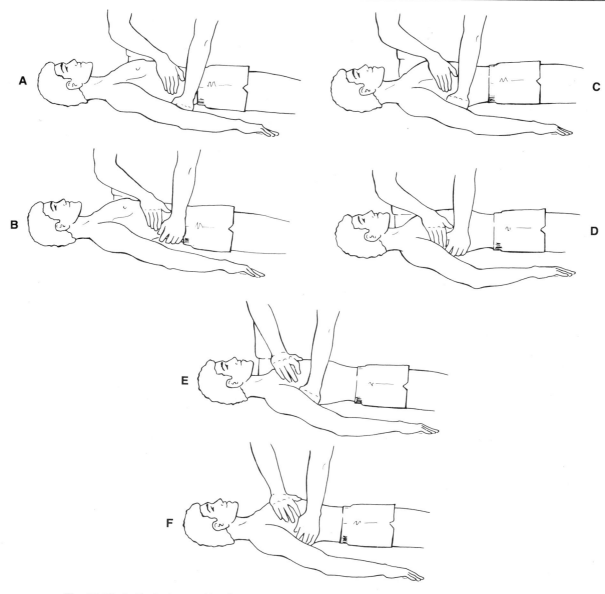

Fig. 21-18. A, Beginning position for manual chest stretch: One hand is placed under ribs with tips of fingers on transverse processes. Place other hand on top of chest with heel of lateral palmar area to the sternum. **B,** Stretching motion: Bring hands together in wringing motion. Do not force on edge of ribs or sternum. Distribute pressure over entire surface of your hands. Progress up the chest, alternating hands. **C,** Beginning position. **D,** Stretching motion. To effectively range the upper chest (**E** and **F**), top hand should be just inferior to the clavicle in the last position. **E,** Beginning position. **F,** Stretching motion.

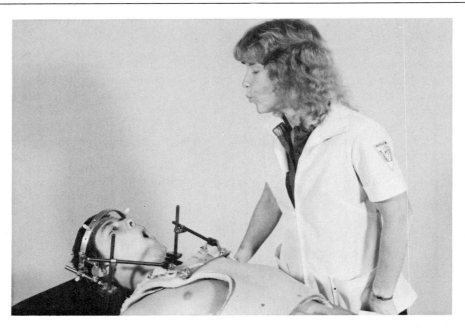

Fig. 21-19. Glossopharyngeal breathing is learned by imitation. Therapist is demonstrating this breathing technique for patient.

alternating use of the manual ventilation bag with abdominal compression.

Manual cough. The manual cough is an excellent method for clearing secretions and maintaining good bronchial hygiene. It is appropriate for any patient with weak cough force as a result of abdominal muscle weakness or paralysis. There are two techniques for manual cough production:

1. The first technique is a maneuver similar to the Heimlich Maneuver taught in cardiopulmonary resuscitation classes. The patient is in the supine position while the assister places his hands over the patient's epigastric area. The heel of one hand is placed over the abdomen, between the umbilicus and 2 inches below the xiphoid process. The other hand is placed on top of the first with the fingers spread apart so that both hands can interlock. The patient is instructed to take as deep a breath as possible and then attempt to cough. The assister pushes down and inward toward the head, compressing the abdomen quickly but with caution to avoid pressure against the xiphoid process. The force of the push should be timed carefully with the patient's attempt to cough (Fig. 21-20).

2. The second technique involves using the assister's hands as a substitute for actual abdominal contraction. The patient should be in the supine position. The assister spreads the fingers apart and places one hand on the upper abdominal area close to the lower ribs. The other hand is placed on the lower abdominal area. The patient should take a full deep breath and then cough. As the patient coughs, the hands are compressed together and thrust downward. The manual compression must be firm, quick, and timed with the patient's effort (Fig. 21-21).

Manual coughing technique may be done with the patient prone, sitting, or standing; however, in other than the supine position it is hard to get the mechanical advantage to correctly compress the abdomen. Any means of cautious but quick abdominal compressions is acceptable during emergency situations when the patient's airway is blocked.

Patients with high cervical injuries find it difficult to achieve sufficient lung volume to produce a forceful manual cough. The vital capacities in these patients are below 1000 cc. To assist the coughing maneuver, one must increase the inspiratory volume either with effective glossopharyngeal breathing (GPB) or with positive-pressure apparatus. For patients who cannot use GPB the manual ventilation bag is used for lung inflation just before a manual cough. These patients will have a tracheostomy and may be able to spend some time detached from the respirator. The ventilation bag is attached with a tracheostomy adapter. Be sure the adapter fits the tracheostomy tube. As the patient inhales, the bag is compressed manually to provide additional inspiratory volume. The bag is removed. The patient should try to hold the air briefly by closing the glottis so that the therapist can effectively assist. Quickly the therapist places the hands on the abdomen and signals the patient to cough as the abdomen is compressed. This technique may be repeated several times until secretions are adequately cleared.

Self-manual cough. Self-manual cough can be taught with the patient in the supine or sitting position. A patient

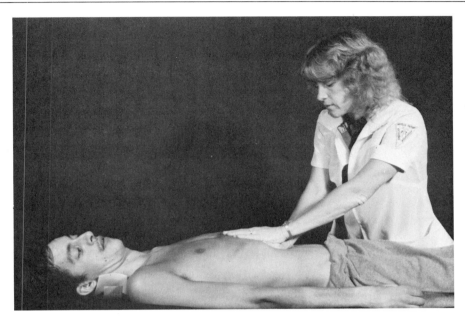

Fig. 21-20. Manual cough technique with therapist's hands one on top of the other.

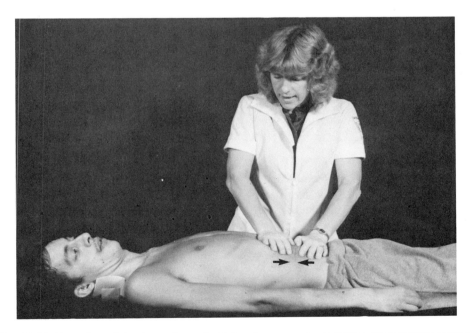

Fig. 21-21. Manual cough is also performed with hand movement substituting for abdominal contraction.

with full upper extremity function can lock the hands together across the epigastric region and push in diagonally toward the head while attempting to cough. Patients with injuries as high as C6 can learn self-manual cough in the sitting position by throwing their arms across the epigastric area and falling forward in time with the cough attempt. Coughing force can be improved in the patient with quadriplegia by placement of a pillow on the lap to increase abdominal compression. GPB will also improve cough force.

Postural drainage. For most patients with paraplegia standard postural drainage positions may be used. Patients with higher injuries may have difficulty breathing in positions that restrict the movement of the diaphragm. All patients must be positioned carefully when there is spinal instability. Auscultation of the chest for adventitious breath sounds should be done for determination of the particular lobes of the lungs that require drainage. The appropriate positions for postural drainage should be selected based on the lobes that require drainage.

Patients with diaphragmatic weakness may not tolerate the Trendelenburg position, since this places the weight of the abdominal contents on the diaphragm. Even patients with a "good" diaphragm may have difficulty tolerating this position, which increases the burden of moving air through the resistance of secretion-filled airways. Upright positions of angles greater than 30 degrees will also increase the demand on the diaphragm. A corset may be necessary in this position. Side-lying positions for posterior segments of the upper lobes require one-fourth turn onto the chest with the arm over a pillow. This semiprone position should be modified to keep pillows from restricting diaphragm movement.

Suctioning. Suctioning is indicated along with postural drainage when there is excessive mucus accumulation in the lungs. The patient with quadriplegia commonly needs to be suctioned because of poor cough function. The therapist should suction these patients before breathing reeducation or GPB lessons to assure clear airways. Be aware of emergency procedures for patients in respiratory distress.

The condition of the tracheostomy may be acute or chronic. The acute form of a tracheostomy condition is most vulnerable to infection for the first 8 weeks. Therefore sterile techniques for suctioning are mandatory. Any patient with known bradycardia should be carefully monitored during suctioning. Suctioning may stimulate the vagus nerve and will further decrease the heart rate. The patient with the chronic form of a tracheostomy condition may be suctioned by use of clean techniques. Portable suction units may accompany the patient to the physical therapy department. Anyone working with the patient should be instructed in suctioning procedures. Patients with paraplegia can learn to suction themselves; however, patients with high spinal cord injuries will usually depend on family or attendant for suctioning at home.

Emergency considerations for respirator-dependent patients

It is important to know adequate emergency procedures in the event of power failure or respirator-equipment malfunction. Essential information to gather before treatment of any respirator-dependent patient includes knowing the patient's abilities, the equipment, and the secondary systems available. The therapist should be skilled in artificial respiration techniques. The patient's ability to breathe without the respirator can be lifesaving in an emergency. Patients who have sustained a C1 or C2 quadriplegia have no diaphragm function but may be able to use glossopharyngeal breathing if the tracheostomy is plugged. Know the endurance of the patient for glossopharyngeal breathing. Patients with weak inspiratory musculature may be able to continue breathing for extended periods of time when detached from the respirator. In the event of a power failure it is important to identify those patients who require immediate attention.

Familiarity with the equipment can also be lifesaving. Know the type of respirator, that is, positive or negative pressure, volume or pressure ventilator. Learn how to ventilate the patient manually. Some respirators will have a hand pump. Make sure the pump attachment is readily available, and know how to assemble it quickly. If there is no manual pump mechanism for the respirator, look for alternative methods for manual ventilation. The manual ventilation bag is primarily used. This bag should go with the patient to all appointments and always be kept within reach of the patient. Know the size of the tracheostomy tube and have the tracheostomy adapters within easy reach.

Each facility should have a preestablished procedure for power failure emergencies. It is advisable to know the philosophy of the facility in the event of life-threatening emergencies. Many facilities will have secondary systems for electrical power operated by an alternate generator. Electrical outlets powered by this generator should be easily recognizable. When there are no alternatives, that is, electrical back-up, manual pump, or manual ventilation bag, and the patient has no time off the respirator, the therapist must use artificial ventilation.

Artificial ventilation is done by mouth or manually. Therefore when using mouth-to-nose, close off both the tracheostomy and the mouth. If mouth-to-mouth is used, close off the nose and tracheostomy. When doing mouth-to-tracheostomy, close off the mouth and nose. Manual ventilation is less efficient, is extremely fatiguing for the person delivering the care, and is used only when mouth breathing is not practical. There are many techniques for manual ventilation; however, abdominal compressions, similar to manual cough, are most readily applied with the patient in any position (Fig. 21-22). An alternative technique is to place the hands laterally on the rib cage with one hand on either side of the lower half of the chest. The ribs are pushed down and released suddenly. Use a normal

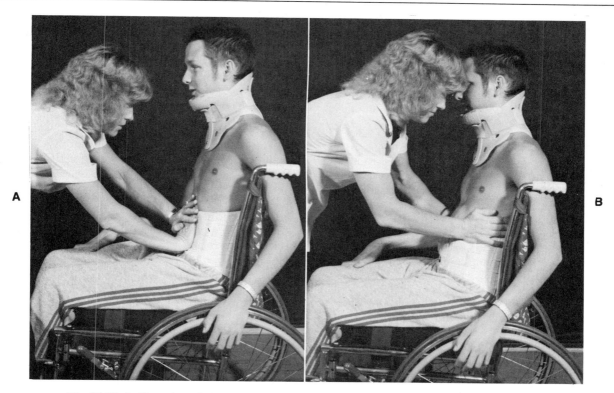

Fig. 21-22. A, Manual ventilation technique using abdominal compression. **B,** Manual ventilation using hands on either side of ribs.

breathing rate with the patient assisting inspiration if possible.

DISCHARGE PLANNING

Preparation for discharge includes a good bronchial hygiene program that will prevent pulmonary complications. The patient should be performing deep breathing with airshifts or glossopharyngeal breathing, or both, daily. If chest expansion is less than 2 inches, the family should be instructed in manual chest-stretching techniques. Daily coughing to prevent an accumulation of secretions in the lungs is necessary at home. The patient and the family should demonstrate the ability to make the cough functionally productive, either with manual assistance or by compensation with increased volume.

The family should be taught how to do postural drainage and manual coughing and be able to recognize the indications for both. Increase in mucus, respiratory infection, and history of pulmonary complications are indications for cough assistance or postural drainage, or both. Emphasize immediate action by the family whenever the patient has even the slightest increase in respiratory symptoms. If the patient has a chronic history of respiratory infections,

IPPB equipment should be provided in the home. Instruct the family in the use of IPPB equipment. IPPB treatments should be administered 30 minutes before postural drainage.

Family members can be taught how to auscultate for significant breath sounds. Instruct the family about drainage positions that have been most productive. Advise them about the frequency of the treatment. Suggest three or four times a day as necessary when the patient is productive. Once in the morning to clear nightly mucus accumulation and once at night are good frequencies to suggest when planning a preventive program.

A patient using a ventilator can go home if the family environment is supportive. Full evaluation of the home setting should be done to aid the patient and family in planning adaptations that will be necessary for the respirator-dependent patient to return home. Any ventilator-dependent patient should have a gasoline-powered emergency generator at home. The family will have to become competent in the operation and maintenance of the equipment and all emergency procedures. Important to successful discharge with this type of patient is family experience with the patient and equipment at home.

CASE STUDY

Bill is a 20 year-old man who was injured April 9, 1977, while diving into a river. He sustained a C5 vertebral teardrop fracture with slight posterior displacement. He was placed in Crutchfield tongs with reduction of the fracture. The third day of his admission to the acute care facility he contracted pneumonia and was placed on a volume-limited respirator. Within 3 weeks the tongs were removed, and he was placed in a halo vest so that he could be mobilized to a rehabilitation center.

The initial physical therapy evaluation (see chart) showed a functional neurological level of C4 quadriplegia. Clinically the patient had a nonfunctional cough and a breathing pattern of 1-neck, 3-diaphragm. The strength of the diaphragm was considered "poor" as demonstrated by an incomplete epigastric rise. The strength of the deltoids bilaterally was consistent with the finding of a weak diaphragm.

Because of recurrent episodes of pneumonia, the first treatment ordered by the physician was postural drainage with sterile suctioning procedures. On fluoroscopy examination the patient was observed to have slight movement of the diaphragm on the right with an excursion of one intercostal space for the diaphragm on the left. His vital capacity was 500 cc. When Bill could tolerate 20 minutes off the ventilator, special attention was paid to his diaphragm function.

Once Bill had confidence in the physical therapist, the therapist began treatment by inclining the bed to 15 degrees before removing Bill from the ventilator. This slightly upright position decreased the force required to move the abdominal contents when the patient inhaled. A large mirror was attached over Bill's bed to allow him to view both the neck muscles and epigastric area. The therapist verified the diaphragm contraction by placing the fingers slightly under the edge of the sixth, seventh, and eighth ribs. Bill was instructed to take a deep breath in an attempt to increase the epigastric rise. While he viewed this movement in the mirror, he could also see if he was using any neck muscles. The therapist could palpate to evaluate the patient's attempt to use the diaphragm. Bill gradually increased his epigastric rise and ceased using his sternocleidomastoid muscles. The treatment time was kept to 5-minute sessions three times a day to avoid fatigue to the diaphragm. Bill felt comfortable off the ventilator for 5 minutes and could concentrate on diaphragmatic breathing.

Diaphragm strength was improving; however Bill was also instructed in isometric neck strengthening to prevent disuse atrophy while in the halo vest. The sigh mechanism on the respirator was used to maintain chest mobility, since routine intermittent positive pressure could not be done with pneumonia present and manual chest stretching was limited by the halo vest.

One month after admission Bill was able to tolerate being without the respirator for several hours during the day. In preparation for early wheelchair activities, thigh-high compression stockings and a corset with a bladder for a pneumobelt was ordered. The stockings were to aid venous return, and the corset was to both reduce splanchnic blood pooling and improve the mechanics of the diaphragm. Once sitting he was trained in the use of the pneumobelt to prevent diaphragm fatigue.

Two weeks later Bill's vital capacity had increased from 500 to 600 cc. The lung congestion had subsided, and he was able to give full attention to learning glossopharyngeal breathing (GPB). Bill's vital capacity with GPB was 700 cc, which increased the

force of his cough. Inspiratory incentive spirometry was added to the diaphragm-strengthening program, since the epigastric rise was still incomplete. Postural drainage, IPPB, and manual cough were decreased in frequency. Eight weeks after admission his epigastric rise reached full excursion. Vital capacity was now 900 cc without GPB and 1100 cc with GPB.

Two months after the injury the halo vest was removed and a cervical orthosis was placed on the patient. Manual resistive exercise was initiated to provide a mild challenge to the diaphragm. Diaphragm weights could not be used, since epigastric rise against external resistance was not full. Bill continued with incentive inspiratory spirometry and learned to do airshifts while the tracheostomy was plugged. Because he was no longer congested, the therapists could initiate routine intermittent positive-pressure breathing through the tracheostomy with a tracheostomy adapter. The RIPP treatments were started at a pressure of 20 cm H_2O. Bill initially tolerated three sets of five breaths each. Meanwhile, he was improving his upright time to 3 hours and tolerating brief periods of mouthstick training from the occupational therapy staff while respiration was assisted by the pneumobelt.

Three months after admission Bill was tolerating a plugged tracheostomy through the night as well as during the day. The tracheostomy sizes were gradually decreased, and finally he was decannulated. Routine intermittent positive pressure and daily use of airshift maneuvers were discontinued to allow healing of the open tracheostomy site. Manual chest stretching was substituted for continued chest mobilization. The patient continued to have difficulty increasing upright and activity tolerance even when using the pneumobelt. His upright tolerance increased from 3 to 4 hours. Strengthening techniques for the diaphragm were limited to incentive spirometry and gentle manual resistance. By the end of the fourth month the tracheostoma had healed, and so routine intermittent positive pressure and airshift maneuvers were reinitiated. At that point the vital capacity was 1200 cc, or 23% of normal. Chest-expansion measurements were taken: without an airshift maneuver expansion was zero; with an airshift expansion was one-fourth inch. He continued short periods of mouthstick training and an active-assistive upper extremity exercise program with occupational therapy. His upper extremities had now improved enough to allow him to use hand controls to operate the electric wheelchair.

In September, 5 months after his admission and a plateau period of 6 weeks, Bill began to again improve his respiratory function. His vital capacity was 1300 cc, or 29% of normal. The patient had full epigastric rise without fatigue. The strengthening program for the diaphragm was altered to begin lifting the weight of the weight pan (1/4 lb). Upright activity tolerance increased to 6 hours, and Bill was able to decrease use of the pneumobelt gradually. He controlled his electric wheelchair well and began feeding and personal hygiene training. Even though the diaphragm strength improved to "fair," as evidenced by a full epigastric rise, Bill still required the pneumobelt, since his tolerance for being upright decreased during activity and his diaphragm would fatigue. His active chest expansion began to show negative values as the diaphragm strength increased. However, with an airshift he improved from −1/2-inch chest expansion to +3/4 inch (xiphoid).

By mid-October, 6 months after his admission, Bill's vital capacity was 41% of normal (1800 cc) and 45% of normal (2000 cc) with GPB. He was completely phased out from the pneumo-

PHYSICAL THERAPY EVALUATION DONE ON 4/21/77

SENSATION EVALUATION:

Key: N = NORMAL
   – = IMPAIRED
   O = ABSENT

	SUPERFICIAL PAIN		LIGHT TOUCH	
	R	L	R	L
C2	N	N	N	N
3	N	N		
4	N	N		
5	N	–	↓	↓
6	O	O	O	↓
7				O
8				
T1				
2				
4				
5				
8				
10				
12				
L1				
2				
3				
4				
5				
S1				
2				
3				
4	↓	↓	↓	↓

PROPRIOCEPTION

	R	L
SHOULDER	N	N
ELBOW	–	O
WRIST	–	O
THUMB	–	O
HIP	O	O
KNEE	↓	↓
ANKLE		
GREAT TOE	↓	↓

76S611 RD241 (R4-79)

RESPIRATORY EVALUATION:

BREATHING PATTERN		DIAPHRAGM FUNCTION	
Neck	I	*Poor*	
Diaph.	3		
Chest	O		Volume ventilator setting
Abdom.	O		Tidal volume—650 cc

COUGH		VC	VC GPB
Functional			
Weak funct.		cc (MA-1)	cc
Nonfunct.		%	%

CHEST EXP. Active   *NT 2° to halo*
(Xiphoid)   c̄ Air shift _____

NECK STRENGTH

Sternocleidomastoids—present*
Extensors—present*

TRUNK MUSCLES

Abdominals—0
Back extensors—0

UPPER EXTREMITY STRENGTH

	R	L
Upper trapezius	P ↑	P ↑
Middeltoid	P ↑	P ↑
Anterior deltoid	P ↑	P ↑
Pectoralis (clavicular and sternal)	0/0	0/0
Biceps	P	P
Triceps	0	0
Wrist extensors (radial and ulnar)	T/0	0/0
Wrist flexors (radial and ulnar)	0/0	0/0
Intrinsics	0	0

LOWER EXTREMITIES—0

---

*Isometric contraction is the only allowable motion.
GPB, Glossopharyngeal breathing.
MA-1, Trade name for a volume respirator.
NT 2° to halo, Not tested; secondary to the patient being in a halo vest.
P ↑, Method of indicating minimal muscle grade when resistance is not allowed; arrow indicates that strength may be greater than given grade.
VC, Vital capacity.

belt. Routine intermittent positive pressure progressed to higher pressures (30-35-40 cm H_2O). The patient progressed over the next 2 weeks from ¼ to 2½ pound weights to the diaphragm. He plateaued at this point, since his vital capacity was 2700 cc and the same from one evaluation to the next. Bill was now close to discharge. He was using the electric wheelchair with a left-hand control and had tried manual propulsion of a wheelchair with hand rim projections. He was independent with feeding and personal hygiene after being set up. The family was instructed in postural drainage and manual cough. They were instructed to do preventive postural drainage to the left lower lobe because Bill's pneumonia history had primarily involved that segment of the lung.

On discharge evaluation, Bill had the following:

RESPIRATORY EVALUATION

BREATHING PATTERN
- Neck   O
- Diaphragm   /
- Chest   O
- Abdomen   O

DIAPHRAGM FUNCTION

Fair +

COUGH		VC	VC GPB
Functional			
Weak funct.	X	cc 2700	cc 3500
Nonfunct.		% 66	% 85

CHEST EXPANSION (Xiphoid)
- Active − ½ inch
- With airshift 2 inches

The strength of the diaphragm improved to fair +. Chest expansion was − ½ inch because of the paradoxical movement of the strong diaphragm but was +2 inches with an airshift. Bill could produce a weak functional cough by compensating with increased volume produced by glossopharyngeal breathing.

REFERENCES

1. Adkins, H.V.: Improvement of breathing ability in children with respiratory muscle paralysis, Phys. Ther. **48**:577-581, 1968.
2. Alvarez, S.E., and others: Respiratory management of the adult patient with spinal cord injury, Phys. Ther. **61**:1737-1745, 1980.
3. Bartlett, R.H., and others: Respiratory maneuvers to prevent postoperative pulmonary complications, J.A.M.A. **224**:1017-1021, 1973.
4. Bergofsky, E.H.: Mechanisms for respiratory insufficiency after cervical cord injury: a source of alveolar hypoventilation, Ann. Intern. Med. **61**:435-437, 1964.
5. Canter, H.G.: Practical pulmonary physiology, GP **35**:104-114, 1967.
6. Carlson, B.: Normal chest excursion, Phys. Ther. **53**:10-14, 1973.
7. Carter, R.E.: Medical management of pulmonary complications of spinal cord injury, Adv. Neurol. **22**:261-269, 1979.
8. Dail, C.W., and others: Glossopharyngeal breathing, Downey, Calif., 1979, Professional Staff Association of the Rancho Los Amigos Hospital, Inc.
9. Dail, C.W.: Muscle breathing patterns, Med. Arts and Sci. **10**:64-70, second quarter, 1956.
10. Dail, C.W.: Respiratory aspects of rehabilitation in neuromuscular conditions, Arch. Phys. Med. Rehabil. **46**:655-675, 1965.
11. Daniels, L., and Worthingham, C.: Muscle testing, ed. 4, Philadelphia, 1980, W.B. Saunders Co.
12. Gayrard, P., and others: The effects of abdominal weights on diaphragmatic position and excursion in man, Clin. Sci. **35**:589-601, 1968.
13. Gray, H.: Anatomy of the human body, ed. 29, Philadelphia, 1973, Lea & Febiger, pp. 412-414.
14. Gross, D., and others: The effect of training on strength and endurance of the diaphragm in quadriplegia, Am. J. Med. **68**:27-34, 1980.
15. Guralnik, D.B., and Friend, J.A.: Webster's new world dictionary of the American language, Cleveland, 1968, The World Publishing Co.
16. Kendall, H.O., Kendall F.S., and Wadsworth G.E.: Muscles, ed. 2, Baltimore, 1971, The Williams & Wilkins Co., pp. 199-235, 264-267.
17. Luce, C.: Respiratory muscle function in health and disease, Chest **81**:82-90, 1982.
18. McMichan, J.C., and others: Pulmonary dysfunction following traumatic quadriplegia—recognition, prevention, and treatment, J.A.M.A. **243**:528-531, 1980.
19. Siebens, A.A., and others: Cough following transection of spinal cord at C-6, Arch. Phys. Med. **45**:1-7, 1964.
20. Stone, D.J., and Keltz, H.: The effect of respiratory muscle dysfunction on pulmonary function, Amer. Rev. Respir. Dis. **88**:621-629, 1964.
21. Wade, O.L.: Movements of the thoracic cage and diaphragm in respiration, J. Appl. Physiol. **124**:193-213, 1954.
22. West, J.B.: Respiratory physiology, Baltimore, 1974, The Williams & Wilkins Co.

GLOSSARY

abruptio placentae Premature separation of the placenta from the uterus, which often leads to hemorrhage.

adrenergic Type of medication or receptor site that stimulates the sympathetic nervous system.

adventitious sounds Breath sounds not normally heard that can be superimposed over normal breath sounds, such as crackles and rhonchi.

aerobic Type of energy produced using oxygen.

afterload The work load during systole applied to the heart by the resistance of the systemic vasculature.

alveolar macrophages Defense cells within the lungs that serve to engulf and digest foreign particles within the alveoli.

alveolar ventilation Amount of air that actually enters the alveolar region of the lungs to take part in gas exchange.

alveolus Smallest distal air sac involved in gas exchange.

anaerobic Type of energy produced without using oxygen.

anastomosis Surgical joining of two tubular structures, such as arteries.

aneurysm A large area of akinetic myocardium that bulges or balloons out when the heart contracts.

angina pectoris Severe chest pain caused by insufficient myocardial oxygen supply.

angiography Examination of the coronary arteries or other blood vessels by use of contrast medium and recording of flow on film.

antiarrhythmics Medications that reduce the incidence and frequency of cardiac arrhythmias, such as quinidine, procaine amide (Procan-SR), disopyramide phosphate (Norpace), and beta blockers.

antibodies A protective substance that plays a role in the immune response to foreign substances including microorganisms.

aortic stenosis Abnormally constricted opening of the aortic valve.

Apgar scores 10-point scoring system to assess newborn status, usually performed at 1 and 5 minutes of life.

apical Referring to the apex or upper portions of the lung.

aplastic anemia Blood disorder characterized by lack of production of blood cells by the bone marrow.

apnea Lack of breathing.

arteriovenous oxygen (a-$\bar{v}o_2$) difference Arterial oxygen content minus central venous oxygen content.

atelectasis Alveolar collapse because of poor lung expansion or complete obstruction of an airway.

atrial fibrillation or flutter High-rate atrial arrhythmias; atrial fibrillation is characterized by the absence of clearly distinguishable P waves and an irregular ventricular response. Atrial flutter is characterized by a pattern of saw-toothed P waves with an atrial rate of 300 and a variable P wave to the ventricular response rate.

auscultation Listening with a stethoscope.

barotrauma Pulmonary trauma associated with high levels of inspiratory pressure from a mechanical ventilator.

basilar Referring to the bases or lower portions of the lung.

beta adrenergic receptor–blocking medications (beta blockers) Medications that inhibit the beta adrenergic receptor–blocking activity of the autonomic nervous system, such as atenolol, nadolol (Corgard), propranolol hydrochloride (Inderal), and timolol hydrogen maleate (Blocadren).

bronchiole Small, distal airway.

respiratory bronchiole Small, distal airway characterized by the appearance of alveoli within the airway wall.

terminal bronchiole Smallest, most distal bronchiole with no obvious alveoli.

bronchodilator Medication that reduces bronchial smooth muscle spasm and thereby increases the size of the bronchial lumen.

bronchoscopy Inspection of a bronchus after passage of a rigid or flexible tube into the airway for either diagnostic or therapeutic procedures.

bronchus Larger more central airways below the trachea characterized by cartilage plates, respiratory epithelium, and glandular elements.

cardiac catheterization Specialized procedure using catheters and opaque dye to analyze heart function and coronary blood flow.

calcium antagonist medications Medications used to control arrhythmias, hypertension, and vasospasm, such as diltiazem (Cardiem, Cardizem, Dilzem), nifedipine (Procardia), and verapamil hydrochloride (Isoptin).

cardiac catheterization Specialized procedure using catheters and opaque dye to analyze heart function and coronary blood flow.

cardiogenic shock A situation in which the heart cannot maintain an adequate cardiac output.

central training effects Training effects that can be measured by changes in cardiac function.

cholinergic Type of medications or receptor sites that stimulate the parasympathetic nervous system.

chronotropic Affecting the rate of the heart beat.

cilia Hairlike projections from respiratory epithelial cells that serve to propel mucus and debris toward the pharynx.

coagulopathy Disorder of clotting.

compliance The ability of tissue (lung or chest wall) to expand. High compliance means easy expandability; low compliance means poor expandability. Measured as ratio of volume change to pressure change.

compliance A patient's adherence to program instructions and to suggestions for risk-factor reduction.

congestive heart failure Inability of the left side of the heart to maintain cardiac output at rest, which results in pulmonary congestion.

cor pulmonale Right-sided heart failure because of pulmonary hypertension secondary to pulmonary disease.

coronary collateralization Development of blood vessels in or around areas of poor blood flow.

coronary insufficiency Inadequate blood flow through the coronary arteries to meet myocardial oxygen demands.

CPK isoenzyme fraction Blood-borne isoenzyme that is released after myocardial necrosis. The isoenzyme of creatine phosphokinase (CPK) is MB.

decubitus posture Side-lying position.

defibrillation Electrical shock of sufficient power to cause a fibrillating heart to resume normal electrical activity.

dehiscence Splitting open of a surgical wound.

diaphoresis Sweating.

diffusion Random movement of gas molecules along a gradient based upon differences in partial pressure of gas. Accounts for the movement of oxygen into and carbon dioxide out of the blood in the pulmonary capillaries.

distribution Dispersion of gas throughout the lung fields.

diuretic Type of medication used to decrease body fluid and thereby decrease blood volume. Often used to control congestive heart failure and hypertension. Examples include furosemide (Lasix), Dyazide (triamterene and hydrochlorothiazide), and the thiazide diuretics.

driving force Force generated by respiratory muscles to move air through the airways.

dysphagia Pain and difficulty during swallowing.

dyspnea Inability to take a normal breath because of labored breathing. The sensation of not being able to catch your breath.

effusion Abnormal collection of fluid (commonly seen in the pleura).

egophony (tragophony) The change in a voice sound from *a* to *e*, somewhat like the bleating of a goat (from Greek *aix, aig-*, 'goat,' and *phōnē*, 'voice').

ejection fraction A hemodynamic measurement of the stroke volume divided by end-diastolic volume. Ejection fraction indicates resting heart function, with normal being 55 to 65 m^2.

endotracheal tube A plastic tube that is inserted orally or nasally to provide direct access into the trachea. These tubes are commonly attached to mechanical ventilators.

eosinophil White blood cell associated with asthma and allergy.

epiglottis Cartilage that protects the trachea from aspirated foodstuff during the normal swallowing process.

esophageal atresia Incomplete development of the esophagus.

extracorporeal oxygenation Use of an artificial membrane outside the body by which to provide for oxygenation in a patient with severe lung disease.

fibrillae The many tiny threads that a striated muscle fiber can be split into.

fibrinolysis Destruction of fibrin by fibrinolysin.

fissure Clearly discernible divisions in lung tissue that separate the lobes of the lungs.

fremitus Vibrations within the thorax that can be palpated.

glycogenolysis Change of glycogen into glucose for use by body tissues.

goblet cells Mucus-producing cells found in the respiratory epithelium.

hemoptysis Pulmonary hemorrhage.

huffing Forced expiration with an open glottis to replace coughing when pain is a major factor that limits coughing.

hydrostatic densitometry Underwater weighing to determine a person's lean to fat body weight.

hypercapnia (hypercarbia) Increased arterial carbon dioxide level.

hyperlipidemia Excessive fat content in the blood, specifically elevated cholesterols and triglycerides.

hyperoxygenation The use of high concentrations of inspired oxygen before and after endotracheal aspiration.

hypertrophic cardiomyopathy Abnormal cardiac hypertrophy having numerous causes that results in poor cardiac function.

hyperventilation Increase in alveolar ventilation resulting in decreased arterial carbon dioxide level.

hypoadaptive blood pressure (see also **hypotension**) Abnormally low blood pressure at rest.

hypocapnia (hypocarbia) Decreased arterial carbon dioxide level.

hypotension (see also **hypoadaptive blood pressure**) A fall in systolic blood pressure with an increase in exertion or heart rate, or both.

hypoventilation Decrease in alveolar ventilation resulting in increased arterial carbon dioxide level.

hypoxemia Low arterial oxygen tension.

immunoglobulins Circulating antibodies that protect against foreign substances including microorganisms.

intermittent mandatory ventilation A mode of mechanical ventilation that guarantees a specific minute volume to the patient but simultaneously permits the patient to breathe spontaneously.

intraventricular conduction defects Loss of the normal electrical conduction system in the ventricles.

ischemia Inadequate blood flow to meet the metabolic demands of tissue.

isocapnic Condition in which the carbon dioxide level remains unchanged despite changing levels of ventilation.

Lambert's canals Channels connecting alveoli with respiratory bronchioles.

lipolysis Destruction of lipids or fats.

meconium The first stool passed by a newborn.

metabolic acidosis Decreased arterial pH secondary to a nonrespiratory disorder.

metabolic alkalosis Increased arterial pH secondary to a nonrespiratory disorder.

minute ventilation The volume of air inspired, or expired, in 1 minute.

mouthstick Mouth-operated control stick for a power wheelchair.

mucociliary transport The process of removal of mucus and debris within the mucus by means of the wavelike motion of cilia lining the respiratory epithelium.

muscle bridging Myocardium bridges over one or more of the large epicardial coronary vessels causing constriction during systole.

MVo₂ Myocardial oxygen consumption.

myocardial infarction Death of heart muscle tissue.

obstructive disease Disorders characterized by obstruction of airways.

osteoarthropathy Swelling and pain within the joints secondary to numerous chronic pulmonary infections and other disorders. Can mimic early rheumatoid arthritis.

osteopenia (osteoporosis) Reduction in the amount of bone substance per unit volume of bone tissue.

oximeter Device used to measure oxygen level.

oxygen toxicity An inflammatory response of the lung tissue to exceedingly high concentrations of inspired oxygen over long periods of time.

parietal pleura That layer of the pleural sac adjacent to the chest wall.

pathophysiology The science of pathological processes and their effects on normal tissue.

pectoriloquy Transmission to the chest of a whispered sound.

pectus carinatum ''Pigeon breast'' deformity, a protrusion of the sternum and costal cartilages.

pectus excavatum ''Funnel chest'' deformity, a sunken sternum and costal cartilages.

perfusion Flow of pulmonary blood or other fluid through the vessels.

pericarditis Inflammation of the pericardium (sac that encloses the heart).

phenotype Inherited blood type. Referred to here in relation to cholesterol levels in the blood.

physiological dead space Areas of the lung that are well ventilated but poorly perfused with blood.

placenta previa Development of the placenta low in the uterus that may cause it to rupture and hemorrhage.

pleura Two-layered sac that encases the lungs.

plexus Group of nerves.

plethysmograph Airtight ''body box'' that is used to measure various pulmonary function values.

pneumomediastinum Leakage of free air into the mediastinum.

pores of Kohn Channels connecting adjacent alveoli.

positive inotropic pertaining to any phenomenon that increases cardiac contractility; most commonly a glycoside medication like digoxin or digitalis.

preload The volume of blood in the left ventricle just before systole, the end-diastolic volume.

progression of coronary artery disease Worsening of the obstructive processes of coronary atherosclerosis.

R-on-T phenomenon An arrhythmia characterized by premature ventricular contraction that occurs on or before the completion of the T wave of the previous beat. Associated with acute ventricular fibrillation and sudden death.

radiolucent Radiographic density that appears very dark, indicating material through which the x-ray beam passes easily, such as air.

radiopaque Radiographic density that appears white indicating material through which the x-ray beam does not pass well, such as bone or metal.

rate-pressure product Heart rate multiplied by systolic blood pressure. A clinical indicator of myocardial oxygen demand.

regression of coronary artery disease Decrease in the obstructive processes of coronary atherosclerosis.

respiratory acidosis Decreased arterial pH secondary to respiratory disorder.

restrictive disease Disorders characterized by restriction of expansion by the lungs or chest wall.

revascularization Ischemic or potentially ischemic areas that are provided, either surgically or naturally, with an alternative blood supply.

stenosis Narrowing of a tube, such as tracheal stenosis.

stroke volume Volume of blood, in millimeters, ejected from the heart with each beat.

subcutaneous emphysema Leakage of free air into the subcutaneous tissue.

subendocardial Pertaining to a nontransmural infarction. Myocardial necrosis is limited to the subendocardium.

surfactant Material produced by type II alveolar cells that serves to reduce surface tension in the alveoli.

sympathomimetic bronchodilators Medications that are useful at reducing bronchial muscle spasm because of their action that mimics the sympathetic nervous system response resulting in reduced smooth muscle spasm.

syncope Sudden, but transient, unconsciousness. (Pronounced sing′ko-pee)

thoracentesis (thoracocentesis) Removal of fluid from the thorax, usually through a wide lumen syringe.

torr Unit name for mm Hg (millimeters of mercury).

tracheoesophageal fistula Abnormal communication between the esophagus and trachea.

tracheomalacia Eroding of the trachea because of excessive pressure from a cuffed endotracheal tube.

transmural infarction Myocardial necrosis that is full thickness in nature. The necrotic tissue extends from the endocardium to the epicardium.

unstable angina pectoris Preinfarction chest pain characterized by discomfort occurring at rest and low levels of activity.

ventilation The process in which air moves into the lungs in preparation for gas exchange.

ventricular dysfunction Myocardial dysfunction within the ventricles that exhibits abnormalities in contraction and wall motion.

ventricular tachycardia Life-threatening arrhythmia usually associated with a high rate and a series of ventricular ectopic beats (three in a row).

visceral pleura The inner layer of pleura that is adjacent to the external lung tissue.

weaning Coordinated effort to remove the patient from dependency on mechanical ventilation.

INDEX

Page numbers in boldface indicate volume in *Physical Therapy* series. **1,** Irwin, S., and Tecklin, J.S.: Cardiopulmonary physical therapy, St. Louis, 1985, The C.V. Mosby Co.; **2,** Gould, J.A., and Davies, G.J.: Orthopaedic and sports physical therapy, St. Louis, 1985, The C.V. Mosby Co.; **3,** Umphred, D.A.: Neurological rehabilitation, St. Louis, 1985, The C.V. Mosby Co.
Page numbers in *italics* indicate boxed material and illustrations.
Page numbers followed by *t* indicate tables.

1, Cardiopulmonary physical therapy; 2, Orthopaedic
and sports physical therapy; 3, Neurological
rehabilitation.

1, Cardiopulmonary physical therapy; **2,** Orthopaedic
and sports physical therapy; **3,** Neurological
rehabilitation.

1, Cardiopulmonary physical therapy; **2,** Orthopaedic
and sports physical therapy; **3,** Neurological
rehabilitation.

1, Cardiopulmonary physical therapy; **2,** Orthopaedic
and sports physical therapy; **3,** Neurological
rehabilitation.

1, Cardiopulmonary physical therapy; **2,** Orthopaedic
and sports physical therapy; **3,** Neurological
rehabilitation.

Exercise(s)—cont'd
  physiology of
    abnormal, **1:**50-62
      anginal responses to, **1:**56-59
      blood pressure response to, **1:**52-56; *see also* Blood pressure, response of, to exercise
      heart rate response to, **1:**50-53; *see also* Heart rate, response of, to exercise
      respiratory limitations to maximum oxygen consumption and, **1:**59-62
    postural, for child with respiratory dysfunction, **1:**358
  prescription of
    based on maximal-exercise test results, **1:**94-96
    in knee rehabilitation, **2:**360
  programs of
    biomechanical principles and, **2:**80-82
    to improve exercise tolerance, **1:**245-246
  progressive resistive, for diaphragm strengthening in spinal cord injury client, **1:**405-406
  relaxation
    in pain management, **3:**613
    to reduce body work, **1:**236
  renal responses to, **2:**260-261
  responses to, evaluation of, objective continuous, in cardiac rehabilitation, **1:**3-4
  for spine, mobility, **2:**544, *547*
  steady-state, cardiorespiratory responses to, **2:**258-260
  strengthening, in pulmonary hygiene for ventilator-dependent client, **1:**299-302
  stress of, adaptation of bone to, **2:**38-39
  sympathetic nervous system response to, **1:**26-28
  tolerance of
    effect of respiratory muscle training programs on, **1:**392
    treatments to improve, **1:**244-246
  and training, specificity of, **2:**267-268
  vasodilation/vasoconstriction in, **1:**25-26
Exercise bicycles in administration of cardiac rehabilitation program, **1:**157
Exercise testing
  contraindications and precautions to, **1:**102
  graded, in respiratory assessment, **1:**227
  in inpatient cardiac rehabilitation, **1:**107-108
  low-level, **1:**80-90; *see also* Low-level exercise testing
  maximal, **1:**90-97; *see also* Maximal exercise testing
  protocols for, **1:**102
  standard evaluative procedures for, **1:**162
  termination of, criteria for, **1:**102
Exercise training
  in phase II cardiac rehabilitation
    intensity of, **1:**110
    program for, **1:**108-110
    results of, **1:**114

Exercise training—cont'd
  in phase III cardiac rehabilitation, program for, **1:**116-117
Exhalation belt for spinal cord injury client, **1:**407, *408*
Expectancy for recovery in psychosocial adjustment to neurological disability **3:**119
Expiratory grunting in respiratory distress in neonate, **1:**317
Expiratory pressure, decreased, in spinal cord injury, **3:**332, 359-360
Expiratory reserve volume (ERV), definition of, **1:**174
Extensor digitorum communis (EDC) tendons, **2:**443
Extensor responses
  bedridden head injury client with, early management of, **3:**274, 276
  moderate, head injury client with, early management of, **3:**277-280
External oblique muscle of abdomen, **2:**523
External stabilization for lumbosacral region, **2:**578-579
External supports in orthopaedic and sports rehabilitation, **2:**182
External survival, homeostasis in, **3:**32-33
Exteroceptive input techniques, **3:**84*t*
Exteroceptive system, cutaneous, treatment techniques using, **3:**82-83
Exteroceptors, treatment techniques using, **3:**81-85
Extracorporeal circulation for cardiac surgery, **1:**251
Extracranial blood vessels, injury to, **3:**251
Extremity(ies)
  ataxia of, in cerebellar lesions, **3:**455-461
  control of, in hemiplegia, reestablishment of, **3:**502-503
  deformed, taping of, for high-risk neonates, **3:**149, *152, 153*
  mobility examination of, in musculoskeletal disorder evaluation, **2:**177
  pain in, acupuncture points for, **2:**201*t*
Eye(s)
  movements of, **3:**555-556
    in cerebellar lesions, **3:**461-463
  range of motion of, in visual screening for adults, **3:**568
Eye-hand coordination in evaluation of learning disabled child with motor deficits, **3:**220

F

F wave, electroneuromyographic studies of, **3:**591
Fabere's test, **2:**565
  in hip evaluation, **2:**387
  in preseason athletic physical evaluation, **2:**634, *635*
Facial agnosia
  assessment of, **3:**567
  identification of, **3:**576
  treatment of, **3:**577
Facial (VII) nerve, evaluation of, in brain tumor therapy, **3:**447

Facilitation
  of movement patterns, orthotics in, **3:**618
  oral motor, in multisensory treatment, **3:**102-104
  posture and, **3:**34
Facilitory and inhibitory techniques
  classification of, **3:**72-114
  influencing total body responses, **3:**89
  for postural extensors, **3:**88-89
  using vestibular system, **3:**87-90
Family
  of cerebral palsied child
    active involvement of, by therapist, **3:**178-179
    consultation with, therapist in, **3:**180
  data on, in head-injury evaluation, **3:**256-257
  factors related to, in head injury evaluation, **3:**261
  of head injury client, psychosocial consideration, **3:**286
  importance of, in care of child with respiratory dysfunction, **1:**335
  in initial physical therapy evaluation, **1:**70
  and loss in psychosocial adjustment to neurological disability, **3:**123-124
  maturation in, in psychosocial adjustment to neurological disability, **3:**124
  needs of, in psychosocial adjustment to neurological disability, **3:**123
  reactions of, to cerebral palsied child, **3:**166-167
  responses of, as predictor of outcome of head injury, **3:**265-266
Fascia, thoracolumbar, **2:**520-521
Fasciculation potentials in muscle at rest, electromyographic studies of, **3:**590
Fast-twitch skeletal muscle fibers, **2:**253-254
Fat, globules of, in synovial fluid, **2:**104
Fat metabolism, conditioning programs and, **2:**244-245
Fat pad(s)
  acetabular, **2:**369
  of elbow, **2:**479
  of synovial joints, **2:**106
    injury to, **2:**106-107
Fatigue
  in conditioning, **2:**265-267
    blood flow and, **2:**267
    electrolyte disturbances and, **2:**67
    fuel-related, **2:**266
    hypoxia and, **2:**267
    lactic acid and, **2:**266-267
    pH and, **2:**266-267
    synaptic, **2:**266
    temperature and, **2:**267
    water disturbances and, **2:**267
  easy, physical therapy for child with respiratory dysfunction and, **1:**335
  fractures from, **2:**30-32
  of materials in sports and orthopaedic therapy, **2:**72-73
Fecal impaction in elderly, confusion and, **3:**524
Feeding
  for hemiplegic, treatment procedures for, **3:**504-505

1, Cardiopulmonary physical therapy; **2,** Orthopaedic
and sports physical therapy; **3,** Neurological
rehabilitation.

1, Cardiopulmonary physical therapy; **2,** Orthopaedic
and sports physical therapy; **3,** Neurological
rehabilitation.

1, Cardiopulmonary physical therapy; 2, Orthopaedic
and sports physical therapy; 3, Neurological
rehabilitation.

1, Cardiopulmonary physical therapy; 2, Orthopaedic
and sports physical therapy; 3, Neurological
rehabilitation.

1, Cardiopulmonary physical therapy; **2,** Orthopaedic
and sports physical therapy; **3,** Neurological
rehabilitation.

1, Cardiopulmonary physical therapy; **2,** Orthopaedic
and sports physical therapy; **3,** Neurological
rehabilitation.

1, Cardiopulmonary physical therapy; 2, Orthopaedic
and sports physical therapy; 3, Neurological
rehabilitation.

Russian technique for muscle stimulation (RTMS) for pain control, 2:203

S

S-P support for lumbosacral region, 2:578-579
Saccade(s)
  definition of, 3:556
  measurement of, in visual screening for adults, 3:568-569
Sacral hiatus, palpation of, in lumbopelvic region assessment, 2:567
Sacral sparing in spinal cord injury, 3:318
Sacral sulcus, palpation of, in lumbopelvic region assessment, 2:567-568
Sacral torsion, left-on-left, correction of, 2:571-573
Sacroiliac joint, 2:550-579; see also Lumbopelvic region
  examination of, for orthopaedic and sports rehabilitation, 2:185
Sacroiliac joint tests, 2:*532, 533*
Sacroiliac ligament, 2:554
Sacrospinalis muscle, 2:522
Sacrospinous ligaments, 2:554
Sacrotuberous ligaments, 2:554
Safety in phase II cardiac rehabilitation, 1:111
Sagittal bands of hand, 2:443
Sarcomere in skeletal muscle, 2:248
Sartorius muscle
  in hip anatomy, 2:373
  in lumbopelvic region, 2:553
Saturational cuing in visuoconstructive disorder treatment, 3:581
Scala tympani, 3:94
Scala vestibuli, 3:94
Scalene muscles, evaluation of, palpation in, 1:216, *217*
Scanning
  speech, in cerebellar lesions, 3:461
  visual, in unilateral spatial inattention treatment, 3:574-575
Scanning eye movements, 3:556
Scaphoid, 2:437
  fracture of, 2:467
Scapula
  borders of, palpation of, 2:508
  muscles positioning, 2:523
Scapulohumeral rhythm of shoulder, 2:499
Scapulothoracic joint, 2:498-499
Schedules, disturbed, physical therapy for child with respiratory dysfunction and, 1:335
Schizophrenia
  communication disorders and, 3:538
  phenothiazines for, tardive dyskinesia from, 3:434
School-aged child with respiratory dysfunction, issues regarding, 1:360
Schools with cerebral palsied child, therapist and, 3:180-181
Sciatic nerve, in hip disorders, 2:370, 372
Sclerosis, multiple, 3:398-414; see also Multiple sclerosis
Scoliosis
  in child, physical therapy for, 1:341
  in genetic disorders in children, 3:193

Scoliosis—cont'd
  in hemiplegia, treatment alternatives for, 3:499
  Milwaukee brace for, 2:286, 301-303
  in myelomeningocele, 3:291, 293
  paralytic, in spinal cord injury, 3:321, 322
Scott-Craig orthosis in spinal cord injury rehabilitation, 3:366, *367*
Scouring in hip evaluation, 2:387
Screening, communication, 3:541
Screening examination in musculoskeletal disorder evaluation, 2:174-175
Secretions, respiratory
  clearance of, treatments to improve, 1:236-244
  retained, complications of, in RICU client, 1:274-275
Segmental breathing in breathing-retraining exercises for ventilator-dependent client, 1:297
Segmental breathing exercises to increase ventilation and oxygenation, 1:234, *235*
Selective neuronal necrosis, neuropathology of, 3:138-139
Self-care
  deficits in, 3:644-645, 646*t*
  evaluation of, in initial physical therapy evaluation, 1:71, *72*
Self-care activities in pulmonary hygiene for ventilator-dependent client, 1:303-304
Self-pressurized hydrostatic lubrication of articular cartilage, 2:11
Self-reinforcing adaptation in psychosocial adjustment to neurological disability, 3:120-121
Self-worth, establishment of, in neurological disability treatment, 3:128-130
Semirigid orthotic devices for foot and ankle disorders, 2:333
  fabrication of, 2:334-336, *337-338*
Sensation
  cutaneous, in palpation of shoulder, 2:507
  in evaluation for orthotics, 3:619
  in shoulder, tests for, 2:510
  testing for, in spinal examination, 2:530
Sensitivity, force, of joint mechanoreceptors, 2:58-59
Sensorimotor area of client profile, 3:20
Sensorimotor dysfunction in multiple sclerosis, treatment of, 3:410-411
Sensorimotor intervention for high-risk neonates, 3:153-154
Sensorimotor system, autonomic and somatic, interaction of, 3:32
Sensorimotor therapy in treatment of learning disabled child with motor deficits, 3:230-231
Sensory changes with aging, 3:520-521
Sensory channels in inflammatory brain disorder evaluation, 3:381-383
Sensory development, 3:65-68
Sensory disturbances in cerebrovascular accident, 3:482

Sensory experience of normal movement, developmental meaning of, for cerebral palsied child, 3:175-176
Sensory function
  evaluation of, in spinal cord injury rehabilitation, 3:353
  in head injury evaluation, 3:258
  as predictor of outcome of head injury, 3:266
Sensory input
  integration of, in inflammatory brain disorder therapy, 3:391-382
  for speech production, 3:532-533
Sensory integration
  dysfunction of
    brain dysfunction and, 3:211
    types of, 3:227-229
  in evaluation of learning disabled child with motor deficits, 3:220
Sensory Integration Tests, Southern California, 3:245-246
Sensory integration theory of Ayres
  learning disorders and
    critque of, 3:229
    effects of, on academic and motor performance research on, 3:229-230
    principles of, 3:229
  in treatment of learning disabled child with motor deficits, 3:227-230
Sensory loss in spinal cord injury, 3:326-327
Sensory modalities, classification of treatment techniques according to, 3:74-98
Sensory receptors and physiology of vestibular system, 3:85-87
Sensory testing in spina bifida evaluation, 3:299-300
Sensory training, orthotics in, 3:618
Sequencing in head injury treatment, 3:269-270
Sequential behavior, normal, changes in, throughout developmental arc, 3:41-69
Sequential development, normal, concept of, 3:5-10
Sequential task motor assessent, in neurological deficit evaluation, 3:6
Serotonin, pain control and, 3:601
Serum lipids, levels of, exercise and, 1:137-138
Set point, autonomic nervous system, inflammatory brain disorder evaluation, 3:380
Set and repetition system in ART program, 2:237
Sets, increased, in overload training, 2:233
Sex, mechanical properties of bone and, 2:35
Sex act, male and female, physiology of, 3:643
Sex chromosome abnormalities in children, 3:187
Sex-linked inherited disorders in children, 3:191-192
Sexual dysfunction, 3:640, 643-644
Sexual functioning, changes in, caused by neurological disorders, 3:643-644, 645*t*

1, Cardiopulmonary physical therapy; **2,** Orthopaedic
and sports physical therapy; **3,** Neurological
rehabilitation.

1, Cardiopulmonary physical therapy; **2,** Orthopaedic
and sports physical therapy; **3,** Neurological
rehabilitation.

1, Cardiopulmonary physical therapy; **2,** Orthopaedic and sports physical therapy; **3,** Neurological rehabilitation.